AGING

Communication Processes and Disorders

Editors

Daniel S. Beasley, Ph.D.

Chairman and Professor
Department of Audiology and Speech Pathology
Director
Memphis Speech and Hearing Center
Memphis State University
Memphis, Tennessee

G. Albyn Davis, Ph.D.

Assistant Professor
Department of Audiology and Speech Pathology
Project Director
Extended Service Program in Aphasia
Memphis Speech and Hearing Center
Memphis State University
Memphis, Tennessee

GRUNE & STRATTON

A Subsidiary of Harcourt Brace Jovanovich, Publishers

New York   London   Toronto   Sydney   San Francisco

Library of Congress Cataloging in Publication Data
Main entry under title:

Aging, communication processes and disorders.

   Includes bibliographies and index.
   1.   Geriatrics.   2.   Communicative disorders.
I.   Beasley, Daniel S.   II.   Davis, George Albyn,
1946-   [DNLM: 1.   Aging.   2.   Communication—
In old age.   3.   Speech disorders—In old age.
4.   Language disorders—In old age.   WM 475 A267]
RC952.5.A45   618.97'6855   80-26597
ISBN 0-8089-1281-X

_T1° 199624_ _2_

Grune & Stratton, Inc.
111 Fifth Avenue ﹨
New York, New York   10003

Distributed in the United Kingdom by
Academic Press, Inc. (London) Ltd.
24/28 Oval Road, London NW 1

Library of Congress Catalog Number 80-84074
International Standard Book Number 0-8089-1281-X
Printed in the United States of America

To our parents Irvin, Mary, George, and Mary Jane:
may we become what they are.

Contents

Acknowledgments

In completing our task, we are indebted to a number of individuals. Foremost, we want to thank each of our contributors for their patience and total willingness to work with us as we "editorialized" on their manuscripts and for their attention to the details and subtleties of their topics throughout several revisions. Indeed, this is their book.

Also, we want to thank our colleagues and students in the Department of Audiology and Speech Pathology at Memphis State University for their thoughts, ideas, and criticisms, and for their willingness to serve as readers whenever called upon, particularly Robyn Cox, David Wark, Louise Ward, Debra Van Ort, Al DeChicchis, Stephanie Allisandratos, Wanda Askew, and Linda Riensche (at the University of New Mexico).

Most importantly, we extend our deep appreciation to Shirley Rias and Lorraine Cooper, not only for their exceptional skills in the typing of the entire manuscript but for using their talents in making sense out of our too often unintelligible and agrammatical scribble. And to Lorraine, a special thanks for making sure that the department remained intact and viable when the chairman's mind was elsewhere and for nurturing this book from beginning to end as though it were her own. That, simply, is her way of doing things.

Foreword

The current emphasis placed on the topic of aging springs from a clear realization on the part of society that the cohort age 65 and above is growing rapidly in numbers. Modern science and technology have contributed substantially to extending the life span, and with this extension there are new potentials as well as new problems emerging. Today many more people reach old age than was true of earlier times.

Although in our youth-oriented society there has been a marked resistance toward recognition of the potentials of aging citizens, there is a growing awareness that older people, even though many no longer are part of the work force, do have contributions to make. There is likewise a greater sensitivity developing for the problems of all kinds faced by older people. The growing consciousness on the part of society of the potentials and needs of the elderly should not necessarily be construed as a basic societal shift in human values toward older people but one which is brought about by the very real presence of some 24 million elders who pay taxes, purchase commodities and services, and exercise pressures on politicians and others in policy making positions.

By its very nature the topic of aging is exceedingly broad because it deals with human beings—human beings in an extended period of life, on into retirement, and with the many variables associated with this extension of life activities. Their growing numbers have made new demands on the ingenuity of those responsible for health care, life-long education, housing, transportation, and the very systems themselves that provide for financial support of retirement plans of one kind or another.

New organizations, associations, and institutions have emerged to help meet the demands of our older citizens. Those who have chosen to articulate the needs of the elderly are little by little effecting change in society's response to them. The existence of the Administration of Aging, the National Institute of Aging, the many programs throughout the United States sponsored by state governments, and local programs developed and supported by the various institutions all bear witness to the fact that older people in many instances must be given special consideration by society.

The editors of this text have skillfully brought together three quite distinct but none-theless related areas of concern. The primary focus, as is obvious from the title of the book, is that of aging—aging in relation to the communication process and the disorders that are observable in that process among older people. Any one of the three topics—

aging, the communication process, and communication disorders—is the topic not only for several books but for major concentrations at graduate levels of education and training. And to add to the complexity, each one of the areas that comprise a part of this edited work is multidisciplinary in nature.

This important work gathers experts from many areas of concentration to include speech pathology, audiology, neurology, psychology, otolaryngology, linguistics, and education. The depth of penetration into the areas of communication disorders related to aging is such that it should increase the understanding of communication disorders of the elderly among a broad range of specialties—students and professionals alike.

The organization of the book provides for viewing speech, language, and hearing changes against the backdrop of the normal processes of aging. Of particular importance is the fact that the relevant research is brought to bear on the discussions, bringing to the reader the very latest in experimental findings. Thus this work lays the groundwork for the scientific development of intervention strategies for the elderly who sustain disorders of communication.

The editors and contributors to this volume have made an outstanding contribution to the rapidly developing literature in the field of communication disorders related to the older person. This text not only serves to increase the visibility of the older person in relation to the disorders of communication that frequently accompany advancing years but also adds substantially to the store of information to be utilized by those many professionals who serve them.

Herbert J. Oyer, Ph.D.
Dean, The Graduate School
Michigan State University

Preface

A certain mythology has developed that characterizes adulthood and old age. The idea that development of physical and mental processes ceases in adolescence and that adulthood is a single vast monotonous plateau has been dispelled in the popular literature by Sheehy's *Passages*. The ideas that the elderly are generally sickly, lonely, depressed, boring, and bored and possessed with shrinking cognitive abilities have all been questioned by sociological, psychological, medical, and educational research. Indeed, any attempt at stereotypic characterization of older individuals is a myth.

In the late 1960s and early 1970s, the immediate and long-term social and economic effects of the decrease in the birth rate and increase in longevity due to medical advances became public issues, most of which are still unresolved. The proportion of the population over the age of 65 in the United States, for example, has increased steadily since 1900, from 4.1 percent to 10.5 percent in 1975. The Department of Health, Education, and Welfare has predicted that by the year 2000, those over 65 years of age will comprise 11.7 percent of the United States population, an increase of 40 percent from 1970, to 31 million people. These population changes have had major effects on all aspects of society, as is evident in the trend towards increased private and public interest in providing services to adults in society. Such services contribute significantly to the quality of life as we grow older, and a vital ingredient in the life-long developmental process is communication. The expanding size of the elderly population alone has necessitated an increase of services for communicatively-impaired adults. Thus, the major thrust of this book is to present current understanding of adult development and aging as they are related to communication processes and disorders. The topic is multidisciplinary by nature and thus the book is represented by contributions from educational, service, and research leaders from audiology, education, medicine, psychology, speech-language pathology, and governmental affairs.

In Section I, discussions of the ramifications of normal aging as these pertain to communication processes are presented. Section II contains several chapters which review the relationships between speech-language disorders and aging, and Section III deals with several topics in clinical and research audiology and their links to aging. Section IV contains discussions which we feel are unique to this type of text, namely, issues pertaining to delivery of services to communicatively-impaired adults.

An attempt has been made to produce an edited work which is comprehensive without deviating too far from the primary theme—aging, communication processes, and disorders. Thus, certain of the contributions are specific to communication disorders, while others will appeal to the related interests of persons in several professional areas. Further, the book was designed to serve as a text for courses dealing with aging as well as a reference for educators, psychologists, gerontologists, and others who are investigating these topics with an adult population. To accomplish these goals, editorial decisions must be made and we are aware that a great deal more could be added to this volume. We hope our selections of original writings have been complete enough to at least provide the naive reader with a sense of direction and a feel for the viability of adult growth and development, and the seasoned professional with information and concepts which would encourage continued interest in understanding the complex relationships between aging and communication processes and disorders.

Daniel S. Beasley
G. Albyn Davis

Contributors

Martin L. Albert, M.D., Ph.D.
Professor of Neurology and
Clinical Director
Aphasia Research Center
Boston University School of Medicine and
Chief, Clinical Neurology Section
Boston Veteran's Administration Medical
  Center
Boston, Massachusetts

Daniel S. Beasley, Ph.D.
Professor and Chairman
Department of Audiology and Speech
  Pathology, and
Director
Memphis Speech and Hearing Center
Memphis State University
Memphis, Tennessee

Robert Burkard, M.S.
Research Assistant
Department of Communicative Disorders
University of Wisconsin
Madison, Wisconsin

G. Albyn Davis, Ph.D.
Assistant Professor and Director
Veterans Administration Education and
  Training Grant in Aphasia
Department of Audiology and Speech
  Pathology
Memphis State University
Memphis, Tennessee

Nancy Wadsworth Denney, Ph.D.
Associate Professor
Department of Psychology
University of Kansas
Lawrence, Kansas

Richard J. Dowling, M.S., J.D.
Executive Director
American Society of Allied Health Professions
Washington, D.C.

Barry A. Freeman, Ph.D.
Memorial Hospital
Clarksville, Tennessee

Audrey M. Fullerton, Ph.D.
Assistant Professor
Department of Psychology
Syracuse University
Syracuse, New York

Dean C. Garstecki, Ph.D.
Associate Professor of Audiology and
  Hearing Impairment
Northwestern University
Evanston, Illinois

Deborah Hayes, Ph.D.
Assistant Professor
Department of Otorhinolaryngology and
  Communicative Sciences
Division of Audiology and Speech Pathology
Baylor College of Medicine
Houston, Texas

Audrey L. Holland, Ph.D.
Research Scientist
American Institutes for Research, and
Professor of Speech
Department of Speech and Theater
University of Pittsburgh
Pittsburgh, Pennsylvania

Joel C. Kahane, Ph.D.
Associate Professor
Department of Audiology and Speech
  Pathology
Memphis State University
Memphis, Tennessee

Raymond D. Kent, Ph.D.
Senior Research Associate
Boys Town Institute for Communication
  Disorders in Children
Omaha, Nebraska

Alan B. Knox, Ed.D.
Professor of Education
Department of Administration, Higher and
  Continuing Education
College of Education
University of Illinois at Urbana-Champaign
Urbana, Illinois

Leonard L. LaPointe, Ph.D.
Coordinator of Instruction for Audiology and
  Speech Pathology
Veterans Administration Medical Center, and
Adjunct Faculty
University of Florida
Gainesville, Florida

Rosemary Lubinski, Ed.D.
Assistant Professor
Department of Communicative Disorders and
  Sciences
State University of New York
Buffalo, New York

Walter H. Manning, Ph.D.
Associate Professor of Speech Pathology
Department of Audiology and Speech
  Pathology
Memphis State University
Memphis, Tennessee

David Marlin, Esq.
Legal Research and Services for the Elderly
National Council of Senior Citizens
Washington, D.C.

Marion D. Meyerson, Ph.D.
Professor
Department of Communicative Disorders
California State University
Fresno, California

Joseph B. Nadol, Jr., M.D.
Assistant Professor in Otolaryngology
Harvard Medical School, and
Assistant Surgeon in Otolaryngology
Massachusetts Eye and Ear Infirmary
Boston, Massachusetts

Marilyn Newhoff, Ph.D.
Assistant Professor of Speech Pathology
Department of Communicative Disorders
San Diego State University
San Diego, California

Daniel J. Orchik, Ph.D.
Chief of Audiology
Shea Clinic and
Memphis Eye and Ear Hospital
Memphis, Tennessee

Loraine K. Obler, Ph.D.
Assistant Professor of Neurology
  (Neurolinguistics)
Aphasia Research Center, and
Department of Neurology
Boston University School of Medicine, and
Boston Veteran's Administration Medical
  Center
Boston, Massachusetts

John C. Rosenbek
Chief
Speech Pathology and Audiology Service
William S. Middleton Memorial Veteran's
  Hospital, and
Adjunct Professor
University of Wisconsin
Madison, Wisconsin

Susan J. Shanks, Ph.D.
Professor
Department of Communicative Disorders
California State University
Fresno, California

Edward A. Shirkey, M.S.
Research Assistant
Department of Audiology and Speech
  Pathology
Memphis State University
Memphis, Tennessee

J. Stephen Sinclair, Ph.D.
Assistant Professor
Department of Communicative Disorders
California State University
Northridge, California

Anderson D. Smith, Ph.D.
Associate Professor of Psychology
School of Psychology
Georgia Institute of Technology
Atlanta, Georgia

Edward Valenstein, M.D.
Associate Professor
Department of Neurology
University of Florida College of Medicine
Gainesville, Florida

Elizabeth J. Webster, Ph.D.
Professor
Department of Audiology and Speech
  Pathology
Memphis State University
Memphis, Tennessee

Erica F. Wood, J.D.
Legal Research and Services for the Elderly
National Council of Senior Citizens
Washington, D.C.

AGING

Section I

Normal Communication Processes and Aging

EDITORS' INTRODUCTION

Speech–language pathology and audiology have a rich tradition of basing understanding and treatment of communication disorders on a foundation of knowledge of normal human development. Much attention has been given to prenatal growth and to development in infancy and early childhood. However, changes in the physiological and psychological processes associated with communication continue throughout adulthood, and the communication problems of young adults and the elderly occur within the context of dynamic changes comprising the aging process. The eight chapters in Section I present current theory and research pertaining to changes throughout adulthood in the organic and psychological structures and processes that are involved in communication. It is hoped that the contents of this section will enrich the understanding of communication disorders and stimulate continued research, especially in determining the impact of normal aging on the nature and treatment of communication disorders.

The organization of chapters in Section I is not arbitrary. After Knox's general overview of issues in the study of adult development, the remaining seven chapters are oriented, first, toward the aging of organic structures and processes involved in speech and hearing and, then, toward the aging of neurological and psychological mechanisms involved in the

use of language. In a sense, these chapters proceed from a focus on peripheral processes to a focus on central processes.

Knox (Chapter 1) establishes the underlying viewpoint of this book, in which aging is considered to be a lifelong process that is not restricted to childhood or old age. He discusses psychosocial development in adulthood, including such topics as adult education and learning; roles in family, occupation, and community; societal context; physical condition; personality; and key change events. The value of this information for practitioners in speech–language pathology and audiology is given repeated attention. Knox believes that practitioners may better serve their adult clientele by being familiar with the dynamic changes occurring within adulthood. His general perspective on adult development provides a context for the more specific topics covered in the rest of this book.

The next chapter directs attention to a specific component of the communication process as Kahane (Chapter 2) reviews investigations of anatomical and physiological changes in the mechanisms used for speech production. The author contributes a comprehensive survey of research on aging of the respiratory system and the laryngeal and supralaryngeal components of speech production. He concludes with the implications of these changes for speech production.

What enables a person to identify the age of

another person by simply listening to him talk? Kent and Burkard (Chapter 3) discuss acoustic correlates of speech production and relate these correlates to the changes in the respiratory—phonatory system, the supralaryngeal or articulatory system, and the neuromuscular control system. To date only general answers to questions in this area have been obtained, and there is plenty of room for further investigation.

Nadol (Chapter 4) turns to hearing with a review of literature on the normal aging of the peripheral hearing mechanism. Hearing loss that accompanies aging of the inner ear is commonly referred to as *presbycusis*. The author defines four types of presbycusis and illustrates each with case studies including audiometric patterns and pathological findings. The patterns of hearing loss can be related to structural changes within the inner ear.

The next chapter leaves peripheral mechanisms behind and focuses on aging of the central nervous system. The central nervous system is responsible for higher levels of communicative function including perception, use of language, and the programming of motor activity. Valenstein (Chapter 5) deals primarily with age-related changes in human brain structure, including its gross morphology and its microscopic neural structure. Certain changes begin in adulthood or middle adulthood and continue throughout life rather than starting only in old age. The author also examines structural changes in Alzheimer's disease, thereby addressing the difficult distinction between normal and pathological aging.

Obler and Albert (Chapter 6) discuss the behavioral changes that may accompany changes in the neurophysiological substrata described by Valenstein. Obler and Albert focus on changes in language behavior and present some previously unpublished research from their preliminary investigation of this area. They also address characteristics of language use in the dementia of Alzheimer's disease. Finally, they look into the development of functional specialization within the cerebral hemispheres, namely, whether left lateralization of language function is a phenomenon of childhood or actually continuous throughout the lifespan.

The last two chapters are concerned with general mental functions in adulthood that are related to communicative behavior, especially language behavior. It is commonly believed that a person's intelligence and memory are necessarily victimized by the aging process. Denny (Chapter 7) examines three traditions in the investigation of adult cognition. These traditions include the use of intelligence tests, the Piagetian model of cognitive structures, and use of problem-solving tasks. The author subsequently explores a variety of approaches used to facilitate the cognitive function of elderly people. This chapter concludes with a theory of cognitive development that outlines stages throughout adulthood.

The naivete of simplistic statements about memory changes as a function of aging becomes obvious after reading Smith and Fullerton's review (Chapter 8) of the extensive research on the subject. Memory itself is a highly differentiated process; therefore, if one were to think accurately about age and memory, one must think about particular components of memory. The authors come to conclusions about aging of sensory memory, short-term memory, and the various aspects of long-term memory. Many of the studies reviewed in this chapter include verbal stimuli and address memory processes used in language behavior.

Hopefully the contributions in Section I will provide the reader with an adequate background in the various dimensions of normal aging as they relate to communication. In turn, this background should permit the interested student to pursue individual interests in this area as well as provide a backdrop to later chapters, which are oriented more specifically to communication problems.

Alan B. Knox

1

Adult Development

Audiologists and speech and language pathologists are dealing increasingly with an adult clientele. Practitioners concerned with communication disorders are thus becoming more interested in psychosocial development during adulthood. A speech pathologist may want to better understand problems of relearning by an older adult following throat surgery. An audiologist may want to better understand likely personality changes of a middle-aged adult who experiences a major hearing loss. An increasing number of practitioners concerned with communication disorders wonder about the influence on therapeutic efforts of the settings of older adults (such as living alone, living in a nursing home, or living with offspring).

This chapter provides an overview of generalizations about adult development along with implications for practitioners. Following the initial section regarding the utility of a comprehensive and developmental perspective on adulthood by practitioners who work with adults, there are sections on developmental trends regarding educative activity; role performance in family, occupation, and community; societal context; physical condition; personality; and change events. The chapter concludes with a section on the professional's role in using such generalizations in the process of professional decision making. The purpose of this chapter is to provide a brief overview of normal adult development and to thus encourage practitioners to become more familiar with the growing literature on adult

development in order to acquire a comprehensive developmental perspective on adulthood (Birren, 1964; Howe, 1977; Hurlock, 1968; Kalish, 1975; Knox, 1977a; Maas & Kuypers, 1974; Troll, 1975).

PERSPECTIVE ON ADULTHOOD

Practitioners concerned with communication disorders during adulthood can be more effective if they have a comprehensive perspective on adult development. Such a perspective includes an understanding of the interplay of personal and situational influences on adult development, of developmental processes related to adaptation and change, and of ways in which practitioners can use these generalizations to help adult clients function more effectively.

Overview

Practitioners engaged in speech pathology and audiology are not alone in their growing interest in psychosocial development during adulthood and old age (*Counseling Psychologist*, 1976). Traditionally practitioners throughout the helping professions (teaching, social work, clergy, and health professions) focused their attention to human development on childhood and adolescence. Adulthood was considered a period of stability.

In recent decades, however, rapid social

change, pluralistic and equalitarian values, and an aging population have shifted our attention to the processes by which adult life unfolds. Practitioners have discovered that adulthood is composed of much outward adaptation and internal change, along with the established interests and activities that appear to be so stable over the years. They have gained useful insights into adult functioning by considering the mix of stability and change that occurs during adulthood. Some changes, such as increased confidence or decreased speed, occur gradually. Others, such as marriage or retirement, occur more abruptly. As a result of changes in physical condition, personality, and environmental conditions, performance evolves as the individual interacts with his or her societal context.

The adult clients themselves are also becoming more aware of their own development and change. This insight has been aided by attention to adult development in the mass media. Radio, television, and the movies deal with issues regarding adult adaptation and change, and newspapers and magazines are giving increasing attention to many aspects of adult development. Some books on this topic have reached a large readership (O'Neill & O'Neill, 1974; Sheehy, 1976). One important task of practitioners is to help adult clients gain a broad and accurate perspective on adult development.

Adult Development

Practitioners who understand age-related trends and processes related to adaptation and growth are more likely to help clients. Many aspects of adult development have implications for practitioners. Included are generalizations about expectations and performance in family, occupation, and community roles throughout the adult life cycle. In addition to adult role performance and influences from the societal context in which it occurs, the professional literature on adult development includes generalizations regarding developmental trends and mechanisms regarding physical condition and personality. Practitioners tend to be especially interested in interactions among the foregoing generalizations that help to predict and explain successful adaptation. The major increase in tested knowledge from research about adult development during recent decades enables practitioners to move beyond a generalized commitment to being responsive to adult clients to apply detailed insight into developmental mechanisms and adaptation by adults (Knox, 1977a). Such organized knowledge can be greatly augmented

through perceptiveness and reflectiveness in daily interactions with individual adults, and it is in this arena that organized knowledge about adult development must be applied if it is to be most useful to practitioners and their clients.

Practitioners with a developmental perspective recognize the important interweaving of stability and change. Such a perspective helps identify more options in the process of coping with changes. In addition, each stage of life tends to have its own values for judging desirable behavior. Such insights can enable practitioners to approach the specific and immediate concerns of adult clients in comprehensive and developmental ways. Adults who recognize developmental changes as normal can approach many changes not as isolated problems but as part of the total life cycle, affected by experiences that preceded them and affecting experiences yet to come. Such a perspective helps the individual to recognize more options.

Application

It is not sufficient for practitioners to gain a comprehensive and developmental perspective on adulthood. They should in turn help clients acquire such a perspective for themselves. This is important because, by definition, the client's active participation is essential for effective practice in the helping professions. Practitioners then can assist adults to recognize likely trends and adjustments. Practitioners also can use generalizations about adult development and learning in several other ways, such as facilitation of client self-directedness, linking of client needs with relevant resources, and articulation of services with those from other specialists.

There are various ways in which practitioners can help adults maintain and enhance their self-directedness in life roles generally and in specific learning activities related to speech and hearing. Adults can be encouraged to revise old dreams and aspirations and to create or adopt new ones to provide a sense of direction (Levinson, 1978). The likelihood that a person will approach adulthood as a period of continued change is enhanced by contact with similar people whose approach to life is growthful. Practitioners can encourage adults to associate with such role models and to be alert to societal expectations and opportunities that foster development. Effective practitioners help adults help themselves (Knowles, 1970). In most instances, forms of assistance that encourage initiative and self-sufficiency are desirable, and forms of assistance that foster dependency on professionals or others are undesirable. Effective practitioners sometimes serve as knowledge brokers and change agents (Havelock, 1969). Such assistance is more likely for practitioners who are aware of relevant resources.

EDUCATIVE ACTIVITY

Practitioners concerned with communication disorders of adulthood tend to deal with educative activity by adults in several ways. One occurs when an adult client seeks the assistance of a speech pathologist or audiologist because a communication disorder (such as hearing loss by an older adult or motor speech disorder due to stroke) interferes with the adult's efforts to engage in educative activity (such as participation in a study–discussion group). Another occurs when the practitioner seeks to help an adult client learn as a part of the therapeutic activity. Examples include learning in order to adjust to the use of a hearing aid and to recover satisfactory speech following a stroke.

This section of the chapter provides an overview of developmental generalizations about adult learning activities, ability, and dynamics. Practitioners with such a perspective on adult learning should be more able to help adults with various characteristics, including age, to learn effectively than practitioners who assume that adults learn best under the conditions children typically confront in school (Belbin & Belbin, 1972; Botwinick, 1967; Gagné, 1972; Houle, 1972; Knowles, 1970; Knox, 1974, 1977a; Parker & Paisley, 1966; Tough, 1978).

Information Seeking

Purposeful and systematic adult learning activities, such as work with a speech therapist or participation in a continuing education course or workshop, are part of a broader range of activity referred to as information seeking (Parker & Paisley, 1966). Information seeking includes instrumental use of mass media and conversation with acquaintances and experts. Information seeking for instrumental purposes by blue-collar adults (those with lower levels of education, income, and occupational prestige) of any age tends to emphasize oral communications with family, friends, and acquaintances and not to include use of the mass media and experts (Knox, 1977a). Practitioners who seek to serve blue-collar adults are therefore more likely to help them with learning activities that fit their life-styles and

information-seeking methods. This might include an oral explanation supplemented by a brief and basic outline of major points to remember.

Similarly, the extent of adult participation in part-time or short-term continuing education activities is largely associated with the level of formal education, age, and sense of educational efficacy. There is a decline with age for major instances of self-directed study and for participation in educational programs sponsored by educational institutions and other types of organizations, such as employers, churches, and professional associations. Better understanding of adults as learners can help practitioners establish more effective linkage between client systems and relevant resource systems and services. Practitioners can use this understanding to decide which type of educational activity to suggest to a specific adult client (Johnstone & Rivera, 1965; Knox, 1977a; Knox & Farmer, 1977; Tough, 1978).

Learning Effectiveness

Practitioners with experience helping adults learn discover that almost any adult is able to learn almost any subject, given sufficient time and attention (Botwinick, 1973; Howe, 1977; Jarvik, Eisdorfer, & Blum, 1973; Knox, 1977a; Tough, 1978). However, both practitioners and their adult clients are sometimes concerned about trends in learning ability during adulthood. This is in part because adults tend to underestimate their learning ability by overemphasizing their early school experiences and underemphasizing their recent informal learning experiences.

Learning effectiveness is also affected by the adult's approach to the learning activity. This approach partly reflects personality characteristics such as self-directedness and preference for structure. It also reflects recency of educational experience. For adults with comparable ability, participants in recent educational activities typically learn more effectively. Learning effectiveness also is difficult to estimate because it is often characterized by bursts of new ideas and insights followed by periods of consolidation. As a result, there is an increasing range of individual differences in learning abilities, at least through the fifties.

For the individual adult, the greatest decline in learning ability with age occurs for tasks that are abstract, fast paced, unusual, and complex. However, for learning tasks that draw from adult experience, such as those related to general information and formal reasoning, performance is stable or improves somewhat during most of adulthood. In combination, this produces a fairly stable ceiling capacity.

Most people perform well below their ceiling capacity. Social class differences in verbal behavior further confound an accurate estimate of learning ability. Practitioners who recognize this can provide newcomers with attractive learning tasks in which they will readily succeed so that they gain realistic estimates of their learning abilities. Evaluation feedback during learning activities can further contribute to effective learning. Practitioners can also emphasize learner abilities and minimize features related to disabilities by drawing upon the learner's experience so that "wisdom" can be substituted for "brilliance."

Learning Dynamics

As practitioners engage in patient education, even more important than optimism about learning ability throughout adulthood is attention to processes and conditions that contribute to learning effectiveness. Included are attention to memory, reinforcement, interference, pacing, search for meaning, adjustment, perception, and creativity.

Short-term memory for moderate amounts of meaningful material with adequate opportunity for acquisition tends to be relatively stable during most of adulthood. Older adults, however, experience an increasing deficit in the ability to register information in memory. This is especially so when older adults try to store new information and recall stored information at the same time (Botwinick, 1967). Older adults become more cautious and make errors due to forgetting (omission) instead of mistakes (commission). Greater accumulation of related information causes older adults to expand the scope of their search in efforts to recall. This may result in greater interference. Conditions that aid meaningful organization facilitate recall, especially for older adults with high verbal ability. Long-term memory is retained even better with age, and the small amount that is forgotten can usually be regained by practice (Botwinick, 1967; Eisdorfer & Lawton, 1973). Practitioners can use advance organizers, summary materials, personal pacing, and reviews of previous material to compensate for inadequate memory.

Learning is facilitated by reinforcement, which encourages the learner to persist in the learning activity and to master learning tasks. One form of reinforcement is practice. Older adults typically require more practice to master new verbal material. Other forms of reinforcement include job advance-

ment and recognition. Practitioners can increase reinforcement by matching program objectives to learner needs, by varying learning tasks to encourage practice, by recognizing educational achievements, by encouraging group support, and by connecting learning activities with opportunities for application (Knowles, 1970).

When an adult studies a topic, some prior learning facilitates new learning, some interferes, and some is unrelated (Knox, 1977a). When prior learning interferes, it may take longer to master a learning task because it is necessary to unlearn the interfering materials as well as to learn the new material. Older adults tend to experience more interference from conflicting prior learning, but they also obtain more assistance from facilitative prior learning, which largely reflects their extent of experience with the topic instead of age itself.

Older adults especially learn most effectively when they set their own pace, when they take a break periodically, and when the distribution of learning episodes is fitted to the context (Knox, 1977a). The speed at which learning occurs is a major age-related influence on learning effectiveness. Much of the decline in educational performance by older adults reflects a speed deficit instead of a decline in learning power. Older adults tend to reduce speed and emphasize accuracy. Sufficient time and personal pacing can help reduce age differences in learning performance.

Effective adult learning is an active search for meaning. Adults seldom learn, remember, and use answers for which they do not already have the question. Practitioners who understand this point seek to involve participants actively in objective setting to increase relevance, in selection and organization of learning activities to fit preferred learning style, and in evaluation to increase responsiveness and use of increased proficiency. The general goal is helping adults to learn how to learn.

In patient education, it is fairly easy for educational activity to be problem and experience centered. Adults tend to accumulate experience and concepts around adult life tasks instead of around the structure of knowledge. A practitioner who wants to build new information on existing understandings can talk with an adult client to identify current understandings and feelings related to the communication disorder. Materials and discussion with a practitioner or other adults with the same health problem can then provide opportunities for the client to actively explore the topic and to consider how to use the concepts in dealing with the problem. Evaluative feedback by the practitioner can also help the client gain a sense of progress in the patient-education activity.

Learning is enhanced by satisfactory adjustment to the physical and social environment of the learning activity. A participant who feels estranged by social relationships or threatened by educational expectations typically has difficulty learning and consequently withdraws. Practitioners who understand this concept seek to create a setting for learning that helps adults achieve important and relevant educational objectives in addition to encouraging them to feel welcome, that provides reassurance to offset a fear of failure, that encourages group support and sharing, and that provides freedom to explore within democratic limits the achievement of objectives and the discovery of additional desirable objectives. An adjustment problem that affects many adults is competing demands from other adult responsibilities that can interfere with patient-education activities. A practitioner who understands this can work out with the adult client arrangements for educative activities that are least likely to conflict with other responsibilities and are most likely to be accomplished.

Especially for older adults, learning can be affected by the interrelated influences of biological systems, mental health, nutrition, and exercise. After age 50, visual acuity and hearing sensitivity decline gradually. An impoverished learning environment and disuse of study skills also affect learning performance. Practitioners can minimize the extent to which these conditions hamper learning by providing appropriate diagnostic and therapeutic services.

It is helpful for practitioners to recognize connections between adaptation and creative activity generally. Creativity is little related to age, although test results on creative intellectual output parallel findings from productivity studies (Knox, 1977a). The more creative adults at any age are more sensitive to external stimuli and more receptive to internal impulses. They are less censoring during the exploratory stage of creative effort. Less creative adults concentrate too earnestly, stifle novelty, and often concentrate on the defects of an approach instead of exploring its potential. Practitioners who understand this can help adults approach change and adaptation in growthful and creative ways.

In general, practitioners can help create circumstances under which adults with various characteristics, including age, learn effectively. Because adults vary in their abilities and disabilities related to learning, educational activities can be designed to minimize features related to disabilities and to emphasize features that build on abilities and experi-ence. Because an understanding of major aspects of a topic enables adults to relate prior knowledge and accumulate additional knowledge, advance organizers (composed of such major aspects as basic concepts, definitions, and rules) facilitate the building of a useful cognitive structure and contribute to progress from basic concepts to more difficult ones. Because affective intensity contributes to strong registration in memory, memorable encounters encourage rehearsal and reinforcement. Because adults learn more effectively when they proceed at their own pace and are able to use preferred resources, effective educational programs provide for individualization. Because feedback enhances learning effectiveness and persistence, program-evaluation procedures are very desirable. An understanding of learning dynamics as well as variations in learning activity with educational level and age can enable practitioners to design effective patient education activities.

ROLE PERFORMANCE

Most practitioners in the helping professions use generalizations about adult development and learning to help clients function or perform effectively. Practitioners concerned with communication disorders help adults with speech or hearing problems to function more effectively in any setting. Thus, an understanding of developmental trends in role performance can contribute to an appreciation of points at which therapeutic activities regarding communication disorders are likely to be affected by major areas of adult role performance.

The following adult-life-cycle trends in performance are grouped around family, occupational, and community roles. Suggestions are also provided regarding ways in which educative activity might facilitate adaptation and growth related to each role area. Some distinctive age trends are associated with each area of role performance. Regarding family role, as adolescents leave home, parents lose satisfaction from active parenting but gain freedom to pursue personal interests. Regarding occupational role, young workers tend to excel in tasks that use speed, strength, memory, and production of novel solutions, in contrast with older workers who tend to excel in tasks that use experience, steadiness, attendance, patience, and conscientiousness. Regarding community roles in recreation, organizations, political affairs, and religious organizations, although the extent of social participation is stable during most of adulthood, the mix of types of activities shifts from active in young adulthood to interpersonal in middle age to introspective in old age (Atchley, 1972; Bengston, 1973; Kimmel, 1974; Neugarten, 1968).

Family

Performance in family roles provides an especially congenial aspect of performance to which to relate therapy regarding communication disorders because such performance is so familiar (Eshleman, 1974; Hill, Foote, Aldous, Carlson, Macdonald, 1970; Hurlock, 1968; Troll, 1975). Almost everyone has some family experience. However, patterns of family life are varied. There is a widespread pattern in which a young couple is married, has children, and remains married until death. Other patterns include childless couples; unmarried parents; couples who marry late and have children late; divorced, widowed, and single adults; and remarried adults. Within each of these patterns, part of the variability is associated with the level of income and education. Among white-collar families that follow the widespread pattern, the husband and wife typically divide responsibilities and power either in generally equalitarian or in somewhat partriarchal ways. This occurs for the majority of both white and black middle-class families (Eshleman, 1974).

There is some evidence of a trend toward more equalitarian marriages and a decrease in sex-role differentiation among young white-collar couples, but among blue-collar couples the emotional allegiance to traditional patterns remains strong. Practitioners who work with adults should recognize these varied patterns of family life and take them into account.

There has been a gradual decline in age of first marriage during the past two generations (especially for white-collar families) followed by a rise during the past decade. For those who follow the widespread pattern, early marital adjustment is associated both with characteristics that the partners bring with them and with evolving interrelationships between them. Personal characteristics associated with marital happiness include personal adjustment, similarity of backgrounds and values, effective interpersonal relationships, complementarity of needs, compatibility of role expectations, and well-adjusted parents. Interpersonal relationships associated with marital happiness include mature and stable love for each other, satisfactory sexual adjustment, adequacy of family finances, participation in family work and activities, and satisfactory relations with in-laws. Blue-collar families tend to experience less satisfactory marital adjustment, which reflects low levels of income, of

occupational stability, and of education. However, more blue-collar families have cohesive extended family systems, which can reduce some in-law problems and increase sources of companionship. Sometimes efforts to assist with communication disorders occur at the same time as major marital adjustments, and in such instances, practitioners who are aware of family-role dynamics can be more effective than those who are unable to interpret symptoms of marital discord.

When the youngest child enters school, a major transition typically occurs, especially for the mother who is not employed outside the home. Many nonworking mothers rethink their interests and activities at this time, and the proportion of employed mothers of young children has been rising rapidly in recent years. Under favorable conditions, maternal employment need not have any major adverse effects on the children. Perhaps the greatest influence on the satisfactoriness of wives' working outside the home is the husbands' attitudes. Societal acceptance of working wives has increased in recent decades. For some women, work satisfaction contributes to an improved quality of family life that compensates for reduced contact and shifts in family responsibilities (Hoffman & Nye, 1974).

The launching of adolescent children as they leave the family for work, marriage, or college constitutes a challenge and transition for the parents as well as the adolescents. Although it may be difficult, it is important that parents accept some adolescent assertiveness as part of the process of establishing adult identity, which is vital to subsequent development. It sometimes helps middle-aged adults to tolerate this challenge to assumptions, authority, and instances in which they do not practice what they preach, if they appreciate that the reassertion of values by the young makes an important contribution to cultural continuity and societal renewal.

The loss of active parent roles tends to be followed by the gain of new roles as grandparents. Especially in white-collar families, grandparents tend to relate to their grandchildren in ways that have been referred to as fun seeking, formal, parent substitute, family wisdom, or distant figure. During the postparental period, there is usually a shift from coping with external changes to interpersonal relationships between the husband and wife.

Retirement brings other adjustments (Atchley, 1975; Binstock & Shanas, 1976; Eisdorfer & Lawton, 1973; Hurlock, 1968; Kalish, 1975; Williams & Wirths, 1965). For many homemakers, an early retirement adjustment occurs when the last child leaves home. This often entails mixed feelings including lost satisfactions from active parenthood and gained freedom to pursue personal interests. When the husband retires from his job, he usually shifts from the role of family provider to a subordinate role in his wife's domain. This role reversal also occurs when aging parents move into the households of their offspring and become dependent on them for financial support and companionship. In general, a mutually satisfactory relationship over the years contributes to a satisfactory relationship in retirement, which brings a greater increase in time together. However, a long-standing frictional relationship is likely to contribute to increased friction and unhappiness with the onset of retirement.

In addition to the foregoing widespread pattern, there are other patterns of the family life cycle. Some couples choose not to have children because of concern about unwanted responsibilities, conflict with careers, or congenital problems. Childless couples realize that today this does not threaten the security of their old age. Those who marry for the first time and have children during their thirties experience about as much marital adjustment and happiness as those who do so during their twenties and more than those who marry in their teens (Eshleman, 1974). The somewhat older parent tends to be more concerned about the child's needs and can become overprotective. Some atypical family patterns include common-law marriage, unmarried parents, and older orphans living together.

Divorce has become more widespread. A few years ago, about one out of six adults who had ever been married had been divorced. Current estimates are that about one out of three current marriages will end in divorce. Divorce and separation rates are higher for blue-collar families than for white-collar families (Epstein, 1974; Eshleman, 1974). Many of those who divorce subsequently remarry or in other ways proceed to very satisfactory lives. The difficult experience of divorce can produce insights into one's self and the marital relationship that can provide the basis for future growth.

Widowhood is one of the most abrupt and difficult adjustments that most people experience. More than half the men and women who are widowed do not marry during the subsequent 5 years, and many never do. Financial and other forms of preparation can reduce some of the problems of widowhood. The great feelings of loss and lack of affection typically constitute the main adjustment problems, which are somewhat reduced if the surviving partner has close and satisfying social relationships with family and friends. The death of a spouse is similar for blue-collar as for white-collar adults, except that financial and social resources are more limited for the former. However, the extended blue-collar family often provides a larger proportion of support and assistance than do white-collar families (Silverman, 1973).

More than one out of five marriages each year is a remarriage for one or both of the new partners. A higher proportion of divorced adults than widowed adults remarry within 5 years, and divorced men remarry sooner than divorced women. About 1 out of 12 adults have never been married, and most of these have remained single by choice. In recent decades women have had a wider range of family-role options. Influences on attitudes toward being a full-time wife and mother include the heavy societal emphasis on self-interest, contractual exchanges, and monetary rewards in the larger society; the giving tasks and intangible rewards of the homemaker role; the shift of former family functions to other institutions; shrinking purchasing power of family income; and an extended postparental period. As a result of such changes and a wider range of options, many women are considering and making choices that formerly seemed unavailable. This is reflected in trends regarding age at marriage, size of family, working mothers, and divorce. Greater self-direction and assertiveness is apparent in work and in the community as well as in family settings.

Occupation

Communication disorders, such as abrupt losses of hearing or speech capability, can be especially disruptive of the worker role for many adults. Such difficulties can have a detrimental effect on self-concept, particularly in view of the fact that one's occupation helps establish one's self-concept as well as one's level of living and prestige. Occupational decisions reflect both personal preferences and available opportunities, and the process of choosing has become more difficult as the variety of occupations has increased (Holland, 1973).

Career development occurs throughout the work life, and it is influenced by attitudes such as assertiveness and willingness to accept new responsibilities. The rapidly changing occupational structure is resulting in multiple careers, for which practitioners can help adults understand and plan. This is especially pertinent when a major communication disorder necessitates a career change.

On some indices of unsatisfactory occupational performance, such as work-related accidents, absenteeism, and unemployment, the average record of young adults is worse than that of middle-aged and older adults. Unemployment rates are mainly affected by general economic conditions and tend to be highest for urban minority youth, blue-collar workers, and women.

People work for many reasons, including money, status, satisfaction, recognition, service, companionship, and self-actualization. More white-collar workers emphasize work itself and deemphasize its benefits than is the case for most blue-collar workers (Herzberg, 1966). Herzberg suggested that this was because the work done by white-collar workers tends to be more interesting. Additionally, there are some shifts in expectations regarding jobs—from income, interesting work, and potential success for young workers to independence from supervision and job security for older workers (Schein, 1978).

Occupational adjustments also have an impact on other life roles. Midcareer occupational changes can reach crisis proportions and adversely affect family life, but they also can present new opportunities and directions. Even though mandatory retirement forces many older workers to terminate employment, this is especially difficult for many white-collar workers whose work satisfaction tends to be high, and thus some persons continue with other forms of economically productive activity (Atchley, 1975).

Practitioners concerned with communication disorders are most likely to deal with occupational adjustments when they are affected by abrupt losses of hearing or speech capability. Practitioners with some understanding of occupational development can refer clients to other practitioners who can provide specialized assistance if needed. However, there are some ways in which speech pathologists and audiologists can contribute directly to occupational adjustment when the occasion arises. They can help clients consider general trends and variability in career development in order to place current adjustment in perspective. Practitioners can help adults recognize satisfactory and unsatisfactory job performance and understand the multiple motives for working, including benefits and the work per se. They can also help clients to consider personal talents and priorities when considering a career change and to locate relevant opportunities to increase occupational satisfaction and performance (Schein, 1978).

Community

Adult role performance also includes community participation in recreation, organizations, political affairs, and religious organizations. Adjustments sometimes occur in participation that practitioners would do well to understand (Hurlock, 1968; Knox, 1977a). Specific types of social participation follow quite different trends during adulthood, which produces a changing mix from young adulthood to middle age and beyond. In spite of the much greater association of social participation with social-class level than with age, there is a developmental shift from activities that are physically vigorous and action oriented in late adolescence and young adulthood to activities that are concerned with interpersonal relations and understanding in middle age to activities that are cultural and introspective beyond middle age.

When the total fabric of participation is analyzed, much of it forms a highly stable plateau for most of adulthood. About half of social-participation variables are quite stable during much of adulthood, and they mainly consist of social relations and solitary activities that reflect such personality characteristics as activity level and values. Examples include informal activities with close friends and religious participation, which tend to be stable until declining health affects activities outside the home. Forms of participation that steadily decline during adulthood reflect differentiation and variety in social relations, as illustrated by the proportion of adults who attend movies or athletic events, participate in outings, or read books. Forms of participation that steadily expand during adulthood reflect informal intimate social relationships with members of primary groups. Interaction with family and close friends tends to increase through middle age. Some forms of social participation follow a cyclical pattern of expansion from young adulthood to middle age followed by reduction of activity. This trend reflects status-related active participation in formal types of interaction, such as the number of organizational memberships or extent of political participation. Participation variables that alternate up and down during adulthood, for example, the frequency of attendance at meetings, reflect changes in roles and statuses in occupation and family. There are also life-cycle shifts in the meanings and satisfactions that leisure activities have for adults; leisure activities of young adults tend to relate to occupation, while for older adults similar activities tend to contrast with occupation.

A little understood but important type of participation is friendship, and making an art of friendship has been identified as a developmental task of adulthood. Most people who fail to establish desired friendships are barred by inadequate understanding of the important functions served by friendship and the effective procedures for making new friends. Practitioners can help adults enter friendship groups and better understand the friend-making process. For example, aspects of close friendships include similarity, reciprocity, compatibility, closeness, and role models. Those who want to make new friends can be helped to acknowledge that their needs for intimacy and relatedness are not being met and to understand that the most enduring and mutually beneficial friendships entail an interdependency in which each member combines self-assertiveness and caring for others (Lowenthal, Thurnher, Chiriboga, Beeson, Giay, Lurie, Pierce, Spencer & Weiss, 1975).

Practitioners can also help adults understand interactions between personal preferences and societal opportunities in relation to likely long-term shifts in participation. This can be especially useful for older adults adapting to communication disorders.

SOCIETAL CONTEXT

Adult performance and adaptation is influenced by expectations, resources, demands, and constraints in the societal context in which he or she functions (Barker, 1968; Maccoby & Jacklin, 1974). Practitioners in the helping professions are more likely to be effective if they understand these major influences and help clients profit from those that are beneficial. Adult development reflects the individual's transactions with the societal context, which includes people, groups, and organizations related to adult roles in family, work, and community. Personal characteristics, such as alertness, accumulated experience, and personality influence the extent to which adults use resources and confront problems in the context of family, community, and world. Such personal characteristics also affect how an adult responds to the problems and opportunities that are encountered.

Social Change

In the United States, rapid social change, widespread mobility, loss of a sense of community, and societal attitudes toward various age groups combine to affect the process of adult development (Toffler, 1970). In a slowly changing society, adolescents and young adults can see in their older relatives and friends the sorts of people they themselves are likely to become. Values and practices are introduced to the young, and the older generations experience little obsolescence. By contrast, in our rapidly changing pluralistic society, young adults confront a world that is different in many ways from the one their grandparents knew as young adults.

Current societal circumstances also affect adult development. For example, poor economic conditions increase unemployment, which adversely affects the self-concept of those who are most likely to be unemployed, such as young men from minority groups, older workers, and women who work part-time.

Gradual shifts in the societal context can also influence adult development. For example, as young people enter adulthood with more formal education and older people with less formal education die, the average level of formal education of adults has risen rapidly. This can affect the occupational prospects of middle-aged workers, especially those who do not keep up with new developments in their field.

Societal Attitudes

Societal attitudes and stereotypes toward various stages of adulthood affect adult development. In actuality, many values and personality characteristics, such as autonomy and nurturance, tend to be quite stable from generation to generation in a family. People's stereotypes of age trends shift from active and outgoing in young adulthood to understanding and restraint in middle age to constricted activity and increased introspection in old age. Such stereotypes partly reflect personal experience as a counterbalance to attitudes acquired from the media and other people. For example, those with more positive attitudes toward the elderly tend to be white collar, to have older living relatives, to have avoided major burdens or conflicts with older adults, and to have strong nurturance needs (Knox, 1977a).

Practitioners can assist adults to gain a broader perspective that includes the distinction between social change and personal change as a basis for interpreting generational differences and guiding adults' own efforts to adapt and change systematically. Some characteristics associated with older adults reflect growing up 60 or 70 years ago. Many adults express a preference for greater control over their lives. A proactive stance toward life and society is enhanced by a sense of security, self-esteem, and direction as the basis for responsible involvement. A recognition of dehumanizing societal influences that discourage responsiveness and frustrate growth helps the individual counteract or at least deflect them. Desirable adjustments can serve as a stimulus for continued development. Small adjustments, such as decisions regarding educational, family, work, and community settings, can increase the likelihood that adults will become the sorts of people they want to become. Supportive attitudes from a reference group can facilitate development.

Social Class

Both problems and opportunities of adulthood are affected by the social-class level of the individual adult, including the life-style and social space associated with white-collar or blue-collar status. Although social-class values and practices have become more intermixed, practitioners can use distinctions between white-collar and blue-collar adults to recognize differences related to participation and information seeking and to minimize thoughtless imposition of middle-class values.

Community participation helps illustrate how social class influences adult development. The blue-collar life-style tends to be neighborhood oriented, and instrumental information is sought mainly through oral communication with family and friends. The white-collar life-style tends to be somewhat more oriented toward activities and ideas in the larger community and beyond, and instrumental information seeking tends to include more use of media and experts. In each stratum, friends and associates serve as opinion leaders and influence choices. Community organizations tend to reflect white-collar orientations toward formal procedures and written communications, which discourages participation by many blue-collar adults.

Encouragement

The setting in which adults live and work can either encourage or discourage development. This is illustrated by influences of college on young people, of the household setting for families, and of living arrangements for older adults.

During the past generation, a higher proportion of young people have attended college full-time than ever before. The college experience has an impact on intellectual and personality change. However, those who attend college are most likely to change anyway,

and personality changes tend to revert unless supported by the postcollege environment. Colleges that are most influential on personality development have images that attract students who are open to the types of changes that the colleges want them to acquire and also accentuate those distinctive characteristics. During the college years students tend to become less authoritarian, dogmatic, prejudiced, conservative toward public issues, and committed to religion. Intellectual interests and capability increase, however, and students become more sensitive to aesthetic experiences and open to multiple aspects of the contemporary world. Similar young adults who do not attend college also show increasing openness to new experience and growing tolerance, but perhaps not to the same extent (Trent & Medsker, 1968). In this context, practitioners can help people to achieve a useful match between personal and institutional characteristics and to continue personality and intellectual development beyond college.

The household setting can influence the attitudes and performance of family members in ways that are similar to the impact of college on students. Functioning families maintain their equilibrium and viability because, in the complex and often delicate balance of interpersonal relationships, the constructive and cohesive forces are greater than the destructive and divisive forces. A home and family setting is more likely to facilitate adult development when it is characterized by qualities such as family acceptance of change during adulthood, familiarity with adult role models who adapt, availability of learning resources for adults in the home, and awareness of educational opportunities for adults. Other facilitative qualities are allocation of family resources for adult learning, willingness of other family members to adapt to change by an adult member, and experience by children with their parents' learning activities so that the children enter adulthood with positive attitudes about lifelong learning.

Living arrangements for older adults that used to consist mainly of maintaining one's own home, moving in with family, or going to the "old folks' home," now also include retirement hotels, nursing homes, public housing for the elderly, and retirement communities. The accessibility and satisfactoriness of these alternative living arrangements vary substantially with the health and wealth of the older adult. Although many older adults live on very limited incomes, most are satisfied with their housing, and resist moves. Most older adults prefer not to live with their grown children unless it is necessitated by financial or health conditions. Each alternative living arrangement for the elderly has its costs and benefits. Residents of retirement communities report less interaction with family but more with friends. Some environments, such as homes for the aged or retirement hotels, tend to encourage dependence. Practitioners can help adults recognize the distinctive features of alternative settings and select a setting that encourages what the adult wants to become (Atchley, 1972; Bengston, 1973; Hill, Foote, Aldous, Carlson, & Macdonald, 1970; Kalish, 1975).

A better understanding of the influence of social-class levels, community settings, and intergenerational relations on adult development also contributes to a perspective that enables adults to recognize some of the major forces that affect their lives. A sense of personal direction can help adults deal with societal attitudes toward various stages of adulthood as well. A more proactive approach to adult life can enable men and women to select and shape living arrangements and community activities so that these interpersonal relationships help them achieve their goals.

For practitioners concerned with communication disorders, an understanding of societal expectations, resources, demands, and constraints is especially important. The attitudes of others regarding a hearing loss or a speech disorder of a client can either compound the problem or contribute to progress toward a solution. Both practioners and their clients can seek to establish such resources as satisfactory sound amplification and acoustics at public meetings, and group activities for adults engaged in speech therapy. A recognition of variations in social class and life-style can enable practitioners to appreciate an individual client's life space, and to help the client function maximally under the circumstances.

PHYSICAL CONDITION

Practitioners concerned with communication disorders during adulthood are very knowledgeable about physiology related to speech and hearing. However, many other aspects of physical condition shift during adulthood and need to be taken into account when working with adults of various ages (Finch & Hayflick, 1977; Kastenbaum, 1965; Timiras, 1972).

One major influence on physical condition is heredity (Maccoby & Jacklin, 1974). There are large variations in living conditions and other environmental influences that also affect appearance and level of physical functioning. Included are health conditions and practices before adulthood, adult nutrition and exercise, disease and emotional stress, and practices such as smoking and drinking.

Heredity and environmental circumstances influence longevity. Most of the increase in average life expectancy occurred during the first half of this century. More people are living to become old, but maximum life span for the human species has been fairly constant. Declining functional capacities interact with each other and with environmental hazards to increase sharply the risk of death with advancing age. Condition and longevity especially are associated with exposure and immunity to disease during middle age. The probability of incurring additional impairment at any time increases with the accumulation of previous impairments. With advanced old age, there appears to be a reduction in immunity (Timiras, 1972). Throughout most of adulthood, regular exercise in which the body is overloaded in graduated increments contributes to strength, endurance, and vitality that add life to the years as well as years to the life (Devries, 1974).

It becomes increasingly difficult for older adults to hear the softest sounds, smell the faintest aromas, and see in the dimmest lights. The aging eye and related nervous system reduce the visual information that is received. However, with corrective lenses and satisfactory illumination, most adults experience few restrictions because of visual impairment. Few visual changes are noted until about age 40. In addition to corrective lenses and illumination, visual impairments other than blindness can be compensated for by longer exposure time, increased print sizes, and combined audio and visual presentation of material, simplified sequences of information, and increased time for adaptation between lighted and darkened surroundings and for recovery from stress.

Hearing impairments increase gradually until the fifties, followed by an increase in the rate of degradation of auditory sensation and perception. Pitch discrimination gradually declines between the twenties and the fifties and then drops more abruptly. Older adults also have more difficulty screening out interfering noises (Bergman, 1971; Ramsdell, 1965). Practitioners can suggest the use of hearing aids and sound amplification to overcome these problems.

The frequency level or pitch of speech declines until middle age and then rises gradually into old age for males but changes little for females (Mysak, 1959). From middle age onward the rate of speech slows. Sensitivity to smell begins to decline after age 40, and most changes in taste sensitivity occur after age 50. The sense of touch increases until the midforties and then becomes less acute, and sensitivity to pain declines.

General slowing during adulthood is widely recognized. The peak in reaction time is about age 20, and by age 50 it has returned to about the average level of age 15. The slowing of reaction time is greater than for movement time. Older adults typically compensate for reduced speed by increased attentiveness and accuracy. Practitioners can use clear instructions and reinforcement procedures to help older adults improve speed and accuracy.

There are many ways in which practitioners might assist adults in preserving good physical condition and health. These include income maintenance as related to the understanding of balanced nutrition and access to and use of health services and health education relative to preventative health care.

The physical health of an adult reflects his or her transaction with the physical and social environment, and this is even more true for mental health. Typical mental health problems shift during adulthood. For example, phobias and tantrums are most likely to occur during youth and hysterical reactions during young adulthood. Obsessive−compulsive reactions are more typical of emotional problems during middle age, when the demands of life can overtax inadequate adaptive mechanisms. Depression for younger adults typically reflects introjection, whereas the more widespread incidence of depression for older adults reflects the external conditions that contribute to feeling depressed. The incidence of hypochondria also increases with age. Although the suicide rate increases with age, it rises steadily for men after retirement but increases only slightly for women through middle age and declines after age 60. Practical assistance related to nutrition, exercise, and preventive health can help most adults add more life to their years.

PERSONALITY

Experienced practitioners realize how important feelings are to adult clients who seek to adjust to communication disorders and to engage in related patient-education activities. To this end, a number of factors need to be emphasized, factors which may have a significant impact on the success of a clinical program.

Stability and Change

Personality characteristics and tendencies provide continuity across specific times and situations that enables us to predict likely thoughts, feelings, and actions. However, in addition to stability and continuity from year to year, there is evidence of substantial change and modification of adult personality from decade to decade (Baltes & Schaie, 1973; Birren & Schaie, 1977; Britton & Britton, 1972; Maddi, 1972; Neugarten & Assoc., 1964; Vaillant, 1977; White, 1961, 1972; Williams & Wirths, 1965).

An understanding of general personality constructs and trends during adulthood can enable practitioners to help adults gain a broader perspective on the variability within each phase of adulthood and the typical trends from phase to phase. Consistency in personal characteristics and societal circumstances helps maintain personality stability. In addition, there are adult-life-cycle shifts in self-concept, decision making, attitudes, moral development, and adaptation. The main impetus for personality change may come from either the individual or society, and change is more likely when facilitated by both personal striving and societal encouragement. In general, the sense of self tends to become more positive until middle age, and then to stabilize or gradually become less positive.

Practitioners can help adult clients resist false stereotypes about age-related personality characteristics, recognize the great variability in adult personality patterns, and understand the extent to which personality change occurs during adulthood. In some instances, practitioners may help clients recognize how other people contribute to their development, and in other instances they may help clients avoid overdependence. Shifts occur between deepening self-understanding and broadening experience through friendship. Practitioners can help clients use an increased understanding of their past interpersonal relations to deal more effectively with the present and plan for the future.

Self-Concept

Self-concept and performance interact during adulthood. Some young people create adolescent dreams that give a sense of direction and aspiration to their lives. As friends are substituted for family and adult commitments are made, the young adult's personality structure and pattern of participation become more complex. In midlife, some of the abstract commitments and aspirations that were formed in adolescence begin to wane. Being one's own person seems to be especially salient. This may be reflected in the transition from having a mentor to being a mentor (Levinson, 1978).

The increasingly widespread midlife transition

entails a reexamination of the relationship between the current sense of self and the structure of participation and commitments that have evolved. Around the forties there is often an increase in stocktaking as the adult realizes that the future is now. Although the stability and integration of self-concept tends to be predictive of subsequent adaptation, there is much variability in midlife adjustments. At any stage, the fragments of the sense of self that result from an identity transition become the building blocks for a reintegration that can allow the individual to become a more fully functioning person. For older adults, the adolescent dream is replaced by protection of gains and an inward shift toward more personal concerns. For many, a shift in time orientation occurs in which time remaining until death becomes more salient than time spent since birth.

Decision Making

An aspect of personality, in addition to self-concept, is the process of making choices or decisions. This executive function of the self entails assertiveness, goal setting, accommodation, and self-directedness. It also includes the mix of proactive and reactive behavior. Adults can become more assertive and decisive in the achievement of personal change. An active and self-directed approach to life entails the addition of commitment to the ability to transcend limitations. Practitioners can assist adults to become more self-directed through activities such as values clarification and priority setting. In addition, people can be helped to deal with change in a growthful way by recognizing that a positive attitude can turn an uncertain situation into success, by putting apprehension about an unknown situation in perspective, by focusing on past successes, and by retaining stability in other aspects of one's life when making a major change. Many adults who participate in patient-education activities want to be self-directed in the learner role as well. Practitioners who understand such generalizations about adult development can appreciate the variability that occurs and can help adults approach specific concerns and change events developmentally by recognizing options and opportunities for growth. For this to occur, however, adults who approach patient-education activities in a very dependent way must be helped to gradually become more self-directed learners.

Interests and Values

Vocational and avocational interests remain relatively stable during young adulthood. Change events are more frequent than for older adults. Those who recognize that they are not going to achieve their adolescent dreams but refuse to accept this conclusion and set more unrealistic goals are likely to experience frustration and depression. Those who achieve their dreams are often able to avoid stagnation by starting a challenging new career.

Adult-life-cycle shifts in value orientations also occur. Young adults emphasize expansiveness and high expectations, middle-aged adults emphasize self-limitation and reduction of frustrations, and older adults emphasize transcendence of self and family to include people generally. Older women stress personal caring and religious life, and older men stress leaving a tangible legacy or contribution to society (Lowenthal et al., 1975).

Happiness, morale, and life satisfaction also fluctuate during adulthood and reflect both objective circumstances and approach to life. Satisfaction is a function of expectation as well as of performance. Happiness is related to feelings of personal security, acceptance by others, personal efficacy, and a belief that life has meaning (Bradburn, 1969). Life satisfaction in old age is little related to age as such but rather to conditions such as illness and poverty that are associated with old age (Butler, 1975).

Adult life-cycle fluctuations in happiness are relatively stable when compared with other characteristics, such as socioeconomic status, self-esteem, physical health, and social participation. Perceived well-being typically rises from late adolescence to young adulthood, drops in early middle age, rises in late middle age before retirement, and then declines in old age (Campbell & Converse, 1975). Happiness tends to be associated with the individual's psychological resources. Reactive behavior tends to decline from late adolescence through middle age, followed by an increase in old age. Many older adults reminisce and weave recollected facts and unresolved conflicts of the past into an acceptable perspective. Often during a transition, a person experiences strong feelings of vulnerability and panic that make it difficult to maintain continuity and a sense of worth. Practitioners can assist adults to recognize the types of adjustments they are likely to confront, to develop realistic and constructive attitudes toward the resultant problems and opportunities, to acquire the needed understanding and competence, and to acquire supportive services (Binstock & Shanas, 1976).

In general, as practitioners work with adults with speech or hearing disorders, an understanding of personality development during adulthood can be useful in several ways. Practitioners can help adult clients to appreciate the extent of personality development that occurs during adulthood, as well as to understand the great variability in personality patterns. Practitioners can assist clients who confront major adjustment problems related to communication disorders to deal with change in positive and growthful ways. This process includes placing apprehension about the unknown in perspective, focusing on past successes, retaining stability in other aspects of one's life when making a major change, and recognizing the value of support groups of people who have gone through similar experiences (Levine & Scotch, 1970; O'Neill & O'Neill, 1974; Silverman, 1973; Toffler, 1970).

CHANGE EVENTS

Practitioners who deal with adult communication disorders can benefit from an understanding of change events during adulthood in at least two ways. One has to do with the abrupt onset of a speech or hearing disorder as a change event itself. The second is the variety of other change events that may affect the client during an extended period in which a practitioner is providing assistance regarding a communication disorder (Binstock & Shanas, 1976; Knox, 1977a).

Adaptation

Adult life is periodically punctuated by such change events as the birth of a child, a move to a new community, or retirement. An adult's approach to a change event is influenced by both personal and situational characteristics. The resulting changes help explain how adults experience so much change over the years in spite of great stability over the months. Because change events entail alterations in role relationships, some adaptation is inescapable. Change events vary regarding whether role relationships are gained, lost, or changed and regarding the extent of voluntariness, predictability, intensity, and stage of adulthood when they are most likely to occur. They tend to be concentrated in young adulthood.

Major change events tend to have great influence on adult development. Practitioners can help adults understand how change events disrupt the stability that is usually maintained by personality, habit, and the expectations of others. Change events may be met with apprehension, regret, and inaction, but they can also present opportunities for growth. The need for adaptation associated with most change events tends to produce heightened readiness to learn. Practitioners can help adults resist the tendency to panic and instead become more proactive through continuing action and contemplation.

Change events such as temporary unemployment or the death of a loved one are associated with feelings of loss. There is a general developmental process that often occurs when adults find out that a loss has or will soon occur. The stages are denial, anger, depression, bargaining, and acceptance. They do not necessarily occur in sequence; several may occur together, and some may not occur at all (Glaser & Strauss, 1968; Kastenbaum & Aisenberg, 1972; Kubler-Ross, 1969; Parkes, 1972; Schoenberg, 1974).

Retirement

Occupational retirement is one form of loss that is part of the social and psychological disengagement process that occurs during old age. Disengagement refers to the general process of withdrawal from society by older adults and the withdrawal of support to older adults by society (Atchley, 1975; Binstock & Shanas, 1976; Butler, 1975; Eisdorfer and Lawton, 1973; Kalish, 1975; Neugarten & Assoc., 1964; Williams & Wirths, 1965). Influences on the structure of participation and the retirement process include the environmental press from role expectations, opportunity system, general values and attitudes about aging, health, income, and personality. Some workers who retire early do so because of health problems or pressure from the employer. An increasing proportion are doing so voluntarily to enjoy their leisure, and a higher proportion of those who plan an early retirement enjoy their leisure than those who retire unexpectedly.

It appears that aging is a complex developmental process in which continuing modifications of activities and preferences reflect past adjustments. Personality characteristics are most predictive of successful aging. Blue-collar workers tend to adapt better to retirement in the short run, whereas white-collar workers adapt better in the long run (Atchley, 1975; Kalish, 1975). In general, life satisfaction results from the match between personality type and structure of participation (Atchley, 1975; Bengston, 1973; Kimmel, 1974; Williams & Wirths, 1965).

PRACTITIONER ROLE

In summary, an understanding of adult development and learning will be useful to practitioners to the extent to which they reflect such understanding in professional decision making. This can occur in relation to transactional influences, change events, relations among practitioners, policy issues, and research approaches. One way to use generalizations about adult development is to recognize likely developmental trends and to help clients do so as well.

Transactional Influences

Another use of developmental generalizations is to help clients understand how growth occurs as the individual adult interacts with people and activities in the societal context. For practitioners in the helping professions, information about contextual influences must typically be combined with information about the individual's outlook and aspirations. For example, the life-style and social space of blue-collar and white-collar adults differs in both prior experience and current problems and opportunities.

Generalizations about contrasting patterns of participation and information seeking in relation to social-class level become more useful to the practitioner when they are combined with insights about the outlook of the individual client. An adult who strongly prefers informal social groups and personalized information sources will probably adjust more successfully to a major role change if a family- or neighborhood-based self-help group rather than a formal organization is available. Likewise an adult whose typical learning strategy is characterized by openness and challenge-seeking is likely to respond to a provocative patient-education program, whereas an adult whose typical learning strategy is characterized by rigidity and defensiveness is likely to respond to a more structured educational program. Effective practitioners are able to match personal preferences of clients with facilitative people, resources, and settings.

Interrelations between personal and historical trends occur during the later part of adulthood. Since the turn of the century, the number and proportion of older adults has increased greatly. During the past generation or two, there has also been an increase in services, legislation, and public awareness related to aging. Regarding life-cycle trends, from middle to old age there tends to be an increase in sensory impairments, especially for hearing and vision. However, increased use of hearing aids, corrective lenses, and cataract surgery during the past generation have favorably influenced the problems and adjustments that individual older adults face.

Change Events

Major role changes are especially important for practitioners to understand. Practitioners can help clients become more self-directed and gain access to opportunities and resources that can facilitate adaptation. Adults can be encouraged to realize their potential more fully and to broaden their perspective on alternatives and on the process of change (Havelock, 1969).

The most fundamental way in which practitioners can assist clients is through broadening their perspective on adult development and learning. As adults better understand the orderly and sequential developmental changes in characteristics and attitudes that have occurred to them and to others in the past, they will become more able to predict and understand their subsequent behavior. A developmental perspective can enable adults to grasp essential current and unfolding features of their own lives and to recognize similarities and differences between their own lives and those of others. This can be difficult because of the great variability among adults and the differences from generation to generation due to rapid social change. A developmental perspective also helps minimize the imposition of value judgments on the changes. Each stage of life tends to have its own values, which are used to judge which combinations of changes are most desirable and constitute progress. The shift from leadership of youth groups in middle age to discussion of social issues in old age can be viewed as an expansion of engagement with mankind as well as a contraction of life space.

Even for desirable change events, adults vary greatly in their outlooks regarding change. Many people fear and resist changes, reacting to them with regret about what might have been and using their regret as an excuse for inaction. They become more vulnerable and less open, and their restriction of experience leads to narrowness. However, change events can also heighten an individual's potential, increase susceptibility to influence, and provide an impetus and an opportunity to grow. Adults who are most open, but have a sense of direction, are able to reconcile contradictions between the old and the new and achieve growth through action and contemplation.

Relations Among Practitioners

Adults are frequently caught in a cross fire of conflicting recommendations from various practitioners who are unaware of each other's efforts to assist the same client with related problems. Some of the ways in which discrepancies can be reduced include comprehensive career and educational counseling, clinics that maintain a common health and medical record for each patient that all specialists may consult, and comprehensive multipurpose senior citizens' centers. However, in any instance a practitioner can alert each adult client to the importance of trying to accommodate varied sources of assistance, obtain information about other practitioners who currently or recently worked with the client, and strive to use referrals to and consultations with other practitioners in ways that treat each client as a whole person.

Policy Issues

There are many ways in which practitioners who deal with communication disorders can take leadership regarding social policy related to adult development. The fundamental way is to enhance their own developmental perspective on adulthood through preparatory and continuing education, professional associations, and collaborative efforts. However, to increase their own proficiency is not enough. As has been emphasized throughout this chapter, members of the helping professions need to help their adult clients actively participate in the process. Therefore, practitioners should work with journalists and educators to increase public understanding of adult development. Part of the process entails awareness and use of community opportunity systems that can contribute to the client's development. To accomplish this objective, practitioners should work with others to increase adult access to such opportunity systems. Even though there is now a rich literature on adult development and learning, much more needs to be known. As a result, practitioners should encourage and support research on adult development.

Research Directions

Some practitioners who deal with communication disorders have conducted research on speech and hearing during adulthood, and it seems likely that many more will do so in the future (Bergman, 1971; Mysak, 1959; Ramsdell, 1965). In some instances

such research will occur as part of graduate study. In the process of formulating a research question and reviewing relevant literature, several recent books will be helpful (Baltes & Schaie, 1973; Binstock & Shanas, 1976; Birren & Schaie, 1977; Eisdorfer & Lawton, 1973; Finch & Hayflick, 1977; Goulet & Baltes, 1970; Havelock 1969; Howe, 1977; Kalish, 1975; Knox, 1977a, 1977b; Troll, 1975). In addition, some volumes contain chapters or appendices that can help in planning procedures for data collection and analysis (Goulet & Baltes, 1970; Knox, 1977a; Nesselroade & Reese, 1973).

An initial decision is whether the emphasis of a study will be on theory building, theory testing, intervention, or comparative analysis. Specific research designs include those that are descriptive (cross-sectional, longitudinal, cross-sequential, time-lag) as well as those that are experimental, in which two or more treatments are used with experimental and control groups. An increasing number of data collection instruments are being developed and refined for the collection of qualitative as well as quantitative data.

CONCLUSION

Practitioners concerned with communication disorders appear to be at the threshold of a major increase in interest in adult development and learning. Although preparation in speech pathology and audiology has traditionally emphasized child development and language acquisition, an increasing proportion of the clientele consists of adults and especially older adults. Growing recognition of this shift in clientele is contributing to an increased readiness by practitioners to become more proficient regarding adult development and learning. This chapter provides a brief overview of the topic. The references constitute recommended professional reading for practitioners who would like to increase their effectiveness in helping adults with speech or hearing disorders. The chapter also outlines the comprehensive and developmental view of adulthood that can contribute to utilization of generalizations from the subsequent chapters of this volume.

REFERENCES

Atchley, R. C. *The social forces in later life: An introduction to social gerontology.* Belmont, Calif.: Wadsworth, 1972.
Atchley, R. C. *The sociology of retirement.* Cambridge, Mass., Schenkman Publishing Co., 1975.

Baltes, P. B., & Schaie, K. W. (Eds.). *Life-span developmental psychology: Personality and socialization.* New York: Academic Press, 1973.

Barker, R. G. *Ecological psychology.* Stanford, Calif.: Stanford University Press, 1968.

Belbin, E., & Belbin, R. M. *Problems in adult retraining.* London: Heinemann, 1972.

Bengston, V. L. *The social psychology of aging.* Indianapolis: Bobbs-Merrill, 1973.

Bergman, M. Changes in hearing with age. *Gerotonlogist,* 1971, *11,* 148−151.

Binstock, R. H., & Shanas, E. (Eds.). *The handbook of aging and the social sciences.* New York: Van Nostrand Reinhold, 1976.

Birren, J. E. *The psychology of aging.* Englewood Cliffs, N.J.: Prentice-Hall, 1964.

Birren, J. E., & Schaie, K. W. (Eds.). *Handbook of the psychology of aging.* New York: Van Nostrand Reinhold, 1977.

Botwinick, J. *Cognitive processes in maturity and old age.* New York: Springer Publishing Co., 1967.

Botwinick, J. *Aging and behavior.* New York: Springer Publishing Co., 1973.

Bradburn, N. M. *The structure of psychological well-being.* Chicago: Aldine Publishing Co., 1969.

Britton, J. H., & Britton, J. O. *Personality changes in aging.* New York: Springer Publishing Co., 1972.

Butler, R. N. *Why survive? Being old in America.* New York: Harper & Row, Publishers, 1975.

Campbell, A., & Converse, P. *Monitoring the perceived quality of life.* New York: Russell Sage Foundation, 1975.

Counseling Psychologist, 1976, 6 (1), Special Issue on counseling adults.

Devries, H. A. *Physiology of exercise* (2nd ed.). Dubuque: William C. Brown, 1974.

Eisdorfer, C., & Lawton, M. P. *The psychology of adult development and aging.* Washington, D.C.: American Psychological Association, 1973.

Epstein, J. *Divorced in America.* New York: E. P. Dutton, 1974.

Eshleman, J. R. *The family.* Boston: Allyn & Bacon, 1974.

Finch, C. B., & Hayflick, L. (Eds.). *Handbook of the biology of aging.* New York: Van Nostrand Reinhold, 1977.

Gagné, R. M. *The conditions of learning.* (Rev. ed.). New York: Holt, Rinehart & Winston, 1972.

Glaser, B. G., & Strauss, A. L. *Time for dying.* Chicago: Aldine Publishing Co., 1968.

Goulet, L. R., & Baltes, P. B. (Eds.). *Life-span developmental psychology: Research and theory.* New York: Academic Press, 1970.

Havelock, R. G. *Planning for innovation.* Ann Arbor: CRUSK, ISR, University of Michigan, 1969.

Herzberg, F. *Work and the nature of man.* Cleveland: World, 1966.

Hill, R., Foote, N., Aldous, J., Carlson, R., & Macdonald, R. *Family development in three generations.* Cambridge, Mass., Schenkman, 1970.

Hoffman, L. W., & Nye, F. I. *Working mothers.* San Francisco: Jossey-Bass, 1974.

Holland, J. L. *Making vocational choices.* Englewood Cliffs, N.J.: Prentice-Hall, 1973.

Houle, C. O. *The design of education.* San Francisco: Jossey-Bass, 1972.

Howe, M. J. A. (Ed.). *Adult learning: Psychological research and applications.* London: John Wiley & Sons, 1977.

Hurlock, E. B. *Developmental psychology* (3rd ed.). New York: McGraw-Hill Book Co., 1968.

Jarvik, L. F., Eisdorfer, C., & Blum, J. (Eds.). *Intellectual functioning in adults.* New York: Springer Publishing Co., 1973.

Johnstone, J. W. C., & Rivera, R. J. *Volunteers for learning.* Chicago: Aldine Publishing Co., 1965.

Kalish, R. A. *Late adulthood: Perspectives on human development.* Monterey, Calif.: Brooks/Cole Publishing Co., 1975.

Kastenbaum, R. (Ed.). *Contributions to the psycho-biology of aging.* New York: Springer Publishing Co., 1965.

Kastenbaum, R., & Aisenberg, R. *The psychology of death.* New York: Springer Publishing Co., 1972.

Kimmel, D. *Adulthood and aging.* New York: John Wiley & Sons, 1974.

Knowles, M. S. *The modern practice of adult education.* New York: Association Press, 1970.

Knox, A. B. Life-long self-directed education. In R.J Blakely (Ed.), *Fostering the growing need to learn.* Rockville, Md: Division of Regional Medical Programs, Bureau of Health Resources Development, 1974.

Knox, A. B. *Adult development and learning.* San Francisco: Jossey-Bass, 1977(a).

Knox, A. B. *Current research needs related to systematic learning by adults.* (Occasional Paper No. 4), Urbana, Ill: University of Illinois, Office for the Study of Continuing Professional Education, 1977 (b).

Knox, A. B., & Farmer, H. S. Overview of counseling and information services for adult learners. *International Reveiw of Education,* 1977, *23,* 387–414.

Kubler-Ross, E. K. *On death and dying.* New York: Macmillan, 1969.

Levine, S., & Scotch, N. A. (Eds.). *Social stress.* Chicago: Aldine Publishing Co., 1970.

Levinson, D. J. *The seasons of a man's life.* New York: Alfred A. Knopf, 1978.

Lowenthal, M. F., Thurnher, M., Chiriboga, D., Beeson, D., Giay, L., Lurie, E., Pierce, R., Spencer, D., & Weiss, L. *Four stages of life: A comparative study of women and men facing transitions.* San Francisco: Jossey-Bass, 1975.

Maas, H. S., & Kuypers, J. A. *From thirty to seventy.* San Francisco: Jossey-Bass, 1974.

Maccoby, E. E., & Jacklin, C. N. *The psychology of sex differences.* Stanford, Calif.: Stanford University Press, 1974.

Maddi, S. R. *Personality theories: A comparative analysis* (Rev. ed.). Homewood, Ill.: Dorsey Press, 1972.

Mysak, E. Pitch and duration characteristics of older males. *Journal of Speech and Hearing Research,* 1959, *2,* 46–54.

Nesselroade, J. R., & Reese, H. W. *Life-span developmental psychology: methodological issues.* New York: Academic Press, 1973.

Neugarten, B. L. (Ed.). *Middle age and aging.* Chicago: University of Chicago Press, 1968.

Neugarten, B. L., & Associates: *Personality in middle and late life.* New York: Atherton, 1964.

O'Neill, N., & O'Neill, G. *Shifting gears.* New York: Avon Books, 1974.

Parker, B., & Paisley, J. *Patterns of adult information seeking.* Stanford, Calif.: Stanford University, 1966. (Final Report on USOE Project NO. 2583)

Parkes, C. M. *Bereavement: Studies of grief in adult life.* New York: International Universities Press, 1972.

Ramsdell, D. A. The psychology of the hard of hearing and deafened adult. In H. Davis & R. Silverman (Eds.), *Hearing and deafness.* New York: Holt Rinehart & Winston, 1965.

Schein, E. H. *Career dynamics: Matching individual and organizational needs.* Reading, Mass.: Addison-Wesley Publishing Co., 1978.

Schoenberg, B. (Ed.). *Anticipatory grief.* New York: Columbia University Press, 1974.

Sheehy, G. *Passages: Predictable crises of adult life.* New York: E. P. Dutton, 1976.

Silverman, P. R. *Widow-to-widow program.* New York: Health Sciences Publishing Corp., 1973.

Timiras, P. S. *Developmental physiology and aging.* New York: Macmillan, 1972.

Toffler, A. *Future shock.* New York: Random House, 1970.

Tough, A. Major learning efforts: recent research and future directions. *Adult Education,* 1978, *28,* 250–263.

Trent, J. W., & Medsker, L. B. *Beyond high school.* San Francisco: Jossey-Bass, 1968.

Troll, L. E. *Early and middle adulthood.* Monterey, Calif.: Brooks/Cole Publishing Co., 1975.

Vaillant, G. *Adaptation to life.* Boston: Little, Brown & Co., 1977.

White, R. W. *Lives in progress.* New York: Holt, Rinehart & Winston, 1961.

White, R. W. *The enterprise of living.* New York: Holt, Rinehart & Winston, 1972.

Williams, R. H., & Wirths, C. G. *Lives through the years.* New York: Atherton Press, 1965.

Joel C. Kahane

2

Anatomic and Physiologic Changes in the Aging Peripheral Speech Mechanism

The purpose of this chapter is to summarize data from a number of disciplines regarding age-related changes in the organs of the peripheral speech mechanism in order to identify the biologic changes that underlie alterations in speech output resulting from aging. To accomplish this goal, it is necessary to understand the effects of aging on the structure and nonspeech functions of the organs utilized in speech production. Such insight provides a data base from which to interpret the functional capacity of the aging speech mechanism.

To date, basic information on the aging of the peripheral speech mechanism has not been synthesized into a single work. This chapter attempts to do so through identification of salient age-related changes in the respiratory system, larynx, and the supralaryngeal system and discussion of the potential effects that these changes may have on basic processes required for speech production.

THE RESPIRATORY SYSTEM

The respiratory system is central to human existence and serves as the power source for speech production. The efficiency of this "pump" depends on a number of anatomic, physiologic, and neurologic relationships. Changes in the thoracic cage, chest wall muscles, and lungs may alter respiratory function.

Rib Cage, Vertebral Column, and Muscles of the Chest Wall

The thorax has been noted to change in shape in old age (McKeown, 1965; Reveille–Parise, 1851) and to become concave ("sunken in"). This results from a narrowing of the anteroposterior dimension. The concave shape of the aging thorax results from one of the most common skeletal deformities in aging, that of senile kyphosis (McKeown, 1965). This condition results in a pronounced curvature of the vertebral column in the upper and middle thoracic regions that exaggerates the normal thoracic curvature of the spine. It is caused by thinning and degeneration of the vertebral discs (Fig. 2–1). The degeneration is typically greatest in the anterior aspect of the disc, which results in a forward tipping of the vertebral column. Thus, vertebrae often are in direct contact with each other or are separated by only a thin layer of degenerated disc. The bodies of the vertebrae also may become compressed into a wedge shape or even fused anteriorly.

There are a number of changes in costovertebral joints (articulation of the head of the ribs with the articular facets of the vertebrae) related to these alterations in the vertebral column. According to Macklin and Macklin (1942), in 1914 Nascher reported that the compression of the vertebrae associated with senile kyphosis causes the articular facets of the vertebrae to become flattened. This

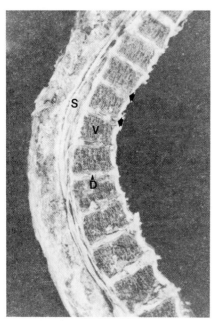

Fig. 2-1. Anatomical preparation exhibiting senile kyphosis (from McKeown, F. *Pathology of the Aged,* London: Butterworth & Company, Ltd., 1965). Note that the curvature is in the thoracic region of the vertebral column and also affects the contour of the spinal cord (*S*). The intervertebral discs (*D*) are thinning and degenerating, the vertebrae (*V*) exhibit some porosity (i.e., osteoporosis), and some are fused anteriorly (*arrows*).

alters the angle of inclination of the necks of the vertebrae (fulcrum in the mechanical system) and results in restriction of movement of the ribs. Macklin and Macklin noted that senile changes in the curvature of the vertebral column crowd the ribs together. The direct effects of these changes on breathing are not completely known. It appears likely that altered rib cage movement could affect the extent to which intrathoracic dimensions could be changed during inspiration and consequently the extent to which the lungs could be inflated.

With increasing age, the thorax becomes more rigid or stiff, yielding less easily to respiratory muscle forces. The increased rigidity results from changes in the ribs, costal joints, and the muscles of the chest wall. Nascher reported that the costal cartilages sometimes become ossified in old age, resulting in reduced mobility in the ribs during elevation and return to rest position. Calcification and ossification also have been reported (Jamieson, 1937; Noback, 1949) in the costal cartilages as early as age 20 (Todd, 1942). Nascher (1914) and Grant (1972) indicated that the manubrium and body of the

sternum fuse with increasing age, resulting in synarthroses (immovable joints) in about 10 percent of adults between 30 and 80 years old. Bates and Christie (1955) suggested that significant differences in vital capacity between young and old adults results from changes in the lung and fixation of the thoracic cage, as well as decreased elasticity and immobility of the costal cartilages.

Little data has been published on changes in the respiratory muscles as a function of aging. Ufland (1933), McKeown (1965), and Dhar, Shastri, and Lenora (1976) reported that respiratory muscles become weakened with increasing age throughout adulthood. Ufland also observed that the respiratory muscles begin to show reduction in strength between 30 and 40 years of age. Nascher (1914), however, stated that he found marked atrophy only in advanced years, although the definition of "advanced" was not specified.

In summary, with increasing age, mobility of the ribs appears to decrease because of a combination of factors that include changes in the structure of the costovertebral and costochondral joints, changes in the shape of the thoracic skeleton, and weakening of the respiratory muscles. These muscular and skeletal changes are likely to contribute to reduced biomechanical efficiency of the aging respiratory system.

Lower Airways and Lung

Merkel (1902), cited in Macklin and Macklin (1942), and Grant (1940) reported that the bronchi and lungs gradually descended to lower levels in the thorax throughout adulthood and into old age. The caudal migration of these structures may result, in part, from weakening of structural support as well as thinning of the intervertebral discs and reduced height of the vertebral bodies. A similar age-related descent for the larynx was reported by Ferreri (1959). He referred to this as *laryngeal ptosis* and said that it was extremely common in older persons. Accordingly, the cricoid cartilage becomes located at a level between the seventh cervical and first thoracic vertebrae as compared to the sixth cervical vertebrae in younger adults.

Nascher (1914) and McKeown (1965) reported that there are demonstrable changes in the pleura of the lungs. The visceral pleura of the aged lung are thinned, often uneven in surface architecture, and lacking color or luster. Pierce and Ebert (1965) studied the arrangement and concentration of collagen and elastin in the lungs and pleura of adults.

They found that the ratios of collagen to elastin (the major fibrous-connective-tissue proteins in the lungs) decrease markedly between young and old adulthood. These changes make the pleural membranes stiffer and less capable of sliding over each other, an activity that is essential to efficient pulmonary function (Comroe, 1965). Thus, if the tensile strength and elasticity of the pleural membranes depreciates with age, the biomechanical advantage of the lungs—thorax linkage may be lessened and respiratory functioning is likely to be less efficient.

This notion is supported by anatomic and physiologic data. McKeown (1965) reported that sclerosis of the bronchi and supporting tissues of the lungs interferes with normal respiratory movements. Pierce and Ebert (1965) and Turner, Mead and Wohl (1968) reported that there is diminished lung recoil with advancing age, particularly at high lung volumes. It is at these high lung volumes that the relaxation pressure, that is, nonmuscular pressures generated by the respiratory system, are most prominent.

Respiratory Function

In the previous sections, several structural changes associated with aging of the respiratory system were noted. Of course, not all of these changes occur in all individuals, and some undoubtedly would exert more restrictive effects on respiratory function than others. Shock (1962) has vividly illustrated the effects of aging on respiratory efficiency by showing that respiratory function (vital capacity, maximum breath capacity, maximum ventilation rates, maximum oxygen uptake during exercise) in a man aged 75 was only 40−55 percent that of a man aged 30.

The results of several physiologic studies (Kaltieider, Fray, & Hyde, 1938; Pierce & Ebert, 1965; Turner et al., 1968) suggest that one major factor contributing to these lowered levels of respiratory functioning is decreased elasticity of the lungs. The marked reduction in lung-recoil force that results directly affects the rate and amount of air that may be expelled from the lungs. Norris, Shock, Landowne and Falzone (1956) observed, however, that, despite these physiologic changes, total lung capacity (i.e., the volume of air contained within the lungs and airways at the end of a maximum inspiration) remained unchanged.

Investigators have tried to explain these age-related respiratory changes by searching for the intrinsic changes in the lungs that accompany aging.

Hieronymi (1960) obtained data on lung dry weight from autopsied subjects between birth and 70 years. He found no appreciable change in the weight of the adult lung after age 20. This finding is supported by other studies (Briscoe, Loring, & McClement, 1959; Pierce & Elbert, 1965) which have shown that structural proteins do not increase with age during adulthood. Thus, increases in lung volumes in aging subjects do not result from increases in the size of the lung and must therefore result from increases in compliance of the lung because of decreases in the elasticity of its structures.

Several investigators (Bickerman, 1952; Turner et al., 1968) have found increases in elastic tissue in the aging lung. Pierce and Ebert (1965) also have shown that the increases in elastic tissue in aging adult lung do not occur uniformly throughout the lung, but rather are confined to the pleura, the septa of the lung, and possibly the bronchi, but not in the respiratory parenchyma (i.e., regions where there is gaseous exchange).

The data from the aforementioned studies, which have demonstrated increased elastic tissue in aging human lungs, appear to be in conflict with physiologic data that have shown that there is diminished recoil in the aging lung. These inconsistencies apparently are resolved by Turner et al. (1968), who showed that increases in the elastic content of aging lungs reflect a progressive breakdown in the number of cross linkages in the elastin fibers. These physical alterations cause an overall loss in extensibility or recoil in the individual fibers. It is believed that this results in diminished capacity to push the air out of the alveoli and alveolar ducts into larger intrapulmonary air spaces, where the forces generated by the chest wall facilitate the movement of air out of the lungs and through the lower airways.

It is this loss of elasticity in the lung that pulmonary physiologists believe has the most deleterious effect on respiratory functioning (Bates & Christie, 1955; Lynne−Davies, 1977; Mead, Turner, Maclem, & Little, 1967; Pierce & Ebert, 1965; Turner et al., 1968). The reduced ability of the lungs to return from the inflated or extended state to resting levels results in greater amounts of air remaining entrapped within the lungs and intrapulmonary airways. This increase in residual volume (Lynne−Davies, 1977; Turner et al., 1968) results in decreased vital capacity (Baldwin, Cournand, & Richards, 1948; Bates & Christie, 1955; Kaltieider et al., 1938; Pemberton & Flanagan, 1956; Pierce & Ebert, 1965; Shock, 1962; Turner et al., 1968) and diminished expiratory flow rates (Bates & Christie,

1955; Lynne-Davies, 1977; Mead et al., 1967) and accounts for the smaller amounts of air that are expelled from the lungs as a person ages (Table 2−1). As a consequence, an individual may increase his respiratory rate in order to supply his body with sufficient amounts of oxygen (Pace, 1970).

It is likely that reduced pulmonary function with increasing age results from a combination of factors, which include decreased elastic recoil pressures of the lungs and conducting airways, smaller vital capacity, and decreased power from the respiratory muscles. Research is needed to determine the relationships among these as they contribute to alterations in speech production.

THE LARYNX

The larynx is an important respiratory organ that also serves as an edge tone generator during sound production. This section will provide a review of data on the aging of laryngeal cartilages, soft tissues, muscles, and nerves.

Cartilages and Joints

Several authors have noted that the structure of adult laryngeal cartilages changes with increasing age.

Opinion among these investigators is divided as to whether the cartilages become calcified (Ardran, 1965; LeGros−Clark, 1952; Negus, 1949; Pressman & Keleman, 1955; Segre, 1971) or ossified with age (Beau, 1939; Chamberlain & Young, 1935; Chievitz, 1882; Ferreri, 1959; Hately, Evison & Samuel, 1965; Hommerich, 1972; Kahane, Stadlan, & Bell, 1979; Keen & Wainwright, 1958; Noback, 1949; Puschel & Nowakowski, 1954; Roncollo, 1948).

In most of the studies in which ossification of the cartilages was found, it was of the endochondral type and progressed in a caudocranial fashion in the cricoid and thyroid cartilages. When sex differences were considered, ossification began slightly earlier in the male than in the female but was identifiable in both sexes during the second decade of life (Chievitz, 1882; Roncollo, 1948; Hommerich, 1972). Hately et al. (1965) found no differences between sexes in the onset of ossification. Most investigators reported that ossification is greater in male cartilages than in female cartilages. The thyroid and cricoid cartilages undergo the most extensive ossification, whereas the epiglottis reportedly never becomes ossified (Ardran, 1965; Kahane et al., 1979; Negus, 1949; Pressman & Kelemann, 1955). Ferreri (1959) and Hommerich (1972) found that elastic fibers in the epiglottis break down with increasing age. They noted that the

Table 2.1

Selected Measurements of Pulmonary Function in American Adults of Average Height[1]

Measure (in liters (L) and liters per second (L/sec)		Age (in years)					
		20	30	40	50	60	70
Total lung Capacity (L)	Male	6.20	6.20	6.20	6.20	6.20	6.20
	Female	4.60	4.60	4.60	4.60	4.60	4.60
Vital capacity (L)	Male	5.19	4.91	4.70	4.48	4.24	4.02
	Female	3.60	3.41	3.25	3.04	2.86	2.68
Residual volume (L)	Male	1.01	1.29	1.50	1.72	1.96	2.18
	Female	1.00	1.19	1.35	1.56	1.74	1.92
Forced expiratory volume at 1 sec (L/sec)	Male	4.35	4.05	3.75	3.50	3.20	2.85
	Female	3.25	3.03	2.80	2.60	2.38	2.18

[1]Measurements derived from prediction normograms of Boren, Kory, and Syner (1966) and Warren E. Collins, Inc., (1965). Average height for men is 173.99 cm (68.7 in.), and for women, 161.29 cm (63.5 in.).

arytenoid cartilage becomes only partially ossified, the apex and vocal processes never ossify, and the body and muscular processes usually become totally ossified. This finding has also been identified (Kahane et al. 1979) in whole-organ histologic sections of male and female larynges ranging in age from the third to the ninth decades.

Little information is available on nonpathologic changes of the aging laryngeal joints. Segre (1971) reported that the joint capsule of the cricoarytenoid joint loosens and the articular surfaces show some erosion with increasing age, although this observation was not supported empirically. Ferreri (1959) showed histologically that the articular surface of the cricoarytenoid joint in an 80-year-old woman was structurally normal but that the elastic ligaments of the joint capsule were thinned. Kahane et al. (1979) did not find light-microscopic evidence of erosion of the articular surfaces of the cricoarytenoid joint in subjects from the third to ninth decades of life.

Epithelia, Connective Tissues, and Glands

The effects of aging on laryngeal epithelia have been studied by several investigators. Eggston and Wolff (1947) and Hommerich (1972) reported that laryngeal epithelia thicken with age. Ryan, McDonald, and Devine (1956), Noell (1962), and Ruckes and Cause (1964) did not find an age-dependent relationship. Ryan et al. reported that laryngeal mucosa in men was innately thicker than in women. Noell found only one mucosal alteration that was demonstrably age dependent, consisting of a loosening of the connective tissue (lamina propria) underlying the mucosa over the vocal folds. In younger adults, this mucosa was usually tightly adherent to the lamina propria.

Ferreri (1959) also found alterations in the submucosal connective tissue in larynges of persons in their ninth decade. These changes consisted of hyalin thickening of collagen in the basement membrane. He also routinely found edema of the mucosa in all aged larynges and considered it to be a characteristic of aging.

Segre (1971) reported that after middle age, the laryngeal mucosa has a thin, yellowish appearance laryngoscopically. He noted that the laryngeal mucosa often underwent nonpathologic metaplastic changes (i.e., transformation of one type of epithelium into a simpler type, specifically, pseudostratified ciliated columnar into cuboidal or stratified). These changes were not accompanied by abnormalities in cell nuclei or by breakdown in basement membranes, which usually accompany pathologic change. Further, changes in surface epithelia of the larynx, such as hyperkeratosis or leukoplakia, should not be viewed as natural results of aging but rather as pathologic changes.

Elastic fibers in the vocal ligament (Ferreri, 1959; Hommerich, 1972; Kofler, 1932) and epiglottis (Ferreri, 1959; Hommerich, 1972) have been shown to break down or become thinned with advancing age, particularly in men (Ferreri, 1959). Whether age-related changes in the vocal ligament and/or epiglottis are indicative of a general pattern of elastic-tissue breakdown in the aging larynx has yet to be determined.

Ruckes and Hohmann (1963) and Hommerich (1972) have found that the mucous glands in the larynx degenerate and atrophy in persons over the age of 70. Hommerich (1972) suggested that these glandular changes result from the cumulative effect of repeated slight infections of the upper respiratory tract that occur over a lifetime. The diminished production of mucus by the laryngeal glands results in drying out of the laryngeal mucosa, which consequently predisposes it to trauma and disease.

Specific age-related changes for glands in the ventricular folds have been noted by Ferreri (1959) and Ruckes and Hohmann (1963). They found that with increasing age, mucus-secreting cells in the ventricular folds became replaced by fat cells, thus reducing the total number of secretory units. This would appear to contribute significantly to atrophy of these glands.

Age-related changes in the laryngeal cartilages, loose and dense connective tissues, and glands have been reported in both sexes. They were more extensive in the male than in the female and had an earlier onset in males. Thus, it is likely that the potential effects of these structural changes on vocal function may also be greater in the male than in the female.

Intrinsic Muscles and Nerves

Several investigators have reported that aging laryngeal muscles undergo degeneration and atrophy. However, there has been disagreement among investigators as to which muscles are most affected. Also, little information is available regarding aging of laryngeal muscles in females. Ferreri (1959) and Segre (1971) contended that changes in the female larynx begin at menopause, although no experimental data were presented to support this claim.

Kofler (1932) and Carnevalle-Ricci (1937) reported that there is atrophy in all the intrinsic muscles of the larynx. Segre (1936) found atrophic changes in all the intrinsic muscles and hypertrophy of the cricothyroid muscle, which he felt was compensatory for deficits in the adductor muscles.

Bach, Lederer, and Dinolt (1941) studied five larynges from persons between 50 and 70 years. They obtained data from each organ by excising small pieces of each intrinsic laryngeal muscle and staining them with selected stains to illustrate general morphology, fat content, and some enzymatic properties. They found that laryngeal muscle changes consisted of slight fatty infiltration in muscles in the oldest specimen (70 years) and progressively increased amounts of connective tissue interspersed between degenerating muscle fibers. Muscle fibers within a given muscle exhibted unusual amounts of variation in cross-sectional area, and also a loss of cross striations, an accumulation of debris in the cytoplasm, and a tendency for nuclei to become grouped and arranged into rows.

Bach et al. found these histologic changes in all the intrinsic laryngeal muscles but reported that they were most pronounced in the posterior cricoarytenoid muscles, moderate in the cricothyroid muscles, and least prominent in the adductor muscles. These results are not in complete agreement with Segre's (1937) findings and were not supported by Ferreri (1959). He found atrophy in all laryngeal muscles but failed to find qualitative or quantitative differences between muscle changes in the posterior cricoarytenoid and other intrinsic muscles.

Investigators have observed specific changes in aging vocal fold musculature. Ferreri (1959) found muscle atrophy, homogenation, and loss of the internal architecture of fibers and occasional thickening of individual fibers. Leutert (1964), as reported by Hommerich (1972), found degeneration of muscle fibers resulting in significant decreases in fiber diameter. Segre (1971) reported that fibers of the thyroarytenoid muscle have an undulent appearance suggesting a breakdown in structural support for the fibers or a breakdown of the muscle fiber itself. Hommerich (1972) reported that the vocal folds became more fragile with increasing age and that they showed progressive accumulation of lipofucsin granules, often called ''aging'' or ''wear and tear'' pigment. The fragility of the aging vocal folds, according to Hommerich, results from disorganization of elastic fibers composing the perpendicular layer of the vocal ligament. These findings were consistent with those of Ferreri (1959) who reported that there was a breakdown of elastic fibers in the submucosa and vocal ligaments near their attachment to the vocal processes.

Aging changes in laryngeal muscles appear to be closely related to disturbances in the vascular supply to the muscles. Ferreri (1959), Leutert (1964), and Hommerich (1972) found that the walls of capillaries supplying the intrinsic muscles were thickened and the diameter of the vessels reduced. These structural changes would decrease the blood supply to the muscles, which in turn would have deleterious effects on the muscle. Leutert found these vascular changes to be present as early as the fifth decade.

Though Bach et al. (1941) proposed that the decreased blood supply to the laryngeal muscles was central in mediating aging changes, they did not find evidence of definitive structural changes in the peripheral blood vessels of the laryngeal muscles. Rather, they maintained that vascular disturbances and consequent undernourishment of the laryngeal muscles result from paralysis of the vasomotor fibers of the sympathetic nerves supplying these vessels.

Kahane et al. (1979) have observed that after the sixth decade of life male muscle fibers exhibit a greater tendency towards separation after fixation than female muscle fibers. This vulnerability has been discussed by Fujisawa (1974) for human skeletal muscle, and Gutmann and Hanzlikova (1972) suggested that it may result from the decreased levels of mitochondrial enzymes and glycogen found in aged muscles. Cautiously interpreted, these findings in laryngeal muscles may suggest reduced metabolic capabilities and consequently reduced biochemical efficiency with increasing age. This relationship must be investigated more completely by means of histochemical studies.

Though age-related changes in laryngeal muscles have been noted, the etiology has not been established. Some characteristics of aging laryngeal muscles have been identified, but they appear to vary slightly from muscle to muscle and a hierarchy of muscle affectedness has not been determined.

Little has been written about the aging of the superior or inferior laryngeal nerves. Ferreri (1959) did not find significant age-related changes in sensory nerves supplying the mucous membranes or in the motor end plates of nerves supplying the intrinsic laryngeal muscles. Segre (1971) reported that muscle spindles and subepithelial receptors become reduced in number in aged larynges. He contended that the reduction in these mechanoreceptors may account for loss of laryngeal control during vocal production. He did not document this statement, however, with neuroanatomic data of his own or of others.

In summary, limited information is available on the aging of the intrinsic laryngeal muscles. Several basic issues remain unresolved, including the nature of sex differences pertaining to such changes and whether all laryngeal muscles age uniformly. On the basis of existing data, it appears justified to infer that with increasing age, laryngeal muscles become biomechanically less efficient. This results from age-related disturbances in the vascular supply to the muscle. Little is known about the neurologic changes that accompany alterations in the laryngeal musculature.

THE SUPRALARYNGEAL SYSTEM

The supralaryngeal component of the peripheral speech mechanism consists of the vocal tract and the articulators used in speech production. Age-related changes in these structures may have measurable effects on articulation, resonation, and speech intelligibility, as well as on the biologic functions served by them.

Craniofacial Skeleton

Disagreement exists among investigators about the extent and pattern of growth in the adult craniofacial skeleton. Hellman (1927) and Goldstein (1936) reported that the dimensions of the craniofacial skeleton continue to increase throughout adulthood and only begin to decrease in size after age 60. Jarcho (1935), Buchi (1950), Hooton and Dupertuis (1951), and Lasker (1953) reported that the dimensions of the craniofacial skeleton increase throughout adulthood. Moore (1955) could find no age-related pattern for growth of the adult craniofacial skeleton.

In spite of these differing appraisals, the aging craniofacial skeleton is stereotypically depicted in textbooks as edentulous (Fig. 2−2), with changes in the mandible typifying the effects of aging on the facial skeleton.

These typical changes were described by Robinson, Boling, and Lisher (1942):

The body is greatly decreased in height by loss of alveolar processes leaving the mylohyoid ridge at or just below the upper surface. The mandibular canal is near the alveolar surface and the mental foramen appears near, or even on the alveolar surface. The ramus is narrowed and thinned with marked diminution of the muscle attachments. The angle of the ramus with the body is increased and approaches the angle of the infant (p. 381).

Robinson et al. noted that the maxilla undergoes little change with advancing age, although there is a

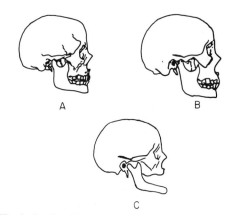

Fig. 2−2. Israel's conception of adult craniofacial growth based on analyses of lateral cephalograms. The craniofacial morphology of young adulthood (*A*, mean = 34 years) and older adulthood (*B*, mean = 55 years) are contrasted with the edentulous skull (*C*), which is representative of aging by textbook standards. (Modified from original by Israel, H., Age factor and the patterns of change in craniofacial structures. *American Journal of Physical Anthropology,* 1973, *39,* 107.)

slight loss in width and depth in aging persons. They did not explain the mechanisms responsible for these changes. Miller and Roth (1940) found that with increasing age, the tori palatini (boney protuberances on the midline of the hard palate at the palatomaxillary suture) and tori mandibulari (boney protuberances on the inner surface of the mandible in the premolar region) increased in size. These changes probably are not clinically or functionally significant except that, in some people, their presence may interfere with denture retention.

There still appears to be a significant need for further research into adult craniofacial development. Krogman (1962) has noted that earlier studies (as exemplified by Hellman, 1927) have not provided a timetable for these craniofacial changes, nor have they produced specific information about how these structures become altered by age. Krogman maintained that such information was not extractable from cross-sectional studies of facial growth. Rather, it is most reliably obtained from longitudinal studies of facial growth using cephalometric techniques.

This longitudinal research approach was used by Israel (1973). In his comprehensive study of craniofacial aging, 36 men and 26 women were followed for periods of 13 to 28 years. A total of 41 measurements were made from the calvarium, cranial base, and facial skeleton from two cephalograms per subject taken at a young adult age (24−48 years, mean = 35.4 years) and at an older adult age (41−64 years, mean = 54.9 years). Thus the mean length of the growth period studied was 19.48 years or almost two decades. The results of this study did not support classical descriptions of aging of the craniofacial skeleton. Israel found that the cranial and facial skeletons continue to grow throughout life. The diminution of craniofacial dimensions in old age reported by Hellman (1927) and Goldstein (1936) was not substantiated. According to Israel, growth of the craniofacial skeleton in later life results from "symmetrical enlargement" of the neural and visceral components, which was, with few exceptions, ". . . uniform in all areas." Thus, growth of the craniofacial skeleton does not change the proportional relationship among the component parts but does result in a modest increase in their absolute size (compare *A* and *B* in Fig. 2−2). The facial skeleton increased in size from 3 to 5 percent and the neurocranium increased in size from 4 to 7 percent for the 20-year period studied, which encompassed the middle third to the sixth decade. The classic textbook description of senile changes in the mandible (see Robinson et al. [1942] and Fig. 2−2C) was not substantiated by measurement data from Israel's study. Israel reported systematic enlargement of the mandible in both sexes (compare *A* and *B* in Fig. 2−2). The total length of the mandible (distance between the condyle and gnathion) increased by 4 percent, the body of the mandible (distance between menton and gonion) showed a mean gain of 5 percent, and there was no tendency for the gonial angle to become more obtuse with age. No significant trend was found for growth in ramus height.

Israel (1973) maintained that the loss of dentition and alveolar bone should not automatically be accepted as typifying aging craniofacial morphology because ". . . there is no evidence to incriminate age alone as responsible for loss of teeth or bone" (p 26). Though Israel's data suggested the need to modify previous conceptions of craniofacial aging, more data are needed from the sixth to ninth decades of life to confirm that the trend he described continues into the oldest age ranges.

In summary, morphologic changes in facial bones may alter the points of attachment for masticatory and facial muscles which may reduce their biomechanical efficiency during speech. Age-related changes in the maxilla and mandible may change the shape of the oral cavity sufficiently to alter oral resonatory characteristics.

Temporomandibular Joint

The temporomandibular joint may undergo extensive changes with aging. These changes largely involve alterations in the mandibular condyle with lesser changes in the glenoid fossa and few changes in the articular disc.

CELL ZONES OF THE MANDIBULAR CONDYLE

Blackwood (1966) has shown that growth of the mandibular condyle is dependent upon the activity of three distinct cellular zones in the condyle. These cells play significantly different and changing roles during postnatal development. Figure 2−3 is a photomicrograph of a section through an adult mandibular condyle that illustrates the articular (outer) zone consisting of the outer or surface cells, the proliferative (or middle) zone and the hypertrophic (or inner) zone. Cells in the articular zone produce a tough, fibrous surface covering for the articular surface of the joint. Cells in the proliferative zone are actively involved in the production of cartilage cells, which increase in number and size. In the hypertrophic zone, cartilage cells hypertrophy (i.e., swell) and secrete a matrix around themselves and between contiguous cell clusters. The matrix hardens (a process called mineralization) and consequently undergo degeneration, as does the cartilage matrix, and are replaced by bone cells (osteocytes) carried into the area by invading blood vessels. These osteocytes grow, secrete matrix, and form bone. The bone that is laid down in the hypertrophic zone results in quantitative increases or growth in the condyle.

With increasing age, the outer (articular) zone becomes progressively more fibrous and the middle (proliferative) zone becomes reduced because of decreased growth activity (Fig. 2−3). The inner (hypertrophic) zone is nonexistent in the adult temporomandibular joint. It is replaced by a layer of fibrocartilage that rests on top of condylar bone. Thus no further new bone growth occurs. The study of cellular maturation of the articular and subarticular areas of the temporomandibular joint serves as a basis for interpreting growth- and age-dependent changes in this joint.

REMODELING OF THE MANDIBULAR CONDYLE

Johnson (1962) and Moffett, Johnson, McCabe, and Askew (1964) have shown that cellular activity in the outer, middle, and inner zones of the condyle represents different responses to changing orofacial physiology. These changes have been called progressive, peripheral, and regressive remodeling, respectively, and are discussed by Blackwood (1966) as adaptive changes in the temporomandibular joints.

Progressive and peripheral remodeling are pro-

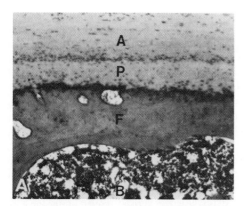

Fig. 2–3. Photomicograph through a normal adult mandibular condyle showing the surface articular zone (*A*), proliferative zone (*P*), and the fibrocartilagenous zone (*F*), which has replaced the hypertrophic zone present in younger developing joints. The fibrocartilage rests on the subarticular bone (*B*) of the condyle. (From Blackwood, H. J. Adaptive changes in the mandibular joints with function. *Dental Clinics of North America,* November 1966, pp. 566–595.)

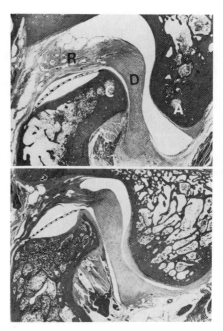

Fig. 2–4. Photomicrographs of the temporomandibular joint of a 49 year old edentulous man (upper) and a 65-year-old edentulous man (lower). Note that resorption or loss of bone (regressive remodeling) on the posterior aspect of the articular surface of the mandibular condyle. Dotted lines (my addition) represent an attempt to approximate the contour of the articular surface as it might have appeared prior to remodeling. *A* = articular tubercle; *C* = mandibular condyle; *D* = articular disc; *R* = retrodiscal pad. (From Blackwood, H. J. Adaptive changes in mandibular joints with function. *Dental Clinics of North America,* November 1966, pp. 566–595.)

cesses that serve to maintain functional alignment of the articular surfaces of the temporomandibular joint (TMJ) during the first two decades of life. This period is characterized by growth that constantly alters craniofacial relationships, particularly the vertical height of the facial skeleton. Increases in the vertical height of the condyle result from added growth near joint surfaces (progressive remodeling) and from increases in the transverse dimensions of the condyle (peripheral remodeling), particularly in the anterior articular margin of the condyle.

Regressive remodeling occurs in edentulous persons and also, according to Blackwood, in some persons in older (unspecified) age groups. It consists of removal of bone from the condyle and glenoid fossa through breakdown of preexisting bone in the subarticular zones (Fig. 2–4). The breakdown of bone in these areas effectively reduces the height of the condyle and reestablishes the articular surface at a lower level. Vaughan (1943) noted gross anatomic changes in the aging TMJ, which consist of a gradual reduction in the size of the mandibular condyle, flattening of the articular surfaces of the joint, and marked thinning of the glenoid fossae with age. Subsequent histologic descriptions of regressive remodeling of the TMJ by Moffett et al. (1964) and Blackwood (1966) supported Vaughan's observations.

Regressive remodeling has been thought to occur because of abnormal forces that are transmitted

to the TMJ in elderly individuals. This may occur because of loss of teeth, malocclusion, and consequent resorption of alveolar bone. Blackwood (1969) maintained that the loss of teeth and supporting tissues results in the direct transmission of masticatory forces to the TMJ. The dentition and supporting tissues normally help to absorb these forces and distribute them through bones of the facial skeleton, thereby shunting them away from the TMJ. Over time, this causes resorption of bone and habitual posterior positioning of the condyle in the glenoid fossa.

Brietner (1940, 1941) documented similar findings in monkeys who had their posterior teeth extracted. Coleman and Kaiser (1966) further hypothesized that abnormal retruded positioning of the mandibular condyle results from reduced proprioceptive feedback from the periodontal ligaments, which are lost when teeth are lost. Intact proprioceptive feedback in dentulous subjects results in more anterior positioning of the mandible. It appears, therefore, that the teeth and supporting structures play a central role in maintaining the structural integrity of the TMJ.

Extensive discussion on the aging temporomandibular joint by Blackwood and Moffett et al. does not include descriptions of changes in the articular discs. Blackwood (1969), in a paper on pathology of the temporomandibular joint, noted that changes in the articular disc are usually not characteristic of the normal aging process of the joint, but rather are more often associated with pathologic changes from degenerative and/or inflammatory diseases.

PHYSIOLOGICAL CHANGES IN THE AGING TEMPOROMANDIBULAR JOINT

Specific information on nonpathologic physiologic changes in the aging TMJ has not been reported. However, Blackwood (1969) reported that in a study of 400 TMJs from cadavers aged 40 and older, 40 percent exhibited histologic evidence of arthritic changes. In pathologic conditions, pain, restricted movements, and ankylosis were commonly reported symptoms (Blackwood, 1969; Mayne & Hatch, 1969).

In summary, age-related changes in the temporomandibular joint may alter the resting position of the mandible and restrict or alter normal patterns of mandibular movement. These biomechanical changes may affect some articulatory features of certain phonemes and/or alter coarticulatory patterns during speech production.

Masticatory and Facial Muscles

Masticatory and facial muscles are essential to mastication and speech production and also are of interest because they contribute to the appearance of aging in the face. Alterations in their structure and in their attachments to the craniofacial skeleton may result in measurable reductions in function. Due to the paucity of research in physiologic studies of the effects of aging on masticatory or facial muscle functioning, the data reported deal almost exclusively with structural changes.

MASTICATORY MUSCLES

The significant effect of aging on the masticatory muscles is a reduction in biting force, which decreases from approximately 300 lb/sq in. in young people to 50 lb/sq in. older individuals (Kaplan,

1971). This may result from weakness of the masticatory musculature because of atrophy (Greenfield, Shy, Alvord, & Berg, 1957; MacMillan, 1936) and from a reduction in biomechanical efficiency due to altered muscular attachments (MacMillan, 1936). MacMillan, using cadaver dissections, found that the attachment of the temporalis and mylohyoid muscles to the mandible are radically altered in edentulous persons as compared to individuals with dentition. The muscles also are atrophic. In edentulous subjects, the mylohyoid muscle is attached to the crest of the alveolar bone rather than to the mylohyoid line, as is customary. MacMillan suggested that this occurred because the vertical height of the alveolar ridge was reduced due to a resorption of bone and lost dentition. These dentoalveolar changes also affect the topography of the mylohyoid line, which decreases in length and becomes positioned relatively higher on the mandible. The fibers of the mylohyoid muscle in the aged individual were found to course more horizontally than in younger persons. This arrangement may reduce the effectiveness with which the muscle may elevate or stabilize the hyoid bone and larynx or facilitate lowering of the mandible.

MacMillan also found that in the endentulous mandible, the temporalis muscle attaches to the mandible more inferiorly. He found that muscle fibers attach extensively to the inner surface of the coronoid process and also extend down to the region of the retromolar triangle.

These muscular changes described by MacMillan are effects of changes in the underlying bone. The resultant differences in muscle orientation to the bone are secondary.

FACIAL MUSCLES

Limited information is available on the effects of aging on specific facial muscles (Gerrero—Santos, 1978; Pitanguy, 1978). Most interest in the aging of facial muscles comes from clinicians involved in "surgical rejuvenation" of the face (Brown, 1953; Fomon, 1961; Gordon, 1978).

Santos reported that the platysma muscle in persons over age 50 becomes flattened, fibrotic, and contractured. The medial fibers of the muscle tend to be affected most, although alterations in the posterolateral fibers occur occasionally. The degree of flaccidity and contracture of the muscle varies among individuals.

Pitanguy (1978) also reported that in persons over age 50 there was a tendency for fat to accumulate in the submandibular region resulting in sagging of the chin and ptosis of the mentalis muscle. The effects of these structural changes, according to Gordon (1978), is a sagging of the skin in the neck with the formation of vertical folds of tissue. The alterations in musculature in the submandibular and chin region appear to be largely cosmetic and would not be likely to have any deleterious effect upon speech production. This is well illustrated by Martone and Edwards (1962, Fig. 2−5).

Losses in muscle tonus and changes in the structure of specific facial muscles may simply be a part of a general pattern of skeletal muscle weakness that accompanies aging (Corso, 1975; Gutmann & Hunzlikova, 1975; Retzlaff & Fontaine, 1965). Facial muscle changes, however, may result directly from histologic changes in the facial nerve nucleus during adulthood. Maleci (1936) studied the changes in the facial nerve nucleus of adults of various ages. He found that there was a decrease in cells with age of approximately 16 cells/year or 0.25 percent of the annual neuronal pool. The subtle changes in facial muscles that occur with aging would not be expected to reflect lower motor neuron disease. However, small neuronal losses over time may cumulatively result in subtle changes and weakness. More definitive research, however, is needed to determine the effect of this cell decrease.

In addition to intrinsic changes in the facial musculature, Brown (1951) noted that a loss of elasticity of the skin of the face and a break down in collagenous fibers in the dermis of the skin result in wrinkles and redundancy of skin over the facial

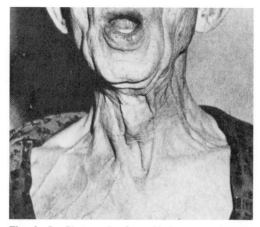

Fig. 2−5. Photograph of an elderly woman (age unspecified) saying the word "lone." Note sagging in the submandibular and chin areas and the vertical folds in the skin of the neck. (From Martone, A. L. & Edwards, L. F. Anatomy of the mouth and related structures. Part II. *Journal of Prosthetic Dentistry*, 1962, *12*, 4−27.)

skeleton. Figure 2−6 (Martone & Edwards, 1962) illustrates this well. Gordon (1978) noted that in aging the subcutaneous layer of fat underlying the skin of the face is also depleted. This tissue normally smooths the contours of the youthful face. In aged persons, as illustrated in Figure 2−7 (Martone & Edwards 1961), the facial region is often accentuated by bony prominences, such as the malor eminence

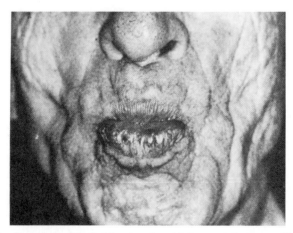

Fig. 2−6. Photograph of the facial region of an elderly woman (age unspecified) saying the word "pooh." Note the wrinkles and redundancy of skin in the face, thought to result from break down in collagen fibers in the dermis of the skin. (From Martone, A. L., & Edwards, L. F. Anatomy of the mouth and related structures. Part II. *Journal of Prosthetic Dentistry*, 1962, *12*, 4−27.)

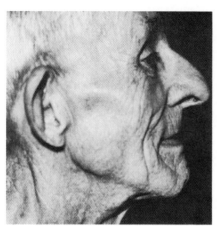

Fig. 2-7. Edentulous older man (age unspecified). Photograph illustrates the accentuation of different regions of the face resulting from facial-muscle atrophy and changes in facial skin and subcutaneous connective tissues. (From Martone, A. L., & Edwards, L. F. Anatomy of the mouth and related structures. Part I. *Journal of Prosthetic Dentistry,* 1961, *11,* 1009–1018.

and chin, and "sinking in" of other areas, such as in the buccal and temporal regions. Gordon also has noted that the connective tissue attaching muscle fibers to the skin undergoes shrinkage that, coupled with reduced muscle tonus, may smooth out some of the natural folds in the face and make it appear less expressive.

Brown (1953) maintained that the appearance of aging in the face results from a disproportionate relationship between the vertical heights of the upper (forehead), middle (frontonasal suture to anterior nasal spine), and lower (anterior nasal spine to mental protuberance) thirds of the face. He maintained that in the youthful looking face, the facial regions are essentially equal in height, while in the aged face, the middle third of the face takes up more than one-third of the facial profile. The distance between the nose and chin (lower third of the face) becomes reduced. This results largely from the wearing down of the dentition, subsequent resorption of alveolar bone in the maxilla and mandible, and atrophy of elastic tissue in the nose. The distance between the chin and nose is shortened because the soft tissue of the nose elongates.

Some preliminary statements can be made about the effects of aging on the facial muscles. The muscles undergo some atrophy, probably resulting from muscle and facial nerve changes. Facial expression and appearance are affected by aging through reduction in fatty and subcutaneous connective tis-

sues as well as by reduced muscle tonus. The changes in the facial musculature, however, do not appear to be sufficient to result in measurable alterations in speech production.

Oral Cavity

Several age-related changes have been observed to take place in the oral cavity involving epithelia, salivary glands, perioral tonsillar tissues, and the oral mucous membranes.

ORAL MUCOSA

Klingsberg and Butcher (1960) and Squier, Johnson, and Hopps (1976) have noted that there are several changes in the structure of the oral mucosa that normally accompany aging. These changes consist of thinning of the mucosa with some loss in elasticity and less firm attachment to underlying connective tissue, muscle, and bone. Squier et al. indicated that this reduction in structural support results from the thinning out of epithelial—connective tissue junctions in the basement membrane and atrophy of the lamina propria, where connective tissue appears to be shrunken or absent. Thinning out of the mucosa makes the oral epithelium quite susceptible to trauma and slow to heal. Decreased amounts of salivary secretions result in drying out of the oral epithelium, which exacerbates the condition.

Several investigators have described surface changes that occur in the oral mucosa in aging persons. Papic and Glickman (1950) studied changes in gingival mucosa in females aged 13 to 54 and reported that, beginning at the third decade, there is a decrease in the protective outer (keratinized) cell layers of the gingiva. Pedriera (1951) found similar changes in the oral mucosa of 50 men, age 60 to 80. Montgomery (1951), however, failed to find significant differences in keratinization[1] on the basis of sex or age. Squier et al. (1976) reported that some nonkeratinized, aging oral epithelium often becomes keratinized and thus creates atypical regions of roughness in the oral cavity. These epithelial changes may reflect alteration in the way food is moved through the oral cavity as a result of loss of teeth and reduced strength in masticatory, facial, and tongue muscles. Changes also occur in oral and pharyngeal epithelium because of exogenous factors such as to-

---

[1]As used here, keratinization refers to the accumulation of scleroprotein by the superficially lying epithelial cells, which serve to protect underlying tissue against mechanical and chemical irritation.

bacco smoke (Radsel & Kambic, 1978). These changes, however, must be differentiated from those that are a result of age-related biological changes.

In addition to structural changes in the oral epithelium proper, data from Truex (1940) has shown that aging oral epithelium may also undergo changes in sensory innervation. He studied ten pairs of Gasserian ganglia (sensory division of the trigeminal nerve that innervates facial and oral epithelium) histologically. Ganglia were obtained from five males (age 2 to 66 years) and five females (26 to 81 years). Truex found that the first-order sensory ganglion cells of individuals beyond the fourth decade underwent fatty degeneration. Associated with these neural changes was thickening of the lining of the small arterioles that supplied the ganglion, likely due, in part at least, to vascular deficiency. Truex concluded that the loss of these sensory cells would result in a reduction of sensitivity in the orofacial area. He maintained that his data also provided the neuroanatomic bases for clinical observations of reduced vibrotactile sensitivity in the oral and facial regions of aged persons.

Grossman and Hattis (1967) reported that investigators have demonstrated the presence of encapsulated endings analogous to Meissner's corpuscles in the oral epithelium. These receptors mediate discriminative touch. Aging of these and other oral epithelial receptors has not been reported. Insight into the potential effect of the aging of Meissner's corpuscles in the oral cavity, however, may be obtained from a study by Ronge (1943, a & b) of these receptors in the skin of the index finger of autopsied subjects ranging in age from 1 to 80 years. Ronge found that there was a substantial decline in the number and concentration of receptors with age. By 70 to 80 years of age, only one-quarter of the receptors remained (1000−1500) and their concentration per square inch was only about 12 percent of the density observed at 1 to 5 years of age. If similar trends obtain for these receptors in the oral cavity, a significant depreciation in discriminative (epicritic) touch may be anticipated. This would have implications for articulation and maneuvering of the food bolus during mastication.

SALIVARY GLANDS

Robinson et al. (1942) and Kaplan (1971) reported that dryness of the oral cavity occurred as a result of diminished function of the major and minor salivary glands with aging. The saliva becomes thick as a result of the decreased concentration of the carbohydrate-splitting enzyme (ptyalin) contained in saliva, and the pH of the saliva becomes more neutral or alkaline. There is a loss of the cleansing action of saliva on the oral mucous membrane, which results in a greater incidence of irritation of the mucosa of older individuals. In turn, decreased salivation has been thought to cause a thinning out of the oral mucous membrane (Robinson et al., 1942).

Andrew (1971) reported that Yamaguchi (1924), Schram (1933), and Andrew (1952) found that the secretory units of the salivary glands (i.e., parenchyma) were replaced by fat cells, but there were no signs of degeneration. The authors were not in agreement as to which salivary gland is most affected by aging.

TONSILLAR TISSUES OF WALDEYER'S RING

The ring of lymphathic tissue surrounding the oral isthmus is known as Waldeyer's ring. It is composed of the pharyngeal tonsil (adenoid), the palatine tonsils, and the lingual tonsils. Rossing (1940) reported that there is a craniocaudal progression in the atrophy of lymphathic tissue in Waldeyer's ring. The pharyngeal tonsils atrophy first (beginning in adolescence), followed by the palatine tonsils, and then the lingual tonsils. Keleman (1945) studied involutional changes in the palatine tonsil from 309 subjects consisting of 50 men and 50 women each in the seventh, eight, and ninth decades, and also nine subjects (sexes unspecified) from age 90 to 103. Descriptive information about size, shape, location, color, and surface changes was obtained by inspection during clinical examination. Keleman found that the palatine tonsils steadily decreased in size from the sixth decade. They rarely completely atrophied and often formed a vertical ridge in the tonsillar fossa, the dimensions of which never changed with increasing age. There were no signs of a degenerative process that accompanied involution of the palatine tonsils.

PHYSIOLOGICAL CHANGES

Although there is a significant body of literature on oral sensation and perception, largely in young adults (Bosma, 1967, 1970), there is a paucity of research dealing with oral sensitivity in aging subjects. A number of investigators have studied the effects of aging on touch and pressure sensibility (Ronge, 1943a, 1943b) and vibratory sensitivity (Cosh, 1953; Dyck, Schultz, & O'Brien, 1972) elsewhere in the body. It appears reasonable to assume that age-related changes in these sense modalities might be generalized to morphologically similar structures in the oral cavity (Grossman, Hattis & Ringel, 1965). Interest in these studies as they relate to oral function is further justified in that experimenters (Ormea, 1956; Ormea & Re, 1959; Strunghold, 1925) have studied pressure and tactile sensitivity in the lips, tongue, and hard palate and vibratory sensitivity (Plumb & Meigs, 1961) in the lips and tongue.

Touch and pressure sensitivity in aging subjects have been found to decrease significantly with age (Ronge, 1943a, 1943b). Ronge found that there was a gradual decrease in touch perception through the sixth decade of life and a perception of generalized spreading of the sensation from the stimulus site, a phenomenon rarely reported by younger subjects. In addition, greater stimulus strengths were required to elicit higher percentages of positive responses in subjects age 60 and older. These data suggest that with advancing age, there is a decrease in the number and sensitivity of the peripheral receptors.

Cosh (1953) reported similar decreases in vibratory sensitivity in aged subjects. Correct responses to vibratory stimuli diminished with age and were most marked after the fifth decade. The results of Dyck et al. (1972) support Cosh and indicate that, after age 40, physiologic responses to vibrotactile stimuli are poorer in men than in women.

If the physiological deficits in pressure, touch, and vibratory modalities exist in significant proportions in the oral cavity, articulatory feedback and other biologic functions may be affected. The nature and extent of such deficits must be studied carefully.

The Tongue

The tongue plays important roles in mastication, swallowing, and speech production. As such, the biologic significance of age-related changes in this structure are of major significance.

EPITHELIUM

Robinson et al. (1942) classified aging changes in the epithelium of the tongue as consisting of atrophy (thinning) of the surface epithelium, which was observed to be greatest in the center of the tongue and varied in degree towards the periphery. Additionally, the sensory papillae of the taste buds have been shown to become reduced in number (El-Baradi & Bourne, 1951; Kaplan, 1971; Robinson et al., 1942) and size (Kaplan, 1972) as a function of aging. These changes appear to occur earlier in women (40–45 years) than in men (50–60 years) (Harris, 1951). Robinson et al. reported that the filiform and fungiform papillae are most affected. Filiform papillae become reduced or entirely absent; fungiform papillae become reduced in number. Kap-

lan indicated that there is a 60 percent decrease in the number of taste buds in senile individuals. The loss of these papillae, according to Robinson et al., results in a smoothed appearance in localized areas on the tongue (Fig. 2–8). Adams (1975) pointed out that after age 60, it is common for the veins on the undersurface of the tongue to become enlarged and vericosed (sometimes referred to as *caviar tongue*). He also noted that fissuring of the dorsal surface of the tongue may occur with increasing age, particularly in those persons with significant reductions in salivary secretions.

MUSCLES

Using histologic techniques, Bucciante and Luria (1934) studied the musculature of the tongue in aged individuals. They found an increase in muscle-fiber size with increases in the amount of interstitial connective tissues indicating atrophy of the tongue muscles. The effects of these changes on specific muscles, however, was not reported. Kaplan (1971) noted that the net effect of these changes is a loss in muscle mass and tonus with no significant decrease in size of the tongue.

SENSORY CHANGES

Despite the gradual involution of the sensory papillae of the taste buds previously noted, Cooper,

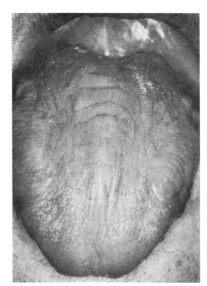

Fig. 2–8. Dorsal surface of the tongue of an 82-year-old subject (sex unspecified). Note the loss of papillae and the smoothed appearance of the lingual surface. (From Adams, D. Age changes in the oral structures. In C. L. Lavelle (Ed.), *Applied physiology of the mouth.* London: John Wright and Sons, Ltd., 1975.)

Bilash, and Zubek (1959) did not find significant losses in sensitivity for salty, sweet, sour, or bitter substances until the fifth decade, followed by a marked decline in sensitivity in the sixth through eighth decades. Cohen and Gitman (1958) found that there are no significant losses in gross taste perception until the middle of the sixth decade. No significant sex differences were reported by either group of investigators.

MOTOR CHANGES

No age-related alterations in tongue mobility during swallowing were reported by Zaino and Benventano (1977) in their extensive cinefluoroscopic studies of upper digestive tract physiology. Ptacek, Sander, Maloney and Jackson (1966), however, reported that lingual diadochokinesis was reduced in geriatic subjects of both sexes aged 66 to 93. This appears to suggest that the neuromuscular mechanism(s) required to produce rapid, alternating movements of the tongue during diadochokinesis, and perhaps also speech production, are different from those operating in more visceral functions such as swallowing. The neuromuscular mechanisms required for articulatory control of the tongue may be more susceptable to age-related changes than those controlling tongue movements for swallowing or mastication.

The Pharynx and Soft Palate

The pharynx and soft palate are centrally involved in swallowing and in resonation during speech production. Data on age-related anatomic and physiologic changes are presented and discussed in terms of their functional significance.

ANATOMICAL CHANGES

Surprisingly little has been written on the aging of pharyngeal and velar musculature. Kiuchi, Sasaki, Arai, and Suzuki (1969) and Zaino and Benventano (1977) noted that the pharyngeal musculature becomes weakened with age and the pharynx becomes dilated. Ferreri (1959) found that with increasing age, the pharyngeal mucosa thins and sensory innervation is reduced.

Bucciante and Luria (1934) studied the uvula muscle histologically and found that after the seventh decade there was hypertrophy of individual fibers and increases in interstitial tissue (collagen and elastic fibers) between muscle fibers, which were interpreted as suggestive of muscular atrophy. Anatomic studies by Azzan and Kuehn (1977) and clinical studies by several investigators (Chaco & Yules, 1969; Croft, Shprintzen, & Daniller, 1978; Pigott, 1969; Pigott, Bensen, & White, 1969) strongly suggest that uvulae muscles play an important facilitating role in velopharyngeal closure during speech. Thus, structural deficiencies in this muscle may contribute to some forms of velopharyngeal insufficiency reported by Hutchinson, Robinson, and Nerbonne (1978) in geriatric speakers.

Information regarding the effects of aging on the tensor veli palatini muscles may be obtained inferentially from data on the aging of the tensor tympani muscles. Tensor veli palatini and tensor tympani are derived from the same embryologic primordium and are innervated by the same cranial nerve (mandibular branch of the trigeminal or fifth cranial nerve). It seems reasonable to assume, therefore, that similar morphological changes may occur in both muscles. Malan (1943) studied the tensor tympani histologically in aging dogs and cats and found striated myofibrils (called *ringbinden*) encircling muscle fibers of tensor tympani. He maintained that ringbinden are caused by a wearing out of myofibrils resulting from continued use of the muscle throughout life. Brain and Walton (1969) explained that ringbinden are probably caused by the fracturing of peripherally situated myofibrils that wind themselves around the larger, intact portion of the fiber. Their presence is often associated with pathology in a muscle. Further experimentation is required to evaluate the frequency of occurrence and the functional significance of ringbinden in velar musculature.

PHYSIOLOGICAL CHANGES

Kiuchi et al. (1969) and Zaino and Benventano (1977) have reported that slow, effortful, and less coordinated swallowing are a typical manifestation of the aging pharynx. These are indicative of some degree of muscular weakening and neural degeneration.

Hutchinson et al. (1978) studied 30 men and 30 women 50 to 80 years old. Each subject produced isolated vowels and read a standard passage containing no nasal consonants. Data were analyzed using an electroacoustic device known as TONAR II (Fletcher & Bishop, 1970), which is designed to compute a ratio (called *nasalance*) of nasal sound-pressure level to total sound-pressure level from oral and nasal channels. Hutchinson et al. found that speakers 50 years of age and older exhibited significantly higher levels of nasalance than younger subjects during connected speech (i.e., reading of the standard passage). No systematic increases in nasalance were observed as a function of age. Both sexes exhibited significantly higher levels of nasalance than their younger counterparts, and this effect was particularly evident in females.

Three patterns of velopharyngeal incompetence were found among geriatric speakers. The most frequent type was a pervasive mild level of hypernasality during speech (pervasive nasalance). The next most frequent pattern was a gradual loss of velar control that became most severe toward the end of the utterance (progressive loss of velar control). The least frequent type was characterized by isolated instances of excessive nasalance that were interspersed throughout speech of normal quality (momentary loss of velar control). The authors speculated that each of the defective patterns of velopharyngeal valving may be related to different neurologic deficits. Pervasive nasalance may be reflective of general neuromuscular weakness, whereas progressive loss of velar control may be the result of reduced stores of neurotransmitters that reach deficient levels after prolonged periods of continuous speech. Momentary loss of velar control may result from neuromotor timing deficits that cause the velum to elevate sluggishly following pauses, junctures, or word boundaries.

Evidence from multiview cinefluoroscopic studies (Skolnick, 1969, 1970) indicates that the lateral pharyngeal walls make essential contributions to adequate velopharyngeal valving. Previously cited research (Ferreri, 1959; Kiuchi et al., 1969; Zaino & Benventano, 1977) has shown that muscular and neural changes in the pharyngeal walls often accompany aging. Such changes may contribute directly to the resonance distortions found by Hutchinson et al. (1978) among aged adult speakers. Further research is required to determine the extent to which the superior constrictor musculature contributes to faulty velopharyngeal valving during speech.

IMPLICATIONS FOR SPEECH

In previous sections, anatomic and physiologic changes in the organs used for speech were discussed. These age-related changes may limit the potential for various structures to perform work during speech production.

The Respiratory Pump

Bouhuys (1977) has stated that the pressures required to drive the vocal apparatus during speech production derive from three sources: (1) elastic recoil forces generated by the lungs and the chest cage, (2) active contraction of the expiratory muscles, and (3) contraction and relaxation of the inspiratory muscles that serve to brake the recoil forces and insure that the driving force is maintained evenly at large lung volumes.

Structural changes in the aging respiratory system may limit or affect the speaker's ability to develop an adequate driving force for all speech situations. Weakening of the respiratory muscles may affect the speaker's ability to produce the slow muscle pressures required to expel air during exhalation. Such muscular weakening may also have a deleterious effect on rapid muscular pressure variations called pulsatile variations. These rapid increases in muscle force result in increases of $1-3$ cm H_2O during conversational speech of normal loudness (Hixon, 1973) and have been shown to be of linguistic significance in stress contrasts (Netsell, 1969). The atrophy and weakness of the respiratory muscles may, therefore, contribute to prosodic changes in the speech of aged talkers.

Speakers try to use the midrange of vital capacity during speech because it requires less speaker (muscular) effort to drive the speech mechanism (Hixon, 1973). The speaker takes advantage of the recoil forces of the respiratory system, which are, for the most part, sufficient to drive the larynx within this lung volume.

Reductions in elastic recoil of the lung and chest wall and in vital capacity are characteristic changes in aging respiratory systems. Alterations in the lungs−thorax linkage also render the system biomechanically disadvantaged; that is, the reduced elasticity and vital capacity of the aging respiratory system may make it difficult for aged speakers to use their respiratory systems efficiently for speech. Because the recoil forces of their systems may not be adequate, they may have to expend more muscle force during speech than younger speakers, and this may be quite fatiguing.

Aging speakers may have difficulties in producing speech of adequate loudness. Hixon (1973) noted that loud speech requires high levels of alveolar pressure and is usually initiated at high lung volumes. Because elastic recoil of the aging lung is reduced, aging speakers may not be able to inflate their lungs sufficiently to speak at a consistently loud level for long periods of time.

Changes in lung volume and flow rates in aging speakers may affect the prosody of their speech. Vital capacity determines the maximum volume of air that can be exhaled for a prolonged utterance. Because vital capacity is reduced in aged speakers, the amount of air available to "speak on" is reduced. Consequently, this may affect the number of words produced per unit time and may determine how frequently speech must be interrupted for air intake.

Decreased maximum expiratory flow rates have been shown to accompany aging in the respiratory system (i.e., air comes out of the lungs more slowly in older people than in younger people). The reduced flow rates may cause speakers to have difficulty maintaining a given flow rate over the full range of their vital capacity. This in turn may result in the need for the speaker to pause more frequently during speech because of an inability to maintain the required flow rate, except at higher lung volumes.

Thus, age-related changes appear to affect the respiratory pump's capacity to perform work. These changes could result in deficits that may reduce a speaker's ability to (1) produce speech of adequate loudness in some speech situations, (2) develop forces sufficient to drive the larynx so that sound production can be maintained for adequate periods of time without interruption, and (3) exhibit variation in prosodic features in speech.

The Sound Generator

Age-related changes in the laryngeal cartilages, muscles, and connective tissues may affect the ability of the larynx to function as a sound generator. Stiffening of the laryngeal cartilages (particularly in the thyroid cartilage) resulting from ossification or calcification may reduce the "spring action" of the thyroid cartilage, which has been described by Zenker (1964), Kotby and Haugen (1970), and Fink (1974). These investigators found that extrinsic laryngeal muscles could compress the thyroid laminae and cause the vocal folds to approximate and lengthen. Relaxation of these muscles causes recoil forces in the cartilage to separate the vocal folds. Such action has been shown to occur in effort closure and swallowing. Zenker has proposed that this mechanism plays a role in phonation, although this concept has not gained wide acceptance to date.

Lauth (1835) noted that fibroelastic tissues of the larynx could produce passive recoil of laryngeal tissues after they have been stretched by muscle forces. Fink (1974) has shown that these fibroelastic tissues, when stretched by intrinsic and extrinsic laryngeal muscles, function to reopen the glottis when the vocal folds are fully adducted, to narrow and widen the glottis, to shorten the vocal folds, and to change the size of the ventricle, functions that are important to phonation.

Hirano (1974) has described the vocal fold as consisting of three layers. The superficial layer, or *cover*, consists of the mucous membrane and the superficial lamina propria. The middle layer, or *transition*, consists of the intermediate and deep layers of the lamina propria which contribute, largely, to the vocal ligament. The deepest layer of the vocal fold, or *body*, is formed by the vocalis muscle. Hirano has shown that the mucous membrane may participate in vocal-fold vibration, depending on the stiffness and tension in the underlying ligament and muscle, a role that may be altered with aging. Thinning (atrophy) of the mucosa, changes in its texture, and loosening of its submucosal connective tissue from the vocal ligament may reduce the combined affect of vocalis muscle contraction and stiffness of the vocal ligament on the mucosa. This could affect the compliance and shape of the medial margins of the vocal folds, which could in turn alter the mode of vibration of the vocal folds. For example, the mucosa may vibrate out of phase with the body of the vocal fold.

Drying out of the mucosal surfaces because of atrophy of mucous and serous glands may affect the texture and surface architecture of the folds. These surface changes may set up eddy currents, which could be sources for noise in the glottal spectrum.

Another age-related factor that may alter vocal-fold function are changes in the structure of the vocal ligament, which have been noted by several investigators (Ferreri, 1959; Hommerich, 1972; Kofler, 1932). This condition could have deleterious affects on vocal functioning since the pattern of vibration of the vocal folds appears to be largely determined by the properties of the vocal ligaments, and these properties are determined by the elastic and collagenous fibers composing the ligaments (van den Berg & Tan, 1959). Longitudinal stability of the vocal fold during vibration has been shown (Titze, 1973) to be largely determined by the vocal ligament. Alterations in the physical properties of the ligament will likely affect how effectively tension can be transmitted to the mucosal covering of the folds as well as influencing vibration of the fold generally.

Age-related changes in the intrinsic laryngeal muscles also have been reported (Bach et al., 1941; Carnevalle-Ricci, 1937; Ferreri, 1959; Hommerich, 1972; Imhofer, 1912; Kofler, 1932; Segre, 1936, 1971). These reductions in muscle strength would probably reduce the effectiveness of these muscles in changing vocal-fold length, tension and mass per unit area. Because the mass of the thyroarytenoid muscle has been shown to decrease with age and because the vocal folds become stiffer, it is likely that fundamental frequency would become elevated. In addition, changes in the cricothyroid muscle may reduce the pitch range. Thus, atrophy of the thyroarytenoid muscle and breakdown in the vocal ligament could affect the ability of the vocal fold to develop isometric tension, which is important in the control of fundamental frequency and in the regulation of glottal resistance.

Overall weakness of the intrinsic muscles may affect vocal efficiency by reducing the degree of glottal resistance. It may also limit the degree of adduction of the vocal folds at the initiation of phonation, thereby permitting air to leak through the glottis, creating turbulence and reduction of subglottal power.

There appear to be several physical changes in the aging larynx that could reduce the capabilities of the larynx as a sound generator. Combined with respiratory changes, it appears likely that aging measurably affects phonatory efforts.

The Supralaryngeal Resonators

Involutional changes have been reported for the pharynx (Ferreri, 1959; Kiuchi et al., 1969; Zaino & Benventano, 1977), velopharyngeal mechanism (Bucciante & Luria, 1934; Hutchinson et al., 1978), and oral cavity (Andrew, 1971; Kaplan, 1971; Klingsberg & Butcher, 1960; Pedriera, 1951; Robinson et al., 1942; Yamaguchi, 1924, as reported in Andrew, 1971). These changes would appear to have measurable effects on the modification of normal vocal-tract function during speech. Weakening and atrophy of the pharyngeal muscles that have been shown to dilate the cavity and reduction in sensory and motor innervation to this region would appear to contribute significantly to these changes.

The muscular changes may alter the resonance characteristics of the pharynx by changing the size of the cavity and by reducing the elasticity of its walls, which may become more energy absorbing. Disturbances in sensory and motor innervation may limit the activity of the pharynx during articulation, an action that has been shown to be notable during the production of vowels (Kelsey, Woodhouse, & Minific, 1969) and consonants (Bell-Berti, 1975). Such pharyngeal adjustments also would alter the diameter of the pharyngeal airway during speech.

Though no age-related data on pharyngeal articulation has been reported, Hutchinson et al. (1978) found three degrees of abnormal nasal resonance in speakers who ranged in age from 50 to 80 years of age. Thus it is not unreasonable to assume that other changes may also exist.

Changes in the size of the oral cavity resulting from loss of teeth, subsequent resorption of alveolar bone, and retrusion of the mandible as a consequence of temporomandibular joint changes may affect oral resonance. Alterations in the oral epithelium may affect the compliance of the walls of the cavity. Restrictions on movement of the temporomandibular joint may restrict or otherwise influence the ability of the speaker to change the size and shape of the oral cavity as dictated by the demands of speech.

Thus there is reason to anticipate that the transfer function of the vocal tract is likely to change as a function of age. The character of this change must await controlled study.

The Articulators

The tongue, facial muscles, temporomandibular joint, and associated musculature constitute a major group of articulatory structures. Their reduced efficiency of performance resulting from age-related changes may have measurable effects on speech adequacy.

Although data are incomplete on age-related muscle changes in the tongue, facial, and masticatory muscles, each of these muscle groups has been shown to undergo some atrophy with aging. Thus, some reduction in the extent and speed of movement of these articulators would be anticipated. There is no information on the circumoral musculature and no specific data on intrinsic and extrinsic tongue muscles. Reduced diadochokinesis, however, has been reported (Mysak, 1959; Ptacek et al., 1966), as have specific velopharyngeal deficiencies in speakers aged 50 to 80 (Hutchinson et al., 1978).

The reported decrease in salivary secretions with aging dries the epithelial surfaces of the tongue and oral cavity. These changes may make movement of the tongue across the palate towards an articulatory target more difficult and sluggish because of increased resistances. In addition, submucosal changes in aging oral epithelium also may bring about alterations in proprioceptors that have been shown to be located there. Changes in the sensory portion of the trigeminal nerve (Truex, 1940) point to the possibility that there may be reduced sensory feedback from these regions, which also may affect the precision of articulation as one ages.

The loss of permanent dentition and wearing of dentures may interfere with articulation with age. These changes are likely to be temporary, and the speaker may adapt to them over time.

The affects of alterations in the articulatory apparatus with age may result in coarticulatory changes or altered prosody of speech. It must be remembered, however, that speech is a continuous process in which articulatory movements are produced synergistically (Daniloff & Hammarberg, 1973). Speech sounds are serially ordered into a flow of speech. Thus, statements regarding limitations of individual articulators may be artificially simplifying the process.

The state of the art regarding aging of the peripheral speech mechanism necessitates developing hypotheses on limited data. Careful documentation of many of these age-related changes is needed.

FUTURE DIRECTIONS

There are numerous facets of aging of the peripheral speech mechanism that must be studied and be more clearly understood. Among these are detailed analyses of speech breathing. Such data would be helpful in explaining the physiologic strategies employed by speakers as they age to compensate or accommodate changes in the respiratory and laryngeal mechanism. The use of body plethysmography as described by Hixon, Mead, and Goldman (1976) would be invaluable in describing static and kinematic aspects of the chest wall, lungs, and abdomen during speech.

Another area of research involves detailed histologic studies on the larynx, tongue, velopharyngeal mechanism, and pharynx using light and electromicroscopic techniques. When possible, histochemical analyses should be performed to determine the nature of biochemical changes in these structures, particularly muscles, that may affect their ability to do work. This basic data would be quite valuable as corroborative information for studies on the kinesthesiological and temporal aspects of articulation.

Functional changes in the larynx with age must be investigated more thoroughly. In addition to anatomic research, investigations into physiology and biomechanics must be undertaken. The use of inverse filtering techniques (Davis, 1976) could provide information regarding changes and properties of the glottal spectrum and information on "jitter" and

"shimmer" characteristics that may be significant in providing distinctive cues to listeners about the age of the voice. High-speed motion picture films of the vocal folds during speech may help to determine the pattern(s) of vocal fold vibration and enable investigators to quantify temporal characteristics of the vibrating cycle that may become altered with age. Aerodynamic techniques (Hirano, Koike, & von Leden, 1968; Koike & Hirano, 1968; Yanagihara & Koike, 1967; Yanagihara & von Leden, 1966) could be used to calculate measures of vocal efficiency such as phonation volume, vocal velocity indices, and glottal resistance. Such data would be invaluable in describing normal and pathologic changes in the aging voice mechanism.

More data are needed regarding alterations in the properties of the vocal tract as a consequence of aging. Information on changes in the physical characteristics of the vocal tract such as cross-sectional area, length, and shape would provide a more substantial basis to evaluate acoustic data. Because hypotonicity and hypokinesis in the pharynx have been shown to be characteristic changes in aging, it is likely that the normative data on young adults will be different from those in middle and old age.

Little information appears to be available on the kinesthesiology of the articulators. Such information is vitally important in order to determine how aging affects the timing, extent, and velocity of movement of the temporomandibular joint, tongue, and velopharyngeal mechanism. Also, the maintenance of coarticulatory strategies as a function of aging needs to be explored.

The assumption that changes in the oral mucosa might also involve reductions in proprioception needs to be tested. This may be difficult to achieve, however, because of the inherent problems of separating cognitive factors from physiologic responses in older people and the reliability of evaluations of psychophysical data from older individuals.

Our knowledge regarding aging of the peripheral speech mechanism is in an embryonic state. Substantial amounts of research into basic processes must be done to provide the yardstick against which speech performance can be measured.

REFERENCES

Adams, D. Age changes in the oral structures. In C. L. Lavelle (Ed.), *Applied physiology of the mouth*. London: John Wright & Sons, 1975.

Andrew, W. *The anatomy of aging in man and animals*. New York: Grune & Stratton, 1971.

Ardran, G. M. Calcification of the epiglottis. *British Journal of Radiology*, 1965, *38*, 592−595.

Azzan, N. A., & Kuehn, D. P. The morphology of musculus uvulae. *Cleft Palate Journal*, 1977, *14*, 78−87.

Bach, A. C., Lederer, F. L., & Dinolt, R. Senile changes in the laryngeal musculature. *Archives of Otolaryngology*, 1941, *34*, 47−56.

Baldwin, E., Cournand, A., & Richards, D. W., Jr. Pulmonary insufficiency. I. Physiological classification, clinical methods of analysis, standard values in normal subjects. *Medicine* (Baltimore), 1948, *27*, 243−278.

Bates, D. V., & Christie, R. V. Effects of aging on respiratory function in man. In G. F. Wolstenholme & M. P. Cameron (Eds.), *Ciba foundation colloquia on aging*, Volume 1. Boston: Little, Brown, & Co., 1955.

Beau, A. Considerations sur le mode d'ossification des cartilages du larynx. *Revue Medicale de Nancy*, 1939, *67*, 127−136.

Bell-Berti, F. Control of pharyngeal cavity size for English voiced and voiceless stops. *Journal of the Acoustical Society of America*, 1975, *57*, 456−461.

Bickerman, H. A. The respiratory system in the aged. In A. I. Lansing (Ed.), *Cowdry's problems of aging*, (3rd ed.). Baltimore: Williams & Wilkins, 1952.

Blackwood, H. J. Adaptive changes in the mandibular joints with function. *Dental Clinics of North America*, November 1966, pp. 559−566.

Blackwood, H. J. Pathology of the temporomandibular joint. *Journal of the American Dental Association*, 1969, *79*, 118−124.

Boren, H. C., Kory, R. C., & Syner, J. C. The Veterans Administration−Army cooperative study of pulmonary function. II. The lung volume and its subdivisions in normal men. *American Journal of Medicine*, 1966, *41*, 96−114.

Bosma, J. F. *Symposium on oral sensation and perception*. Springfield, Ill.: Charles C. Thomas, Publisher, 1967.

Bosma, J. F. *Second symposium on oral sensation and perception*. Springfield, Ill.: Charles C. Thomas, Publisher, 1970.

Bouhuys, A. *The physiology of breathing*. New York: Grune & Stratton, 1977.

Brain, W. R., & Walton, J. N. *Diseases of the nervous system*. London: Oxford University Press, 1969.

Brietner, C. Bone changes resulting from experimental orthodontic treatment. *American Journal of Orthodontics and Oral Surgery*, 1940, *26*, 521−546.

Brietner, C. Further investigations of bone changes resulting from experimental orthodontic treatment. *American Journal of Orthodontics and Oral Surgery*, 1941, *27*, 605−632.

Briscoe, A. M., Loring, W. E., & McClement, J. H. Changes in human collagen and lipids with age. *Proceedings of the Society for Experimental Biology and Medicine*, 1959, *102*, 71−74.

Brown, A. M. Surgical restorative art for the aging face: Note on artistic anatomy. *Journal of Gerontology*, 1951, *8*, 173−190.

Bucciante, L., & Luria, S. Trasformazioni nella struttura dei muscoli voluntari dell'uoma nella senescenza. *Archivio Italiano di Anatomia e di Embriologia*, 1934, *33*, 110−187.

Buchi, E. C. Anderungen des Korperform beim Erwachsamen Menschen. *Anthropologischer Forschungen Anthropologischer Gesellschaft Wein*, 1950, *1*, 1−44.

Carnevalle-Ricci, F. Osservazioni isopathologiche sulla laringe nells senescenza. *Archivo Italiano di Otologia, Rinologia e Laringologia*, 1937, *49*, 1.

Chaco, J., & Yules, R. B. Velopharyngeal incompetence post tonselloadenoidectomy. *Acta Otolaryngologica*, 1969, *68*, 276−278

Chamberlain, W. E., & Young, B. R. Ossification (so-called "calcification") of normal laryngeal cartilages mistaken for foreign bodies. *American Journal of Roentgenology*, 1935, *33*, 441−450.

Chievitz, H. Untersuchungen uber die Verknocherung der Kehlkopf-Knorpel. *Archieve fuer Anatomischer und Physiologie*, 1882, 303−349.

Cohen, T. & Gitman, L. Taste perception in the aged. *Journal of Gerontology*, 1958, *13*, 441. (Abstract)

Coleman, D. R., & Kaiser, W. F. Anatomy. In Shapiro, M. (Ed.), *The scientific bases of dentistry.* Philadelphia: W. B. Saunders, 1966.

Comroe, J. H. Mechanical factors in breathing. In Comroe, J. H., *Physiology of respiration.* Chicago: Year Book Medical Publishers, 1965.

Cooper, R. M., Bilash, I., & Zubek, J. P. The effect of age on taste sensitivity. *Journal of Gerontology,* 1959, *14*, 56−58.

Corso, J. F. Sensory processes in man during maturity and senescence. In Ordy, J. M., & Brizzee, K. R. (Eds.), *Neurobiology of aging—An interdisciplinary life span approach.* New York: Plenum Press, 1975.

Cosh, J. A. Studies on the nature of vibration sense. *Clinical Science,* 1953, *12*, 131−151.

Croft, C. B., Shprintzen, R. J., & Daniller, A. The occult submucous cleft palate and the musculus uvulae. *Cleft Palate Journal,* 1978, *15*, 150−154.

Daniloff, R. G., & Hammarberg, R. F. On defining coarticulation. *Journal of Phonetics,* 1973, *1*, 239−248.

Davis, S. B. Computer evaluation of laryngeal pathology based on inverse filtering of speech. *Speech Communications Research Laboratory (SCRL) Monograph,* 13, 1976, 1−247.

Dhar, S., Shastri, S. R., & Lenora, R. A. K. Aging and the respiratory system. *Medical Clinics of North America,* 1976, *60*, 1121−1139.

Dyck, P. J., Schultz, P. W., & O'Brien, P. C. Quantitation of touch-pressure sensation. *Archives of Neurology,* 1972, *26*, 465−473.

Eggston, A. A., & Wolff, D. *Histopathology of the ear, nose and throat.* Baltimore: Williams & Wilkins, 1947, 587.

El-Baradi, A. F., & Bourne, G. H. Theory of tastes and odors. *Science,* 1951, *113*, 660−661.

Ferreri, G. Senescence of the larynx. *Italian General Review of Oto-Rhino-Laryngology,* 1959, *1*, 640−709.

Fink, B. R. Spring mechanisms in the human larynx. *Acta Otolaryngologica,* 1974, *77*, 295−304.

Fletcher, S. G., & Bishop, M. E. Measurement of nasality with TONAR. *Cleft Palate Journal,* 1970, *7*, 610−621.

Fomon, S., Bell, J. W., Schattner, A., & Syracuse, V. Aging face: Surgical management. *Archives of Otolaryngology,* 1961, *73*, 153−168.

Fujisawa, K. Some observations on the skeletal musculature of aged rats. II. *Journal of the Neurological Sciences,* 1974, *24*, 447−469.

Gerrero-Santos, J. The role of the platysma muscle in rhytidoplasty. *Clinics in Plastic Surgery,* 1978, *5*, 29−49.

Goldstein, M. S. Changes in dimensions and form of the face and head with age. *American Journal of Physical Anthropology,* 1936, *22*, 37−89.

Gordon, H. L. Rhytidectomy. *Clinics in plastic surgery,* 1978, *5*, 97−109.

Grant, J. C. B. *Method of anatomy* (2nd ed.). Baltimore: Williams & Wilkins, 1940.

Grant, J. C. B. *Grant's atlas of anatomy.* Baltimore: Williams & Wilkins, 1972.

Greenfield, J. C., Shy, G. M., Alvord, E. C., & Berg, L. *Atlas of muscle pathology in neuromuscular diseases.* Edinburgh: Livingstone, 1957.

Grossman, R. C., Hattis, B. F., & Ringel, R. L. Oral tactile experience. *Archives of Oral Biology,* 1965, *10*, 691−705.

Grossman, R. C., & Hattis, B. F. Oral mucosal sensory innervation and sensory experience. In J. F. Bosma (Ed.), *Symposium on oral sensation and perception.* Springfield, Ill.: Charles C. Thomas Publisher, 1967.

Gutmann, E. & Hanzlikova, V. Old-age changes in the muscle. In E. Gutmann & V. Hanzlikova (Eds.), *Age changes in the neuromuscular system.* Bristol: Scientechnica Ltd, 1972.

Gutmann, E., & Hunzlikova, V. Changes in neuromuscular relationships in aging. In J. M. Ordy & K. R. Brizzee (Eds.), *Neurobiology of aging—An interdisciplinary life-span approach.* New York: Plenum Press, 1975.

Harris, W. The fifth and seventh cranial nerves in relation to the nervous mechanism of taste sensation. *British Medical Journal,* 1951, *1*, 831−836.

Hately, B. W., Evison, G., & Samuel, E. The pattern of ossification in the laryngeal cartilages: A radiological study. *British Journal of Radiology,* 1965, *38,* 585–591.

Hellman, M. Changes in the human face brought about by development. *International Journal of Orthodontics,* 1927, *13,* 475–516.

Hieronymi, G. On the change in the morphology of the human lung due to aging. *Verhandlungen der Deutschen Gesellschaft fur Pathologie,* 1960, *44,* 128–130.

Hirano, M. Morphological structure of the vocal cord as a vibrator and its variations. *Folia Phoniatrica,* 1974, *26,* 89–94.

Hirano, M., Koike, Y., & von Leden, H. Maximum phonation time and air usage during phonation. *Folia Phoniatrica,* 1968, *20,* 185–201.

Hixon, T. J. Respiratory function in speech. In F. D. Minifie, T. J. Hixon, & F. Williams (Eds.), *Normal aspects of speech, hearing and language.* Englewood Cliffs, N.J.: Prentice-Hall, 1973.

Hixon, T. J., Mead, J., & Goldman, M. D. Dynamics of the chest wall during speech production: Function of the thorax, rib cage, diaphragm and abdomen. *Journal of Speech and Hearing Research,* 1976, *19,* 297–356.

Hommerich, K. W. Der alternde Larynx: Morphologische Aspekte. *Hals Nasen Ohrenaerzte,* 1972, *20,* 115–120.

Hooton, E. A., & Dupertuis, C. W. Age changes and selective survival in Irish males. In *American association of physical anthropology, studies in physical anthropology, no. 2.* New York: Wenner-Gren Foundation, 1951.

Hutchinson, J. M., Robinson, K. L., & Nerbonne, M. A. Patterns of nasalance in a sample of normal gerontologic subjects. *Journal of Communication Disorders,* 1978, *11,* 469–481.

Imhofer, F. Ueber das Abnutzungspigment in der Muskulatur der Stimmbander. *Zeitschrift fuer Laryngologie, Rhinologie, Otologie und Ihre Grenzebiete,* 1912, *5,* 389.

Israel, H. Age factor and the pattern of change in craniofacial structures. *American Journal of Physical Anthropology,* 1973, *39,* 111–128.

Jamieson, E. B. Osteology. In J. C. Brash & E. B. Jamieson (Eds.), *Cunningham's textbook of anatomy* (7th ed.). London: Oxford Medical Publications, 1937.

Jarcho, A. Die Altersveranderungen der Rassenmerkmale bei den Erwachsensen. *Anthropologischer Anzeiger,* 1935, *12,* 173–179.

Johnson, L. C. Joint remodelling as the basis for osteoarthritis. *Journal of the American Veterinary Medical Association,* 1962, *141,* 1237–1241.

Kahane, J. C., Stadlan, E. M., & Bell, J. S. A histological study of the aging human larynx. Scientific Exhibit, American Speech, Language and Hearing Association Meeting, Atlanta, 1979.

Kaltieider, N. L., Fray, W. W., & Hyde, H. The effect of age on the total pulmonary capacity and its subdivisions. *American Review of Tuberculosis,* 1938, *37,* 662–689.

Kaplan, H. The oral cavity in geriatrics. *Geriatrics,* 1971, *26,* 96–102.

Keen, J. A., & Wainwright, J. Ossification of the thyroid, cricoid, and arytenoid cartilages. *South African Journal of Laboratory and Clinical Medicine,* 1958, *4,* 83–108.

Keleman, G. Clinical observations on the palatine tonsil. *Annals of Otology, Rhinology and Laryngology,* 1945, *54,* 421–438.

Kelsey, C. A., Woodhouse, R. N., & Minifie, F. D. Ultrasonic observations of coarticulation in the pharynx. *Journal of the Acoustical Society of America,* 1969, *46,* 1016–1018.

Kiuchi, S., Sasaki, J., Arai, T., & Suzuki, T. Functional disorders of the pharynx and esophagus. *Acta Oto-laryngologica,* 1969. *Supplementum 256.*

Klingsberg, J., & Butcher, E. O. Comparative histology of age changes in oral tissues of rat, hamster and monkey. *Journal of Dental Research,* 1960, *39,* 158–169.

Kofler, K. Die Altersveranderungen in Larynx. *Monatsschrift fuer Ohrenheilkunde und Laryngo-Rhinologie (Wein),* 1932, *66,* 1468.

Koike, Y., & Hirano, M. Significance of vocal velocity index. *Folia Phoniatrica,* 1968, *20,* 285–296.

Kotby, M. N., & Haugen, L. K. Attempts at evaluation of the function of various laryngeal muscles in the light of muscle and nerve stimulation experiments in man. *Acta Oto-laryngologica,* 1970, *70,* 419−427.

Krogman, W. M. Geriatric research and prosthodontics. *Journal of Prosthetic Dentistry,* 1962, *12,* 493−515.

Lasker, G. W. The age factor in bodily measurements of adult male and female Mexicans. *Human Biology,* 1953, *25,* 50−63.

Lauth, E. A. Remarques sur la structure du larynx et de la trachee-artere. *Memoires de l'Academie Royale de Medecine de Belgique,* 1835, *4,* 95−116.

LeGros-Clark, W. E. *The tissues of the body* (3rd ed.). Oxford: Clarendon Press, 1952.

Lynne-Davies, P. Influence of age on the respiratory system. *Geriatrics,* 1977, *32,* 57−60.

Macklin, C. C., & Macklin, M. T. Respiratory system. In E. V. Cowdry (Ed.), *Problems of aging* (2nd ed.). Baltimore: Williams & Wilkins, 1942.

Maleci, O. Sul rapporto numerico tra le cellule dei nuclei di origine e le fibre di nervi motor encefalici dell'uoma, con osservazioni sulle differenze qualitative delle dette fibre. *Archives Italiano di Anatomia e di Embriologia,* 1936, *35,* 559−583.

Macmillan, H. W. Anatomy of the throat, mylohyoid region and mandible in relation to retention of mandibular artificial dentures. *Journal of the American Dental Association,* 1936, *23,* 1435−1442.

Malan, E. Etude d'histologie comparee sur quelques modifications particulieres des fibres du tensor tympani dues a la senescence. *Archives de Biologie* (Paris), 1934, *45,* 355−375.

Martone, A. L., & Edwards, L. F. Anatomy of the mouth and related structures. Part I. *Journal of Prosthetic Dentistry,* 1961, *11,* 1009−1018.

Martone, A. L., & Edwards, L. F. Anatomy of the mouth and related structures. Part II. *Journal of Prosthetic Dentistry,* 1962, *12,* 4−27.

Mayne, J. G., & Hatch, G. S. Arthritis of the temporomandibular joint. *Journal of the American Dental Association,* 1969, *79,* 125−130.

McKeown, F. *Pathology of the aged.* London: Butterworths, 1965.

Mead, J., Turner, J. M., Macklem, P. T., & Little, J. B. Significance of the relationship between lung recoil and maximum expiratory flow. *Journal of Applied Physiology,* 1967, *22,* 95−108.

Miller, S. C., & Roth, H. Torus palatinus: a statistical study. *Journal of the American Dental Association,* 1940, *27,* 1950−1957.

Moffett, B. C., Jr., Johnson, L. C., McCabe, J. B., & Askew, H. C. Articular remodeling in the adult human temporomandibular joint. *American Journal of Anatomy,* 1964, *115,* 119−142.

Montgomery, P. W. A study of exfoliative cytology of normal human oral mucosa. *Journal of Dental Research,* 1951, *30,* 12−18.

Moore, S. *Hyperostosis Cranii.* Springfield. Ill.: Charles C. Thomas, Publisher, 1955.

Mysak, E. D. Pitch and duration characteristics of older males. *Journal of Speech and Hearing Research,* 1959, *2,* 46−54.

Nascher, I. L. *Geriatrics.* Philadelphia: Blakiston's Son and Co., 1914.

Negus, V. E. *The comparative anatomy and physiology of the larynx.* London: W. Heinemann Medical Books, 1949.

Netsell, R. A perceptual−acoustic−physiological study of syllable stress. Doctoral dissertation, University of Iowa, 1969.

Noback, G. J. Correlation of stages of ossification of the laryngeal cartilages and morphologic age changes in other tissues and organs. *Journal of Gerontology,* 1949, *4,* 329. (Abstract)

Noell, G. On the problem of age related changes of the laryngeal mucosa. *Archiv fuer klinische and experimentelle Ohren-, Nasen- und Kehlkopfheilkunde,* 1962, *179,* 361−365.

Norris, A. H., Shock, N. W., Landowne, M., & Falzone, J. A. Pulmonary function studies: Age differences in lung volumes and bellows functions. *Gerontologia,* 1956, *11,* 379−387.

Ormea, F. La cute quale organo di senso. I. Sui rapporti tra recettore e localizzazeone della sensibilita. *Minerva Dermatologica,* 1956, *31,* 323−326.

Ormea, F., & Re, G. Strutture nervose e funzione nervose della regione buccale. *Minerva Dermatologica,* 1959, *34,* 611−631.

Pace, W. R. *Pulmonary physiology in clinical practice* (2nd ed.). Philadelphia: F. A. Davis, 1970.

Papic, M., & Glickman, I. Keratinization of the human gingiva in the menstrual cycle and menopause. *Oral Surgery, Oral Medicine and Oral Pathology,* 1950, *3,* 504−516.

Pedriera, R. A. A study of keratinization of the oral mucosa of aged males. *Journal of Dental Medicine,* 1951, *6,* 88−91.

Pemberton, J., & Flanagan, E. G. Vital capacity and timed vital capacity in normal men over forty. *Journal of Applied Physiology,* 1956, *9,* 291−296.

Pierce, J. A., & Ebert, R. V. Fibrous network of the lung and its change with age. *Thorax,* 1965, *20,* 469−476.

Pigott, R. W. The nasendoscopic appearance of the normal velopharyngeal mechanism. *Plastic Reconstructive Surgery,* 1969, *43,* 19−24.

Pigott, R. W., Bensen, J. F., & White, F. D. Nasendoscopy in the diagnosis of velopharyngeal incompetency. *Plastic Reconstructive Surgery,* 1969, *43,* 141−147.

Pitanguy, I. Ancillary procedures in face lifting. *Clinics in Plastic Surgery,* 1978, *5,* 51−70.

Plumb, C. S., & Meigs, J. W. Human vibration perception. Part I. Vibration perception at different ages. *Archives of General Psychiatry,* 1961, *4,* 611−614.

Pressman, J. J., & Keleman, G. Physiology of the larynx. *Physiological Review,* 1955, *35,* 506−554.

Ptacek, P. H., Sander, E. K., Maloney, W. H., & Jackson, C. C. R. Phonatory and related changes with advanced age. *Journal of Speech and Hearing Research,* 1966, *9,* 353−360.

Puschel, L., & Nowakowski, H. The effects of androgens on ossification of the laryngeal skeleton. *Archiv für Ohren-Nasen und Kehlkopheilkunde,* 1954, *166,* 255−274.

Radsel, Z., & Kambic, V. The influence of cigarette smoke on pharyngeal mucosa. *Acta Oto-laryngologica,* 1978, *85,* 128−134.

Retzlaff, E., & Fontaine, J. Functional and structural changes in motor neurons with age. In A. I. Welford & J. E. Birren (Eds.), *Behavior, aging and the nervous system.* Springfield, Ill.: Charles C. Thomas Publisher, 1965.

Reveille-Parise, M. Modifications seniles des organes de la respiration; sont-elles le point de depart de la vieillesse? *Gazette Medicale de Paris,* 1851, *3,* 200−205.

Robinson, H. B., Boling, L. R., & Lisher, B. E. Teeth and jaws. In E. V. Cowdry (Ed.), *Problems of aging* (2nd ed.). Baltimore: Williams & Wilkins, 1942.

Roncollo, P. Researches about ossification and conformation of the thyroid cartilage in men. *Acta Oto-laryngologica,* 1948, *36,* 110−134.

Ronge, H. Alterveranderungen des Beruhrungssinnes. I Druckpunktschwellen und Druckpunktfrequenz. *Acta Physiologica Scandinavica,* 1943, *6,* 343−352. (a)

Ronge, H. Altersueranderungen der Meissnerschen Korperchen in der Fingerhaut. *Zeitschrift Fuer Mikroskopisch-Anatomische Forschung,* 1943, *54,* 167−177. (b)

Rossing, F. Histologische Unterlagen zum kraniokaudalen Entwicklungsgang des Waldeyerschen, Rachenringes. *Zeitschrift Fuer Betriebswirtschaft,* 1940, *105,* 17.

Ruckes, J., & Cause, A. Extent and presence of squamous epithelium in the human ventricular band. *Zeitschrift fur laryngologie, rhinologie, otologie, und ihre grenzgebiete,* 1964, *43,* 197−206.

Ruckes, J., & Hohmann, M. On the topography and presence of fatty tissue in the human superior vocal cord in relation to age, weight, and disease. *Anatomischer Anzeiger,* 1963, *112,* 405−425.

Ryan, R. F., McDonald, J. R., & Devine, K. D. Changes in laryngeal epithelium: Relation to age, sex and certain other factors. *Mayo Clinic Proceedings,* 1956, *31,* 47−52.

Segre, R. La laringe senile. *Valsalva,* 1936, *14,* 15.

Segre, R. Senescence of the voice. *Eye, Ear, Nose and Throat Monthly,* 1971, *50,* 62−68.

Shock, N. W. The physiology of aging. *Scientific American,* 1962, *206,* 100−110.

Skolnick, M. L. Video velopharyngography in patients with nasal speech with emphasis on lateral pharyngeal motion in velopharyngeal closure. *Radiology,* 1969, *93,* 747−755.

Skolnick, M. L. Videofluoroscopic examination of the velopharyngeal portal during phonation in lateral and base projections. A new technique for studying the mechanics of closure. *Cleft Palate Journal,* 1970, *7,* 803−816.

Squier, C. A., Johnson, N. W., & Hopps, R. M. *Human oral mucosa*. London: Blackwell Scientific Publications, 1976.

Strunghold, H. Die topographic des Kaltesinnes in der Mundhohle. *Zeitschrift fur Biologie*, 1925, *83*, 515–534.

Titze, I. R. The human vocal cords: A mathematical model. Part I. *Phonetica*, 1973, *28*, 129–170.

Todd, T. W. Skeleton, locomotor system and teeth. In E. V. Cowdry (Ed.), *Cowdry's problems of aging*. Baltimore: Williams & Wilkins, 1942.

Truex, R. Morphological alterations in the Gasserian ganglion cells and their association with senescence in man. *American Journal of Pathology*, 1940, *16*, 255–268.

Turner, J. M., Mead, J., & Wohl, M. E. Elasticity of human lungs in relation to age. *Journal of Applied Physiology*, 1968, *25*, 664–671.

Ufland, J. M. Einfluss des Lebensalters, Geschlechts, der Konstitution und des Berufs auf die Kraft Verschiedener Muskelgruppen. I. Mitteilungen uber den Einfluss des Lebensalfers auf die Muskelfraft. *Arbeitsphysiologie*, 1933, *6*, 653–663.

United States National Center for Health Statistics. Average heights and weights by age and sex: 1960–1962 and 1971–1974 (Table 185). *Statistical abstracts of the United States*, 1976.

van den Berg, J., & Tan, T. S. Results of experiments with human larynges. *Practica Oto-Rhino-Laryngologica*, 1959, *21*, 425–450.

Vaughan, H. C. Study of the temporomandibular articulation. *Journal of the American Dental Association*, 1943, *30*, 1501–1507.

Warren E. Collins, Inc. *Spirometry in normal females: prediction normograms*. Cat. No. P465-A. Braintree, Mass, 1967.

Yanagihara, N., & Koike, Y. The regulation of sustained phonation. *Folia Phoniatrica*, 1967, *19*, 1–18.

Yanagihara, N., & von Leden, H. The cricothyroid muscle during phonation. Electromyographic aerodynamic and acoustic studies. *Annals of Otology, Rhinology and Laryngology*, 1966, *75*, 987–1006.

Zaino, C., & Benventano, T. C. Functional, involutional and degenerative disorders. In Zaino, C, & Benventano, T. C. (eds.), *Radiologic examination of the oropharynx and esophagus*. New York: Springer-Verlag, 1977.

Zenker, W. Questions regarding the function of extrinsic laryngeal muscles. In Brewer. D. W. (Ed.), *Research potentials in voice physiology*. Syracuse: State University of New York, 1964.

Raymond D. Kent
Robert Burkard

3

Changes in the Acoustic Correlates of Speech Production

When listening to an unfamiliar speaker who is not visible, for example, someone speaking over a telephone, a person often draws inferences about the speaker's age. Although the estimates of speaker age may be in error, many people believe that they can differentiate elderly speakers from younger adults. To the extent that such differentiation is possible, then there must be differences in the acoustic speech signal between aged persons and younger adults. This chapter reviews evidence on the perceptual identification of aged speech and considers various acoustic features that might relate to such judgments. In addition, the acoustic features are discussed with respect to the underlying physiological aspects of speech production. Perceptual–acoustic descriptions of aged speech may lead to a better understanding of several issues, including listener reactions to elderly speakers, communication problems of the elderly, and generalized changes in perceptual–motor capabilities of the aged.

PERCEPTUAL AGE IDENTIFICATION

Several studies have determined how accurately listeners can estimate the age of a speaker. Ptacek and Sander (1966) investigated the ability of auditors to differentiate the speech of young (under 35) from old (over 65) individuals. Speech samples included a prolonged vowel and an orally read passage that was played both forward and backward to the listeners. The authors attempted to control the variable of vocal pitch in the vowel prolongation task by having the speakers phonate at a fundamental frequency of 130 ± 20 Hz for men and 210 ± 30 Hz for women. The rate of correct age identification was 78 percent for the vowel prolongations, 87 percent for the backward-played speech and 99 percent for the forward-played speech. These differences in age identification probably can be explained by reference to the cues that are available in the three tasks. In vowel prolongation, the primary cues are voice quality, voice stability (that is, the degree of frequency and amplitude fluctuations), and, depending upon the adequacy of the control for fundamental frequency, the pitch of the voice. As will be discussed later, (see section on Acoustic Studies related to Supralaryngeal Speech Function) the vowel-formant frequencies also might be a consideration in perceptual age identification, but for the most part, the cues available in sustained vowel phonation are related to laryngeal function. In backward-played speech, the listener can detect the additional cues of short-term phonetic variation (that is, changes in spectrum related to some segmental aspects), prosodic variation, and speaking rate. Although backward-played speech is presumed to eliminate articulation as a prime cue, some segmental information probably is present. Forward-played speech gives the listener the full range of segmental and suprasegmental acoustic cues, together with a meaningful linguistic message. The increase in age identification from vowel prolongation to backward-played speech to forward-played speech indicates that the cues for age identification are not simply those found in a static phonatory task. However, the fairly high rate of age identification for the sustained vowels must be taken to mean that laryngeal function, even in a relatively static task, carries strong information about speaker age (see also Ryan & Burk, 1974).

Shipp and Hollien (1969) investigated more refined age identifications by audition. Male speakers ranging in age from 20 to 89 years prolonged a vowel, spoke extemporaneously for 1 minute, and read aloud the first paragraph of the Rainbow Passage (Fairbanks, 1960). Listeners were randomly assigned to one of three groups. The first group judged speaker age on a three-point scale: 1, young; 2, middle-aged; and 3, old. The second group used a seven-point rating scale, assigning a number from 2 to 8 to indicate the age of the speaker in decades. The third group directly estimated the age of the speaker. As shown in Figure 3−1, there was a direct monotonic relationship with chronologic age for the mean values of all three scales. In a similar study, Ryan and Capadano (1978) evaluated age-estimation for speakers grouped according to sex. Female speakers ranged in age from 12 to 71 years and male speakers ranged from 17 to 68 years of age. For both sexes,

the Pearson correlation coefficient relating chronologic and estimated ages was significant, as was Kendall's coefficient of concordance. The R^2 coefficients of determination were 0.86 for the female voices and 0.66 for the male voices, indicating a strong relationship between the perceived and actual age of the speakers.

The perceptual studies clearly show that aging speech can be reliably identified. These investigations point the way toward acoustic studies that attempt to determine which aspects of the speech-signal change with age. In this chapter, these acoustic studies are reviewed within three categories of speech systems: respiratory−phonatory, supralaryngeal, and neuromuscular control.

THE RESPIRATORY−PHONATORY SYSTEM

This section briefly reviews anatomic and physiologic changes that occur with aging of the respiratory−phonatory system. With this background, consideration is given to acoustic measures of respiratory and phonatory performance in speech. Examples of these measures are maximum vowel-phonation time, vocal fundamental frequency, vocal intensity, and indices of irregularity in vocal-fold vibration.

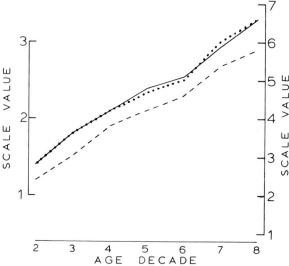

Fig. 3−1. Relationship between actual speaker age and perceived speaker age using three different rating scales: Dashed line = three-point scale; solid line = seven-point scale; dotted line = transformed data from direction estimation to seven-point scale. (Based on data from Shipp and Hollien, 1969.)

Anatomic and Physiologic Changes

With increased age, there is generally a reduction of the vital capacity, or the total amount of air that can be moved in a maximal inspiration and expiration. Vital capacity measurements for aged subjects have been reported by Muiesan, Sorbini, and Grassi (1971), Jalavisto (1965), and Ptacek, Sander, Maloney, & Jackson, (1966). In a factorial study, Jalavisto concluded that the reduction of vital capacity does not depend on the well-known reduction of height with advanced age, and added, "Whether this finding should be interpreted to mean that respiratory function is impaired in the old to such an extent that it affects the performance of mental and speed tests is not clear" (p. 362). Shock and Yiengst (1955) reported that with increasing age, basal-heat production and carbon dioxide elimination are significantly reduced, but they did not see evidence for age-related changes in respiratory rate, total ventilation volume, or tidal volume. One complicating factor in studies of the aged lung is that emphysematous lesions may exist even when the subjects present no symptoms of respiratory disease (Pump, 1971). Whether because of senescent degeneration or late effects of injury and disease, it appears common for elderly people to have a weakening and stretching of the alveolar septal membranes, which causes a dilatation of individual alveoli. In addition, increasing rigidity of collagenous tissue in the lung with advanced age (Cander & Moyer, 1964, p. 47) reduces the mobility of the respiratory system.

Probably the major consequence of aging on the larynx is the calcification and ossification of the hyaline cartilages that make up most of this structure (Kirchner, 1970; Malinowski, 1967; Roncallo, 1948). As these mineralization processes occur, the larynx becomes more rigid. Ossification can be detected by the age of 20 years (Roncallo, 1948), and it has been concluded that complete calcification or ossification generally has occurred by age 65 (Kirchner, 1970; Zemlin, 1968). Degenerative changes related to aging have been observed in the laryngeal muscles (Bach, Lederer, & Dinolt, 1941) and in the laryngeal ligaments (Luchsinger & Arnold, 1965). Published descriptions of the aged larynx include ossification or calcification of the cartilages; atrophy of muscles, glands, and other soft tissues; laxity, thinning, and bowing of the vocal folds; reduction of vascular supply; and changes in mucus secretion (Keleman & Pressman, 1955; Luchsinger, 1962; Meyerson, 1976; Zemlin, 1968).

Acoustic Studies Related to Respiratory-Phonatory Function

One simple measure that has differentiated aged and younger speakers is that of vowel duration in a task of maximally prolonging a vowel sound. Ptacek et al. (1966) compared vowel prolongations of males and females in two age groups, those under 40 years and those over 65 years. Maximum vowel duration of sustained /ɑ/ for the male subjects declined by about 26 percent between the young and old age groups. For the females, this measure declined by about 32 percent with advanced age. The mean duration for males under 40 years was 24.6 sec and that for males over 65 years was 18.1 sec. For the females, the younger group had a mean duration of 20.9 sec and the older group a mean duration of 14.2 sec. Similar results in comparing young and elderly subjects were reported by Kreul (1972). He determined maximum vowel phonations for young adults (18 to 26 years) to be 18.2 sec for /ɑ/, 18.5 sec for /o/ and 22.8 sec for /i/. The mean durations for elderly subjects (65 to 75 years) were, for the same vowels, 14.6 sec, 14.6 sec, and 15.8 sec. The elderly subjects had vowel prolongations that were from 19 to 26 percent shorter than those for the younger subjects.

Duration of vowel prolongation sometimes is taken as an index of respiratory support for speech. From the data of Ptacek et al. (1966) and Kreul (1972), it appears that respiratory support declines with age. However, this interpretation must be regarded cautiously because measurements of vowel prolongation are influenced by the respiratory volume available for phonation and the mean air flow during phonation. Conceivably, two subjects with the same respiratory volume for speech could have different durations of vowel phonation if one of the subjects had greater flow, which would expend the available air sooner. Data on the durations of vowel prolongation are fully interpretable only if the mean flow also is reported. The Subcommittee on Human Communication and Its Disorders (1970) expressed the belief that air wastage because of inefficient laryngeal or articulatory valving is of more importance to voice production than is reduced vital capacity.

Although phonatory air flow apparently has not been investigated in a large-scale study of elderly subjects, there are several published studies of fundamental frequency and vocal intensity that might offer some insights into laryngeal function in the aged. Fundamental frequency (f_o) perhaps has been studied more than any other acoustic correlate of aging speech, but only a modestly secure generalization can be made on the basis of the available data. Mysak and Hanley (1958) and Mysak (1959) reported increases in f_0 across three age groups (32−62, 65−79, and 80−92 years) for both impromptu speaking and oral reading. Moreover, f_0 increases with advancing age were substantial: for example, the median f_0 in oral reading for the three age groups were 110, 125, and 143 Hz respectively.

More recent studies are disparate in their conclusions. McGlone and Hollien (1963) did not observe a significant difference in mean f_0 between women aged 65 to 79 and 80 to 94 years. Endres, Bambach, and Flosser (1967) reported reductions in f_0 over the span of a 13- to 15-year longitudinal study of individuals aged 29 to 42 years when the study began. Hollien and Shipp (1972) observed for men a decline in mean f_0 from the second to the fourth decade (120−107 Hz) followed by an increase through the eighth decade (at which time a mean f_0 of 146 Hz was obtained). Similarly, Horii and Ryan (1975) determined that the mean f_0 of adult male speakers was positively correlated with perceived age obtained in a direct estimation experiment. If mean f_0 alone contributes significantly to judgments of perceived age, then it should be possible to demonstrate an f_0-related bias in perceived-age judgments even for a single age-group, perhaps with the extreme mean f_0 values being associated with more judgments of advanced age. Finally, Kelley (1977) and Stoicheff (personal

communication, 1978) concluded that for female speakers there was a decrease in f_0 with advanced age.

These disparate results do not permit a simple generalization about the relationship between f_0 and aging. Additional studies, with careful control over variables such as smoking (Gilbert & Weismer, 1974) and subject state, are required. However, the existing data can be described tentatively by two conclusions: (1) For males, f_0 decreases into middle age, then increases into senescence, and (2) for females, f_0 is stable during adulthood until the geriatric years, when it decreases. The pattern for males is illustrated in Figure 3−2, which is based on various reports of f_0 in male subjects aged 10 to 90 years. After a sharp reduction during adolescence, f_0 gradually lowers during early and middle adulthood. The f_0 curve then assumes an upward swing with an inflection point at middle age. This pattern of change is consistent with a slight thickening or lengthening of the vocal folds up to middle age and then a progressive thinning or shortening into the geriatric years, as was suggested by Mysak and Hanley (1959). On the other hand, the data for females, at least in the unpublished studies of Kelley (1977) and Stoicheff (personal communication, 1978) imply a progressive thickening or lengthening.

Intrasubject f_0 variability also has been investigated in the aging. One common measure of this variability is pitch sigma, the intrasubject standard deviation about an individual's mean f_0. In males,

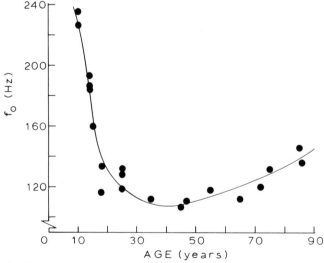

Fig. 3−2. Fundamental frequency (f_0) of voice for males as a function of age. The data points are a composite of means and medians from various published studies. Sources for adult data are included in text and sources for children's data are listed by Kent (1976).

there is evidence of a trend of increasing pitch sigma with increasing age (Mysak, 1959; Mysak & Hanley, 1959), whereas women show a trend of reduced pitch sigma with increasing age (McGlone & Hollien, 1963). Endres et al. (1967), in a longitudinal study of vocal characteristics of six male and female speakers over a period of 13 to 15 years, observed a decrease in pitch sigma with increasing age. No statement was made regarding a difference in pitch sigma as a function of sex. Horii and Ryan (1975) reported that for their sample of 57 adult males, the mean f_o was correlated with perceived speaker age but f_o variability was not. The discrepancy between these studies has yet to be resolved.

Studies of vocal intensity as a function of age were reported by Ptacek et al. (1966) and Ryan (1972). Ptacek et al., comparing persons younger than 40 with those older than 65, determined a 5.3 dB reduction in vowel intensity between young and old males and a 7.6 dB reduction between young and old females. All subjects studied by Ryan were males, grouped by age in decades from the fourth to the seventh, with tonal thresholds for unspecified frequencies of 30 dB HL or better in the better ear. The speech sample consisted of both extemporaneous speech and a reading of the first paragraph of the Rainbow Passage (Fairbanks, 1960). There was a significant difference in vocal intensity across age groups, but a post hoc procedure showed that the only significant difference was between the septuagenarians and the other three groups, with the septuagenarians having significantly greater vocal intensity.

It is of interest to compare the acoustic changes of the aging voice to the cues reportedly used by listeners in an age-identification task. Listeners have reported using vocal pitch and vocal tone quality as cues in age identification, with both males (Ptacek & Sander, 1966; Ryan & Capadano, 1978); and females (Ptacek & Sander, 1966) judged as having a lower vocal pitch with increasing age. Two-fifths of the aged speakers engaged by Ptacek and Sander reported that the pitch of their voices became lower as they got older, although several reported an increase in pitch. Of ten listeners engaged by Ptacek and Sander (1966), five reported hoarseness or strain and three reported pitch breaks as characteristics of the aging voice. In a study of the characteristic perceptual features for four perceived age decades, Hartman and Danhauer (1976) isolated the vocal features of low pitch and hoarseness for the decades of 40 to 50 and 50 to 60 years of age. Ryan and Burk (1974) reported that among the speech characteristics most predictive of age were voice tremor, laryngeal tension, and air loss. Some listeners in the Ptacek and Sander (1966) study specifically mentioned reduced pitch variability as a characteristic of the aging voice, and listeners also have reported reduced vocal loudness (or volume) as a sign of aging (Ptacek & Sander, 1966; Ryan & Capadano, 1978). Obviously, listener intuitions about the features of aged speech are not easily reconciled with acoustic data.

Among the perceptual characteristics, then, that appear to be associated with voice production in the aging speaker are roughness, breathiness, hoarseness, and tremor. Roughness is associated with irregularities in the vibratory pattern of the larynx and can be studied acoustically. These irregularities may be of two forms, affecting either the frequency or amplitude of vibration. Irregularities in frequency (or, to say the same thing in the time domain, irregularities in the fundamental period of vocal-fold vibration) are referred to as jitter or pitch perturbation. Irregularities in amplitude are referred to as shimmer or amplitude perturbation. A voice with a large amount of jitter is one that has a substantial variation in fundamental period from one cycle of vocal-fold vibration to the next. An example is shown in the first spectrogram in Figure 3−3, which is a wide-band (300Hz) spectrogram of the word *light* produced by a 60-year-old woman with Friedreich's ataxia (a neurological disorder). The fundamental period is represented by the distance between adjacent vertical striations, each such striation marking a pulse of air from the larynx. In the interval marked by the arrows, the fundamental period changes abruptly, first increasing and then decreasing. Over just a few cycles of vocal-fold vibration, the fundamental frequency (the reciprocal of the fundamental period) changes by a factor of three. When such irregularities in fundamental period occur over a brief, confined interval, the percept is one of a "break," "skip," or "catch" in the voice. When the fundamental period varies excessively over a long period of voiced speech, the percept is one of roughness. The spectrogram does not reveal as clearly the variations in amplitude of vocal-fold vibration (a waveform display is preferable to the spectrogram for this purpose), but a crude indication of amplitude irregularity, or shimmer, can be seen in the fact that some striations are darker or more pronounced than others. Both jitter and shimmer are deviations from the smoothly varying, quasi-periodic vibratory pattern of the normal larynx, and it is quite likely that they are useful descriptors of the aged voice. Computer methods for the evaluation of these irregularities (re-

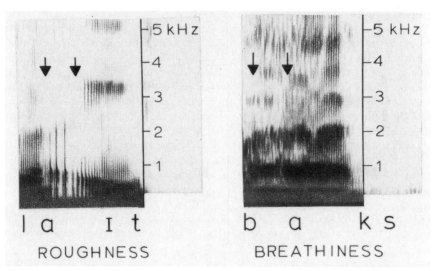

Fig. 3–3. Spectrograms of rough and breathy voice quality. The intervals marked by double arrows are particularly illustrative of the feature in question.

viewed by Davis, 1979) should facilitate investigation of these acoustic indices of vocal function in the aged.

Breathiness is noise resulting from excessive air loss during phonation. The noise is generated because the vocal folds do not close completely between the opening phases of the vibratory cycle. As a consequence of the incomplete closure, air escapes between the folds and generates a turbulence noise rather like aspiration. On a spectrogram, the noise associated with breathiness appears as diffuse spectral energy, with random fine structure in time. An example of a breathy voice is shown in the second spectrogram in Figure 3–3. The sample word is *box*, spoken by an aged man who was perceived as having frequent periods of air wastage in speech. The noise of breathiness is particularly noticeable in the interval marked by the arrows.

Hoarseness is a combination of roughness and breathiness. The spectrographic appearance of hoarseness, as described by Yanigahara (1967), includes noise components in the main vowel formants, noise components above 3000 Hz, and loss of high-frequency harmonic components. As mentioned above, the noise components arise in part because of incomplete glottal closure, allowing wastage of air and glottal turbulence noise. The reduction in the high-frequency harmonics is related to a change in the glottal waveform in which the amplitude peaks are rounded and the closure phase absent or only approximating the zero-axis. The disappearance of abrupt or sharp changes in the glottal waveform is associated with an attenuation of the high-frequency

periodic components in a Fourier (spectral) analysis. These acoustic features of voice disorders have proved helpful in clinical evaluation of voice problems and in documenting recovery from such disorders (Cooper, 1974; Gould, 1975; Laguaite & Waldrop, 1964; Rontal, 1975).

Vocal tremor is a periodic interruption or modulation of the fundamental frequency or amplitude of the glottal wave. Figure 3–4 is an analysis of the cry of a premature infant, who has a mean f_o of about 430 Hz. The tremor is evident as a wavering in the laryngeal harmonics. The wavering is especially marked for the higher harmonics (e.g., the tenth harmonic, indicated by the number 10 on the spectrogram). For this infant, the tremor has a frequency of about 16 Hz, meaning that the fundamental frequency of laryngeal vibration is modulated at the rate of 16 Hz. Tremor is illustrated in Figure 3–5 for a man in his late sixties diagnosed as having idiopathic tremor. Spectrograms are shown for the isolated vowel /ɝ/, the isolated diphthong /ai/, and the word *rainbow* /reinbou/ in sentence context. The tremor appears as a marked variation in f_o, most clearly visible in a higher harmonic such as the fifth or seventh, and has a frequency of about 5 Hz.

SUPRALARYNGEAL SYSTEM

This section deals with the parts of the speech mechanism lying above the level of the larynx. It begins with a short summary of anatomic and physiologic changes associated with aging and then

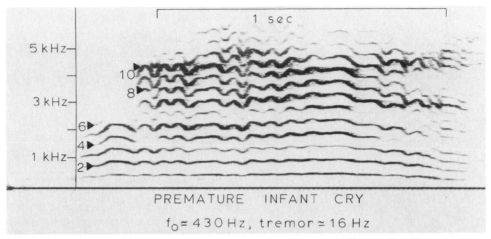

Fig. 3–4. Spectrogram of cry of premature infant, showing vocal tremor. Even-numbered laryngeal harmonics are labeled.

turns to related acoustic studies of speech behavior. The acoustic variables of primary interest are formant frequencies for vowels, syllable repetition rates, speaking rates, and dysfluencies.

Anatomic and Physiologic Changes

Many aged individuals experience degenerative changes in the bony or soft tissues. Loss of dental structures, because of dental or periodontal disease, tooth abrasion, gum retraction, or reduction of salivary and mucous secretions, may have direct effects on speech-sound articulation. Moreover, these dental changes may lead to an eventual collapse of facial form (Silverman, 1972) and to further disruptions of speech articulation. As a consequence of changes in orofacial skeletal support, the oral musculature may become hypertonic, with excessive contracture in speech or deglutition and even an increase in the size of the tongue (Balogh and Lelkes, 1961; Silverman, 1972). Certain atrophic changes also are fairly common in the oral structures of the elderly. Cohen and Gitman (1959) described atrophy of the lips and oral mucosa, as well as a reduction of tonus in lingual muscle. Massler (1971) noted that among the "characteristic changes" in the oral tissues of the elderly was a lingual atrophy marked by a smooth or fissured surface. The oral mucosae are particularly subject to senescent degeneration, becoming thin, relatively less moist, and easily damaged by abrasion (Massler, 1971; Miles, 1972). Another common effect of aging is the development of vascular nodules on the undersurface of the tongue and lips (Bean, 1956; Miles, 1972). Of course, it is the loss of denti-

tion that is most noticeable and often of greatest consequence to speech. Miles (1972), adding to the adage that we are as old as our neurons (which do not exhibit mitosis and therefore do not reproduce), suggested that we also are as old as the formative cells of the dentin crown.

Although individual structures, such as the mandible, may become smaller with age as the consequence of bone resorption (Silverman, 1972; Zemlin, 1968), there is evidence that the craniofacial complex as a whole grows throughout life, even into the geriatric years (Buchi, 1950; Hooton & Dupertuis, 1951; Israel, 1968, 1973; Lasker, 1953). On the basis of his anatomic measurements, Israel (1973) concluded, "unlike changes in early life from birth to adulthood where the two segments do not mirror each other, the later life changes follow a relationship that could best be described as symmetrical enlargement" (p. 125). Two patterns of craniofacial alteration with advanced age are depicted in Figure 3–6. One pattern shown in *a*, is a progressive and symmetrical enlargement of the craniofacial complex, as described by Israel (1968, 1973). The other pattern, in *b*, represents the alternative view that the major change in craniofacial structure with advanced age is resorption of bone causing a loss of mandibular mass.

Acoustic Studies Related to Supralaryngeal Speech Function

Longitudinal data on acoustic properties of speech are extremely rare, but the report of Endres et al. (1967) is one source of information on both vowel formants and fundamental frequency. Six individu-

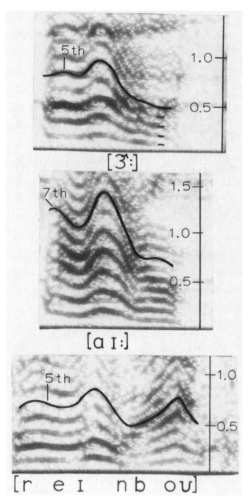

[ɜˑ]

[aɪˑ]

[r e ɪ n b oʊ]

Fig. 3—5. Spectrograms showing vocal tremor in an elderly man diagnosed as having idiopathic tremor. The fifth or seventh harmonic is highlighted to show the f_o variation.

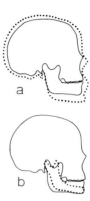

Fig. 3—6. Two patterns of craniofacial change in advanced age: Pattern *a* is one of progressive, symmetrical enlargement and pattern *b* is one of selective size reduction occurring through bone resorption. (Adapted with permission from Israel, H. Age factor and the pattern of change in craniofacial structures. *American Journal of Physical Anthropology,* 1973, *39,* 111—128.

Such lengthening could occur with a descent of the larynx within the neck or with a relative descent of the vocal folds within the larynx. We are not aware of anatomical data to substantiate these possibilities. However, as noted above, there are anatomical data to show that the craniofacial complex grows throughout life (Buchi, 1950; Hooton & Dupertuis, 1951; Lasker, 1953; Israel, 1968, 1973). The reduction in formant frequencies reported by Endres et al. is compatible with a gradual increase in the size of the craniofacial structures. Thus, individual development is marked by a continuous reduction of formant frequencies, with a rapid change in the growing years of childhood and a slower change during adulthood.

The gradual reductions in formant frequency with growth and aging can be summarized with "isovowel lines" in the $F_1 - F_2$ plane, that is, a graph having the first (F_1) and second (F_2) formant frequencies as its axes (Fig. 3—7). The isovowel lines show the ranges of F_1 and F_2 values that speakers of different sizes (hence, different age—sex groups) might use to produce the same vowel. Speakers with small vocal tracts would have $F_1 - F_2$ values on the high-frequency end of each line and speakers with large vocal tracts would have $F_1 - F_2$ values on the low-frequency end of each line. Thus, each isovowel line is a sort of "acoustic lifeline" for vocal tract growth. Details of the isovowel lines are discussed by Kent (1978, 1979) and Kent and Forner (1979).

With respect to the dynamic properties of speech, maximum diadochokinetic rate (the maximal rate of syllable repetition) has been investigated as a function of age by Ptacek et al. (1966), Shanks

als, aged from 29 to 42 years at the beginning of recording, were studied over an interval of 13 to 15 years. At the end of this period, both formant frequencies and fundamental frequencies assumed lower values. Most of the data on formants were presented as "points of formant concentration," for the first four formants. However, from the one graph of individual formant frequencies that the authors provided, it is evident that all of the first four formant frequencies were lowered with age. For the speaker in question, the approximate downward shifts of the formants of vowel /e/ were 166 Hz for F_1, 150 Hz for F_2, 166 Hz for F_3, and 155 Hz for F_4. One explanation for reductions in the formant frequencies is a progressive lengthening of the vocal tract with age.

(1970), and Kreul (1972). In comparing individuals over 65 and those under 40 years of age, Ptacek et al. reported that the average diadochokinetic rate for /pʌ/, /tʌ/, and /kʌ/ syllable repetitions was reduced by 22 percent for the aged men and 20 percent for the aged women. For example, whereas the young men had rates of 7.0, 6.9, and 6.2 repetitions per second for /pʌ/, /tʌ/, and /kʌ/, respectively, the aged men achieved rates of only 5.4, 5.3, and 4.9 for the same syllables. However, the authors allowed that the performance of the aged subjects might have been improved by increased motivation and a better understanding of the task. On the other hand, results obtained by Kreul (1972) for comparisons of young (18–26 years) and old (65–76 years) speakers showed that diadochokinetic rates for /pʌ/, /tʌ/, /kʌ/, and interrupted /i/ did not differentiate the two age groups of speakers. There was evidence of an age–sex interaction, however, with young men having faster rates than young women but elderly women

having faster rates than elderly men. In fact, the mean data show that elderly women had the fastest rates of any group, with young men, young women, and elderly men having nearly the same values. Finally, Shanks (1970) reported that young and old female subjects performed similarly in a vocal diadochokinetic task. Given these mixed results, it must be concluded that diadochokinetic rate does not distinguish reliably between young and aged speakers.

Several studies have shown that the rate of speaking decreases with increases in age (Hartman and Danhauer, 1976; Mysak, 1959; Mysak & Hanley, 1959; Ryan, 1972; Ryan & Capadano, 1978). In addition, reduced speaking rate was one trait attributed to advanced age by listeners engaged in age-identification tasks. It can be argued that the decrease in rate of speech is related to increased cautiousness or related psychosocial factors that accompany advanced age (Mysak, 1959; Mysak & Hanley, 1959;

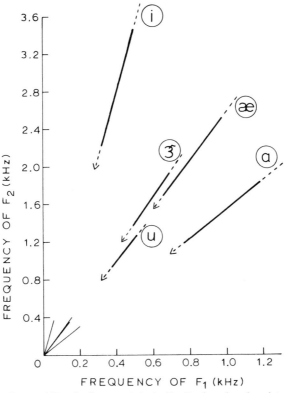

Fig. 3–7. Isovowel lines for five vowels in the F_1–F_2 plane, based on data from Kent (1978) and Kent and Forner (1979). The solid midsegment of each line indicates the range of F_1–F_2 values for which data were obtained, and the broken lines are extrapolations to larger and smaller vocal tracts. With growth of the vocal tract, the formant frequencies roughly follow the lines to assume progressively smaller values.

Schow, Christensen, Hutchinson & Nerbonne, 1978) rather than a general reduction in neuromuscular activity. Hollien and Shipp (1972) reported an increased silence time in total reading duration, particularly for intrasentence pauses, for their elderly subjects. They considered that these pauses might have been related to fatigue, oxygen replacement, or visual acuity problems in reading. Hartman and Danhauer (1976) also noted that slow rate and long pauses were prominent perceptual features used to describe the speech patterns of men in the higher age decades. Mysak and Hanley (1959) compared the rates of oral reading and impromptu speaking and discovered little or no difference between these two tasks as performed by aged subjects. Given the complicated interactions of factors that might influence measures of speaking rate, it is wise to forgo strong interpretations of the data at this point.

Quantitative studies of articulatory ability in senescence are few, but it is interesting to note that listeners in an age-identification task have reported an impression that hesitancy and "less-clear" speech are characteristics of advancing age (Ptacek & Sander, 1966). Hartman and Danhauer (1976) reported that their listeners associated the feature of imprecise articulation with speakers in the perceived age decades of 40 to 50 and 50 to 60. Possibly, an increased tendency to misarticulate causes the aged speaker to decrease his rate in an attempt to reduce the likelihood of an error. Data relevant to this issue are the dysfluency counts reported by Ptacek and Sander (1966) indicating fewer dysfluencies for young than for old speakers in reading a 53-word passage. During extemporaneous speech, younger males had 8.5 dysfluencies per 100 words compared to 9.8 for older male speakers, and younger females had 5.4 dysfluencies per 100 words compared to 9 for older females. Similarly, Yairi and Clifton (1972) reported more frequent dysfluencies for nonstuttering geriatric subjects than for nonstuttering high school subjects. The dysfluencies of the aged individuals were like those of nonstuttering younger individuals, that is, they were characterized by interjections, revisions, and incomplete phrases. Smith and Tierney (1971), in an investigation of the effects of delayed feedback and age on oral reading, determined that the older subjects (42 to 68 years) were more affected by the delayed feedback than were younger subjects. The greater frequency of errors (repetitions, mispronunciations, pauses or blocks) for the older subjects was seen as evidence for a reduction in the capability of ". . . reacting to variable-feedback space and time compliances" (p. 218).

NEUROMUSCULAR CONTROL SYSTEM

This section, although not totally independent of the preceding sections, concentrates on aspects of neuromuscular control, beginning with a brief summary of anatomic and physiologic changes affecting neural and muscle tissues, and concluding with a review of acoustic measures that may be useful in identifying or describing the neuromuscular control of speech. To a degree, aging effects on neuromuscular control may be separable from effects on the flesh and bone periphery.

Anatomic and Physiologic Changes

Anatomic and physiologic studies of aging have revealed a number of changes affecting the nervous and muscular systems. Among these changes are degeneration of the sense organs of hearing and vision (Smith & Sethi, 1975), reductions of nerve conduction velocities (Wagman & Lesse, 1952), decrease of muscle mass (Rowe, 1969), a possible decrease in the number of central nervous system neurons (Kent, 1976) and spinal cord axons (Barrett, 1972), reduction of brain weight (Bondareff, 1964; Minckler, 1972), and changes in the availability of neurotransmitter substances (McGeer, Fibiger, McGeer, & Wiskson, 1971; McGeer & McGeer, 1975a, 1975b). A number of physiologic changes with age have been noted, including a reduction of tremor frequency (Marshall, 1961) and slight alteration of the electroencephalogram (Obrist, 1965).

Neuromotor Control of Selected Nonspeech Behavior

Research on motor performance of several kinds, but especially speed of response, has shown that normal aged subjects do less well than normal young adults. Of particular note are the many studies that show increases in simple reaction time (SRT) and decision reaction time (DRT) as a function of age (Botwinick, 1973; Spirduso, 1975). Some investigators have proposed that speed of perception, rather than speed of the motor component, is the critical factor in this change of performance. Changes in the sense organ of hearing and vision (Smith & Sethi, 1975) are evidence that reaction time may be increased because of a diminishing efficiency of the acoustic—photic-to-neural transduction process. But changes in the effectors also may be involved. Spirduso (1975) has reported changes in movement time (MT) that parallel changes in SRT and DRT with increasing age. Thus, increased time of response may be the combined result of sensory, motor, and central factors. Whatever the various factors may be, increases in SRT and DRT with age reflect changes in the nervous system. However, it appears that automated movements are less affected by aging than movements performed infrequently (Smith & Green, 1962) and that reaction time decreases on repeated trials in the aged (Botwinick & Thompson, 1967). These results are of interest in relation to the effects of aging on speech because speech is a highly rehearsed motor behavior. Therefore, speech, as a highly practiced and frequently used motor behavior, may be resistant to many degenerative effects of aging.

Acoustic Methods for Examining the Neuromuscular Control of Speech

Data on geriatric changes in the neuromuscular control of speech are fragmentary. The limited experimental work in this area is explained partly by the fact that most geriatric persons maintain functional speech communication. Of course, not all of the aged share this fortune: Many suffer aphasia, dysarthria, dysphonia, or articulation problems related to hearing impairment. Very few reports have been published to describe changes in speech motor function that might normally accompany the aging process. Although such changes may be subtle, they could be important in understanding the aging process and diseases that are most commonly seen in aged persons. For example, Petajan and Jarcho (1975) observed similarities between parkinson patients and normal elderly subjects with respect to the control of motor unit firing. They hypothesized that one consequence of aging may be the atrophy of dopaminergic brain or noradrenergic spinal pathways. In addition, studies (McGeer et al., 1971; McGeer & McGeer, 1975a, 1975b) have revealed changes in the availability of neurotransmitter substances. These changes in the nervous system might have consequences on speech motor control.

A link between the normal aging process and neuromuscular disease is supported to some degree by the perceptual study of Ryan and Burk (1974), who concluded that the five speech and voice characteristics most predictive of aged speech were voice tremor, laryngeal tension, air loss, imprecise consonants, and slow rate of articulation (see also Hartman & Danhauer, 1976). Because these characteristics also apply to some categories of neuromuscular disease (Darley, Aronson, & Brown, 1969), Ryan and Burk considered it possible that older speakers lie at the mild end of a continuum of dysarthria. Direct evidence of similarities between aging speakers and speakers with diagnosed neuromuscular disease is scant. Kreul (1972) reported that normal aged subjects and subjects with parkinsonism share a reduction of vowel-prolongation time and a slowing of reading rate. The mean age of the normal subjects was 70 years and that of the subjects with parkinsonism was 56 years, so it is difficult to reject aging as a factor in the performance of both groups. In a cinefluorographic, perceptual, and acoustic study of ten individuals with parkinsonism, ten with essential tremor, and ten neurologically normal geriatric subjects, Blonsky, Logemann, Boshes, and Fisher (1975) concluded that the normal geriatric subjects ". . . maintained a normal neuromuscular control of speech" (p. 302), with no occurrences of abnormalities of vocal tract control (hoarseness/roughness, lingual dysfunction, labial dysfunction, voice tremor, dysfluencies/stuttering).

Given the subtlety of the possible acoustic correlates of aging speech, it seems appropriate to consider measures that focus on finer aspects of speech motor control. For example, future investigations might include measures of both jitter and shimmer (Deal & Emanuel, 1978; Horii, 1979; Lieberman, 1963; Smith, Weinberg, Beth, & Horii, 1978), vowel spectrum noise level (Sansone & Emanuel, 1970), shape of gottal waveform (Monsen & Engebretson, 1977), and segment duration (Klatt, 1975, 1976; Tingley & Allen, 1975). With these additional acoustic measures, it is possible to study aspects of speech behavior that have not yet been addressed in the literature on aging. Moreover, these measures would permit more confident interpretations regarding age-related changes in the different systems of speech production.

It also may prove profitable to explore possible dimensions of similarity between the normal aging process and neurologic disorders like Parkinson's disease (Petajan & Jarcho, 1975). Parkinson's disease frequently is accompanied by a dysarthria that is notable for its abnormal phonatory components (Darley, Aronson, & Brown, 1969). Given that aging also seems to have effects on phonatory function, a careful parallel study of parkinsonism and normal aging may reveal important similarities and dissimilarities. For example, although aging speech and the hypokinetic dysarthria in parkinsonism may have in common certain phonatory abnormalities, the frequent reports of slow speaking rate in normal geriatric speech are not easily squared with the fast speaking rate (short rushes or accelerations) sometimes observed in Parkinson's disease. Some dimensions of dysarthria in parkinsonism that also might apply to aged speech include monopitch and monoloudness; imprecise consonants; inappropriate silences; harsh, breathy, or hoarse voice; and inappropriate vocal pitch.

Some possible acoustic−phonetic correlates of parkinsonian dysarthria are illustrated by the spectrogram in Figure 3−8. This spectrogram was made from a recording of the Rainbow Passage read by a man with Parkinson's disease. Some features of interest are identified by the numbers at the top of the spectrogram. These features are as follows:

1. The diphthong /aɪ/ in *sunlight* has high-frequency noise components above 4 kHz, apparently related to breathy voice quality.
2. The formant patterns for the liquid-diphthong combination /raɪ/ in *strikes* are somewhat abnormal in that the third-formant frequency is atypically high for the /r/ segment.
3. The velar stop /k/ is spirantized (made with frication noise), as evidenced by the high-frequency noise during the intended stop segment. (A slight spirantization also can be seen for the /t/ in *strikes*).
4. The formant pattern for the liquid-diphthong combination /reɪ/ in *raindrops* is possibly abnormal because of the high initial values of the second and third formant frequencies during the /r/.

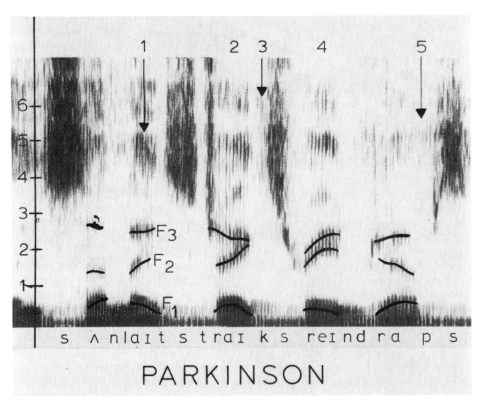

Fig. 3−8. Wide-band (300 Hz) spectrogram of an excerpt from the Rainbow Passage as read by a man with Parkinson's disease. The excerpt is "sunlight strikes raindrops." Frequency in kHz is shown on the scale at the left, and the numbers at the top identify features of interest (see text). For convenience of interpretation, the first three formants have been highlighted in ink and a phonetic transcription of the target utterance is shown at the bottom.

5. The /p/ in *raindrops* is spirantized, as evidenced by the high-frequency noise during the intended stop segment.

Similar acoustic—phonetic features have been observed for other individuals with parkinsonian dysarthria (Kent & Netsell, 1979). In addition, spectrograms reveal other abnormalities such as vocal tremor, irregular glottal vibration, nasalization, and voicing errors. Whether similar features characterize senescent speech is a matter for research. It would be of particular interest to discover frequent occurrences of irregular glottal vibration, glottal air loss, reduced formant movements, nasalization, and spirantization.

SUMMARY

Acoustic studies of aging speech not only are few in number but they have tended to use relatively gross measures, frequently focusing on performance extremes (e.g., vowel prolongation time, maximum diadochokinetic rate, and maximal vocal intensity). Even when measures of fine grading, such as f_o, have been used, the interest typically has been to derive a group average for isolated vowels or for connected speech. The finer aspects of speech have not been investigated well enough to permit any conclusion at this time.

Studies of perceptual identification of speaker age show that listeners can use information in the acoustic speech signal to make such judgments. The acoustic studies conducted to date do not allow a definitive description of the relevant acoustic dimensions or their relative weightings. Because age identification is fairly accurate even with sustained vowels as stimuli, acoustic cues related to respiratory—phonatory function are strongly implicated. However, the increases in accuracy of age identification that occur with the additional cues in connected speech indicate that a variety of acoustic properties can contribute to perception of aging speech. It is likely that aging eventually affects most if not all aspects of speech production to some degree, but the perceptual salience of these effects is not uniform. Many of the effects may be subtle, particularly so because speech is a highly rehearsed motor behavior that gives rise to a highly redundant message.

REFERENCES

Bach, A., Lederer, F., & Dinolt, R. Senile changes in the laryngeal musculature. *Archives of Otolaryngology,* 1941, *34,* 47−56.

Balogh, K., & Lelkes, K. The tongue in old age. *Gerontologia Clinica,* 1961, *3,* (Supplement), 38−54.

Barrett, J. *Gerontological psychology.* Springfield, Ill.: Charles C. Thomas Publisher, 1972.

Bean, W. The changing incidence of certain vascular lesions of the skin with aging. *Geriatrics,* 1956, *11,* 97−102.

Blonsky, R., Logemann, J., Boshes, B., & Fisher, H. Comparison of speech and swallowing function in patients with tremor disorders and in normal geriatric patients: A cinefluorographic study. *Journal of Gerontology,* 1975, *30,* 299−303.

Bondareff, W. Histophysiology of the aging nervous system. *Advances in Gerontological Research,* 1964, *1,* 1−22.

Botwinick, J. *Aging and behavior.* New York: Springer Publishing Co., 1973.

Botwinick, J., & Thompson, L. Practice of speeded response in relation to age, sex, and set. *Journal of Gerontology,* 1967, *22,* 72−76.

Buchi, E. Anderungen der Korperform beim Erwashsamen Menschen. *Anthropologische Forschunger der Anthropologische Gesellschaft Wien,* 1950, *1,* 1−44.

Cander, L., & Moyer, J. *Aging of the lung.* New York: Grune & Stratton, 1964.

Cohen, T., & Gitman, L. Oral complaints and taste perception in the aged. *Journal of Gerontology,* 1959, *14,* 294−298.

Cooper, M. Spectrographic analysis of fundamental frequency and hoarseness before and after vocal rehabilitation. *Journal of Speech and Hearing Research,* 1974, *39,* 286−297.

Darley, F., Aronson, A., & Brown, J. Differential diagnostic patterns of dysarthria. *Journal of Speech and Hearing Research,* 1969, *12,* 246−269.

Davis, S. Computer evaluation of laryngeal pathology based on inverse filtering of speech. SCRL Monograph No. 13, Speech Communications Research Lab, Santa Barbara, Calif., September 1976.

Davis, S. Acoustic characteristics of normal and pathological voices. In N. Lass (ed): *Speech and language: Advances in basic research and practice (vol 1).* New York: Academic Press, 1979, pp 273−338.

Deal, R., & Emanuel, F. Some waveform and spectral features of vowel roughness. *Journal of Speech and Hearing Research,* 1978, *21,* 250−264.

Endres, W., Bambach, W., & Flosser, G. Voice spectrograms as a function of age, voice disguise, and voice imitation. *Journal of the Acoustical Society of America,* 1967, *49,* 1842−1848.

Fairbanks, G. *Voice and articulation drillbook* (2nd ed.). New York: Harper & Row, 1960.

Gilbert, H., & Weismer, G. The effects of smoking on the speaking fundamental frequency of adult women. *Journal of Psycholinguistic Research,* 1974, *3,* 225−231.

Gould, W. Quantitative assessment of voice function in microlaryngology. *Folia Phoniatrica,* 1975, *27,* 157−165.

Hartman, D., & Danhauer, J. Perceptual features of speech for males in four perceived age decades. *Journal of the Acoustical Society of America,* 1976, *59,* 713−715.

Hollien, H., & Shipp, T. Speaking fundamental frequency and chronologic age in males. *Journal of Speech and Hearing Research,* 1972, *15,* 155−159.

Hooton, E., & Dupertuis, C. Age changes and selective survival in Irish males. In American Association of Physical Anthropology, *Studies in Physical Anthropology,* No. 2. New York: Wenner-Gren Foundation, 1951.

Horii, Y., & Ryan, W. Fundamental frequency characteristics and perceived age of adult male speakers. Paper presented at 89th Meeting of Acoustical Society of America, Austin, Tex., 1975.

Horii, Y. Fundamental frequency perturbation observed in sustained phonation. *Journal of Speech and Hearing Research,* 1979, *22,* 5−19.

Israel, H. Continuing growth in the human cranial skeleton. *Archives of Oral Biology,* 1968, *13,* 133−137.

Israel, H. Age factor and the pattern of change in craniofacial structures. *American Journal of Physical Anthropology,* 1973, *39,* 111−128.

Jalavisto, E. The role of simple tests measuring speed of performance in the assessment of biological vigor: A factorial study in elderly women. In A. Welfard & J. Birren (Eds.), *Behavior, aging and the nervous system.* Springfield, Ill.: Charles C. Thomas Publisher, 1965.

Keleman, G., & Pressman, J. Physiology of the larynx. *Physiological Review,* 1955, *35,* 506−554.

Kelley, A. Fundamental frequency measurements of female voices with aging. Paper presented at American Speech and Hearing Association Convention, Chicago, Illinois, 1977.

Kent, R. Imitation of synthesized vowels by preschool children. *Journal of the Acoustical Society of America,* 1978, *63,* 1193−1198.

Kent, R. Isovowel lines for the evaluation of vowel formant structure in speech disorders. *Journal of Speech and Hearing Disorders,* 1979, *44,* 513−521.

Kent, R., & Forner, L. Developmental study of vowel formant frequencies in an imitation task. *Journal of the Acoustical Society of America,* 1979, *65,* 208−217.

Kent, R., & Netsell, R. Acoustic-phonetic features of parkinsonian dysarthria. Paper presented to Annual Convention of the American Speech and Hearing Association, Atlanta, Georgia, November, 1979.

Kent, S. Scientists count brain cells to figure theory of aging. *Geriatrics,* 1976, *31,* 114−123.

Kirchner, J. *Pressman and Keleman's physiology of the larynx.* Rochester, Minn.: American Academy of Opthalmology and Otolaryngology, 1970.

Klatt, D. The duration of [s] in English words. *Journal of Speech and Hearing Research,* 1974, *17,* 51−63.

Klatt, D. Voice onset time, frication, and aspiration in word−initial consonant clusters. *Journal of Speech and Hearing Research,* 1975, *18,* 686−706.

Klatt, D. Linguistic uses of segmental duration in English: Acoustical and perceptual evidence. *Journal of the Acoustical Society of America*, 1976, *59*, 1208−1221.

Kreul, E. Neuromuscular control examination (NMC) for parkinsonism: Vowel prolongations and diadochokinetic and reading rates. *Journal of Speech and Hearing Research*, 1972, *15*, 72−83.

Lasker, G. The age factor in bodily measurements of adult male and female Mexicans. *Human Biology*, 1953, *25*, 50−63.

Laguaite, J., & Waldrop, W. Acoustic analysis of fundamental frequency of voice before and after therapy. *Folia Phoniatrica*, 1964, 183−192.

Lieberman, P. Some acoustic measures of the fundamental periodicity of normal and pathological larynges. *Journal of the Acoustical Society of America*, 1963, *35*, 344−353.

Luchsinger, R. Voice disturbances on an endocrine basis. In N. Levin (Ed.), *Voice and speech disorders: Medical aspects.* Springfield, Ill.: Charles C. Thomas Publisher, 1962.

Luchsinger, R., & Arnold, G. *Voice-speech-language.* Belmont, Calif.: Wadsworth Publishing Co., 1965.

Malinowski, A. The shape, dimensions, and process of calcification of the cartilaginous framework of the larynx in relation to age and sex in the Polish population. *Folia Morphologica*, 1967, *26*, 118−128.

Marshall, J. The effect of aging upon physiological tremor. *Journal of Neurology, Neurosurgery and Psychiatry*, 1961, *24*, 14−17.

Massler, M. Oral aspects of aging. *Postgraduate Medicine*, 1971, *49*, 179−183.

McGeer, E., Fibiger, H., McGeer, P., & Wiskson, V. Aging and brain enzymes. *Experimental Gerontology*, 1971, *6*, 391.

McGeer, E., & McGeer, P. Age changes in the human for some enzymes associated with metabolism of colecholamines, GABA, and acetylcholine. In J. Ordy and K. Brizzee (Eds.), *Neurobiology of aging.* New York: Plenum Publishing Corp., 1975(a).

McGeer, P., & McGeer, E. Aging and neurotransmitter synthetic enzymes in the brain. In *Abstracts of the Tenth International Congress of Gerontology* (Vol. 1), Jerusalem, 1975. (b)

McGlone, R., & Hollien, H. Vocal pitch characteristics of aged white men. *Journal of Speech and Hearing Research*, 1963, *6*, 164−170.

Meyerson, M. The effects of aging on communication. *Journal of Gerontology*, 1976, *3*, 29−38.

Miles, A. "Sans teeth": Changes in oral tissues with advancing age. *Proceedings of the Royal Society of Medicine*, 1972, *65*, 801−829.

Minckler, T. Growth, biometrics, and aging. In J. Minckler (Ed.), *Introduction to neuroscience.* St. Louis, Mo.: C. V. Mosby, 1972.

Monsen, R., & Engebretson, A. A study of variations in the male and female glottal wave. *Journal of the Acoustical Society of America*, 1977, *62*, 981−993.

Muiesan, G., Sorbini, C., & Grassi, V. Respiratory function in the aged. *Bulletin of Physio-Pathology in Respiration*, 1971, *1*, 973−1009.

Mysak, E. Pitch and duration characteristics of older males. *Journal of Speech and Hearing Research*, 1959, *2*, 46−54.

Mysak, E., & Hanley, T. Aging processes in speech: Pitch and duration characteristics. *Journal of Gerontology*, 1958, *13*, 309−313.

Mysak, E., & Hanley, T. Vocal aging. *Geriatrics*, 1959, *14*, 652−656.

Obrist, W. Electroencephalographic approach to age changes in response speed. In A. Welford & J. Birren (Eds.): *Behavior, aging and the nervous system.* Springfield, Ill.: Charles C. Thomas Publisher, 1965.

Petajan, J., & Jarcho, L. Motor unit control in Parkinson's disease and the influence of levadopa. *Neurology*, 1975, *25*, 866−869.

Pump, K. The aged lung. *Chest*, 1971, *60*, 571−577.

Ptacek, P., & Sander, E. Age recognition from voice. *Journal of Speech and Hearing Research*, 1966, *9*, 273−277.

Ptacek, P., Sander, E., Maloney, W., & Jackson, C. Phonatory and related changes with advanced age. *Journal of Speech and Hearing Research*, 1966, *9*, 353−360.

Robinson, D., Nies, A., Davis, S., Bunney, W., Davis, J., Colburn, R., Bourne, H., Shaw, D., &

Coppen, A. Aging, monoamines and monoamineoxidase levels. *Lancet,* 1972, *1,* 290–291.

Roncallo, P. Researches about ossification and conformation of the thyroid cartilage in men. *Acta Oto-laryngologica,* 1948, *36,* 110–134.

Rontal, E. "Picturing" vocal cord therapy results. *Journal of the American Medical Association,* 1975, *233,* 1149–1150.

Rowe, R. The effect of senility on skeletal muscles in the mouse. *Experimental Gerontology,* 1969, *4,* 119–126.

Ryan, W. Acoustic aspects of the aging voice. *Journal of Gerontology,* 1972, *27,* 265–268.

Ryan, W., & Burk, K. Perceptual and acoustic correlates of aging in the speech of males. *Journal of Communication Disorders,* 1974, *7,* 181–192.

Ryan, W., & Capadano, N. Age perceptions and evaluative reactions toward adult speakers. *Journal of Gerontology,* 1978, *33,* 98–102.

Sansone, F., & Emanuel, F. Spectral noise levels and roughness severity ratings for normal and simulated rough vowels produced by adult males. *Journal of Speech and Hearing Research,* 1970, *13,* 489–502.

Schow, R., Christensen, J., Hutchinson, J., & Nerbonne, M. *Communication disorders of the aged.* Baltimore, Md: University Park Press, 1978.

Shanks, S. Effects of aging upon rapid syllable repetition. *Perceptual and Motor Skills,* 1970, *30,* 687–690.

Shipp, T., & Hollien, H. Perception of the aging male voice. *Journal of Speech and Hearing Research,* 1969, *13,* 703–710.

Shock, N., & Yiengst, M. Age changes in basal respiratory measurements and metabolism in males. *Journal of Gerontology,* 1955, *10,* 31–40.

Silverman, S. Degeneration of dental and orofacial structures. In *Orofacial function: Clinical research in dentistry and speech pathology.* ASHA Reports No. 7. Washington, D.C.: American Speech and Hearing Association, 1972.

Smith, K., & Green, D. Scientific motion study and aging process in performance. *Ergonomics,* 1962, *5,* 155–164.

Smith, B., & Sethi, P. Aging and the nervous system. *Geriatrics,* 1975, *30,* 109–115.

Smith, K., & Tierney, D. Delayed speech feedback and age. *Journal of Speech and Hearing Research,* 1971, *14,* 214–219.

Smith, B., Weinberg, B. Beth, L., & Horii, Y. Vocal roughness and jitter characteristics of vowels produced by esophageal speakers. *Journal of Speech and Hearing Research,* 1978, *21,* 240–249.

Spiriduso, W. Reaction and movement time as a function of age and physical activity level. *Journal of Gerontology,* 1975, *30,* 435–440.

Stoicheff, M., 1978. Personal communication.

Subcommittee on Human Communication and Its Disorders: *Human communication and its disorders: An overview.* Washington, D.C.: National Institute of Neurological Diseases and Stroke, 1970.

Tingley, B., & Allen, G. Development of speech timing control in children. *Child Development,* 1975, *46,* 186–194.

Wagman, I., & Lesse, N. Maximum conduction velocities of motor fibers of ulnar nerve in human subjects of various ages and sizes. *Journal of Neurophysiology,* 1952, *15,* 235–244.

Yairi, E., & Clifton, N. Disfluent speech behavior of preschool children, high school seniors, and geriatric persons. *Journal of Speech and Hearing Research,* 1972, *15,* 714–719.

Yanigahara, N. Significance of harmonic changes and noise components in hoarseness. *Journal of Speech and Hearing Research,* 1967, *10,* 531–541.

Zemlin, W. *Speech and hearing science.* Englewood Cliffs, N.J., Prentice-Hall, 1968.

Joseph B. Nadol, Jr.

4

The Aging Peripheral Hearing Mechanism

INTRODUCTION

Presbycusis is the descriptive term used to denote a common but not universal deterioration of auditory function coincident with aging. Approximately 35 percent of the American population over the age of 70 has a handicapping hearing loss (National Center for Vital and Health Statistics, 1967). However, Rosen, Bergman, Plester, El-Moffey, & Salti (1962) demonstrated that presbycusis is not strictly related to age alone. In their study they found that the Mabaans of the Sudan possessed better hearing acuity than their western contemporaries, and it was suggested that this difference in hearing might be attributed in part to a significantly different noise exposure over time. Rather than the result of a single detrimental influence such as acoustic trauma, presbycusis is probably best understood as the cumulative effect of a number of disorders or insults contributing to the degeneration of the auditory mechanism.

Many of the causes of progressive hearing impairment are well known. These include inherited genetic defects, acoustic trauma, ototoxic substances, disorders of circulation, and true cellular aging. Progressive forms of genetically determined sensorineural hearing loss (Nance & McConnell, 1973) are easily recognized when they occur in large kindreds or in association with other syndromic defects. It is difficult or impossible, however, to eliminate genetic causes in other cases even in the absence of a suggestive family history. The effect of

acute and chronic noise exposure on the ear and its relationship with the "aging process" have also been recognized (Glorig & Davis, 1961). Many drugs are known or are thought to adversely affect the hearing mechanism (Worthington, Lunin, Heath & Catlin, 1973), and the variables associated with these interactions are innumerable. For example, synergism between drugs, genetic predisposition to drug effect, synergism of drugs and other causes of degeneration of the auditory system, idiosyncratic reactions, intercurrent disease processes such as renal dysfunction, and the delayed effect of drug toxicity, to name a few variables, have been described as having deleterious effects on hearing, thereby making difficult the precise evaluation of the role of ototoxicity in presbycusis. The contribution of vascular disease to degeneration of the auditory system is controversial. Although a relationship between arteriosclerosis and presbycusis appeals to the intuitive sense and was suggested over four decades ago (Saxen, 1937), no study to date has satisfactorily correlated these two phenomena as more than coincident events.

The discussion of the aging phenomenon in the auditory mechanism must include correlation with the pertinent neuropathology of the aging central nervous system (see Chap. 5). The sensory and neural structures of the auditory pathway share with central neural cells the characteristics of the postmitotic state. That is, as part of the differentiation process of these specialized cells, there is a programmed arrest of mitosis and hence a lack of replacement of aging cells. Although presumably this has some evolutionary survival value, it does subject these cells to the cummulative effect of cellular insults and decreased function. The process of aging of individual cells has been the subject of extensive research but is still incompletely understood. There is evidence, however, to suggest that cells "age" by the accumulation over time of acquired errors in nucleic acids including that portion of DNA which encodes ribosomal RNA. This in turn results in attrition of ribosomal RNA and a progressive inefficiency in synthesis of essential proteins and hence in cell function (Andrew, 1952; Johnson, Chrisp, & Strehler, 1972; Strehler, 1976). Among the best studied age-related forms of sensory degeneration is the progressive degradation of visual acuity as measured by several parameters (Birren, 1959). Similar and multiple defects in the aging auditory system, particularly a decrement of proficiency in discrimination tasks, also have been described (Kirikae, Sato, & Shitara, 1964; Matzker, 1958; Jerger, Shedd, and Harford, 1959).

The histologic correlates of aging in the central nervous system are not fully agreed on, and the findings are not specific for a single etiology. There is some evidence for changes in the volume and number of nerve cells in the aging brain (Brody, 1955; Hanley, 1974; Konigsmark & Murphy, 1970). Subcellular changes include neurofibrillary tangles (Alzheimer, 1907; Wisniewski, Terry, & Hirano, 1970), senile plaques (Wisniewski, Ghetti, & Terry, 1973), loss of dendritic spines and hence intercellular connections (Feldman & Dowd, 1975), the accumulation of lipofuscin pigment (Reichel, Hollander, Clark, & Strehler, 1968), and a decrease in ribosomal RNA (Andrew, 1952). As in the central nervous system, the histologic study of the aging peripheral auditory system is hampered by lack of specificity. That is, the histologic patterns of degeneration of the sensory and neural structures of the inner ear due to a wide variety of etiologies possess many similarities. This fact prevents a precise designation of the etiology of presbycusis based on histopathology alone. Nevertheless, histologic study gives us the clearest insight into the mechanism, if not the causes, of presbycusis.

THE MIDDLE EAR

The effect of aging on the sound-conductive mechanism of the middle ear has been studied by Nixon, Glorig, and High (1962). They found a slight impairment of transmission of sound in the frequencies above 2 kHz with a maximum effect of 12 dB at 4 kHz. They suggested that this inefficiency of sound transmission was due to alterations in the elasticity of

the tympanic membrane and changes in the ossicular joints and tendons. Histologic study of the aging middle ear (Belal & Stewart, 1974) has demonstrated that arthritic changes, including fibrous and bony ankylosis of ossicular articulations, do occur, but that these changes seem to have no significant effect on hearing. Therefore, the significant alterations in the degeneration of the peripheral hearing mechanism seem to be limited to the inner ear.

THE INNER EAR

Schuknecht (1964) has categorized the clinical types of presbycusis and their histopathologic correlates into four varieties: (1) degeneration and loss of hair cells, or "sensory presbycusis"; (2) degeneration and loss of neural cells, or "neural presbycusis"; (3) an inner ear conductive defect, or "mechanical presbycusis"; and (4) an inner ear biochemical defect, or "metabolic presbycusis". These categories provide a convenient framework with which to evaluate the variable clinical presentations of presbycusis and a way to understand the underlying degenerative phenomena. Characteristics common to all four varieties include interaural symmetry and slow progression with age. These categories comprise pure forms, but considerable overlap or admixture of two or more types may exist in individual cases. In addition, in some cases central auditory degenerative phenomena may exist.

Degeneration and Loss of Hair Cells: Sensory Presbycusis

The usual audiometric pattern in this form of degeneration is a high-frequency hearing loss starting at 2 to 3 kHz. There is interaural symmetry and good discrimination. Recruitment may be present. The hearing loss may begin in childhood and slowly progress with age (Guild, 1950). The histologic characteristics can be reviewed by reference to actual case histories.

CASE 1.

This 70-year-old man died of carcinoma of the floor of the mouth. An audiogram performed several hours before death demonstrated a high-frequency hearing loss in the right ear (Fig. 4–1). The audiogram of the left ear could not be completed because of deterioration of the patient's condition. Serial sections and reconstruction of the pathologic findings of both ears revealed essentially identical pathology. There was moderate to severe loss of hair cells in the basal 10 mm of the cochlea (Figs. 4–1, 4–2) and good preservation of hair cells in the remainder of the

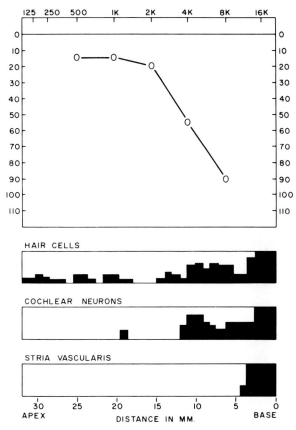

HAIR CELLS

COCHLEAR NEURONS

STRIA VASCULARIS

Fig. 4−1. Sensory presbycusis. Audiogram and histogram of right ear in Case 1, on the day of death.

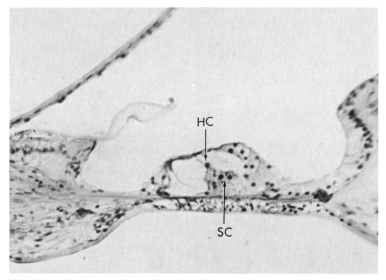

Fig. 4−2. Sensory presbycusis. Section of lower basal turn in right ear in Case 1. Although supporting cells *(SC)* in the organ of Corti are present, there has been severe loss of hair cells *(HC)*. (55 ×)

cochlea (Fig. 4−1, 4−3). There was a coincident decrease in the cochlear neuronal population that corresponded to areas of hair-cell loss.

CASE 2.

This patient died at the age of 83 of cerebral infarction and pulmonary emboli. He was exposed to considerable noise during World War I at age 22 and 23 years. However, he first complained of a slowly progressive hearing loss at age 64. Audiometric evaluation performed at ages 69, 71, and 81 documented a bilateral progressive sensorineural hearing loss with a downsloping threshold (Figs. 4−4, 4−5). SISI scores at 2 kHz were 90 percent on

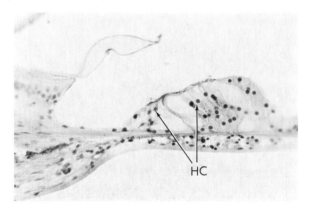

Fig. 4−3. Sensory presbycusis. Upper basal turn in Case 1. The organ of Corti including its complement of hair cells (*HC*) is normal. (240×)

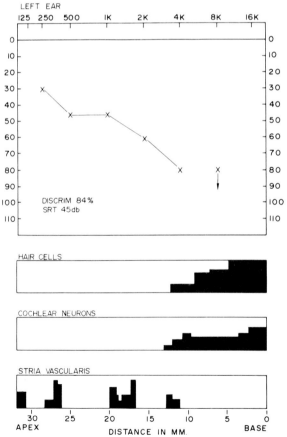

Fig. 4−4. Sensory presbycusis. Audiogram and histogram of left ear in Case 2, 2 years before death.

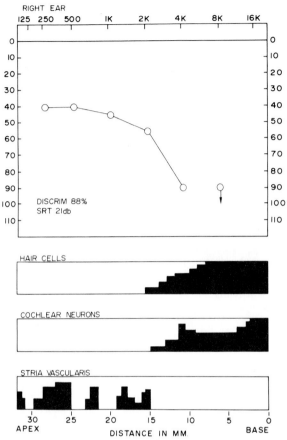

Fig. 4−5. Sensory presbycusis. Audiogram and histogram of right ear in Case 2, 2 years before death.

the right and 100 percent on the left. Histologic study of the temporal bones revealed severe atrophy of the hair and supporting cells of the organ of Corti in the basal 15 mm of the cochlea bilaterally (Figs. 4−4, 4−5, 4−6) and a corresponding loss of cochlear neurons in the same area (Figs. 4−4, 4−5). In addition, there was atrophy of areas of the stria vascularis (Figs. 4−4, 4−5).

As demonstrated in these two case reports, the prominent histologic alteration in this form of presbycusis is loss of hair cells, particularly in the lower basal turn. Ultrastructural analysis of the organ of Corti in such cases further defines the pattern of cellular degeneration. Hair cells only may be missing (Figs. 4−7a, 4−7b), or in severe atrophy of the organ of Corti, supporting and pillar cells may be missing and the organ of Corti replaced by a single layer of epithelial cells (Fig. 4−8). It appears that despite severe loss of cells of the organ of Corti, including pillar and other supporting cells, a permeability barrier between endolymph and perilymph is maintained. This consists of a series of tight junc-

tions, or zonvlae occludentes, between squamous epithelial cells on the scala vestibuli side of the basilar membrane (Nadol, 1978, 1979a, 1979b) (Fig. 4−8b). Within remaining hair cells in the aging inner ear the only abnormality so far recognized is the accumulation of lipofuscin granules (Ishli, Murakami, Kimura, & Balogh, 1967) (Fig. 4−9). Products of cell degeneration may also be found as inclusions in supporting cells of the degenerating organ of Corti (Fig. 4−10). The cause of cellular degeneration and loss is not clarified by the histopathology.

Cochlear neuronal degeneration is commonly found in areas of the cochlea where there has been significant degeneration of the organ of Corti. Schuknecht (1964) has stated that this neural degeneration is secondary to degeneration of the organ of Corti and seems to coincide best with loss of supporting elements. Bredberg (1968), on the other hand, concluded that neuronal degeneration coincides best with loss of the inner hair cells. Spoendlin (1978) found that damage to the unmyelinated dendrites in

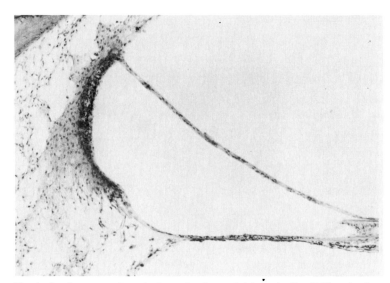

Fig. 4-6. Sensory presbycusis. Lower basal turn of right ear in Case 2. There has been total loss of the organ of Corti. (95×)

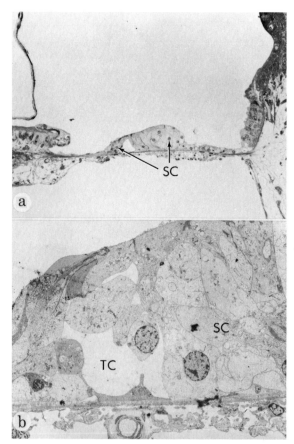

Fig. 4-7. *a)* Upper basal turn in a human ear with severe hair-cell loss. No hair cells are present, although supporting cells *(SC)* appear normal. (115×) *b)* Electron micrograph of organ of Corti shown in Figure *a*. Supporting cells *(SC)* and the tunnel of Corti *(TC)* are present, but no hair cells remain. (1240×)

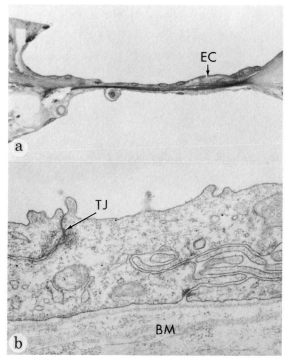

Fig. 4–8. *a)* Lower basal turn of a human ear with severe atrophy of the organ of Corti. Only a single layer of squamous epithelial cells (*EC*) line the scale media side of the basilar membrane. (210×) *b)* Electron micrograph of same ear shown in Figure *a*. The epithelial cells on the scala media side of the basilar membrane (*BM*) are joined by tight junctions (*TJ*), which serve as a permeability barrier between endolymph and perilymph. (2500×)

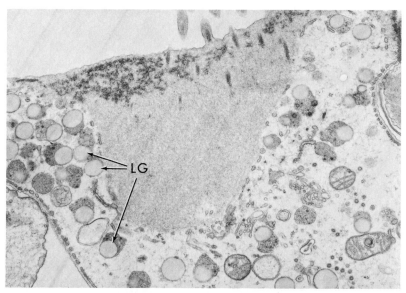

Fig. 4–9. Electron micrograph of apical end of an outer hair cell in the basal turn of a man that died at the age of 64. There are many lipofuscin granules (LG) or "pigment of aging," within the cytoplasm. (17,500×)

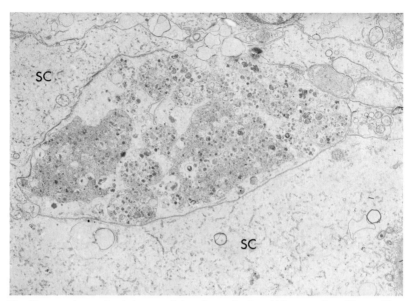

Fig. 4—10. Electron micrograph of the outer hair cell area in the middle turn of an 81-year-old man who demonstrated both sensory and neural forms of presbycusis. There are large intracellular collections of cellular debris among otherwise normal supporting cells (*SC*). This material is presumably the product of cell degeneration and death in the organ of Corti. (4650×)

the organ of Corti was the most consistent coincident finding in areas with neuronal loss, rather than loss of either hair cells or supporting elements. Whatever the initiating factors, the structural alterations among remaining fibers in such areas of secondary neuronal degeneration are striking. The myelin sheaths of such fibers show disruption of the normal lamellar pattern particularly at Schmidt-Lantermann's clefts and the nodes of Ranvier (Nadol, 1979a) (Fig. 4—11). The structural abnormalities may cause dysfunction in the remaining neural fibers before complete degeneration and loss of fibers has occurred.

Loss of Neural Fibers: Neural Presbycusis

The typical audiometric pattern in this form of presbycusic degeneration is a bilaterally symmetrical descending threshold curve with reduced discrimination scores, termed phonemic regression by Gaeth (1948). The relatively greater decrement in discrimination ability compared to pure tone thresholds is explained by a greater requirement for neural integration in encoding speech compared to pure tone signals. That is, more neural fibers are needed to allow accurate interpretation of a complex acoustic stimulus such as speech than are needed for the detection of a relatively simple acoustic stimulus such as a pure tone. This form of hearing loss may begin at any age. Clinically, it is more likely to be

considered "genetically determined" if it begins in early life and "presbycusis" if the onset is later in life. However, there is no obvious distinction between these mechanisms of nerve-cell loss based on audiometric or histologic findings, nor indeed should it be expected in view of the multifactorial etiology of "presbycusis." Three case reports will illustrate the histologic pattern of degeneration in this form of presbycusis.

CASE 3.

This patient died at age 81 of cardiac failure. He wore bilateral hearing aids starting at the age of 70 years. Audiometry at age 80 years revealed a bilateral symmetrical sensorineural loss (Fig. 4—12). The principal histologic correlate of this hearing loss was severe loss of spiral ganglion cells in the basal turn (Figs. 4—12, 4—13). In addition, there was degeneration of the organ of Corti in limited areas of the basal turn. The neuronal degeneration was considered primary since it was not limited to areas in which there was also degeneration of the organ of Corti.

CASE 4.

This man died at age 75 years of myocardial infarction. There had been a progressive hearing loss for at least 10 years. An audiogram at age 67 is shown in Figs. 4—14. 4—15. The histologic findings were almost identical in the two ears. There was

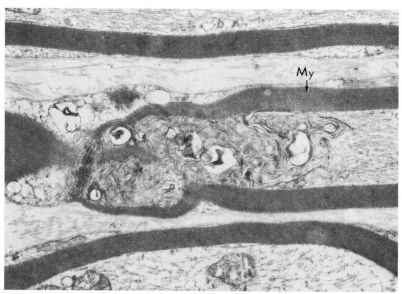

Fig. 4–11. An 8 mm area of the organ of Corti of a 51-year-old man with sensory presbycusis and secondary cochlear neuronal loss. The lamellae of the myelin sheath (*My*) of a remaining axon in Rosenthal's canal is disrupted near a node of Ranvier. (7750×)

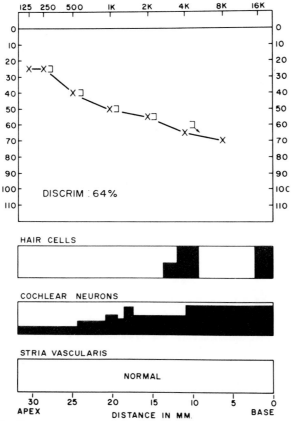

Fig. 4–12. Neural presbycusis. Audiogram and histogram of the left ear in Case 3, one year before death.

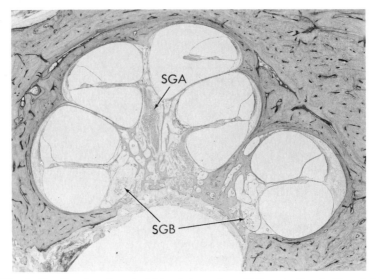

Fig. 4−13. Neural presbycusis. Midmodiolar section of left ear in Case 3. The spiral ganglion population is greatly decreased in the basal turn (*SGB*) and nearly normal in more apical areas of the cochlea (*SGA*). (15×)

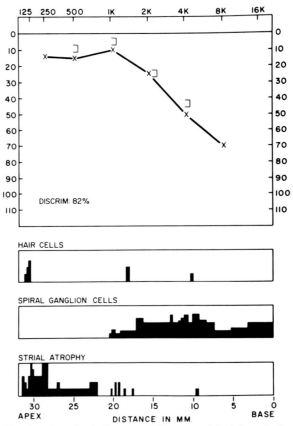

Fig. 4−14. Neural presbycusis. Audiogram and histogram of the left ear in Case 4, 8 years before death.

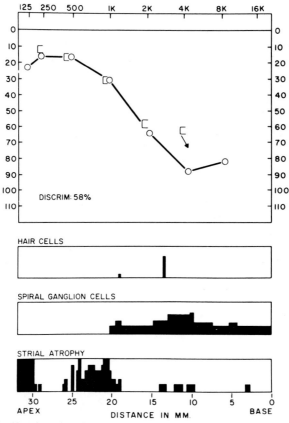

Fig. 4–15. Neural presbycusis. Audiogram and histogram of right ear in Case 4, 8 years before death.

significant loss of cochlear neurons in the basal 15 mm of the organ of Corti (Figs. 4–16, 4–17). In addition, there was patchy atrophy of the stria vascularis in the apical turn.

CASE 5.

This man died of uremia and pneumonia at age 51 years. He had suffered a total hearing loss in the left ear at about age 21 and a slowly progressive loss in the right ear for many years. An audiogram 2 months before death revealed no hearing in the left ear and a downsloping threshold curve on the right with good discrimination (Fig. 4–18). Serial reconstruction demonstrated that the principal abnormality on the right was loss of cochlear neurons in the basal turn (Fig. 4–18). In addition, electron microscopic examination revealed abnormalities in the myelin sheath of the remaining dendrites in the osseous spiral lamina (Fig. 4–19), similar to the pathologic changes seen in secondary neural degeneration in sensory presbycusis. Other changes included

lysosomal-like inclusions along the course of the unmyelinated afferent fibers (Fig. 4–20), amorphous deposits in cell bodies of the spiral ganglion (Fig. 4–21), and degeneration of myelin of the afferent axons, consistent with degeneration along the entire course of the first order neuron. The cause of degeneration and eventual loss of the first order neuron cannot be determined by the pathologic changes.

Inner Ear Conductive Loss: Mechanical Presbycusis

This is perhaps the most controversial type of presbycusis. Its hypothetical existence is based on the clinical finding of a group of aging ears that demonstrate a symmetrical descending audiometric pattern, usually with good discrimination, and in which the loss of hair cells, neurons, and stria vascularis at a light microscopic level is insufficient to explain the degree of hearing loss. Mayer (1919–1920) suggested that alterations in the mechanical prop-

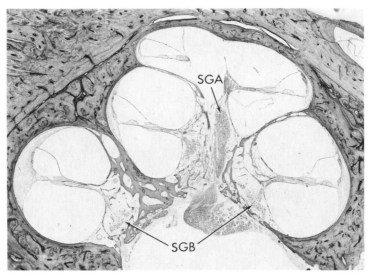

Fig. 4–16. Neural presbycusis. Midmodiolar section of right ear in Case 4. There has been considerable loss of spiral ganglion cells in the basal turn (*SGB*), whereas the ganglion population of the apical turn (*SGA*) is normal. (15×)

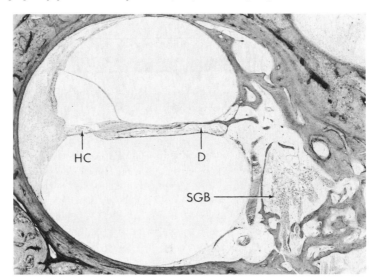

Fig. 4–17. Neural presbycusis. Basal turn of organ of Corti of Case 4. The number of spiral ganglion cells (*SGB*) and dendrites (*D*) in the osseous spiral lamina are reduced to approximately 50% of normal. The hair cells (*HC*) are normal in number. (31×)

erties of the cochlea may be the cause of some cases. There is some histologic evidence to support the thesis of an inner ear conductive etiology. Alterations in both the basilar membrane (Crowe, Guild, & Polvogt, 1934; Nomura, 1970; Kraus, 1970; Wright & Schuknecht, 1972) and spiral ligament (Takahashi, 1971) have been described and are illustrated by the following two case reports.

CASE 6.

This patient died at age 53 of coronary thrombosis. At age 49 an audiogram (Fig. 4–22) demonstrated bilateral high-frequency hearing loss. Speech discrimination was 72 percent in the right ear and 68 percent in the left ear. Serial reconstruction of both ears demonstrated no significant alterations of the hair cells, cochlear neurons, and stria vascularis (Fig.

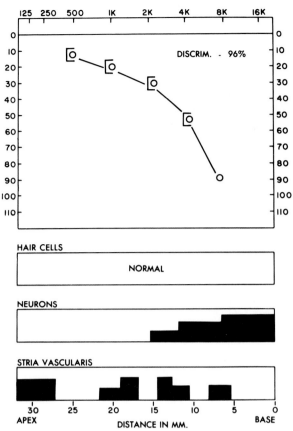

Fig. 4—18. Neural presbycusis. Audiogram and histogram of right ear in Case 5, 2 months before death.

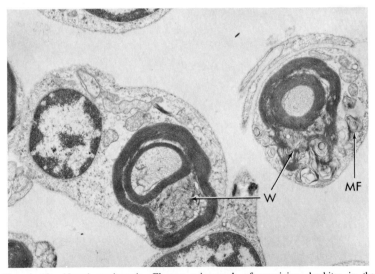

Fig. 4—19. Neural presbycusis. Electron micrograph of remaining dendrites in the osseous spiral lamina in the 8 mm region of the organ of Corti in Case 5. The normal lamellar pattern of the myelin sheaths is disrupted by whorls of apparently degenerating myelin (*W*), and myelin figures (*MF*) are present within the surrounding supporting-cell cytoplasm. (7500×)

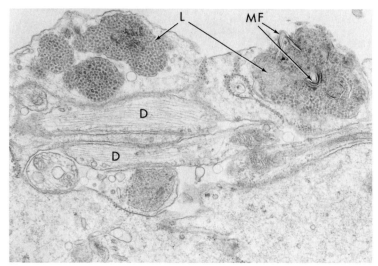

Fig. 4−20. Neural presbycusis. Electron micrograph of unmyelinated afferent dendrites (*D*) in the outer hair-cell area of the 8 mm region of the organ of Corti in Case 5. Large intracellular vacuoles of lysosomal-like material (*L*) and myelin figures (*MF*) suggest an active degenerative process. (19,000×)

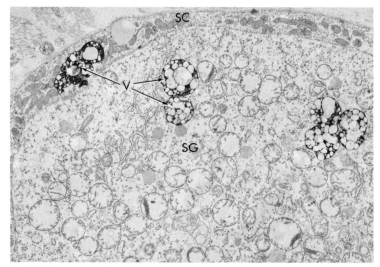

Fig. 4−21. Neural presbycusis. Electron micrograph of a spiral ganglion cell in the 8 mm region of the organ of Corti in Case 5. Vacuoles (*V*) of amorphous material within the cytoplasm of the ganglion cell (*SG*) and supporting cell (*SC*) are consistent with products of degeneration. (4850×)

4−23). Both ears demonstrated decreased cellularity and cystic degeneration of the spiral ligament in the basal turn. The relationship, if any, between this degenerative change of the spiral ligament and the hearing loss is unknown.

CASE 7.

This patient died at the age of 75 of myocardial infarction. She had a bilateral hearing loss for many years. The patient described a sudden deterioration in hearing 4 months before death. The audiogram for the right ear performed at that time is shown in Figure 4−24. Serial reconstruction of the cochlea demonstrated significant loss of cochlear neurons in the basal 15 mm, sufficient to explain the increased threshold. In addition, there was marked atrophy of the spiral ligament in the apical 20 mm and actual separation of the spiral ligament from the lateral

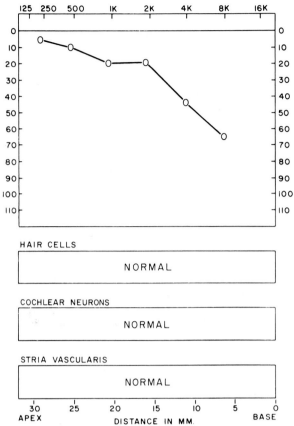

HAIR CELLS

NORMAL

COCHLEAR NEURONS

NORMAL

STRIA VASCULARIS

NORMAL

Fig. 4–22. Mechanical presbycusis. Audiogram and histogram of right ear in Case 6, 4 years before death.

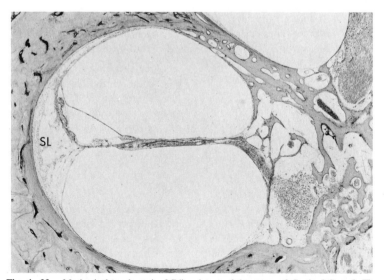

Fig. 4–23. Mechanical presbycusis. Midbasal turn of the organ of Corti of Case 6. The organ of Corti and neuronal population show no significant abnormalities. The spiral ligament (*SL*), however, shows moderate cystic degeneration. (31×)

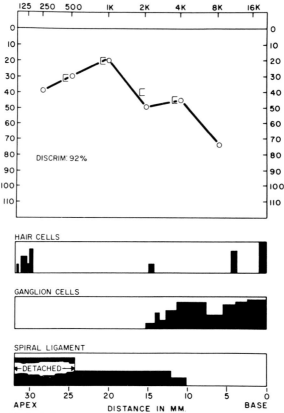

Fig. 4—24. Mechanical presbycusis. Audiogram and histogram of right ear in Case 7, 4 months before death.

cochlear wall in the apical 10 mm of the cochlea (Fig. 4—25, 4—26). There is sufficient correlation of the high-frequency hearing loss and the loss of basal neurons to classify this case as primary neural degeneration. However, the low-frequency hearing loss has no correlate in the loss of neurons, hair cells, or stria vascularis. The possible relationship between the low-frequency hearing loss and the change in the spiral ligament of the apical turn is hypothetical.

In addition to this suggestive light microscopic evidence, a case demonstrating significant thickening of the basilar membrane in the basal turn has been studied by electron microscopy (Nadol, 1979a). Marked thickening of the basilar membrane was due to an increase in the number of fibrils (Fig. 4—27 a—d). In this case, however, the loss of hair cells and neurons in the basal turn was sufficient to explain the hearing loss. Nevertheless, it does demonstrate that significant alterations in supporting structures may occur in association with presbycusis.

Atrophy of the Stria Vascularis: Metabolic Presbycusis

The audiometric pattern in this form of presbycusis is characteristically flat, that is with equal loss of threshold at all frequencies. The discrimination score typically is excellent. The usual onset of hearing loss is in the third to sixth decades and slow progression is characteristic. The histopathology is illustrated by a case report.

CASE 8.

This patient died at age 77 years of carcinoma of the pancreas. A bilateral, slowly progressive hearing loss was present for at least 8 years before death. Audiometry performed 3 years before death showed a bilateral sensorineural loss of 30 to 50 dB at all frequencies tested. Serial reconstruction of the cochlea demonstrated that the most significant pathologi-

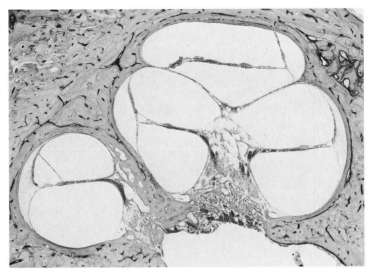

Fig. 4−25. Mechanical presbycusis. Midmodiolar section of the organ of Corti in Case 7. There is marked atrophy of the spiral ligament in the apical 20 mm of the cochlea (17×)

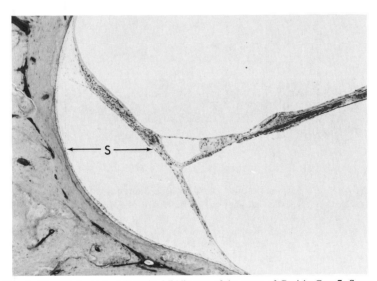

Fig. 4−26. Mechanical presbycusis. Middle turn of the organ of Corti in Case 7. Severe atrophy of the spiral ligament has resulted in its separation (S) from the bony lateral cochlear wall. (54×)

cal alteration was atrophy of the stria vascularis (Figs. 4−28, 4−29, 4−30, 4−31). In addition to loss of cells in the stria vascularis, concretions of presumed degenerative material are often found in the strial or substrial tissue (Figs. 4−31, 4−32).

The most consistent histologic finding in this form of presbycusis is atrophy of the stria vascularis. This may be quite unequal from turn to turn and even from millimeter to millimeter of the cochlea but is usually most severe in the apical and lower basal turns (Takahashi, 1971). Kimura and Schuknecht (1970) have demonstrated at an electron microscopic level that all three cell layers of the stria vascularis are affected, but that the most severe changes are found in the marginal cells, which become flattened and lose their basal infoldings (Fig. 4−33). The theoretical consequences of atrophy of the stria vascularis include disordered production of endolymph

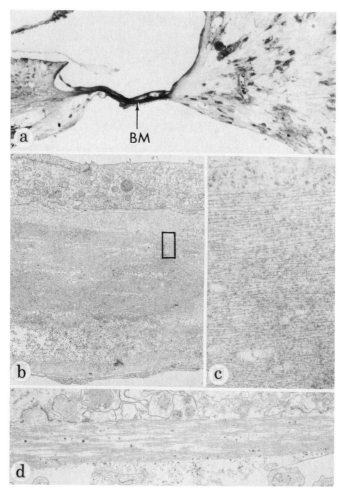

Fig. 4–27. *a)* Basal turn (3 mm) of the organ of Corti of an 81-year-old man with a combined sensory and neural presbycusis. The basilar membrane *(BM)* appears thicker and more densely staining than normal. (160×) *b)* Electron micrograph of 3 mm region of the thickened basilar membrane shown in Figure 4–27. (3500×) *c)* Electron micrograph of a small portion of the thickened basilar membrane corresponding to the boxed area in Figure 4–28. The increase in thickness is due to an increase in the number of fibril layers within the acellular portion of the basilar membrane. (26,500×) *d)* Electron micrograph of the basilar membrane of the upper basal turn (17 mm) of the same ear. The basilar membrane is normal in thickness. (6200×)

(Smith, 1957) or an adverse effect on oxidative enzymes (Vosteen, 1961) and hence on the metabolism of the cochlea, resulting in an alteration of the endocochlear potential (Davis, Deatherage, Rosenblat, Fernandez, Kimura, & Smith, 1958).

SUMMARY

Presbycusis is the term used by clinicians to describe hearing loss that seems to have no other obvious cause or correlate except progressive age of the patient. It is likely, however, that presbycusis represents the cummulative effect of a number of disorders and insults. Probable contributing causes of hearing loss include acoustic trauma, ototoxic substances, genetic defects, and true cellular aging. Histopathology at light and electron microscopic levels demonstrate that most cases of presbycusis can be satisfactorily correlated with cell degeneration and loss of structural integrity in the peripheral auditory system, although undoubtedly alterations in the cen-

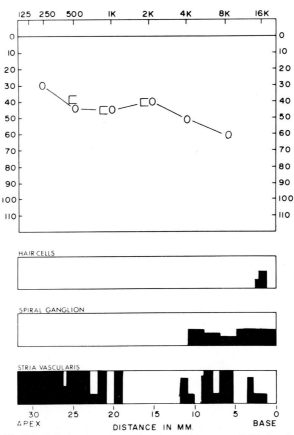

Fig. 4-28. Metabolic presbycusis. Audiogram and histogram of right ear in Case 8, 3 years before death.

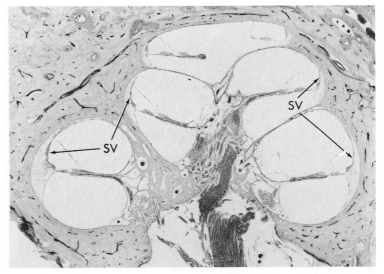

Fig. 4-29. Metabolic presbycusis. Midmodiolar section of the organ of Corti in Case 8. Changes in the neuronal and hair cell populations are insufficient to explain the degree of hearing loss. The most striking abnormality is marked atrophy of the stria vascularis (*SV*). (15×)

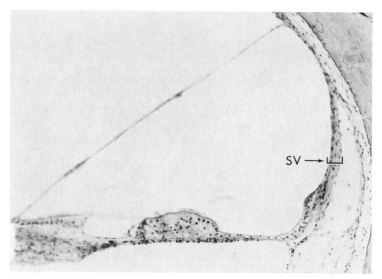

Fig. 4–30. Metabolic presbycusis. Middle turn of the organ of Corti in Case 8. There is marked atrophy of the stria vascularis (*SV*). (115×)

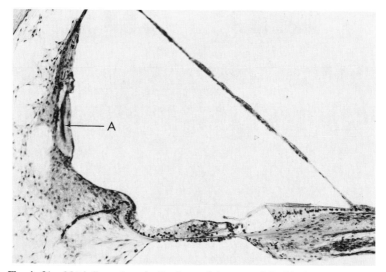

Fig. 4–31. Metabolic presbycusis. Basal turn of the organ of Corti in Case 8. Part of the stria vascularis has been replaced by amorphous material (*A*), which may represent products of degeneration. (117×)

tral auditory pathways contribute to the hearing deficit and in a few cases may represent the principal pathology. The histologic correlates of presbycusis in the peripheral auditory system include degeneration and loss of sensory cells, or sensory presbycusis, degeneration and loss of first order neurons, or neural presbycusis, and atrophy of the stria vascularis, or metabolic presbycusis. In addition, alterations in supportive elements in the organ of Corti, such as the basilar membrane and spiral ligament, may cause mechanical presbycusis. However, histopathology does not clarify fully the etiology of presbycusis

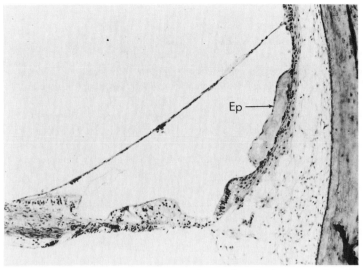

Fig. 4–32. Metabolic presbycusis. Upper basal turn of another human ear demonstrating severe atrophy of the stria vascularis. Amorphous material is encapsulated by a single layer of epithelial cells *(Ep)* (105×)

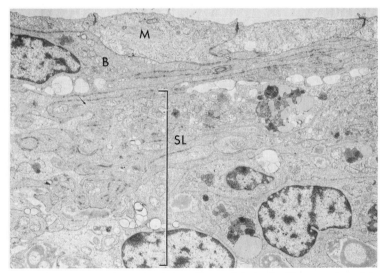

Fig. 4–33. Electron micrograph of the stria vascularis in the 23 mm region of the cochlea of an 81-year-old man. There is moderate strial atrophy. The marginal cells *(M)* have lost their basal infoldings. In this area there are no remaining intermediate cells above the basal cells *(B)* and spiral ligament *(SL)*. (900×)

because these patterns of degeneration are not specific to any one etiologic factor. Productive areas for future investigation include ultrastructural histopathologic analysis with the hope that observations concerning degenerating structural elements before their complete loss may clarify mechanisms of degeneration. Biochemical and histochemical analysis of the aging human inner ear, clarification of the role and mechanisms of central auditory neuropathology, and systemic evaluation of animal models of aging and genetically determined degeneration of the auditory apparatus also need to be undertaken.

REFERENCES

Alzheimer, A. Ueber eine eigenartige Erkrankung der Hirnrinde. *Zentralblatt fur die gesamte Neurologie und Psychiatrie,* 1907, *18,* 177–179.

Andrew, W. *Cellular changes with age.* Springfield, Ill.: Charles C. Thomas, Publisher, 1952.

Belal, A., & Stewart, T. J. Pathological changes in the middle ear joints. *Annals of Otology, Rhinology and Laryngology,* 1974, *83,* 159–167.

Birren, J. E. *Handbook of aging and the individual.* Chicago, University of Chicago Press, 1959.

Bredberg, G. Cellular pattern and nerve supply of the human organ of Corti. *Acta Oto-laryngologica,* Supplement 236, 1968.

Brody, H. Organization of the cerebral cortex. Study of aging in human cerebral cortex. *Journal of Comparative Neurology,* 1955, *102,* 511–556.

Crowe, S., Guild, S., & Polvogt, L. Observations on pathology of high-tone deafness. *Bulletin of Johns Hopkins Hospital,* 1934, *54,* 315.

Davis, H., Deatherage, B. H., Rosenblut, B., Fernandez, C., Kimura, R., & Smith, C. Modification of cochlear potentials produced by streptomycin poisoning and by extensive venous obstruction. *Laryngoscope,* 1958, *68,* 596–627.

Feldman, M. L., & Dowd, C. Loss of dendritic spines in aging cerebral cortex. *Anatomy and Embryology* (Berlin), 1975, *148,* 279–301.

Gaeth, J. H. Study of phonemic regression in relation to hearing loss. Thesis, Northwestern University, Chicago, 1948.

Glorig, A., & Davis, H. Age, noise and hearing loss. *Transactions of the American Otologic Society,* 1961, *49,* 262–280.

Guild, S. R. The progression of impaired hearing for high tones during childhood. *Laryngoscope,* 1950, *60,* 885–911.

Hanley, T. "Neuronal fall-out" in the aging brain: A critical review of the quantitiative data. *Age and Ageing,* 1974, *3,* 133–151.

Ishii, T., Murakami, Y., Kimura, R. S., & Balogh, K. Electron microscopic and histochemical identification of lipofuscin in the human inner ear. *Acta Oto-laryngologica,* 1967, *64,* 17–29.

Jerger, J., Shedd, J. L., & Harford, E. On the detection of extremely small changes in sound intensity. *Archives of Otolaryngology,* 1959, *69,* 200–211.

Johnson, R., Chrisp, C., & Strehler, B. L. Selective loss of ribosomal RNA genes during the aging of post-mitotic tissues. *Mechanisms of Ageing and Development,* 1972, *1,* 183–198.

Kimura, R. S., & Schuknecht, H. F. The ultrastructure of the human stria vascularis. Part II. *Acta Oto-laryngologica,* 1970, *70,* 301–318.

Kirikae, I., Sato, T., & Shitara, T. A study of hearing in advanced age. *Laryngoscope,* 1964, *74,* 205–220.

Konigsmark, B. W., & Murphy, E. A. Neuronal populations in the human brain. *Nature,* 1970, *228,* 1335–1336.

Kraus, H. Quantitativ-cytochemische Untersuchungen am Innenohr junger und seniler Meerschweinchen. *Acta Oto-laryngologica,* Supplement 278, 1970.

Matzker, J. Ein binauraler Horsynthese—Test zum Nachweis zerebraler Horstorungen. Stuttgart, Georg Thieme Verlag, 1958.

Mayer, O. Das anatomische Substrat der Alterschwerhorigkeit. *Archiv fur Ohren- Nasen- und Kehlkopfheilkunde,* 1919–1920, *105,* 1.

Nadol, J. B., Jr. Electron microscopic findings in presbycusic degeneration of the basal turn of the human cochlea. *Head and Neck Surgery,* 1979, *87,* 818–836.

Nadol, J. B., Jr. Intercellular fluid pathways in the organ of Corti of cat and man. *Annals of Otology, Rhinology and Laryngology,* 1979, *88,* 2–11. (b)

Nadol, J. B., Jr. Intercellular junctions in the organ of Corti. *Annals of Otology, Rhinology and Laryngology,* 1978, *87,* 70–80.

Nance, W. E., & McConnell, F. E. Status and prospects of research in hereditary deafness. *Advances in Human Genetics,* 1973, *4,* 173–250.

National Center for Vital and Health Statistics. Characteristics of persons with impaired hearing. United States, July 1962—June 1963, Series 10, No. 35, 1967, pp. 1—64.

Nixon, J. C., Glorig, A., & High, W. S. Changes in air and bone conduction thresholds as a function of age. *Journal of Laryngology*, 1962, *76*, 288—298.

Nomura, Y. Lipidosis of the basilar membrane. *Acta Oto-laryngologica*, 1970, *69*, 352—357.

Reichel, W., Hollander, J., Clark, J. H., & Strehler, B. L. Lipofuscin pigment accumulation as a function of age and distribution in the rodent brain. *Journal of Gerontology*, 1968, *23*, 71—78.

Rosen, S., Bergman, M., Plester, D., El-Moffey, A., & Salti, M. Presbycusis: Study of a relatively noise free population in the Sudan. *Annals of Otology, Rhinology and Laryngology*, 1962, *71*, 727—743.

Saxen, A. Pathologie und Klinik der Altersschwerhorigkeit. *Acta Oto-laryngologica*, 1937, Supplement 23.

Schuknecht, H. F. Further observations on the pathology of presbycusis. *Archives of Otolaryngology*, 1964, *80*, 369—382.

Smith, C. A. Structure of the stria vascularis and the spiral prominence. *Annals of Otology, Rhinology and Laryngology*, 1957, *66*, 521—536.

Spoendlin, H. H. Personal communication, 1978.

Strehler, B. L. Introduction: Theories of aging. In D. Platt (Ed.), *Third Geissen Symposium on Experimental Gerontology*. Stuttgart, New York: Schattauer, 1976.

Takahashi, T. The ultrastructure of the pathologic stria vascularis and spiral prominence in man. *Annals of Otology, Rhinology and Laryngology*, 1971, *80*, 721—735.

Vosteen, K. H. Neue Aspekte zur Biologie und Pathologie des Innenohres. *Arch Ohr Nas-KehlkHeilk*, 1961, *178*, 1—104.

Wisniewski, H. M., Terry, R. D., & Hirano, A. Neurofibrillary pathology. *Journal of Neuropathology and Experimental Neurology*, 1970, *29*, 163—176.

Wisniewski, H. M., Ghetti, B., & Terry, R. D. Neuritic (senile) plaques and filamentous changes in aged Rhesus monkeys. *Journal of Neuropathology and Experimental Neurology*, 1973, *32*, 566—584.

Worthington, E. L., Lunin, L. F., Heath, M., & Catlin, F. I. *Index—Handbook of ototoxic agents, 1966—1971*. Baltimore: Johns Hopkins University Press, 1973.

Wright, J. L., & Schuknecht, H. F. Atrophy of the spiral ligament. *Archives of Otolaryngology*, 1972, *96*, 16—21.

Edward Valenstein

5

Age-Related Changes in the Human Central Nervous System

Age-related changes in human brain structure fall into two classes: developmental and involutional. The major developmental changes occur in the first 3 years of life when brain weight more than triples (Dekaban & Sadowsky, 1978), neuronal processes grow (Schade & van Groenigen, 1961), neurons form more synaptic connections with other neurons (Purpura, 1974), and myelination progresses (Yakovlev & Lecours, 1967). These and other morphological changes allow for rapid development of perceptual, motor, and cognitive abilities. Further development occurs at a slower pace. There is a modest increase in brain weight between the ages of 3 and 18 years (Dekaban & Sadowsky, 1978), presumably reflecting similar growth processes. Myelination of phylogenetically newer cortical areas continues into the fourth decade (Yakovlev & Lecours, 1967). It is not known at what age such "developmental" changes cease, or indeed if they continue into old age.

Involutional changes have been described predominately in old age; however, some are apparent earlier. Lipofuscin may begin to accumulate as early as the first decade (Brizzee, Harkin, Ordy, & Kaack, 1975) and loss of nerve cells may begin by middle age. Clinical findings suggest a progressive diminution of plasticity throughout life; recovery from severe head injury is inversely correlated with age (Carlsson, von Essen, & Lofgren, 1968) and the incidence of nonfluent aphasia and the probability of

making a good recovery from aphasia both decrease with increasing age. The morphological correlates of behavioral plasticity may be neuronal sprouting and synapse formation, which has been observed in animals in response to brain injury (Cotman, 1978). Scheff, Bernardo, & Cotman (1978) demonstrated that axonal sprouting induced by brain lesions is less vigorous in senescent than in young adult rats. It would be attractive to hypothesize that in humans also the ability of neurons to form new synapses diminishes with age; however, there are many problems in applying animal research on aging to the human aging process (Himwich, 1973). The rat, for example, has a much shorter life span, its brain weight does not diminish with age, and its brain does not undergo all of the pathologic changes seen in aging human brains.

While there is little data on age-related changes in the human brain during young adulthood and middle age, there is abundant documentation of involutional changes occurring in old age. Since most old people suffer from one or more diseases, many factors other than age and genetic programming contribute to these involutional changes. To the extent that pathologic factors are involved, these changes cannot be regarded as normal or obligatory accompaniments of aging. At this time, however, we do not know the causes of any of the changes that accompany aging, and we can only speculate as to which of them are "normal." Nevertheless, there are a number of morphological changes that occur with fair regularity among aging brains, and these will be reviewed in this chapter. In addition, selected aspects of neurochemistry and physiology will be reviewed as they relate to aging. Only aging changes in humans will be discussed, but the interested reader is urged to consult recent reviews for an introduction to the extensive literature on aging in other animals (Bondareff, 1977; Brizzee, Ordy, Hofer, & Kaack, 1978).

MORPHOLOGICAL CHANGES IN NORMAL AGING

Gross Morphology of the Brain

BRAIN WEIGHT

Brain weight increases rapidly in the first 3 years of life, and then increases slowly, reaching a plateau at about age 18. It remains stable for the next three decades and then slowly declines, so that the average brain weight in persons over 86 is 11 percent less than the mean brain weight for young adults (Dekaban & Sadowsky, 1978) (See Fig. 5–1). It is possible that some or all of this decline with age results from the inclusion of brains of demented patients. Tomlinson, Blessed, and Roth (1968) reported the only series of patients tested psychologically shortly before death. They found that brain weight was only slightly diminished in subjects over 62 when compared to the brain weight of normals under 50, but this difference was only significant for males. Further, within the group aged 62 to 95, there was no correlation of brain weight with age. There were only 28 brains in this series, so that small differences could have been missed.

VENTRICULAR SIZE

Until recently, measurements of ventricular size could only be made at autopsy or from invasive procedures such as pneumoencephalography (PEG) or angiography. Both autopsy and PEG themselves affect ventricular size, and PEG and angiography cannot be used to study normal patients (Messert, Wannamaker, & Dudley, 1972). The use of computerized tomography as shown in Figure 5–2 however, has obviated these problems. Barron, Jacobs, and Kinkel (1976) studied 135 "normal" volunteers, 15 in each decade from birth to 90 years. No psychologic assessment was made. A gradual in-

crease in ventricular size was found between the third and seventh decades, and a more rapid increase was found thereafter. Roberts and Caird (1976) studied 66 subjects age 62 to 90, using a geriatric behavioral rating score plus a memory and information test. Seventeen of these subjects were found to be psychologically normal. The ventricular size of these non-demented elderly subjects was significantly larger than that of normal young adults. In the total group, there was a modest correlation of ventricular size with scores on the memory and information test ($r = 0.489$, $p < .01$) and the behavioral test ($r = 0.313$, $p = 0.01$). It appears, then, that there is a modest increase in ventricular size with age, and that more severe ventricular enlargement occurs with dementia.

CORTICAL ATROPHY

Autopsy material has generated the impression that the cerebral cortex atrophies with increasing age, (McMenemey, 1963). The gyri appear thinner and the sulci are widened, particularly in the frontal lobes. Pneumoencephalographic studies have similarly demonstrated increased cortical atrophy with age (Willanger, Thygesen, Nielsen & Petersen, 1968). These findings have been confirmed in computerized tomographic (CT) scan studies of "normal" elderly subjects (Barron et al., 1976). It is of interest that in the studies of Barron et al., the degree of cortical atrophy did not correlate with the amount of ventricular dilatation. The authors suggest that ventricular enlargement might therefore reflect selective white-matter atrophy. If this were the case, one might expect that the degree of senile dementia (a process usually thought to affect cortical more than subcortical areas) would correlate better with cortical atrophy than with ventricular dilatation. However, in the study of Roberts and Caird (1976) the reverse was the case: intellectual decline was correlated with ventricular atrophy but not with cortical atrophy. Further study of this question is warranted, using better radiological resolution and a larger number of patients. Nevertheless, Roberts and Caird (1976) did make the important observation that moderate cortical atrophy as demonstrated by CT scan is compatible with normal intellectual function. This was confirmed by Kaszniak, Garron, Fox, Bergen, & Huckman (1979), who found that measurements of cerebral atrophy (ventricular enlargement and cortical atrophy) correlated better with age than with measures of intellectual function, although there was an effect of cerebral atrophy on verbal memory that was independent of age.

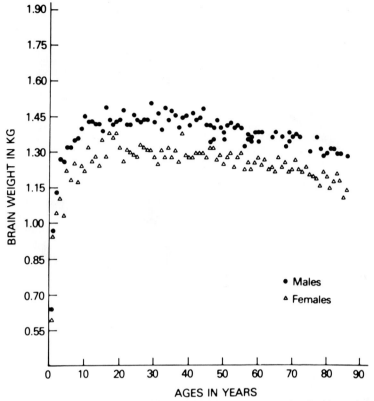

Fig. 5-1. Scattergram of means of brain weights by years. Reproduced with permission from Dekaban, A. S., & Sadowsky, D. Changes in brain weights during the span of human life: Relation of brain weights to body heights and body weights. *Annals of Neurology*, 1978, *4*, 345–356.

Microscopic Anatomy of the Brain

NEURONAL DROPOUT

Until recently, the principal evidence for age-associated loss of neurons in man was the work of Brody (1955), who studied the brains of 20 patients who had died from causes not associated with central nervous system disorder, ranging in age from new-born to 95 years. Comparing neuron counts from the brains of nine subjects over 70 years old to those from the brains of seven adults under 48 years old, Brody demonstrated that there was a significant loss of neurons in the superior temporal gyrus, the precentral gyrus, and the striate cortex (in order of decreasing loss), but not in the postcentral gyrus. The loss was greater for small neurons (granular cells) than for large ones (pyramidal cells). This study has been criticized because of allegedly inadequate sampling,

statistical error, and fixation shrinkage (Berlin & Wallace, 1976; Hanley, 1974; Tomasch, 1972), but it appears unlikely that any of these problems substantially affected the validity of the results (Hanley, 1974).

Much skepticism about neuronal dropout resulted from studies that failed to show any age-associated neuronal loss in regions of the human brainstem, such as the ventral cochlear nucleus (Konigsmark & Murphy, 1972) and the inferior olive (Monagle & Brody, 1974). Studies of the human cerebral cortex, however, generally have been in agreement with Brody's findings. Shefer (1973) demonstrated a decrease in layer III neurons between the third and eighth decades, which varied from 12 percent to 29 percent, depending on the cortical region. Colon (1972) showed a 44 percent loss of neurons in the cortex of two nondemented patients in their ninth decade. Ball (1977) found a 27 percent

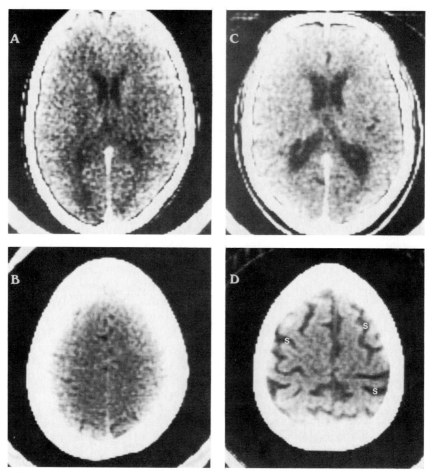

Fig. 5–2. *(A* and *B)* Computerized tomographic *(CT)* scans of a normal elderly person. *C* demonstrates ventricular enlargement (compare with *A*), while *D* demonstrates moderate cortical atrophy (compare with *B*). Note that the cerebral sulci *(s)* that are so apparent in *D* are barely visible in *B*.

decrease in the numbers of hippocampal pyramidal neurons between the ages of 47 and 89.

Not all brainstem nuclei are exempt from cell loss. Brody (1978) has demonstrated age-associated cell loss in the human locus ceruleus, a brainstem structure important for the rapid eye movement (REM) phase of sleep. Neuronal loss has also been demonstrated in the cerebellum by Hall, Miller and Corsellis (1975), who found that 25 percent of Purkinje cells are lost between birth and 100 years of age.

Only a few studies using neurochemical methods have been published, and so far there is little agreement. Bowen, White, Spillane, Goodhardt, Curzon, Igwanoff, Meier-Ruge & Davison (1979) found no loss of nerve cells in the temporal lobes of normal aging subjects. DeKosky and Bass (1979),

however, found a 30 percent loss of small neurons in the prefrontal cortex, without any loss of larger neurons (pyramidal cells), a result in striking agreement with the work of Brody (1955).

Most studies of the morphology of normal aging define their ''normal'' population on the basis of an absence of a clinical history of central nervous system disease. But a moderate degree of dementia can easily go unrecognized, both by family and by medical personnel, particularly in a retired person of whom little is demanded. It is likely, therefore, that in many studies, the ''normal'' aging population contains some demented subjects. To some extent, this problem can be circumvented by interviewing persons who have known the patient. Ideally, objective measures of intellectual function should be available. The work of Tomlinson and his colleagues (reviewed by Tomlinson, 1977) has provided valuable information in this area, because patients were tested shortly before death. In intellectually normal subjects, Tomlinson and Henderon (1976) have shown a decline in the population of neurons in various cortical areas to 50 percent of their young adult numbers.

In summary, the evidence presented suggests that neuronal loss does occur with normal aging in humans, but only in specific areas of the brain. Certain areas of neocortex, the hippocampus, and the locus ceruleus demonstrate considerable loss of neurons, while other cortical areas, and various other brainstem nuclei (such as the ventral cochlear nucleus) show little or no loss. Further study of regional differences in the rate of neuronal loss may help to clarify the relationship between neuronal loss and intellectual function.

INVOLUTION OF NEURONS

Neurons are large and complex structures. With routine histologic staining, only the cell body is defined. Special staining techniques, such as Golgi's stain, demonstrate both the cell body and the extensive neuronal processes (dendrites and axons) (see Fig. 5−3). Although Golgi studies have been performed in brains of normal aged humans, insufficient numbers of brains have been examined to reach definite conclusions about changes in neuronal processes with age (Scheibel, Lindsay, Tomiyasu, & Scheibel, 1975, 1976; Scheibel, 1978), even though extensive changes are seen in demented patients. Cragg (1975) counted numbers of synapses in the brains of normal young adults and seven normal elderly subjects, and found no differences. Cragg, however, did find an inverse correlation of the number of synapses with age in seven biopsy cases, suggesting the need for further research.

LIPOFUSCIN ACCUMULATION IN NEURONS

Lipofuscin is a yellow-brown pigment, composed principally of lipid and protein, that accumulates in the cytoplasm of neurons. Although structural (Samorajski, Keefe, & Ordy, 1964) and enzymatic (Siakotos & Koppang, 1973) similarities to lysosomes* have supported the prevalent view that lipofuscin is derived from lysosomes (see Bondareff, 1977), others have favored the hypothesis that they derive from mitochondria, or the Golgi apparatus, or

_____

*Subcellular vacuolar structures associated with hydrolytic catabolism and excretion.

a combination of subcellular organelles (Brizzee et al., 1975). Although the accumulation of lipofuscin increases with chronological age, the degree of lipofuscin accumulation varies among neuronal populations. For example, the Purkinje cells of the cerebellum show little or no lipofuscin accumulation, while the neurons of the inferior olive contain lipofuscin early in life and accumulate large amounts with increasing age (Brizzee et al., 1978). Since Purkinje cells are lost with age (Hall et al., 1975) but neurons of the inferior olive are not (Monagle and Brody, 1974), it is certain that lipofuscin accumulation alone does not lead to neuronal death. In fact, it is not known if it has any detrimental effect on cell function. Further, lipofuscin accumulation is not specific for aging and is seen as a nonspecific finding in many diseases.

GRANULOVACUOLAR DEGENERATION

Simchowitz (1911) described small, clear vacuoles with a smaller central granule in hippocampal pyramidal cells of patients with senile dementia (see Fig. 5−4). Although granulovacuolar degeneration (GVD) has since been described in cortical neurons in Alzheimer's disease and in the basal ganglia in supranuclear palsy, it is only found with regularity in hippocampal neurons. It is present in this area in the normal aged population, as shown in 14 of 25 cases reported by Tomlinson et al. (1968) and 100 percent of the 18 normal brains (minimum age 47 years) studied by Ball and Lo (1977). Ball and Lo also demonstrated a slight but significant increase in GVD with age.

NEUROFIBRILLARY TANGLES

Neurofibrillary tangles were first described by Alzheimer in 1906 in a case of presenile dementia. Under the light microscope, tangles appear as thick fibrous bands arranged irregularly in the cytoplasm of neurons (see Fig. 5−5). Under the electron microscope, neurofibrillary tangles are seen to be composed of double helical filaments originally thought to be twisted tubules. Although the helical filaments are composed of protein elements that appear electrophoretically similar to normal neurofilament protein and to the beta monomer of the neurotubule (beta tubulin) (Iqbal, Grundke-Iqbal, Wisniewski, & Terry, 1978), double helical filaments are not present in normal neurons (Terry, 1971; Wisniewski & Terry, 1973; Wisniewski, Terry, & Hirano, 1970).

Tomlinson et al. (1968) found small numbers of neurons containing neurofibrillary tangles almost ex-

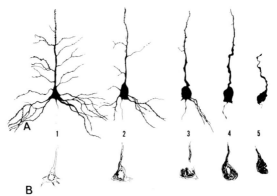

Fig. 5–3. Summary of the progression of senile changes in human cortical pyramidal cells as seen with Golgi impregnations (*A*) and Bielschowsky's stains (*B*). The former shows the progressive loss of the dendritic domain, whereas the latter shows the progressive development of the neurofibrillary changes of Alzheimer. Reproduced with permission from Scheibel, M. E., & Scheibel, A. B., Structural changes in the aging brain. In Brody, H., Harman, D., & Ordy, J. M., eds): *Aging* (Vol 1); *Clinical, morphologic, and neurochemical aspects in the aging nervous system.* New York: Raven Press, 1975.

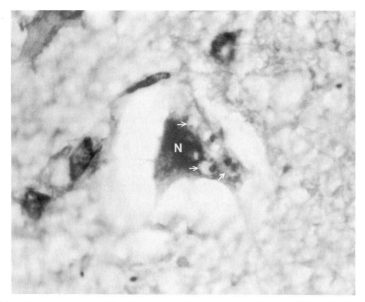

Fig. 5–4. Granulovacuolar degeneration in a hippocampal pyramidal cell. *Arrows* indicate vacuoles with dark inclusions. *N* = nucleus. Hematoxylin and eosin stain. Original magnification = 1000×.

clusively in the hippocampus in the brains of 22 of 28 nondemented old people. Similar findings were reported by Dayan (1970a), while Ball (1977) found at least an occasional neurofibrillary tangle in the hippocampus in all 18 brains of normal persons over 47 years old. Matsuyama and Nakamura (1978) have demonstrated an increase in the number of neurofibrillary tangles with increasing age in normals.

Neurofibrillary tangles are not specific for aging

or Alzheimer's disease. Typical tangles (with double helical filaments) have been documented in young persons with a variety of diseases including lead encephalopathy, Down's syndrome, tuberous sclerosis, subacute sclerosing panencephalitis, Hallervorden-Spatz disease and lipofuscinosis (Wisniewski, Jervis, Moretz, & Wisniewski, 1979). Lead poisoning produced neurofibrillary tangles in animals, and although most of the filaments that make

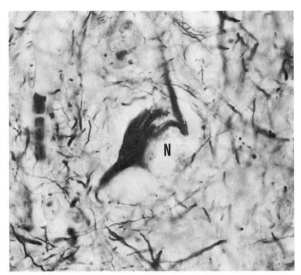

Fig. 5–5. A cortical neuron demonstrating neurofibrillary tangles. The dark-staining neurofibrillary tangles arch around the lightly staining nucleus (*N*). Modified Sevier-Mungen stain. Original magnification = 1000×.

up these tangles are straight, a few are twisted (Nicklowitz, 1975). Apart from this, however, typical double helical filaments have only been found in human brains.

In the brains of both normal elderly patients and patients with Alzheimer's disease, neurons with neurofibrillary tangles have a much higher concentration of aluminum than histologically normal neurons (Perl and Brody, 1980). Since the brains of patients with Alzheimer's disease contain more neurofibrillary tangles than the brains of non-demented aging persons (see the section on the pathology of Alzheimer disease below), they should have higher concentrations of aluminum. This was found by Crapper and his colleagues (Crapper, Karlik, & DeBoni, 1978; Crapper, Krishnan, & Dalton, 1973; Crapper, Krishnan, & Quittkat, 1976), but not by McDermott, Smith, Iqbal, & Wisniewski (1979), who found that brain aluminum concentration was related to age but not to the presence of dementia. Experimentally, aluminum produces neurofibrillary tangles in animals; however, no double helical filaments are seen. Neurofibrillary tangles are not seen in the brains of patients dying of dialysis dementia, despite usually high concentrations of aluminum (Alfrey, Le Gendre, & Kaehny, 1976).

NEURITIC ("SENILE") PLAQUES

These structures were originally described by Blocq and Marinesco in 1892. They are found in the neuropil, which are areas of brain made up principally of neuronal processes and supporting cells, rather than in the nerve cell bodies. The classical neuritic plaque appears under the light microscope to be composed of a central core of amyloid, surrounded by granules, filamentous material, and reactive cells (see Fig. 5–6). Under the electron microscope, it has been shown that the filamentous and granular material of the plaque represent degenerating neuronal processes. Amyloid deposition and cellular infiltration are thought to be secondary events (Wisniewski & Terry, 1973; Wisniewski, Terry, & Hirano, 1970). Neuritic plaques are present in the brains of normal aging persons (Dayan, 1970a; Tomlinson et al., 1968), but they are also present in disease states in persons under 65 (Down's syndrome, Alzheimer's disease) and have been found in normal aged dogs and monkeys (Wisniewski & Terry, 1973).

Neuritic plaques are distributed differently from neurofibrillary tangles. Whereas tangles are found (in normals) principally in the hippocampus, neuritic plaques most often have been observed in the amygdala, but have also been found in cortex, hippocampus, and basal ganglia (Tomlinson et al., 1968). With aging (Dayan, 1970a) and in pathologic processes (Corsellis, 1978), neurofibrillary tangles may be seen without much plaque formation, and vice versa, making it appear unlikely that plaques form in response to the neuronal dysfunction caused by neurofibrillary tangles.

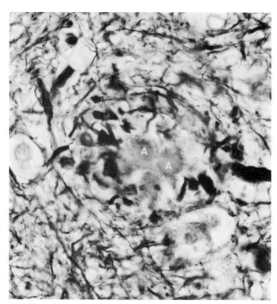

Fig. 5—6. Neuritic ("senile") plaque. Thickened, dark-staining, degenerating neural processes are seen surrounding a central amyloid core (*A*). Modified Sevier-Munger stain. Original magnification = 1000×.

MISCELLANEOUS CHANGES

With increasing age, a number of other nonspecific changes are seen. Other types of neuronal inclusions such as Hirano bodies and Lewy bodies (Wisniewski & Terry, 1973) are seen, and binucleated neurons and axonal spheroids have been observed. Corpora amylacea have been found in glial processes (Adler, 1953; Averbach & Langevin, 1978), although an age-associated increase in the numbers of glial cells has been questioned (Bondareff, 1977). In addition to the increased incidence of atherosclerotic and hypertensive vascular disease with age, congophilic (amyloid) angiopathy has been described in the brains of normal old people (Mandybur, 1975).

THE RELATIONSHIP OF ALZHEIMER'S DISEASE TO NORMAL AGING

Definition

The term dementia refers to acquired deficits in intellectual and emotional behavior. Many aspects of behavior may be affected including memory, cognitive processes (such as language and visuospatial processes), motivation, and emotional behavior. The extent to which each of these is affected depends on the nature, extent, and location of the pathologic process producing the dementia. As the term is generally used, conditions affecting only one process, such as language or memory, are not included among the dementias. Although the term dementia often connotes progression and irreversibility, there are many disorders of intellectual and emotional behavior that are not progressive, and many that improve with treatment. For further discussion of these issues, the reader is referred to Wells (1977).

The custom of dividing the dementias according to age of onset into presenile (onset before 65) and senile forms has met with the difficulty that the most common form of senile dementia has the same clinical presentation and the same pathology as the form of presenile dementia described by Alzheimer (Katzman, 1976; Neumann & Cohn, 1953; Newton, 1948; Wisniewski & Terry, 1973). Although it is still debated whether or not there is a separate presenile form of Alzheimer's disease, it has become common practice to use the term Alzheimer's disease to refer to any dementia that has the characteristic clinical and pathologic findings, regardless of the age of the patient. Although there are many other conditions that cause dementia, the following discussion will be limited to Alzheimer's disease because of its special relationship to the problem of aging.

Clinical Features of Alzheimer's Disease

Alzheimer's disease is the most common cause of dementia, accounting for half of the cases in several autopsy series (Freemon, 1976; Jellinger, 1976; Marsden & Harrison, 1972). Women are affected more often than men, even when the excess of females in the geriatric population is accounted for (Constantinidis, 1978). The patient with Alzheimer's disease usually presents with a disturbance of recent memory, combined with verbal and nonverbal cognitive deficits, such as aphasia, apraxia, and visuospatial and constructional disorders (Coblentz, Mattis, Zingesser, Kasoff, Wiesniewski, & Katzman, 1973; Sjögren, Sjögren, & Lindgren, 1952). Mild disturbances of frontal lobe function, such as loss of motivation and failure to plan, may be seen early in the disease, but prominent frontal lobe disturbances such as akinesia, gait apraxia, and urinary incontinence are usually seen only late in the disease. Seizures and myoclonic jerks may be encountered, but elementary neurological disturbances, such as weakness and sensory loss, are not seen. Progression is slow but relentless, and life expectancy is reduced (Katzman, 1976).

Laboratory evaluation of Alzheimer's disease is usually unremarkable. The electroencephalogram (EEG) is commonly normal in the early stages of the disease. Later, nonspecific slowing is seen, sometimes associated with paroxysmal activity. The computerized tomographic scan can be normal or show mild atrophy early in the disease; later, considerable cortical atrophy usually is demonstrated. The cerebrospinal fluid (CSF) protein content may be slightly elevated, but the CSF is otherwise normal. The diagnosis rests on the history, the typical clinical findings, and the exclusion of other causes of dementia by appropriate tests.

The Pathology of Alzheimer's Disease

There is no pathologic change associated with Alzheimer's disease that is not also seen in the "normal" aging human brain. The classical changes of Alzheimer's disease have therefore already been described in this chapter. They include neurofibrillary degeneration, development of neuritic ("senile") plaques, and granulovacuolar degeneration. Hirano bodies and congophilic angiopathy have also been described.

Even though there are no known *qualitative* differences between the brains of normal old people and the brains of patients with Alzheimer's disease, there are dramatic quantitative differences. Corsellis (1962) found that the severity of Alzheimer-type changes correlated with the presence of dementia, and Tomlinson and his colleagues (as summarized by Tomlinson, 1977), using psychologic data collected shortly prior to death, found a strong correlation between the number of senile plaques and the degree of dementia. They also found that neurofibrillary tangles were more common in patients with dementia, and more commonly affected the cerebral neocortex, instead of just the hippocampus. Furthermore, the degree of granulovacuolar degeneration in the hippocampus was highly correlated with the presence of dementia. These findings are consistent with a substantial number of studies using retrospective data to determine the presence of dementia (Ball, 1976, 1977; Ball & Lo, 1977; Corsellis, 1962; Dayan, 1970b; Woodward, 1966)). Scheibel and his colleagues (Scheibel, 1978; Scheibel et al., 1975, 1976) demonstrated progressive loss of dendritic and axonal branches and of dendritic spines in human cerebral cortex, which correlated better with poor intellectual function than with age. Scheibel (1978) speculated that this involution of neurons may correlate with neurofibrillary degeneration in the cell body.

Alzheimer's Disease versus Normal Aging

Matsuyama and Nakamura (1978) found at least minimal Alzheimer-type changes (neuritic plaques and neurofibrillary tangles) in about 50 percent of nondemented patients in their sixth decade, and in nearly 100 percent in their eighth decade, while all patients over 80 had at least moderate changes. The presence of Alzheimer-type changes in the vast majority of elderly persons' brains has led some to suggest that Alzheimer's disease is the extreme of a spectrum of pathologic changes associated with aging (Terry, 1978). The implication is that Alzheimer's disease may be the expression of aging in the central nervous system. Even if this were true, it would still be necessary to ask why some people get Alzheimer's disease decades before others. Why should there be a predisposition toward "aging"?

The neurohistological changes common to aging and Alzheimer's disease do not necessarily prove the identity of these conditions. It is more likely that these changes are the only way the brain can react to several different types of insult. As discussed in the section on Microscopic Anatomy, each of the three common neurohistological changes (neurofibrillary tangles, neuritic plaques and granulovacuolar degeneration) can occur in other conditions, some of which affect young persons. Since these changes are non-specific, it is possible that Alzheimer's disease itself may turn out to have several different etiologies.

If Alzheimer's disease is different from aging, it should be possible to demonstrate a qualitative difference between the brains in these conditions. As noted in the section on The Pathology of Alzheimer's Disease, Alzheimer-type changes in the brains of demented patients affect areas not usually affected in non-demented patients of similar age. Another possible difference relates to cell loss. If neurons are lost with increasing age, and if Alzheimer's disease were simply an acceleration of the aging process, neuronal loss would be a prominent feature of Alzheimer's disease. If cells were not lost with dementia, this would represent an important difference between dementia and the aging process. The evidence is conflicting. Several studies have demonstrated a dramatic difference in neuron counts between non-demented and Alzheimer patients of similar age, demented patients suffering 50 to 80 percent greater loss than normals (Ball, 1977; Bowen, Smith, White, Flack, Carrasco, Gedye, & Davison, 1977; Shefer, 1973); however, other studies have failed to find any difference between these two groups, even when counting was performed by neurochemical techniques (DeKosky & Bass, 1979) or automated counters (Terry, 1979; Terry, Fitzgerald, Peck, Millner, & Farmer, 1977; Tomlinson & Henderson, 1976). In addition to differences in counting technique, differences in site of sampling (hippocampus versus neocortex) and the failure to correct for a possible decrease in brain volume with dementia may account for some of this discrepancy.

The most dramatic difference between patients with Alzheimer-type senile dementia and normal elderly persons is in the chemical composition of the brain, as discussed in the following section. Complete resolution of the problem of the relation of Alzheimer's disease to normal aging must await better understanding of the pathogenesis of Alzheimer's disease, as well as the events contributing to the aging process. It is certainly of pragmatic value to consider Alzheimer's dementia a disease, rather than an inevitable accompaniment of aging, since investigation and treatment are better served by this approach. This is also in accord with clinical evidence that psychologic decline is not inevitable with

advanced age (Keevil-Rogers & Schnore, 1969; Palmore, 1974).

NEUROCHEMICAL CHANGES: NEUROTRANSMITTER ACTIVITY

A full review of the neurochemical changes in the aging brain and in dementia is beyond the scope of this chapter. The reader may consult reviews for an introduction to this extensive area (Dhopeshwarkar & Mead, 1975; Ordy, Kaack, & Brizzee, 1975; Shelanski, 1976). Neurochemical techniques are powerful tools for the study of quantitative changes in brain structure. Because certain organic substances are concentrated in specific structures, they can be used as markers for these structures. For example, DNA can be used as a marker for cell nuclei, and cerebrosides as a marker for myelin. Combining neurochemical and histologic analyses, estimates can be made of cell concentration (neurons versus glia) and of the extent of cellular processes, among other things (Hess & Pope, 1972). Using these techniques, DeKosky and Bass (1979) confirmed Brody's histologic studies demonstrating the loss of small neurons from human cortex with age. DeKosky and Bass also provided evidence that dementia is associated with shrinkage of the axodendritic tree (as Scheibel and his colleagues [1978] demonstrated using the Golgi technique) and not with loss of neurons.

In addition to supplementing histologic studies, neurochemical analysis permits investigation of specific chemical changes in the brain, among them changes in neurotransmitters and related molecules. Neurons communicate with each other via chemicals called neurotransmitters. At this time, evidence regarding the relationship of aging to neurotransmitters is fragmentary, and at times contradictory. Concentrations of neurotransmitter, of enzymes required for neurotransmitter synthesis and degradation, and of neurotransmitter receptor sites, have been measured. Some authors report loss of synthetic capacity in cholinergic, monoaminergic, and gamma-aminobutyric acid (GABA) systems (Davies, 1978b; McGeer, 1978; McGeer & McGeer, 1976) while others find no decrease in the concentration of choline acetyltransferase (CAT), the enzyme required for synthesis of acetylcholine (ACh) (Bowen et al., 1979). The concentration of ACh receptor sites, however, has been reported to decrease in normal aged brains (White, Hiley, Goodhardt, Carrasco, Keet, Williams, & Bowen, 1977). Bowen, Smith, White, Goodhardt, Spillane, Flack, & Davison (1977) found that the only glutamic acid decarboxylase (GAD), a synthetic enzyme for GABA, decreased with age. Decreases in glial cells and serotonin receptors (Bowen et al., 1979) and increases in monoamine oxidase (MAO) (Robinson, Davies, & Nies, 1972) have also been reported. Other changes are summarized in recent reviews (McGeer, 1978; McGeer & McGeer, 1976; Samorajski, 1977). In addition to differences in technique, size of sample, case selection, and other variables, differences in site of sampling may account for some of the discrepancies noted (McGeer & McGeer, 1976).

While there is little agreement about the changes in neurotransmitter metabolism with age alone, there is considerable evidence that choline acetyltransferase (CAT) is selectively diminished in Alzheimer's disease (Bowen, Smith, White, & Davison, 1976; Bowen, White, Spillane, et al., 1979; Davies, 1978a, 1978b; Perry, Tomlinson, Blessed, et al., 1977; White et al, 1977). Furthermore, in Alzheimer's disease, the level of CAT correlates with the degree of dementia and with the number of senile plaques (Perry, Tomlinson, Blessed, et al., 1978). A decrease in the concentration of acetylcholinesterase, the degradative enzyme for ACh, has also been found (Davies, 1978b), whereas the concentration of ACh receptor sites apparently remains normal (Davies, 1978a, 1978b; White et al., 1977). These findings indicate that in Alzheimer's disease there may be a selective decrease in the metabolic activity (if not the actual numbers) of cholinergic neurons. Since a disturbance of recent memory is a prominent finding in Alzheimer's disease, it is especially relevant that ACh appears to be an important neurotransmitter for normal memory function. Centrally acting anticholinergic drugs, such as scopolamine, produce an amnestic state (Drachman & Leavitt, 1974), while substances that increase ACh activity, such as choline and physostigmine, have been reported to have beneficial effects on memory in normal people (Davis, Mohs, Tinklenberg, Pfefferbaum, Hollister, & Kopell, 1978; Sitaram, Weingartner, & Gillin, 1978). Oral administration of choline and of lecithin (the major source of choline in the diet) increases ACh concentrations in the brain of rats (Hirsch & Wurtman, 1978). Treatment of patients with Alzheimer's disease with choline has not yet been shown to improve memory (Boyd, Graham-White, Blackwood, Glenn, & McQueen, 1977; Ferris, Santhananthan, Gershon, & Clark, 1977).

PHYSIOLOGICAL MEASURES IN AGING

Cerebral Blood Flow

In addition to the increased prevalence of atherosclerosis and of hypertensive vascular changes in old age, progressive vascular changes are noted in normal aging. Large vessels show loss of resiliency and opacification (Fang, 1976), while small vessels demonstrate increased tortuosity (Fang, 1976; Hunziker, Abdel'Al, Frey, Veteau, & Meier-Ruge, 1978). Atherosclerosis and arteriolosclerosis, both significantly related to hypertension, can result in focal death of brain tissue (infarction).

Although multiple infarction is probably the second most common cause of dementia in old age, it is unlikely that vascular disease plays an important part in the pathogenesis of the commonest form of dementia, Alzheimer's disease. The studies of Tomlinson and his colleagues (summarized by Tomlinson, 1977) provide persuasive evidence. Careful pathologic investigation of 50 demented patients revealed that in only 18 percent of the group, multiple infarction was the only pathologic finding that correlated with dementia, while 50 percent had severe Alzheimer's disease without evidence of infarction (to a degree greater than nondemented controls). In only 18 percent of demented patients did these two pathologic conditions (Alzheimer's disease and multiple infarction) coexist. If vascular disease was an important factor in the development of Alzheimer's disease, one would expect that most brains with Alzheimer-type changes would also demonstrate evidence of vascular disease, whereas in fact only 24 percent did. It is in this light that the literature on cerebral blood flow in dementia should be approached.

Cerebral blood flow (CBF) can be measured by various techniques. Most involve the administration of an inert, usually radioactive, substance. The substance can be given intra-arterially (which presents some hazard to the patient) or by intravenous injection or inhalation. Total CBF can be measured, or multiple detectors can be placed over the head to estimate regional cerebral blood flow.

Most studies of normal subjects reveal progressive diminution of total CBF with age (Kety, 1956; Lavy, Melamed, Bentin, Cooper, & Rirrot, 1978; Obrist, 1978; Wang & Busse, 1975). However, when care is taken to exclude patients with even minimal dementia or significant systemic disease, including atherosclerosis, the CBF and the cerebral rate of oxygen consumption (CMRO2) do not differ from young adult levels, although in hypertensive subjects there is an increase in cerebrovascular resistance (Dastur, Lane, Hansen, Kety, Butler, Perlin, & Sokoloff, 1963; Sokoloff, 1975, 1978).

Cerebral blood flow and CMRO2 are both reduced in patients with severe dementia, regardless of etiology. Several studies demonstrate that early in the course of dementia, it may be possible to distinguish multi-infarct dementia from Alzheimer's disease on the basis of the CBF. The CBF is decreased in multi-infarct dementia, but not in comparably demented patients with Alzheimer's disease (Hachinski, 1978; Hachinski, Iliff, Zilkha, DuBoulay, McAllister, Marshall, Ross-Russe, & Symon, 1975; Hoyer, 1978; O'Brien & Mallett, 1970). Other investigators, however, have failed to find this difference (Ingvar, Brun, Hagberg, & Gustafson, 1978; Ingvar & Gustafson, 1970; Lavy et al., 1978), although it is possible that they were investigating patients with more severe disease. The decline of CBF and CMRO2 in Alzheimer's disease is probably due to lowered metabolic demand and not to vascular disease.

Studies of regional cerebral blood flow have demonstrated that the major decrease in blood flow in Alzheimer's disease is in the temporal and parietal regions and the frontal lobes (Ingvar et al., 1978; Ingvar & Gustafson, 1970; Meyer, Welch, Titus, Suzuki, Kim, Perez, Mathew, Gedye, Hrastnik, Miyakawa, Achar, & Dodson, 1976; Obrist, Chivian, Cronqvist & Ingvar, 1970; Simard, Olesen, Paulson, Lassen, & Skinhj, 1971). This distribution coincides with the regions of maximal atrophy in Alzheimer's disease (Ingvar et al., 1978; Ingvar & Gustafson, 1970). Gustafson, Hagberg, & Ingvar (1978) demonstrated that the type of language disturbance in women with Alzheimer's disease correlated with the distribution of diminished CBF. That is, patients with decreased temporoparietooccipital CBF demonstrated poor comprehension with other "receptive" disorders such as alexia, whereas patients with frontal reductions in CBF had "expressive" language disturbances.

Electroencephalographic Changes with Aging

THE ELECTROENCEPHALOGRAM (EEG)

The EEG is the record of the electrical activity of the brain (principally of the slow potentials of cortical dendrites) obtained from electrodes placed on the scalp. The EEG can be described in terms of the dominant frequencies of the voltage oscillations recorded. Normal adults, in the nonalerted awake state, usually have a dominant 8 to 13 Hz background rhythm (called alpha rhythm), seen best over the posterior regions of the head, and a faster, less regular activity (beta rhythms), observed particularly over the anterior regions of the head. In the older population, certain deviations from the normal adult EEG pattern are increasingly likely to occur (Marsh & Thompson, 1977; Obrist & Busse, 1965; Thompson, 1976).

Four types of change have been described, as follows:

1. Alpha (8 – 13 Hz) activity decreases from a mean of 10 to 10.5 Hz in normal young adults to a mean of 8.0 to 9.7 Hz in a population over 60. Longitudinal studies (Wang & Busse, 1969) showed a modest decline in alpha frequency with each decade over the age of 60, although there were patients whose alpha frequency remained the same or even increased. Slow alpha activity has been correlated with a larger verbal-performance gap on the Wechsler Adult Intelligence Scale (WAIS) and has been used as a predictor of intellectual decline (Wang, Obrist & Busse, 1970).

2. Activity faster than the alpha range (beta activity) may become more prevalent during later middle age; however, it is less evident over the age of 70 and in older patients with intellectual deterioration (Busse & Obrist, 1965; Wang, Obrist & Busse, 1970).

3. Diffuse slow activity (frequencies below alpha activity) is seen in about 20 percent of normals over the age of 75. Within this group, it correlates with poor intellectual function and, in longitudinal studies, with a higher incidence of intellectual decline.

4. Finally, 30 to 50 percent of normal old persons have episodic high-voltage slow activity in the temporal region sometimes associated with sharp waves in the left hemisphere. Although some authors have found this focal EEG finding to correlate with poorer performance on the WAIS (Drachman & Hughes, 1971) and to be a predictor of verbal deterioration (Wang, Obrist, & Busse, 1970), others have not found any correlation with intellectual function (Obrist, 1971). The cause of this intriguing EEG finding remains unknown.

AVERAGED EVENT-RELATED POTENTIALS

In the normal alert subject, a single sensory stimulus produces such a small change in the EEG that it is usually indistinguishable from the background EEG activity. Superimposition of segments of the EEG that are time-locked to a repeated stimulus may reveal a pattern of response to the sensory stimulus. This pattern is more evident if these segments of EEG are averaged by a computer. As the EEG "responses" to more stimuli are averaged, random EEG activity (that is, activity not time-locked to the stimulus) will average out and approach zero amplitude, while the portion of the EEG signal that is time-locked to the stimulus will be progressively easier to distinguish from the background. The resulting potential is called the averaged evoked potential.

Averaged evoked responses can be divided into early and late components. The early components (generally occurring within 180 msec of the stimulus) can themselves be divided into two groups: (1) very early, far-field recorded potentials that reflect events in the spinal cord and brainstem, and (2) longer-latency potentials best recorded over the appropriate primary sensory areas, which are presumed to reflect cortical sensory processing. Late components (with latencies over 150 msec) are usually of largest amplitude over the parietal and posterior frontal regions and have been associated with higher-order processing an decision making (Goodin, Squires, & Starr, 1978; Marsh & Thompson, 1977).

Several studies have documented a small increase in latency of the early cortical components of the evoked potential with increasing age for somatosensory potentials (Shagass & Schwartz, 1965), auditory potentials (Goodin, Squires, Henderson, & Starr, 1978), and visual potentials (Celesia & Daly, 1977). Amplitude changes are less uniform. Shagass and Schwartz (1965) reported an increase in the amplitude of early somatosensory potentials with age, whereas Goodin, Squires, Henderson, & Starr (1978) showed a slight decrease in the amplitude of early components.

Of the late components, the third major positive deflection (P3 component) of the auditory evoked response has been the most thoroughly studied. Goodin, Squires and Starr (1978) demonstrated that between the ages of 15 and 76, the latency of the P3 component increased 1.64 msec per year. Marsh and Thompson (1972) reported a similar change. An increase in the latency of the visual-evoked P3 response in old persons has also been reported (see Marsh & Thompson, 1977). Of interest is the recent demonstration that the latency of the auditory P3 component (but not that of the P2 wave) is selectively prolonged in demented subjects when compared to comparably aged normals (Goodin, Squires, & Starr, 1978). These authors proposed that the evoked response may contribute to the clinical assessment of dementia.

Another event-related potential that has been studied in aging is the contingent negative variation (CNV), a slow negative potential shift that occurs prior to an expected signal. In the usual paradigm, a warning stimulus (S1) is given, and the patient must make a motor or mental response to a second stimulus (S2). The CNV occurs prior to the second stimulus. The more attention the subject pays to the task, the larger the CNV (Tecce, 1972). Loveless and Sanford (1974) showed that as the S1−S2 interval is increased, old subjects develop a progressively smaller CNV when compared to young subjects.

Sleep Studies

It is commonly appreciated that sleep habits change with age. These changes have been documented by Feinberg (1969, 1976) who found that, compared with young adults, elderly subjects (aged 65 to 96 years) showed increases in the number of awakenings and the percent of time spent awake in bed. There was a decline in time spent in stage 4 of sleep (as defined electroencephalographically), and there was a decline in the amount of rapid-eye-movement (REM) sleep. In this connection, it is of interest (as noted in the section on Neuronal Dropout) that Brody (1978) has documented a decrease in the numbers of neurons in the locus ceruleus with age in humans, since the locus ceruleus, a small brainstem nucleus from which extensive and important noradrenergic pathways originate, has been demonstrated to be important for the maintenance of REM sleep.

SUMMARY AND CONCLUSIONS

There are numerous morphological changes in the brains of aged humans, many of which correlate with intellectual function. It is still not clear which of these changes are obligatory effects of aging and which can be considered manifestations of disease. Most of the morphological changes reviewed show a striking regional distribution. Neuronal dropout does not occur in most brainstem nuclei, but occurs prominently in the locus ceruleus. Cortical neuronal loss has been more difficult to study, but appears also to be nonuniform. Granulovacuolar degeneration and neurofibrillary tangles have a predilection for neurons of the hippocampus, while neuritic ("senile") plaques are distributed more widely. The regional distribution of these and other morphological changes must in part determine the nature of the intellectual deficits acquired with aging. It is premature to say what the "normal" changes have to do with language function; however, prominent morphological changes have been described in the superior temporal gyrus (Brody, 1955), an area important in language processing. In Alzheimer's disease, language deficits probably result from lesions in the parietotemporal cortex.

Biochemical changes have just begun to be explored, with the exciting result that choline acetyltransferase has been found to be selectively diminished in Alzheimer's disease. It is hoped that these and similar investigations may lead the way toward rational pharmacological therapy for previ-ously untreatable dementias, just as L-dopa provided a treatment for Parkinson's disease. Biochemical methods should enhance our ability to correlate behavior with brain anatomy and physiology, especially as regional differences in chemical and physiologic processes are explored. No information currently available relates biochemical events to language.

Physiologic studies have shown modest changes in the EEG of normal subjects with aging. Because the physiology underlying the EEG is poorly understood, these EEG changes tell us little about the pathophysiology of aging. Averaged event-related potentials are somewhat easier to correlate with specific behavioral variables, and the later components of these potentials (as well as the contingent negative variation) correlate with cognitive and attentional processes. Further application of these methods may well be helpful in understanding the changes in the brain that accompany both normal and pathologic aging.

REFERENCES

Alder, N. On the nature, origin and distribution of the corpora amylacea of the brain with observations on some new staining reactions. *Journal of Mental Science,* 1953, *99,* 689–697.

Alfrey, A. C., Le Gendre, G. R., & Kaehny, W. D. The dialysis encephalopathy syndrome: Possible aluminum intoxication. *New England Journal of Medicine,* 1976, *294,* 184–188.

Averbach, P., & Langevin, H. Corpora amylacea of the lumbar spinal cord and peripheral nervous system. *Archives of Neurology,* 1978, *35,* 95–96.

Ball, M. J. Neurofibillary tangles and the pathogenesis of dementia. *Neuropathology and Applied Neurobiology,* 1976, *2,* 395–410.

Ball, M. J. Neuronal loss, neurofibrillary tangles and granulovacuolar degeneration in the hippocampus with aging and dementia. A quantitative study. *Acta Neuropathologica (Berlin),* 1977, *37,* 111–118.

Ball, M. J., & Lo, P. Granulovacuolar degeneration in the aging brain and in dementia. *Journal of Neuropathology and Experimental Neurology,* 1977, *36,* 474–487.

Barron, S. A., Jacobs, L., & Kinkel, W. R. Changes in size of normal lateral ventricles during aging determined by computerized tomography. *Neurology,* 1976, *26,* 1011–1013.

Berlin, M. & Wallace, R. B. Aging and the central nervous system. *Experimental Aging Research,* 1976, *2,* 125–164.

Bondareff, W. The neural basis of aging. In J. E. Birren & K. W. Schaie (Eds.), *Handbook of the psychology of aging.* New York: Van Nostrand Reinhold, 1977.

Bowen, D. M., Smith, C. B., White, P., & Davison, A. N. Neurotransmitter-related enzymes and indices of hypoxia in senile dementia and other abiotrophies. *Brain,* 1976, *99,* 459–496.

Bowen, D. M., Smith, C. B., White, P., Flack, R. H. A., Carrasco, L., Gedye, J. L., & Davison, A. N. Chemical pathology of the organic dementias. II. Quantitative estimation of cellular changes in post-mortem brains. *Brain,* 1977, *100,* 427–453.

Bowen, D. M., Smith, C. B., White, P., Goodhardt, M. J., Spillane, J. A., Flack, R. H. A., & Davison, A. N. Chemical pathology of the organic dementias. I. Validity of biochemical measurements on human post-mortem brain specimens. *Brain,* 1977, *100,* 397–426.

Bowen, D. M., White, P., Spillane, J. A., Goodhardt, M. J., Curzon, G., Igwanoff, P.,

Meier-Ruge, W., & Davison, A. N. Accelerated aging or selective neuronal loss as an important cause of dementia. *Lancet*, 1979, *1*, 11−14.

Boyd, W. D., Graham-White, J., Blackwood, G., Glen, I., McQueen, J. Clinical effects of choline in Alzheimer senile dementia. *Lancet*, 1977, *2*, 711.

Brizzee, K. R., Harkin, J. C., Ordy, J. M., & Kaack, B. Accumulation and distribution of lipofuscin, amyloid and senile plaques in the aging nervous system. In H. Brody, D. Harman & J. M. Ordy (Eds.), *Clinical, morphologic, and neurochemical aspects in the aging nervous system*. New York: Raven Press, 1975.

Brizzee, K. R., Ordy, J. M., Hofer, H., & Kaack, B. Animal models for the study of senile brain disease and aging changes in the brain. In R. Katzman, R. D. Terry, & K. L. Bick (Eds.), *Alzheimer's disease: Senile dementia and related disorders*. New York: Raven Press, 1978.

Brody, H. Organization of the cerebral cortex. III. A study of aging in the human cerebral cortex. *Journal of Comparative Neurology*, 1955, *102*, 511−556.

Brody, H. Cell counts in cerebral cortex and brainstem in Alzheimer's disease: Senile dementia and related disorders. In R. Katzman, R. D. Terry, & K. L. Bick (Eds.), *Alzheimer's disease: Senile dementia and related disorders*. New York: Raven Press, 1978.

Busse, E. W., & Obrist, W. D. Pre-senescent electroencephalographic changes in normal subjects. *Journal of Gerontology*, 1965, *20*, 315−320.

Carlsson, C. A., von Essen, C., & Lofgren, J. Factors affecting the clinical course of patients with severe head injuries. Part 1. Influence of biological factors. Part 2. Significance of post-traumatic coma. *Journal of Neurosurgery*, 1968, *29*, 242−251.

Celesia, G. G., & Daly, R. F. Effects of aging on visual evoked responses. *Archives of Neurology*, 1977, *34*, 403−407.

Coblentz, J. M., Mattis, S., Zingesser, L. H., Kasoff, S. S., Wisniewski, H. M., & Katzman, R. Presenile dementia: Clinical aspects and evaluation of cerebrospinal fluid dynamics. *Archives of Neurology*, 1973, *29*, 299−308.

Colon, E. J. The elderly brain—a quantitative analysis in the cerebral cortex in two cases. *Psychiatria, Neurologia, and Neurochirurgia (Amsterdam)*, 1972, *75*, 261−270.

Constantinidis, J. Is Alzheimer's disease a major form of senile dementia? Clinical, anatomical, and genetic data. In R. Katzman, R. D. Terry, & K. L. Bick (Eds.), *Alzheimer's disease: Senile dementia and related disorders*. New York: Raven Press, 1978.

Corsellis, J. A. N. *Mental illness and the aging brain*. London: Oxford University Press, 1962.

Corsellis, J. A. N. Post-traumatic dementia. In R. Katzman, R. D. Terry, & K. L. Bick (Eds.), *Alzheimer's disease: Senile dementia and related disorders*. New York: Raven Press, 1978.

Cotman, C. W. (Ed.). *Neuronal plasticity*. New York: Raven Press, 1978.

Cragg, B. G. The density of synapses and neurons in normal, mentally defective, and aging human brains. *Brain*, 1975, *98*, 81−90.

Crapper, D. R., Karlik, S., & DeBoni, U. Aluminum and other metals in senile (Alzheimer) dementia. In R. Katzman, R. D. Terry, & K. L. Bick (Eds.), *Alzheimer's disease: Senile dementia and related disorders*. New York: Raven Press, 1978.

Crapper, D. R., Krishnan, S. S., & Dalton, A. J. Brain aluminum distribution in Alzheimer's disease and experimental neurofibrillary degeneration. *Science*, 1973, *180*, 511−513.

Crapper, D. R., Krishnan, S. S. & Quittkat, S. Aluminum, neurofibrillary degeneration and Alzheimer's disease. *Brain*, 1976, *99*, 67−80.

Dastur, D. K., Lane, M. H., Hansen, D. B., Kety, S. S., Butler, R. N., Perlin, S., & Sokoloff, L. Effects of aging on the cerebral circulation and metabolism in man. In J. E. Birren, R. N. Butler, S. W. Greenhouse, L. Sokoloff, & M. R. Yarrow (Eds.), *Human aging–A biological and behavioral study*. Washington, D. C., 1963, PHS no. 986, pp. 59−76.

Davies, P. Aging of specific neurotransmitter systems and their involvement in senile dementia. *Journal of Neuropathology and Experimental Neurology*, 1978, *37*, 573. (a)

Davies, P. Studies on the neurochemistry of central cholinergic systems in Alzheimer's disease. In R. Katzman, R. D. Terry, & K. L. Bick (Eds.), *Alzheimer's disease: Senile dementia and related disorders*. New York: Raven Press, 1978. (b)

Davis, K. L., Mohs, R. C., Tinklenberg, J. R., Pfefferbaum, A., Hollister, L. E., & Kopell, B. S. Physostigmine: Improvement of long-term memory processes in normal humans. *Science,* 1978, *201,* 272–274.

Dayan, A. D. Quantitative histological studies on the aged human brain. I. Senile plaques and neurofibrillary tangles in "normal" patients. *Acta Neuropathologic (Berlin),* 1970, *16,* 85–94. (a)

Dayan, A. D. Quantitative histological studies on the aged human brain. II. Senile plaques and neurofibrillary tangles in "normal" patients. *Acta Neuropatholica (Berlin),* 1970, *16,* 95–102. (b)

Dekaban, A. S., & Sadowsky, D. Changes in brain weights during the span of human life: Relation of brain weights to body heights and body weights. *Annals of Neurology,* 1978, *4,* 345–356.

DeKosky, S. T., & Bass, N. H. Microchemical studies of cerebral cortex during aging and senile dementia. Defective neuronal arborization associated with intellectual deterioration. Paper presented at the meeting of the Academy of Neurology, Chicago, April 1979.

Dhopeshwarkar, G. A., & Mead, J. F. Age and lipids of the central nervous system: Lipid metabolism in the developing brain. In H. Brody, D. Harman, & J. M. Ordy (Eds.), *Clinical, morphologic and neurochemical aspects in the aging central nervous system.* New York: Raven Press, 1975.

Drachman, D. A., & Hughes, J. R. Memory and the hippocampal complexes: III. Aging and temporal EEG abnormalities. *Neurology,* 1971, *21,* 1–14.

Drachman, D. A., & Leavitt, J. Human memory and the cholinergic system. *Archives of Neurology,* 1974, *30,* 113–131.

Fang, H. C. H. Observations on aging characteristics of cerebral blood vessels, macroscopic and microscopic features. In R. D. Terry & S. Gershon (Eds.), *Neurobiology of aging.* New York: Raven Press, 1976.

Feinberg, I. Effects of age on human sleep patterns. In H. Kales (Ed.), *Sleep: Physiology and pathology.* Philadelphia: J. B. Lippincott, 1969.

Feinberg, I. Functional implications of changes in sleep physiology with age. In R. D. Terry & S. Gershon (Eds.), *Neurobiology of aging.* New York: Raven Press, 1976.

Ferris, S. N., Santhananthan, G., Gershon, S., & Clark, C. Senile dementia: Treatment with deanol. *Journal of the American Geriatrics Society,* 1977, *25,* 241–245.

Freemon, F. R. Evaluation of patients with progressive intellectual deterioration. *Archives of Neurology,* 1976, *33,* 658–659.

Goodin, D. C., Squires, K. C., Henderson, B., & Starr, A. Age-related variations in evoked potentials to auditory stimuli in normal human subjects. *Electrencephalographic and Clinical Neurophysiology,* 1978, *44,* 447–458.

Goodin, D. C., Squires, K. C., & Starr, A. Long latency event-related components of the auditory evoked potential in dementia. *Brain,* 1978, *101,* 635–648.

Gustafson, L., Hagberg, B., & Ingvar, D. H. Speech disturbances in presenile dementia related to local cerebral blood flow abnormalities in the dominant hemisphere. *Brain and Language,* 1978, *5,* 103–118.

Hachinski, V. C. Cerebral blood flow: Differentiation of Alzheimer's disease from multi-infarct dementia. In R. Katzman, R. D. Terry, & K. L. Bick (Eds.), *Alzheimer's disease: Senile dementia and related disorders.* New York: Raven Press, 1978.

Hachinski, V. C., Iliff, L. D., Zilkha, E., DuBoulay, G. H., McAllister, V. L., Marshall, J., Ross-Russe, R. W., & Symon, L. Cerebral blood flow in dementia. *Archives of Neurology,* 1975, *32,* 632–637.

Hall, T. C., Miller, A. K. H., & Corsellis, J. A. N. Variations in the human Purkinje cell population according to age and sex. *Neuropathology and Applied Neurobiology,* 1975, *1,* 267–292.

Hanley, T. Neuronal fallout in the aging brain: A critical review of the quantitative data. *Age and Ageing,* 1974, *3,* 133–151.

Hess, H. H., & Pope, A. Quantitative neurochemical histology. In A. Lajtha (Ed.), *Handbook of* neurochemistry. Vol. 7: Pathological chemistry of the nervous system. New York: Plenum Press, 1972.

Himwich, W. A. Problems in interpreting neurochemical changes occurring in developing and aging animals. In D. H. Ford (Ed.), Neurobiological aspects of maturation and aging. Amsterdam: Elsevier, 1973.

Hirsch, M. J., & Wurtman, R. J. Lecithin consumption increases acetylcholine concentrations in rat brain and adrenal gland. Science, 1978, 202, 223−225.

Hoyer, S. Blood flow and oxidative metabolism of the brain in different phases of dementia. In R. Katzman, R. D. Terry, & K. L. Bick (eds.), Alzheimer's disease: Senile dementia and related disorders. New York: Raven Press, 1978.

Hunziker, O., Abdel'Al, S., Frey, H., Veteau, M. J., & Meier-Ruge, W. Quantitative studies in the cerebral cortex of aging humans. Gerontology, 1978, 24, 27−31.

Ingvar, D. H., Brun. A., Hagberg, B., & Gustafson, L. Regional cerebral blood flow in the dominant hemisphere in confirmed cases of Alzheimer's disease, Pick's disease, and multi-infarct dementia: Relationship to clinical symptomatology and neuropathological findings. In R. Katzman, R. D. Terry, & K. L. Bick (Eds.), Alzheimer's disease: Senile dementia and related disorders. New York: Raven Press, 1978.

Ingvar, D. H., & Gustafson, L. Regional cerebral blood flow in organic dementia with early onset. Acta Neurologica Scandanavica, 1970, 46 (Supplement No. 43), 42−73.

Iqbal, K. Discussion. In R. Katzman, R. D. Terry, & K. L. Bick (Eds.), Alzheimer's disease: Senile dementia and related disorders. New York: Raven Press, 1978.

Iqbal, K., Grundke-Iqbal, I., Wisniewski, H. M., & Terry, R. D. Chemical relationship of the paired helical filaments of Alzheimer's dementia to normal human neurofilaments and neurotubules. Brain Research, 1978, 142, 321−332.

Jellinger, K. Neuropathological aspects of dementias resulting from abnormal blood and cerebospinal fluid dynamics. Acta Neurological Belgica, 1976, 76, 83−102.

Katzman, R. The prevalence and malignancy of Alzheimer's disease. Archives of Neurology, 1976, 33, 217−218.

Kaszniak, A. W., Garron, D. C., Fox, J. H., Bergen, D., & Huckman, M. Cerebral atrophy, EEG slowing, age, education, and cognitive functioning in suspected dementia. Neurology, 1979, 29, 1273−1279.

Keevil-Rogers, P. & Schnore, M. M. Short-term memory as a function of age in persons of above-average intelligence. Journal of Gerontology, 1969, 24, 184−188.

Kety, S. S. Human cerebral blood flow and oxygen consumption as related to aging. Research Publications of the Association for Research in Nervous and Mental Disorders, 1956, 35, 31−45.

Konigsmark, B. W., & Murphy, E. A. Volume of the ventral cochlear nucleus in man: Its relationship to neuronal population with age. Journal of Neuropathology and Experimental Neurology, 1972, 31, 304−316.

Lavy, S., Melamed, E., Bentin, S., Cooper, G., & Rirrot, Y. Bihemisphere decreases of regional cerebral blood flow in dementia: Correlation with age-matched normal controls. Annals of Neurology, 1978, 4, 445−450.

Loveless, N. E., & Sanford, A. J. Effects of age on the contingent negative variation and preparatory set in a reaction-time task. Journal of Gerontology, 1974, 29, 52−63.

Mandybur, T. I. Incidence of cerebral amyloid angiopathy in Alzheimer's disease. Neurology, 1975, 24, 120−126.

Marsden, C. D., & Harrison, M. J. G. Outcome of investigation of patients with presenile dementia. British Medical Journal, 1972, 2, 249−252.

Marsh, G. R., & Thompson, L. W. Age differences in evoked potentials during an auditory discrimination task. Gerontologist, 1972, 12, 44.

Marsh, G. R., & Thompson, L. W. Psychophysiology of aging. In J. E. Birren & K. W. Schaie (Eds.), Handbook of the psychology of aging. New York: Van Nostrand Reinhold, 1977.

Matsuyama, H., & Nakamura, S. Senile changes in the brain in the Japanese: incidence of

Alzheimer's neurofibrillary change and senile plaques. In R. Katzman, R. D. Terry, & K. L. Bick (Eds.), *Alzheimer's disease: Senile dementia and related disorders*. New York: Raven Press, 1978.

McDermott, J. R., Smith, A. I., Iqbal, K., & Wisniewski, H. M. Brain aluminum in aging and Alzheimer disease. *Neurology*, 1979, *29*, 809—814.

McGeer, E. Aging and neurotransmitter metabolism in the human brain. In R. Katzman, R. D. Terry, & K. L. Bick (Eds.), *Alzheimer's disease: Senile dementia and related disorders*. New York: Raven Press, 1978.

McGeer, E., & McGeer, P. L. Neurotransmitter metabolism in the aging brain. In R. D. Terry & S. Gershon (Eds.), *Neurobiology of aging*. New York: Raven Press, 1976.

McMenemey, W. H. The dementias and progressive diseases of the basal ganglia. In H. Blackwood (Ed.), *Greenfield's neuropathology*. London: Edward Arnold Ltd., 1963.

Messert, B., Wannamaker, B. B., & Dudley, A. W. Re-evaluation of the size of the lateral ventricles of the brain. *Neurology*, 1972, *22*, 941—951.

Meyer, J. S., Welch, K. M. A., Titus, J. L., Suzuki, M., Kim, H. S., Perez, F. I., Mathew, N. T., Gedye, J. L., Hrastnik, F., Miyakawa, Y., Achar, V. S., & Dodson, R. F. Neurotransmitter failure in cerebral infarction. In R. D. Terry & S. Gershon (Eds.), *Neurobiology of aging*. New York: Raven Press, 1976.

Monagle, R. D., & Brody, H. The effects of age upon the main nucleus of the inferior olive in the human. *Journal of Comparative Neurology*, 1974, *155*, 61—66.

Neumann, M. A., & Cohn, R. Incidence of Alzheimer's disease in a large mental hospital. *Archives of Neurology*, 1953, *69*, 615—636.

Newton, R. D. The identity of Alzheimer's disease and senile dementia and their relationship to senility. *British Journal of Psychiatry*, 1948, *94*, 225—249.

Nicklowitz, W. J. Neurofibrillary changes after acute experimental lead poisoning. *Neurology*, 1975, *25*, 927—934.

O'Brien, M. D., & Mallett, B. L. Cerebral cortex perfusion rates in dementia. *Journal of Neurology, Neurosurgery and Psychiatry*, 1970, *33*, 497—500.

Obrist, W. D. EEG and intellectual function in the aged. Paper presented at the 25th annual meeting of the American EEG Society, Minneapolis, September 1971.

Obrist, W. D., Noninvasive studies of cerebral blood flow in aging and dementia. In R. Katzman, R. D. Terry, & K. L. Bick (Eds.), *Alzheimer's disease: Senile dementia and related disorders*. New York: Raven Press, 1978.

Obrist, W. D., & Busse, E. W. The electroencephalogram in old age. In W. P. Wildon (Ed.), *Application of electroencephalography in psychiatry*. Durham, N. C.: Duke University Press, 1965.

Obrist, W. D., Chivian, E., Cronqvist, S., & Ingvar, D. H. Regional cerebral blood flow in senile and presenile dementia. *Neurology*, 1970, *20*, 315—322.

Ordy, J. M., Kaack, B., & Brizzee, K. R. Life-span neurochemical changes in the human and non-human primate brain. In H. Brody, D. Harman, & J. M. Ordy (Eds.), *Clinical, morphologic, and neurochemical aspects in the aging central nervous system*. New York: Raven Press, 1975.

Palmore, E. R. *Normal aging. Report from the Duke longitudinal study*. Durham, N. C.: Duke University Press, 1974.

Perl, D. P., & Brody, A. R. Alzheimer's disease: X-ray spectrometric evidence of aluminum accumulation in neurofibrillary tangle-bearing neurons. *Science*, 1980, *208*, 297—299.

Perry, E. K., Perry, R. H., Blessed, G., & Tomlinson, B. E. Necropsy evidence of central cholinergic deficits in senile dementia. *Lancet*, 1977, *1*, 189.

Perry, E. K., Tomlinson, B. E., Blessed, G., Bergmann, K., Gibson, P. H., & Perry, R. H. Correlation of cholinergic abnormalities with senile plaques and mental test scores in senile dementia. *British Medical Journal*, 1978, *2*, 1457—1459.

Purpura, D. P. Dendritic spine "dysgenesis" and mental retardation. *Science*, 1974, *186*, 1126—1128.

Roberts, M. A., & Caird, F. L. Computerized tomography and intellectual impairment in the elderly. *Journal of Neurology, Neurosurgery and Psychiatry*, 1976, *39*, 986–989.

Robinson, D. S., Davies, J. M., & Nies, A. Aging, monoamines and monoamine oxidase levels. *Lancet*, 1972, *1*, 290–291.

Samorajski, T. Central neurotransmitter substances and aging: A review. *Journal of the American Geriatrics Society*, 1977, *25*, 337–348.

Samorajski, R., Keefe, J. R., & Ordy, J. M. Intracellular localization of lipofuscin age pigments in the nervous system. *Journal of Gerontology*, 1964, *19*, 262–276.

Schade, J. P., & van Groenigen, W. B. Structural organization of the human cerebral cortex. I. Maturation of the middle frontal gyrus. *Acta Anatomica*, 1961, *47*, 74–111.

Scheff, S. W., Bernardo, L. S., & Cotman, C. W. Decrease in adrenergic axon sprouting in the senescent rat. *Science*, 1978, *202*, 775–778.

Scheibel, A. B. Structural aspects of the aging brain: Spine systems and the dendritic arbor. In Katzman, R., Terry, R. D., Bick, K. L., (eds.), *Alzheimer's disease: Senile dementia and related disorders*. New York: Raven Press, 1978.

Scheibel, M. E., Lindsay, R. D., Tomiyasu, U., & Scheibel, A. B. Progressive dendritic changes in aging human cortex. *Experimental Neurology*, 1975, *47*, 392–403.

Scheibel, M. E., Lindsay, R. D., Tomiyasu, U., & Scheibel, A. B. Progressive dendritic changes in the aging human limbic system. *Experimental Neurology*, 1976, *53*, 420–430.

Scheibel, A. B., & Tomiyasu, U. Dendritic sprouting in Alzheimer's presenile dementia. *Experimental Neurology*, 1978, *60*, 1–8.

Shagass, C., & Schwartz, M. Age, personality and somatosensory cerebral evoked responses. *Science*, 1965, *148*, 1359–1361.

Shefer, V. F. Absolute number of neurons and thickness of the cerebral cortex during aging, senile and vascular dementia and Pick's and Alzheimer's disease. *Neuroscience and Behavioral Psychology*, 1973, *6*, 319–324.

Shelanski, M. L. Neurochemistry of aging: Review and prospectus. In R. D. Terry & S. Gershon (Eds.), *Neurobiology of aging*. New York: Raven Press, 1976.

Siakotos, A. N., & Koppang, N. Procedures for the isolation of lipopigments from brain, heart and liver and their properties: A review. *Mechanisms of Ageing and Development*, 1973, *2*, 177–200.

Simard, D., Olesen, J., Paulson, O., Lassen, N.Q., & Skinhj, E. Regional cerebral blood flow in senile and presenile dementia. *Neurology*, 1971, *20*, 315–322.

Sitaram, N., Weingartner, H., & Gillin, J. C. Human serial learning enhancement with arecholine and choline and impairment with scopolamine. *Science*, 1978, *201*, 274–276.

Sjögren, T., Sjögren, H., & Lindgren, A. G. H. Morbus Alzheimer and Morbus Pick: A genetic, clinical and pathoanatomical study. *Acta Psychiatrica et Neurologica Scandanavica* (Supplementum), 1952, *82*, 1–152.

Sokoloff, L. Cerebral circulation and metabolism in the aged. In S. Gershon & A. Raskin (Eds.), *Genesis and treatment of psychologic disorders in the elderly*. New York: Raven Press, 1975.

Sokoloff, L. Cerebral blood flow and metabolism in the differentiation of dementias: General considerations. In R. Katzman, R. D. Terry, & K. L. Bick (Eds.), *Alzheimer's disease: Senile dementia and related disorders*. New York: Raven Press, 1978.

Tecce, J. J. Contingent negative variation (CNV) and psychological processes in man. *Psychophysiology*, 1972, *1*, 272–276.

Terry, R. D. Neuronal fibrous protein in human pathology. *Journal of Neuropathology and Experimental Neurology*, 1971, *30*, 8–19.

Terry, R. D. Aging, senile dementia, and Alzheimer's disease. In R. Katzman, R. D. Terry, & K. L. Bick (Eds.), *Alzheimer's disease: Senile dementia and related disorders*. New York: Raven Press, 1978.

Terry, R. D., Fitzgerald, C., Peck, A., Millner, J., & Farmer, P. Cortical cell counts in senile dementia. Abstract No. 118, 53rd Annual Meeting of the American Association of Neuropathologists, Chicago, 1977.

Thompson, L. W. Cerebral blood flow, EEG, and behavior in aging. In R. D. Terry & S. Gershon (Eds.), *Neurobiology of aging*. New York: Raven Press, 1976.

Tomasch, J. Gibt es einen altersbedingten kontinuierlichen Neuronenverlust? *Wiener Klinische Wochenschrift*, 1972, *84*, 169–170.

Tomlinson, B. E. Morphological changes and dementia in old age. In W. Lynn Smith & M. Kinsbourne (Eds.), *Aging and dementia*. New York: Spectrum Publications, 1977.

Tomlinson, B. E., Blessed, G., & Roth, M. Observations on the brains of nondemented old people. *Journal of Neurological Sciences*, 1968, *7*, 331–356.

Tomlinson, B. E., & Henderson, G. Some quantitative cerebral findings in normal and demented old people. In R. D. Terry & S. Gershon (Eds.), *Neurobiology of aging*. New York: Raven Press, 1976.

Wang, H. S., & Busse, E. W. EEG of healthy old persons—A longitudinal study: I. Dominant background activity and occipital rhythm. *Journal of Gerontology*, 1969, *24*, 419–426.

Wang, H. S., & Busse, E. W. Correlates of regional cerebral blood flow in elderly community residents. In A. M. Harper, W. B. Jennett, J. D. Miller, & J. O. Rowan (Eds.), *Blood flow and metabolism in the brain*. London: Churchill Livingstone, 1975.

Wang, H. S., Obrist, W. D., & Busse, E. W. Neurophysiological correlates of the intellectual function of elderly persons living in the community. *American Journal of Psychiatry*, 1970, *126*, 1205–1212.

Wells, C. E. Dementia: Definition and description. In C. E. Wells (Ed.). *Dementia*. Philadelphia: F. A. Davis, 1977.

White, P., Hiley, C. R., Goodhardt, M. J., Carrasco, L. H., Keet, J. P., Williams, I. E. I., & Bowen, D. M. Neocortical cholinergic neurons in elderly people. *Lancet*, 1977, *1*, 668–671.

Willanger, R., Thygesen, P., Nielsen, R., & Peterson, O. Intellectual impairment and cerebral atrophy: A psychological, neurological and radiological investigation. *Danish Medical Bulletin*, 1968, *15*, 63–93.

Wisniewski, K., Jervis, G. A., Moretz, R. C., & Wisniewski, H. M. Alzheimer neurofibillary tangles in diseases other than senile and presenile dementia. *Annals of Neurology*, 1979, *5*, 288–294.

Wisniewski, H. M., & Terry, R. D. Morphology of the aging brain, human and animal. In D. H. Ford (Ed.), *Neurobiological aspects of maturation and aging*. Amsterdam: Elsevier Scientific Publishing Co., 1973.

Wisniewski, H., Terry, R. D., & Hirano, A. Neurofibrillary pathology. *Journal of Neuropathology and Experimental Neurology*, 1970, *29*, 163–176.

Woodard, J. S. Alzheimer's disease in late adult life. *American Journal of Pathology*, 1966, *49*, 1157–1166.

Yakovlev, P., & Lecours, A. R. The myelogenetic cycles of regional maturation of the brain. In A. Minkowski (Ed.), *Regional development of the brain in early life*. Oxford: Blackwell Scientific Publications, 1967.

Loraine K. Obler
Martin L. Albert

6

Language and Aging: A Neurobehavioral Analysis

It is generally held that language functions are the least likely of the neurobehavioral functions to deteriorate with aging. Compared to perceptual and time-constrained motor activities, which clearly deteriorate with aging, linguistic skills may indeed appear to remain stable. However, on certain tests that involve language, such as list learning, elderly subjects tend to perform worse than younger adults. Insofar as there appears to be mild deterioration in certain language abilities, it then becomes important to examine precisely how this deterioration is manifested and to determine if the deterioration is primarily of linguistic function or if linguistic impairment in aging is secondary to other neurologic and neuropsychologic changes, such as memory deficit or general slowness.

Deterioration, it must be stressed, is not the only possible change that language skills may undergo in the process of aging; with healthy children, for example, one would not expect to find linguistic deterioration. At least certain language capabilities potentially may develop throughout the life span. Improvement in narrative skills or style, for example, may be observed as in the ability to encode thought into language, to communicate effectively, and to understand what others intend. Dementia or other neurologic illness, however, may interrupt or reverse this development. Again, if we could demonstrate such developmental language change, we would then want to consider how it relates to underlying neuroanatomic and neuropsychologic changes.

In this chapter we shall attempt to document the patterns of development and of deterioration of language skills that occur in both healthy elderly and dementing individuals and to discuss the evidence that these changes correlate with neurologic changes in the brain. First we shall consider language in healthy elderly individuals, including differences in their abilities to use lexicon, employ discourse, and comprehend speech. Subsequently we shall discuss language associated with the dementias: both the subcortical dementias, which may parallel healthy aging to some extent (Albert, 1978), and the cortical dementias, in particular, Alzheimer's disease. We shall attempt to determine if the language changes are primary or if they may be explained by other cognitive changes, such as those related to intelligence or memory, or by other more basic neurologic changes, such as those related to attention or timing. Finally, we shall consider the possibility that the brain substrate for language itself undergoes continual reorganization throughout the course of the life span.

LANGUAGE SKILLS IN THE HEALTHY ELDERLY

To date three realms of language use have served as the focus for study of cognitively healthy elderly populations: speech comprehension, discourse production, and lexicon. We shall consider them in that order.

Comprehension

For our purposes comprehension serves as an umbrella term to include all processes involved in the reception and understanding of linguistic input. Phoneme discrimination, for example, is considered to be a comprehension function. Since no one claims that comprehension improves with advanced age, we shall consider factors that may contribute to the possibility of deteriorating comprehension of language. We shall also examine the strategies the elderly use to compensate for the deterioration.

Hearing loss accounts for some, though not all, changes in comprehension abilities in the elderly. In modern technological society, aging is associated with hearing loss due, in part at least, to accumulated experiences of exposure to noise (Corso, 1977b). Not only is there a decrease in pure-tone acuity (Goetzinger, Proud, Dirks, & Embrey, 1963), particularly in the high frequencies, but there also are deficits in speech processing, such as increased thresholds for speech discrimination and speech reception (Corso, 1977a). Some of these deficits appear to be associated with sensorineural hearing loss that may be evidenced at any age (Kasden, 1970), although the incidence of sensorineural loss increases with age. On a careful test of phoneme discrimination, Stevenson (1975) demonstrated that elderly subjects made more phonemic confusions, although of the same type, than did younger controls. Front phonemes were perceptually confused for back ones in both groups of people, and the members of fricative classes were confused for each other. But hearing difficulties alone cannot account for all the comprehension difficulties that may come with aging. For example, in elderly subjects with an intact cochlea, auditory comprehension measured by an auditory cloze test was found to be reduced (Nash & Wepman, 1973).

Thus, in seeking explanation for the changes in comprehension abilities in the elderly, we must also consider the general neurologic concomitants of aging. Slower timing or pacing, attentional deficits, difficulty in switching set, short-term memory deficits, and distractibility may make comprehension more difficult. If these factors still do not explain all the data on impaired speech comprehension in the elderly, it may be that some other sort of cognitive decline is contributing to comprehension difficulties. In the fourth section of this paper we shall discuss the possibility that changes in brain substrate for language comprehension occur with aging. It is also of interest to observe the alternate strategies that aging, and particularly hard-of-hearing elderly, individuals develop to cope with their comprehension problems.

Certainly, general slowness of neurologic response is a major factor in comprehension impairment. For example, in a simple measure of response time to tones (Feldman & Reger, 1967; Corso, 1977a), response time increased gradually from young adulthood through the sixties, but then increased dramatically in the seventies. Time-distorted speech also poses additional problems for the elderly. Elderly subjects have been tested with time-compressed speech (Konkle, Beasley, & Bess, 1977; Sticht & Gray, 1969) and expanded speech (DiCarlo & Taub, 1972) and have been found to have more difficulty than younger subjects in processing either type of distorted speech. One might have predicted that electronically time-expanded speech would increase comprehensibility of speech for the elderly, since their information processing rate is slower than that of young adults. Perhaps the results can be explained by the way in which the stimuli were time-expanded. In the case of word lists presented by Schon (1968) and the sentences presented by Bergman, Blumenfeld, Cascardo, Dash, Levitt, & Margulies (1976) stimuli were expanded electronically, so presumably tape was inserted both within and between words. Expansion of speech by only increasing interword intervals or by only extending individual words might provide different results, since one could facilitate lexical processing and the other syntactic processing.

In addition to time-dependent problems associated with aging, attentional changes have also been documented (e.g., Rabbitt, 1965). By means of these we may explain the otherwise paradoxical results of Posner and Ventry (1977), who instructed 45 elderly individuals with sensorineural loss to adjust the volume controls so that a taped radio broadcast was heard *most comfortably*. The adjusted mean intensity level was 56 dB. When they instructed subjects to adjust the controls so that they felt they were best able to *comprehend* the material, however, the mean level was 37 dB. It may be that with a softer auditory stimulus, which may be subjectively difficult to hear, subjects compensate by concentrating more in order to perceive the signal and, as a result, they comprehend better.

Various sorts of speech masking (speech interference through superimposition of some sort of noise over the auditory stimulus) have been shown to differentially impair comprehension in elderly people. Masking by superposition of noise has been used to test phoneme discrimination in aging individuals

(Groen, 1969; Smith & Prather, 1971), and elderly subjects consistently perform more poorly than younger subjects. We may speculate that, since the high-frequency hearing loss of aging is associated with the buzzing noise of tinnitus, part of the difficulty in comprehension may arise from the subject providing her or his own speech masking.

Another sort of masking involves setting up competing stimuli. In the study by Bergman and his colleagues (1976), subjects listened to competing speech signals and were instructed to attend to only one; the elderly performed more poorly than the younger controls. The studies of Maccoby (1971) suggest that such impaired performance may arise when the two voices are presented through the same earphone, in which case the elderly subjects (aged 59−81) perform as poorly as children of third and fourth grades. When the stimuli arrived to separate ears, on the other hand, elderly individuals performed better than ninth-grade students. Unfortunately no intermediate-aged individuals were tested. Moreover the elderly in the study made errors of the sort in which stimuli from one ear were reported as having been heard in the other ear.

When Maccoby's elderly subjects were asked to report messages from both ears in a fixed order, they performed better than the ninth graders on the first message reported and worse on the second message. The authors interpreted this result as a sign that older subjects do not divide their attention as well as do younger subjects. Certain elderly subjects, however, claimed that the act of reporting the first voice seemed to interfere with the memory of the second voice. Thus self-distraction may be operating in the elderly.

Masking to the contralateral ear may also differentially disturb hearing comprehension in the elderly. When Marston and Goetzinger (1972) played a series of time-expanded sentences to younger (mean age 28) and older (mean age 48) adults under two masking conditions, they found the older group to be impaired relative to the younger group when the masking took the form of a competing message to the other ear. The discrepancy between the two age groups on this task, however, was not so severe as it was when the masking was simple noise masking to the contralateral ear.

Certain linguistic characteristics of the messages themselves interact with perceptual difficulties in comprehension. Decreased redundancy of message seems to produce impairments in normal-hearing elderly adults relative to younger adults. Scholes (1978) presented a sentence that required careful discrimination of article location (e.g., "He shows her bird the seed.") and asked subjects to choose which of four pictures best represented the sentence. His group of normal elderly people (mean age 69) performed as well as his group of nonaphasic stroke victims (mean age 60) and a group of 9-year-old children, each achieving scores of 86 percent correct. The performances of 11- and 13-year olds and 27-year-olds tended to be somewhat-better, performing at greater than 90 percent correct.

When we consider the strategies that elderly people employ to compensate for decreased comprehension, we must keep in mind that the ability to develop strategies itself may reflect cognitive flexibility. The ability to employ lipreading or speech-reading skills, for example, may conceivably develop spontaneously as hearing difficulty proceeds. Sanders and Coscarelli (1970) have demonstrated that the ability to succeed in lipreading tasks correlates positively with an ability for what they called "visual synthesis," which they measured by means of three tests. One of these was the Visual Closure Speed Test, in which subjects had to identify 24 incomplete pictures. A second test requires subjects to complete words that were printed without vowels. The third test requires subjects to complete sentences by writing consonants when given only vowels, punctuation, and blanks for the number of words. Good performance on these "visual synthesis" tasks corresponded to success in lipreading.

Studies of the verbal-transformation effect provide further evidence that the elderly use characteristic strategies in the comprehension process itself. To test for this effect, a tape loop repeating the same word is played to subjects, who are asked to call out what they hear each time they hear a new word, that is, when a verbal transformation occurs. Normal adult subjects report verbal transformations at a standard rate. Children below age 8 do not consistently hear transformations, and elderly people, both healthy and dementing, report fewer than young adults (Obusek & Warren, 1973) but more than young children. The sorts of changes that the elderly do report are much closer to the target items (i.e., they involve fewer phonemic substitutions) than those reported by grade-school and junior-college students. Indeed when Clegg (1971) ran a similar study it appeared that elderly subjects reported changes that were meaningful words, while young adults reported nonsense words that conformed to English morphophonological constraints, and children reported changes that included English phonemes but not necessarily in acceptable sequence. Since Warren

(1961) and Warren and Warren (1966) have suggested elsewhere that the verbal-transformation effect reflects the reorganizational mechanisms that one uses to correct misprocessing while listening to continued discourse, we may speculate that elderly individuals are in some sense *monitoring input at a word-by-word level,* at least, while younger subjects are using a more analytic approach at the phonemic level.

We may conclude that, according to several measures, language comprehension appears both to deteriorate and to change with aging. Reduction in auditory acuity is but one cause. Certain general cognitive abilities, such as memory, attention, and timing, attenuate with age and may affect language comprehension. Although in numerous instances of reported comprehension deficit we may be able to posit general underlying neuropsychologic mechanisms that could account for them, we are not able to exclude the possibility that specific neuroanatomic and neurophysiologic changes in brain substrate for language also contribute to the deficits in comprehension seen in aging populations.

Both cortical and subcortical mechanisms relating to the perception and processing of speech may also be implicated. For example, we know that acoustic parameters of the voice, for which subcortical mechanisms play a major role, change consistently with aging (e.g., Meyerson, 1976). It may be that these changes bring about comprehension difficulties. According to the motor theory of speech perception (Liberman, Cooper, Shankweiler, & Studdert-Kennedy, 1967), comprehension relies in part on subvocal processing of incoming speech. If this subvocal processing were slowed down or otherwise impaired, we might logically expect disturbances in comprehension.

Discourse

Fluency of speech is a concept that has many meanings for neuropsychologists and speech pathologists. One standard neurobehavioral measure of "verbal fluency" asks subjects to name as many items within a certain semantic category or beginning with a certain letter as they can in a fixed time period. By this measure elderly people perform worse than younger ones (Spreen & Benton, 1969). We have discovered that given unlimited time for this task, certain elderly individuals may produce as many items, and with as few repetitions, as younger subjects. In such a test, it is difficult to discover if it is

naming facility that is lost or delayed or the ability to generate concepts or simply timing.

Broader measures of fluency may be employed in analysis of continuous discourse. We analyzed the performance of 19 parkinsonian and 18 healthy 50- and 60-year-olds on a written description of the Cookie-Theft picture used in the *Boston Diagnostic Aphasia Examination* (Goodglass & Kaplan, 1972). It became clear that of the two strategies, namely, fluent use of full sentences (e.g., "The boy is standing on a stool.") or use of partial sentences (e.g., "Boy standing on stool"), it was the younger and healthier patients who preferred the abbreviated style (Obler, Mildworf, & Albert, 1977). The 60-year-olds of both healthy and dementing groups used more words for this task than did the 50-year-olds. Yet, although they used more words, the older subjects had fewer total sentences; this resulted in part from the fact that they employed more embedded sentences than the middle-aged groups. The older subjects, however, did not perform better in the task, in that they reported fewer themes in response to the instruction, "Tell what is happening in this picture." In evaluating the quality of their word usage we found that the older groups produced results similar to those found with patients suffering from Wernicke's aphasia (Gleason, Goodglass, Green, Obler, Weintraub, & Hyde, 1977) in that they were more likely than controls to modify nouns and their verb-to-noun ratio was higher. Furthermore, parallel to what Riegel (1968) found on his word association test, only the 60-year-olds used evaluative terms (e.g., *apparently, unfortunately, hectic young family,* and so on).

In a second stage of analysis we considered the written descriptions of the Cookie-Theft picture that Goodglass had elicited from 105 healthy adults ranging in age from their thirties to their seventies. Unpublished results parallel to those of our previous study were seen across the three oldest decades, that is, more older subjects used a full-sentence strategy, and sentence length increased from 6 words to 12.8 words for those subjects who used full sentences. Curiously, however, on these two measures (type of strategy and words per sentence) the 70-year-olds looked most like the 30- and 40-year-olds. In this nonhospitalized population, unlike the previous population, the number of themes actually increased with age from the fifties to the seventies, so that the 70-year-olds obtained a score between that of the 30- and 40-year-olds. Similarly, the number of words per theme remained constant across the entire age span.

Verb-to-noun ratio actually decreased between the fifties and seventies so that for this parameter, too, the score of the 70-year-olds was closest to that of the 30- and 40-year-olds.

A parallel pattern, wherein the oldest group (over 74 years old) produced discourse most like a younger group (55 to 64), was seen for several analyses in a second study, which we carried out with Drs. Edith Kaplan and Amy Veroff. In this study we analyzed the immediate and delayed oral-recall responses to the Wechsler Memory Paragraph on dogs saving the wounded in wartime. We found the over-75-year-old and the 55-to-64-year-old groups to use more repetition, making fewer additions to the story and using less paraphrase than the 65-to-74-year-old group. The use of vague or indefinite words (like *something* or *one*) increased with age, as did the number of comments made to questions asked in response to the task.

If one measures fluency by sentence length in spontaneous (as opposed to recalled) speech, the elderly perform no differently from younger adults (Gordon, Hutchinson, & Allen, 1976) and in most instances are reported to increase unit lengths (Obler et al., 1977; Smith, 1955). By measures of dysfluency, such as counting interjections, filler syllables, and incomplete phrases, however, it would appear that elderly subjects are more dysfluent than young adults (Gordon et al., 1976; Yairi & Clifton, 1972). It is unclear whether sentence length was evaluated in these studies; if not, one possible conclusion is that the elderly produce more dysfluencies because they talk more. Yet the dysfluencies reported by Yairi and Clifton (1972), namely dysrhythmias and phonation dysfluencies, could not be so easily accounted for by this explanation.

Not infrequently, intuitions about linguistic phenomena are not borne out by experimentation. In the case of the popularly alleged loquaciousness of the elderly, however, we have seen that numerous experimental measures document it. This is not to discount individual variation and the possibility that a subgroup of elderly people, perhaps those with certain forms of dementing illness, become more taciturn. On our gross word count for the writing sample, for example, it was the elderly people who provided both the highest and the lowest scores. Although they may be slower at generating concepts than a younger or middle-aged group, the elderly compensate with well-structured, full, and complex syntax. Yet this fluent syntactic frame may be interrupted with speech dysfluencies. Finally, an attitudi-

nal change toward topics may be discerned in the language of the elderly inasmuch as evaluative and modificatory items are more frequent in their discourse.

We can speculate that increased quantity of speech and attitudinal changes may be related to a general tendency toward disinhibition due to age-dependent changes in the frontolimbic system. Anatomic modifications of cortical regions, particularly in or near Wernicke's area, may also be implicated in increased loquaciousness, since damage to that area in older adults regularly results in a fluent aphasia with intact syntactic structures and sometimes with increased speech tempo as well (Brody, 1976). Taciturnity, on the other hand, in those cases where it develops, might relate to a subcortical impairment.

Lexicon

Conflicting reports have been published on the "vocabulary skill" of the elderly. Psychologists working with the geriatric population often boast that it is one of the few skills that improves with aging, while at the same time elderly individuals themselves complain that they forget more words as they grow older. Schow, Christensen, Hutchinson, & Nerbonne (1978) have reviewed the research controversy on this point.

Part of the contradiction may be resolved if we consider how many different ways there are to measure lexical skills. One might count the number of different words a subject uses or recognizes or is able to define. One may evaluate the quality of the definitions or the frequency or correctness of the words used. Pictures or objects may be displayed and subjects' naming responses judged for accuracy and/or reaction time. Subjects may be given various word lists or word pairs to recall or semantic tasks to carry out (e.g., finding synonyms, completing lexical analogies). Certain of these tasks will involve more or fewer components of general cognitive abilities such as speed and memory, which have been shown to deteriorate with aging. Moreover, those scores that rely on judgment of "quality" of response may suffer from societal biases that somehow the responses of the younger group are more "normal".

In relaxed conditions it would appear that elderly subjects have a wider range of vocabulary than do young adults. Smith (1957) considered vocabulary distribution in the writings (journals, letters) of two individuals from their teens through their eighties.

She demonstrated an increase in different words employed (as well as in average letter length of words) through at least the fifties and some diminution of both after the sixties. For one subject the variety of words in her seventies exceeded that of her thirties, but was seen to drop in her eighties. As Smith pointed out, variety of vocabulary in letters and journals may reflect interesting periods in one's life, so the vocabulary limitations she documents for advanced age may result from restricted lifestyle, rather than from linguistic changes. Riegel's (1968) more rigorous study of free word associations supports Smith's basic hypothesis, however, that vocabulary may increase with age. In his group of 500 subjects ranging from 55 to over 75 years of age, Riegel found a wider variety of association responses among the older individuals. Moreover, for those 200 subjects who were retested 5 years later, the oldest subjects were least consistent in producing the same association to the same stimulus item. While it is impossible to rule out the increasingly standardizing effects of twentieth century education, these data may also be read to suggest either a broader vocabulary among older individuals or else freer associations.

Certain characteristics of word stimuli themselves interact with performance, and the interaction is different for the elderly and for younger groups. When Riegel (1968) measured the response time to read words, the word frequency and word length of the item were less important for the young group than was the concreteness of the reference. For the elderly, on the other hand, word length (as measured by the number of letters) increased response time more than did either low frequency or lack of concreteness.

The ability to define words, as vocabulary is measured on the Wechsler Adult Intelligence Scale (WAIS), is generally held to remain stable from early adulthood throughout the lifespan. Thus the peer-scaled scores, which compensate for age-related changes in raw scores on most subtests of the WAIS, do not indicate the need to raise vocabulary scores of the elderly by way of compensation. A similar result was found by Fox (1947), who tested a group of subjects in their seventies and another group in their forties, asking first for an oral definition of a word and then for selection of a definition among four written choices. For the oral definitions subjects were scored as making correct, incorrect, or half-correct answers. No difference was found between the two groups in either condition, either for number of correct responses or number of half-correct responses, which latter measure Fox took to be a sign of quality of response.

On the other hand, Botwinick, West, and Storandt (1975) defined "quality of response" more explicitly and argued that quality of definition declines with aging. Thus synonyms were considered by them to be "best responses" on the WAIS vocabulary subtest, and the elderly individuals were less likely to give synonyms than were young adults. It must be noted that while the largest decline in best responses occurred between the seventh and eighth decades, the second largest decline occurred between the third and fourth decades. Since "good explanations" (presumably consisting of more than one word) were considered inferior to synonyms, we suspect that the increased loquaciousness associated with aging may account in part for the "poorer" responses of older subjects on this task.

When given the *Boston Naming Test* (Kaplan & Goodglass, 1976), in which subjects are asked to name line drawings of objects, elderly subjects tended to give several-word responses when single-word ones are standard with younger normals (unpublished data). These responses sometimes consisted of greater specification than younger subjects feel called upon to give (e.g., *tennis racquet* for what is not specifically that, but rather is a *racquet*). On this naming task, it must also be noted, elderly subjects made numerous errors due to misperception (e.g., they would label *flippers* as *aprons*) and often cued themselves into the correct word by talking, either by providing a syntactic context, or by pronouncing phonologically related forms.

This deliberate use by the elderly of syntactic context is reflected in Riegel's (1968) association test by a predominance of syntagmatically related first responses to the stimuli (e.g., *bark* to *dog*) as compared to the primary paradigmatic responses of younger adults (e.g., *cat* to *dog*). In this behavior the elderly might conceivably be compared to children whose association responses develop from syntagmatic to paradigmatic as they get older (Entwisle, Forsyth, & Muus, 1964). Riegel additionally noted that response times for common responses increased with age. Thus the habit of repetition of syntactic structures may result in syntagmatic responses among the elderly, similar to those observed in young children.

Elderly subjects, Riegel continued, were most likely to give emotional and evaluative responses in his association task than were younger subjects. The parallel phenomenon in patients with dementia was cited in our section on Discourse.

It would appear that *active* vocabulary skills, such as naming objects presented visually, may start to decline with advanced age, while *passsive* vocabulary skills (e.g., definition, word recognition) may remain intact. The strategies for processing lexical items, however, may become increasingly syntagmatic with advanced age.

Conclusions

In reviewing what is known about language skills in healthy elderly people, we have discovered that for the elderly group as a whole comprehension of language may be disturbed, discourse may become more elaborate syntactically yet less fluent in its utterance, and active use of lexicon may falter although passive use is preserved. There is a wide range of individual variation on these skills, perhaps even more than in children, and even with a single elderly person there may be a wide range of language behaviors. This individual variability may account for some of the contradictions in the literature on language in the aging, while problems of definition and method may account for other apparent paradoxes. Life-span changes in both cortical and subcortical mechanisms for speech and language would appear to play a part in the changes of language use associated with aging.

LINGUISTIC BEHAVIOR IN DEMENTIA

Dementia is a term used to describe a constellation of behavioral signs and symptoms of intellectual dysfunction due to widely varying etiologies and dependent on separate neurophysiologic mechanisms. A variety of classification schemes has been offered for the dementing illnesses. Although many studies of language in dementing individuals have been conducted, these studies have often suffered in clarity because no definition or classification scheme for dementia was provided. Because the term dementia covers such a wide variety of diseases and behaviors, it is crucial to know which form of dementia is being considered in order to form a clear neurobehavioral picture of language use.

We have found it useful to apply the operational definitions of subcortical and cortical dementia (Albert, 1978). These labels correspond to two major forms of dementia that can be distinguished on clinical neurobehavioral grounds. Subcortical dementia refers to a behavioral syndrome found in patients with a variety of neurologic illnesses (e.g., progres-

sive supranuclear palsy, Parkinson's disease) in which prominent pathologic changes are seen in subcortical nuclear structures. Clinically this syndrome is manifested by emotional or personality changes, memory disorder, defective ability to manipulate acquired knowledge, and striking slowness in the rate of information processing. Vocabulary and general facility with language are thought to be preserved.

The subcortical dementias may be contrasted clinically with the cortical dementias, in which pathologic changes are prominent in cortical association areas (e.g., Alzheimer-senile dementia complex). These changes lead to aphasias, apraxias, and agnosias that are present in varying combinations with the signs and symptoms of subcortical dementia.

Certain characteristics of language use are reported for dementing individuals of any sort. These include perseveration, a lack of initiative in speech, and naming difficulties. These are broad categories, however, and if we consider different sorts of dementia, we find different manifestations of these phenomena.

Language in Subcortical Dementia

Speech with subcortical lesions is characterized by a slow rate, low volume, and disturbances in rhythm, pitch, and articulation (dysarthria) (Riklan and Levita, 1969). The patient may begin a sentence at an acceptable volume and then trail off towards the end of the sentence. This diminution of volume may be associated with an acceleration of speech rate following electrical stimulation of the ventrolateral thalamus during stereotactic procedures in patients with Parkinson's disease (Botez & Barbeau, 1971). Even in the same patient, however, such stimulation may result in speech arrest or hesitations, which are the more likely consequence of surgical lesions in this area. One 64-year-old patient we saw who had progressive supranuclear palsy sounded like a record played on low speed. Each word was extended, and phrases (as marked by accent and separated from each other by long pauses) contained no more than two words. When medicated with levodopa, his pace picked up and his phrases were in the three-to-four word range, which permitted more normal prosody.

Naming abilities may be impaired in subcortical dementias. Mildworf (1978) tested 38 patients with Parkinson's disease (average age 60), 10 patients with Huntington's chorea (average age 53), and 42 normal controls (average age 60) on a neuropsychologic battery that included selected items from the *Boston Naming Test* (Kaplan & Goodglass, 1976) and from the body-part naming subtest of the *Boston Diagnostic Aphasia Exam* (Goodglass & Kaplan, 1972). On both tests the parkinsonians performed worse than normals but not significantly so, while the Huntington's patients performed significantly worse than both of the other groups. In his study of naming errors under conditions of thalamic stimulation, Ojemann (1975) reported the naming errors of subcortical lesions to be mostly omissions with a few jargon misnamings. Perseveration of one response to another trial was seen only during anterior thalamic stimulation. With further research in dementing patients it may become clear how their "anomia" resembles that produced by electrical stimulation.

Using two tests of word fluency (i.e., "Name as many animals as you can," and "Name as many words beginning with the letter *F* [then *A*, then *S*] as you can") with scores corrected for age and education, Mildworf (1978) and Albert (1978) again demonstrated a trend for parkinsonians to perform worse than normals, whereas patients with Huntington's chorea performed significantly worse than either of the other groups. Certainly the time pressures of this test put dementing patients at a disadvantage, but qualitative analysis of the results remains to be done to determine if other factors contributed to the impaired performance of the subcortically dementing groups.

On a test of serial speech requiring recitation of the months of the year, Mildworf and Albert noted an inability of the dementing patients to stop at the end of the series. Thus, after *December* they would continue with *January* again. When asked to name the months in reverse order, several Huntington's patients and parkinsonian patients simply could not perform the task. Others would start out and, after mentioning several months, revert to the more automatic forward order. All the controls, it should be noted, were able to perform the task.

Reading and writing skills and naming orally spelled words were impaired in the Huntington's patients as compared to the normals, but not in the parkinsonian patients. When asked to write about the Cookie Theft picture (Goodglass & Kaplan, 1972), those Huntington's patients who could perform the task wrote telegrammatic sentences. The parkinsonian patients scored the same as normals by the standard scoring procedure but in fact used more words than did the normals to describe the same number of themes. They tended to use fuller sentences with complex embeddings, as did the older subjects among the normal controls. Moreover the parkinsonians had a higher verb-to-noun ratio, as Wernicke's aphasics did by comparison to normals (Gleason et al. 1977). Yet the dementing subjects differed from the Wernicke's aphasics in that the parkinsonians employed many more substantive nouns and verbs than did the aphasics. Finally it must be noted that the parkinsonian patients used print or a mixture of print and script much more frequently than did the normals. While this may be a strategy to compensate for motor difficulties, other explanations involving hemisphericity of control for the different writing types should be considered (Bryden & Allard, 1976).

Finally we point to an example of high-level language impairment with subcortical damage. It must be stressed that this picture of language impairment in subcortical dementia does not comform to any of the classical aphasic syndromes. Before our patient with progressive supranuclear palsy received medication, proverb interpretation was seen to be impaired (concrete). When he was treated with the levodopa, his proverb interpretation became more abstract. This task is certainly not a purely linguistic one, but rather displays the interaction of language and cognition. More clear-cut instances of language disturbance were seen in the patient's written language. In writing to dictation, letters were omitted and added. When asked to write what goes on in his house at Christmas, he wrote, "The tree gets up, the grandchildren comes around, and gets a new cane (shillelagh)." In addition to the inappropriate person or number agreement between *grandchildren* and *comes* and between the omitted *I* and *gets,* the patient has omitted either *put* or *set* in the first clause.

We may conclude that it is not only speech that is affected in the subcortical dementias, but language as well. Although subcortical nuclear structures have not been traditionally included among the language areas of the brain, recent attempts to come to terms with the data from stimulation, ablation, and natural lesion studies in subcortical areas must lead to the conclusion that subcortical areas are involved in at least the productive language process. It may be that the necessary involvement of the thalamus in normal language production becomes increasingly important throughout the life span, since Darley, Brown, and Swenson (1975) observed that language decrements resulting from neurosurgery for parkinsonian and other movement disorders were more likely in older patients than in middle-aged ones.

Language in Alzheimer–Senile Dementia Complex

In clinical neurobehavioral terms, the Alzheimer–senile dementia complex (ASDC) can be distinguished from both healthy aging and the subcortical dementias. Though ASDC may include all the behaviors of the subcortical dementias, superimposed on these are perceptual problems (agnosias), praxis problems (apraxias), and language problems (aphasias). The language problems that have been documented in the cortical dementias have been, for the most part, problems of production. Comprehension skills are difficult to test in a dementing patient because an incorrect or inappropriate response may be the result of the general cognitive decline rather than the result of impairment of linguistic functioning for comprehension per se. In this section we will first describe the characteristic language and communication patterns of ASDC patients and then compare their language to that of aphasics.

As in the subcortical dementias, dysarthric speech may accompany ASDC (Gustafson, Hagberg, & Ingvar, 1978). Paraphasias (substitution for words or of phonemes within a word), which rarely occur in their whole-word type in subcortical dementias, are common in the speech and written language of ASDC patients. Moreover, both phonemic and verbal paraphasias are evident (Tissot, Richard, Duval, & DeAjuriaguerra, 1967; Whitaker, 1976), but even the whole-word paraphasias may contain elements of the target words (Seglas, 1892). Although the paraphasias may result in incoherent discourse (Albert, Goodglass, Helm, & Rubens, forthcoming), it must be stressed that the syntactic frame for them is relatively complex (Irigaray, 1967).

The preceding elements characterizing language in dementia may not always be observed because contradictory elements occur. Dementing individuals can be mute or effusive, for example, probably depending on which anatomic structures have been affected by disease. Tissot et al. (1967), moreover, pointed to the paradox that a given dementing patient may be both elliptical and redundant in her or his speech. They connected this to a loss of linguistic sensitivity and a reduction, or deterioration, to base-level language with little communicative intent. This disturbed use of language, according to Stengel (1964), results from the patient's not caring if the name she or he gives an item corresponds to the standard one.

The questions as to whether aphasia can or must occur in dementia have been argued several ways. If one defines aphasia as any acquired disturbance in the language system resulting from cerebral dysfunction, then of course aphasia is likely to be found in dementia. If one looks for classic aphasic syndromes in dementing patients, however, one will find that dementing patients most closely resemble two types, anomic and Wernicke's. Certain pragmatic defects (difficulties in communication per se by dementing individuals), however, are less likely to occur in aphasic patients and may serve as one way to distinguish the dementing from aphasic individuals.

Irigaray (1973) has tested a sizable group of dementing patients on a series of psycholinguistic tasks and has detailed the sorts of responses they gave. Many of these tasks are tasks at which aphasic, nondementing patients would also fail, but the types of responses the dementing individuals gave also serve to distinguish them from the various aphasic groups. For example, on a task in which subjects were given a group of two to five words and were instructed to incorporate them into a sentence, dementing subjects who responded generally used only two of the target items and connected them in more than one sentence by means of acceptable syntax but with deviant semantics. The dementing individuals were sensitive to word-class categories, having particular difficulty incorporating adjectives and consecutive words of the same type (e.g., two nouns). Aphasics, on the other hand, would either string the substantive words together telegrammatically (anterior aphasics) or string some or all of them together with reasonable syntactic structures but empty content (posterior aphasics).

Thus, in certain respects the speech and language of ASDC patients resemble that of healthy elderly and subcortically dementing patients. Their communication, however, is generally more bizarrely inappropriate than that of either anomic or Wernicke's aphasics, which groups they most resemble.

Conclusions

Speech disturbances are characteristic of the subcortical dementias. These include dysarthria, timing irregularities, and disturbance in the ability to initiate, maintain, and cease speaking. The anomic problems reported for subcortical lesions include whole-word paraphasias, perseveration, stuttering, and omissions. Comprehension is strikingly preserved.

In cortical dementias, on the other hand, comprehension is impaired. The anomic errors that occur include frequent literal and verbal paraphasias. Speech fluency is generally intact, and syntax is preserved. In the cortically dementing patient inappropriate discourse is characteristic, whereas in the subcortically dementing patient communicative intent is preserved.

NEUROLOGIC SUBTRATE FOR LANGUAGE: A LIFE-SPAN PERSPECTIVE

When one speaks of developmental changes in the brain substrate for language, one usually refers to development during childhood. Since we focus here on language changes at the other end of the development scale, we will, after a brief review of theories of development of brain substrate for language in childhood, consider four models for change in brain substrate for language with aging. Two of these have been proposed by Brown and Jaffe (1975), who hypothesized (1) that left lateralization for language is a process that continues throughout the life span and (2) that within the left hemispheric speech zone itself there is increasing specification throughout life. We will also consider our own hypotheses: (1) that differential cerebral atrophy may contribute to the changes in language we have documented, and (2) that language maintenance requires different brain organization from language development.

There is evidence of anatomical asymmetries of the two hemispheres that may relate to left hemispheric dominance for language (Geschwind & Levitsky, 1968; Teszner, Tzavaras, Gruner, & Hecaen, 1972). Cortical areas of the left hemisphere bordering the sylvian fissure, it would appear, are distinctly appropriate, or are available, for language before birth (Wada, Clarke, & Hamm, 1975; Witelson and Pallie, 1973). With healthy maturation and the appropriate environment, the developing child will acquire at least one native language (Dennis & Whitaker, 1976; Hecaen, 1976). From age 2 until some time before puberty it would appear that the left hemisphere of the normal child becomes dominant for language. This is evident from the dichotic studies (Kimura, 1967; Krashen, 1976) that show a development from no lateralization to right-ear dominance. Not only does the left hemisphere become dominant for language during this period, Lenneberg (1967) argues, but also this period is the

interval during which language acquisition is possible. After the early teens, he continues, many components of the language acquisition system are no longer available to the individual. He takes his evidence from observation of (1) retarded children, (2) people learning a second language, and (3) aphasics. For Lenneberg, in fact, everybody from the late teens through senescence can be classed in one group, since all mature brain functions (except certain ones in myelination and the EEG spectrum) are completed by the early teens. It seems correct to state that the left hemisphere of most right-handers appears to become dominant for language at some point before puberty. We must disagree, however, with the implication based on Lenneberg's critical age theory that after puberty there simply is no further development of brain organization for language.

Brown has proposed a hypothesis opposed to that of Lenneberg in a series of articles (Brown, 1976, 1978; Brown & Jaffe, 1975) in which he suggests that the brain becomes increasingly left-lateralized for language throughout the life span (Brown & Jaffe, 1975) and that this increasing specialization may even account for some of the apparent cognitive deficits observed in senescence (Brown, 1978). Brown extended the common clinical observation that a left posterior lesion will lead to nonfluent aphasia in a child but to fluent aphasia in an adult and speculated that the posterior lesion that leads to nonfluency or mutism in the young child will present as agrammatic aphasia in an older child, with phonemic articulatory errors in a slightly older child. With adolescent aphasics, true phonemic paraphasia and anomia may be seen, he maintained, while in young adults verbal or semantic paraphasias obtain, and in older adults true semantic and neologistic jargon are prominent.

Although this developmental speculation is attractive, Brown never compellingly argues what this notion of life-span development has to do with the alleged increase in left lateralization for language, nor is there as yet convincing evidence to support his speculation. It is equally possible to explain the appearance of different forms of aphasia that result from the same lesion at different ages by suggesting that a left hemisphere lateralized for language by age 5 continually reorganizes that language *within* its "language area" throughout the life span. Brown and Jaffe (1975) propose such a hypothesis also, but they see it as a modification of the hypothesis of increasing left lateralization. The notion of life-span development of brain substrate for language does not logically necessitate increasing left lateralization. Furthermore, even if Brown's lateralization hypothesis were correct, it would be necessary to determine if progressive lateralization were due to a true shift of language skills from right to left, or a deterioration (or relative deterioration) of right hemisphere brain substrate for language as compared to left hemisphere brain substrate, or to shifts in cognitive style.

That aphasia type changes with age, even within the over-50 population, is confirmed by a study of 367 right-handed male stroke victims with unilateral lesions resulting in aphasia (Obler, Albert, Goodglass, & Benson, 1978). Within this group 161 cases with "classical" symptomatology for one or another of the major aphasic syndromes were selected, and an 11-year age difference between the ages of patients with Broca's aphasia (mean 52 years) and those with Wernicke's aphasia (mean 63 years) was found. Thus it would appear that the clinical observation of increasing fluency of aphasia from childhood to adulthood is substantially confirmed even within the older age groups.

With respect to changes in lateralization with aging, however, the evidence is less clear. Molfese, Freeman, and Palermo (1975) show a decrease in degree of lateralization for speech between later childhood and young adulthood, for example, on the basis of auditory evoked response data. They did not, however, check to see if an elderly group would show a decrease. With dichotic listening procedures Clark and Knowles (1973) observed what may be increased left lateralization for language in the elderly. Their older subjects performed even worse, relative to younger adult subjects, in reporting digits to their left ear than in reporting those to their right ear. Goodglass (personal communication) has pointed out that uncontrolled order of report may have influenced the Clark and Knowles data, and so, with Borod, he is now completing another dichotic study with elderly subjects. Their preliminary analysis suggests no change in lateralization for digits with age. Thus while the issue of whether lateralization for language increases with age remains unresolved, the fact that brain substrate for language changes with age is clearly supported by our data on aging and aphasia type.

In order to demonstrate that this change results from a reorganization of functions within the language area, evidence that precisely the same lesion regularly resulted in a different sort of aphasia in older as opposed to younger patients would be necessary. While this can be observed to occur if we compare young children with older adults (Brown & Jaffe, 1975), it is less obvious within the range of adult ages (Carter, 1978).

Even age-related differences in severity of aphasia are difficult to document. At present there is controversy as to whether aphasic syndromes are more severe and/or aphasic patients are slower to recover with increasing age. If, as Smith (1971) argued, the severity of language deficits in aphasia increases with advanced age, one might hypothesize that the general cell loss by atrophy associated with aging gives the older brain fewer areas in which to reassign or reactivate language skills. Atrophy alone cannot explain this loss of plasticity, however, since as Smith pointed out, among left-handers at any age aphasia is less likely to be severe and recovery is apt to be more rapid. Thus some interaction between plasticity and lateralization would have to be posited. Smith's data on increased severity of aphasia in elderly individuals, it must be noted, have been called into question by Culton (1971), who actually saw a trend to greater improvement in his older patients.

The effects of education on brain organization must not be ignored. Smith (1971), for example, reported that residual language functions in aphasics who had been highly educated were greater than in those who had been less well educated. Our own work with E. Kaplan and A. Veroff on recall memory for discourse passages, reported above, saw weighty effects of education level. The adult will, of course, have had many more years of both formal and informal education than the child, and these must be represented somehow in the brain. The automatic habit of continual repetition may be what helps preserve syntactic forms in the elderly aphasic, for example, while recovered child aphasics may have difficulty on an analogy task like (dog:dogs::horse:?) (Geschwind, 1972). Moreover, at all ages, words that occur more frequently will be better recalled. That this recall is related more to long-term than short-term practice is suggested by our study of polyglot aphasics (Obler & Albert, 1977), which demonstrated that the language that had been used most in the period before the accident would likely return first in adult aphasics under age 60, but that this was not the case for the aphasic group aged 60 or older.

We may conclude that brain substrate for language does change with aging, since different aphasic syndromes and different recovery patterns will occur in patients of different ages who have similar lesions. Whether this change may be related to increased left lateralization for language and/or to selective atrophy of certain brain areas, or to some other kind of cortical—cortical or cortical—subcortical reorganization, however, remains to be determined.

CONCLUSIONS

Similarities and differences in language behavior have been documented among the three groups we have discussed: healthy elderly, subcortically dementing, and cortically dementing individuals. Certain changes we have described for language in the healthy elderly may be seen in exaggerated form in dementing individuals. Naming skills, for example, may deteriorate both in the healthy elderly and in patients with subcortical and cortical dementias. The healthy elderly, however, unlike the dementing patients, respond to their disability by developing a strategy of providing a syntactic context in order to cue themselves to the appropriate name. Severely dementing individuals, on the other hand, will unconsciously provide a paraphasic name, or will give up and claim they do not know the name for an item. Similarly, it appears that the healthy elderly have developed some strategies to cope with those comprehension difficulties that appear in both the healthy elderly and in the dementing elderly. In terms of discourse, the healthy elderly and ASDC groups perform closest to each other, inasmuch as their speech becomes more elaborate at a syntactic level. Individuals with subcortical dementia, on the other hand, are likely to lose the initiative to speak and tend toward muteness. This muteness, however, may be related to the difficulty of producing speech, rather than to any changes in language ability per se.

All the language changes we have confirmed may be understood in terms of the neuropsychologic functions that underlie them. Thus memory, timing, and attentional processes will enter into naming abilities, into comprehension, and into maintenance of coherent discourse. Other components of intelligence must also interact with language functioning. Yet given the aphasiological evidence for changes with aging in brain substrate for language, we should not ascribe all the changes we see in language in the elderly to these neuropsychologic factors. It would, however, certainly be premature at this stage to postulate a causal relation between the changes in neurologic substrate and behavioral changes in the language of the elderly.

As we stressed initially, it must be kept in mind that the language changes of aging are not all ones of deterioration. We hypothesize that those age-related changes that must be seen as deterioration in function (e.g., comprehension or naming difficulties) may represent limitations on available alternative strategies resulting from deterioration of the total neurobehavioral cognitive system or limitations on access to these alternative strategies. Those changes that do not represent deterioration, however, (e.g., increased elaborateness in discourse or improved narrative skill) may reflect strategies resulting from reorganization of brain structure in response to lifelong education and experience.

Several avenues of approach suggest themselves for constructively employing the material we have surveyed. Those successful language strategies employed by healthy elderly for production or perception of speech may be incorporated into speech and cognitive therapy programs for elderly persons, both healthy and dementing, who have not spontaneously developed them. For those patients whose behavior suggests subcortical impairment, administration of subcortically active drugs may enhance language abilities. Finally, attitudes of people who communicate with the healthy and dementing elderly may be enlightened, and strategies suggested to them that will make for effective and rewarding communication.

REFERENCES

Albert, M. Subcortical dementia. In R. Katzman, R. Terry, K. Bick (Eds.), *Alzheimer's disease, senile dementia, and related disorders.* New York: Raven Press, 1978.

Albert, M., Goodglass, H., Helm, N., Rubens, A., & Alexander, M. *Clinical aspects of aphasia.* New York: Springer-Verlag, in press.

Bergman, M., Blumenfeld, V., Cascardo, D., Dash, B., Levitt, H., & Margulies, M. Age-related decrement in hearing for speech. *Journal of Gerontology,* 1976, *31, 533—538.*

Botez, M., & Barbeau, A. Role of subcortical structures, and particularly of the thalamus, in the mechanisms of speech and language. *International Journal of Neurology*, 1971, *8*, 300−320.

Botwinick, J., West. R., & Storandt, M. Qualitative vocabulary responses and age. *Journal of Gerontology*, 1975, *30*, 574−577.

Brody, H. An examination of cerebral cortex and brain stem aging. In R. Terry & S. Gershon (Eds.), *Neurobiology of aging*. New York: Raven Press, 1976.

Brown, J. The neural organization of language: Aphasia and lateralization. *Brain and Language*, 1976, *3*, 482−494.

Brown, J. Lateralization: A brain model. *Brain and Language*, 1978, *5*, 258−261.

Brown, J., & Jaffe, J. Hypothesis on cerebral dominance. *Neuropsychologia*, 1975, *13*, 107−110.

Bryden, M., & Allard, F. Visual hemifield differences depend on typeface. *Brain and Language*, 1976, *3*, 192−200.

Carter, J. Letter to *Archives of Neurology*, 1978, *35*, 619.

Clark, L., & Knowles, J. Age differences in dichotic listening performance. *Journal of Gerontology*, 1973, *28*, 173−178.

Clegg, J. Verbal transformations on repeated listening to some English consonants. *British Journal of Psychology*, 1971, *62*, 303−309.

Corso, J. Auditory perception and communication. In J. Birren & K. W. Schaie (Eds.), *The psychology of aging*. New York: Van Nostrand Reinhold, 1977. (a)

Corso, J. Presbycusis, hearing aids and aging. *Audiology*, 1977, *16*, 146−163. (b)

Culton, G. Reaction to age as a factor in chronic aphasia in stroke patients (a letter). *Journal of Speech and Hearing Disorders*, 1971, *36*, 563−564.

Darley, F., Brown. J., & Swenson, W. Language changes after neurosurgery for parkinsonism. *Brain and Language*, 1975, *2*, 65−69.

Dennis, M., & Whitaker, H. Language acquisition following hemidecortication: Linguistic superiority of the left over the right hemisphere. *Brain and Language*, 1976, *3*, 404−433.

DiCarlo, L., & Taub, H. The influence of compression and expansion on the intelligibility of speech by young and aged aphasic (demonstrated CVA) individuals. *Journal of Communication Disorders*, 1972, *5*, 299−306.

Entwisle, D., Forsyth, D., & Muus, R. The syntagmatic−paradigmatic shift in children's word associations. *Journal of Verbal Learning and Verbal Behavior*, 1964, *3*, 19−29.

Feldman, R., & Reger, S. Relations among hearing, reaction time, and age. *Journal of Speech and Hearing Research*, 1967, *10*, 479−495.

Fox, C. Vocabulary ability in later maturity. *Journal of Educational Psychology*, 1947, *38*, 482−492.

Geschwind, N. Disorders of higher cortical function in children. *Clinical Proceedings, Children's Hospital National Medical Center*, 1972, *28*, 261−272.

Geschwind, N., & Levitsky, W. Human brain: Left-right asymmetries in temporal speech regions. *Science*, 1968, *161*, 186−187.

Gleason, J., Goodglass, H., Green, E., Obler, L., Weintraub, S., & Hyde, M. Narrative strategies in aphasic and normal subjects. Paper presented at the meeting of the Academy of Aphasia, Montreal, 1977.

Goetzinger, C., Proud, G., Dirks, D., & Embrey, J. A study of hearing in advanced age. *Archives of Otolaryngology*, 1963, *73*, 662−673.

Goodglass, H., & Kaplan, E. *Assessment of aphasia and related disorders*. Philadelphia: Lea & Febiger, 1972.

Gordon, K., Hutchinson, J., & Allen, C. An evaluation of selected discourse characteristics among the elderly. *Research laboratory report*, Department of Speech Pathology and Audiology, Idaho State University, Pocatello, Idaho, 1976.

Groen. J. Social hearing handicap: Its measurement by speech audiometry in noise. *International Audiology*, 1969, *8*, 182−183.

Gustafson, L., Hagberg, B., & Ingvar, D. Speech disturbances in presenile dementia related to local cerebral blood flow abnormalities in the dominant hemisphere. *Brain and Language,* 1978, *5,* 103−118.

Hécaen, H. Acquired aphasia in children and the ontogenesis of hemispheric functional specialization. *Brain and Language,* 1976, *3,* 114−134.

Irigaray, L. La production de phrase chez les déments. *Languages.* 1967, *5,* 49−66.

Irigaray, L. *Le langage des déments.* The Hague: Mouton, 1973.

Kaplan, E., & Goodglass, H. *Boston naming test* (Experimental Edition). Boston: Boston Veterans Administration Medical Center, 1976.

Kasden, S. Speech discrimination in two age groups matched for hearing loss. *Journal of Auditory Research,* 1970, *10,* 210−212.

Kimura, D. Functional asymmetry of the brain in dichotic listening. *Cortex,* 1967, *3,* 163−178.

Konkle, D., Beasley, D., Bess, F. Intelligibility of time-altered speech in relation to chronological aging. *Journal of Speech and Hearing Research,* 1977, *20,* 108−115.

Krashen, S. Cerebral asymmetry. In H. Whitaker & H. Whitaker (Eds.), *Studies in neurolinguistics (Vol. 2).* New York: Academic Press, 1976.

Lenneberg, E. *Biological foundations of language.* New York: John Wiley & Sons, 1967.

Liberman, A., Cooper, F., Shankweiler, D., & Studdert-Kennedy, M. Perception of the speech code. *Psychological Review,* 1967, *74,* 431−461.

Maccoby, E. Age changes in the selective perception of verbal materials. In D. Horton & J. Jenkins (Eds.), *The Perception of language.* Columbus, Ohio: Charles E. Merrill Publishing Co., 1971.

Marston, L., & Goetzinger, C. A comparison of sensitized words and sentences for distinguishing nonperipheral auditory changes as a function of aging. *Cortex,* 1972, *8,* 213−223.

Myerson, M. The effects of aging on communication. *Journal of Gerontology,* 1976, *31,* 29−38.

Mildworf, B. Cognitive function in elderly patients. Masters Thesis, Hebrew University, 1978.

Molfese, D., Freeman, R., & Palermo, D. The ontogeny of brain lateralization for speech and nonspeech stimuli. *Brain and Language,* 1975, *2,* 356−368.

Nash, M., & Wepman, J. Auditory comprehension and age. *Gerontologist,* 1973, 243−247.

Obler, L., & Albert, M. Influence of aging on recovery from aphasia in polyglots. *Brain and Language,* 1977, *4,* 460−463.

Obler, L., Albert, M., Goodglass, H., & Benson, D. Aging and aphasia type. *Brain and Language,* 1978, *6,* 318−322.

Obler, L., Mildworf, B., & Albert, M. *Writing style in the elderly.* Montreal: Academy of Aphasia Abstracts, 1977.

Obusek, C. & Warren, R. A comparison of speech perception in senile and well-preserved aged by means of the verbal transformation effect. *Journal of Gerontology,* 1973, *28,* 184−188.

Ojemann, G. Language and the thalmus: Object naming and recall during and after thalamic stimulation. *Brain and Language,* 1975, *2,* 101−120.

Posner, J., & Ventry, I. Relationships between comfortable loudness levels for speech and speech discrimination in sensorineural hearing loss. *Journal of Speech and Hearing Disorders,* 1977, *42,* 370−375.

Rabbitt, P. An age decrement in the ability to ignore irrelevant information. *Journal of Gerontology,* 1965, *20,* 233−238.

Riegel, K. Changes in psycholinguistic performances with age. In G. Talland (Ed.), *Human aging and behavior.* New York: Academic Press, 1968.

Riklan, M., & Levita, E. *Subcortical correlates of human behavior.* Baltimore: Williams & Wilkins, 1969.

Sanders, J., & Coscarelli, J. The relationship of visual synthesis skill in lipreading. *American Annals of the Deaf,* 1970, *115,* 23−26.

Scholes, R. Syntactic and lexical components of sentence comprehension. In A. Caramazza & E. Zurif (Eds.), *Language acquisition and language breakdown.* Baltimore: Johns Hopkins University Press, 1978.

Schon, T. The effects of speech compression and expansion on normal hearing, hard of hearing, and aged males. Doctoral dissertation, 1968, Syracuse University (cited in DiCarlo & Taub, 1972).

Schow, R., Christensen, J., Hutchinson, J., & Nerbonne, M. *Communication disorders of the aged: A guide for health professionals*. Baltimore: University Park Press, 1978 (Chapter 5: Speech and language changes among the aging, pp. 95–105).

Seglas, J. Les troubles du langage chez les aliénés. Paris: Rueff, 1892.

Smith, A. Objective indices of severity of chronic aphasia in stroke patients. *Journal of Speech and Hearing Disorders*, 1971, *36*, 167–207.

Smith, M. Linguistic constancy in individuals when long periods of time are covered and different types of material are sampled. *Journal of Genetic Psychology*, 1955, *106*, 109–143.

Smith, M. Relation between word variety and mean letter length of words with chronological and mental ages. *Journal of General Psychology*, 1957, *56*, 27–43.

Smith, R., & Prather, W. Phoneme discrimination in older persons under varying signal-to-noise conditions. *Journal of Speech and Hearing Research*, 1971, *14*, 630–638.

Spreen, O., & Benton, A. *Neurosensory Center comprehensive examination for aphasia*. Victoria, B.C.: Neuropsychology Laboratory, Dept. of Psychology, University of Victoria, 1969.

Stengel, E. Psychopathology of dementia. *Proceedings of the Royal Society of Medicine*, 1964, *57*, 911–914.

Stevenson, P. Responses to speech audiometry and phonemic discrimination patterns in the elderly. *Audiology*, 1975, *14*, 183–231.

Sticht, T., & Gray, B. The intelligibility of time compressed words as a function of age and hearing loss. *Journal of Speech and Hearing Research*, 1969, *12*, 443–448.

Teszner, D., Tzavaras, A., Gruner, J., & Hécaen, H. L'asymetrie droite-gauche du planum temporale, a propos de l'étude anatomique de 100 cervaux. *Révue Neurologique*, 1972, *126*, 444–449.

Tissot, R., Richard, J., Duval, F., & DeAjuriaguerra, J. Quelques aspects du langage des démences dégénératives du grand age. *Acta Neurologica et Psychiatrica Belgica*, 1967, *67*, 911–923.

Wada, J., Clarke, A., & Hamm, A. Cerebral hemispheric asymmetry in humans. Cortical speech zones in 100 adults and 100 infant brains. *Archives of Neurology*, 1975, *32*, 239–246.

Warren, R. M. Illusory changes in repeated words: Differences between young adults and the aged, *American Journal of Psychology*, 1961, *74*, 506–516.

Warren, R. M., & Warren, R. P. A comparison of speech perception in childhood, maturity, and old age by means of the verbal transformation effect. *Journal of Verbal Learning and Verbal Behavior*, 1966, *5*, 142–146.

Whitaker, H. A case of the isolation of the language function. In H. Whitaker & H. Whitaker (Eds.), *Studies in neurolinguistics (Vol. 2)*. New York: Academic Press, 1976.

Witelson, S., & Pallie, W. Left hemisphere specialization for language in the newborn. *Brain*, 1973, *96*, 641–646.

Yairi, E., & Clifton, N. Dysfluent speech behavior of preschool children, high school seniors, and geriatric persons. *Journal of Speech and Hearing Research*, 1972, *15*, 714–719.

Nancy Wadsworth Denney

7
Adult Cognitive Development

Although it was at first assumed by many investigators and theorists in the area of cognitive development that there were no major changes in cognition beyond adolescence (e.g., Flavell, 1970), more recent research indicates that there may be a number of changes in cognition beyond adolescence. The descriptive research from three major research traditions that suggest the possibility of cognitive change during the adult years will be presented. The three traditions are the psychometric tradition, the Piagetian tradition, and the problem-solving tradition. Additionally, intervention research aimed at exploring the extent to which cognitive abilities in adults are modifiable also will be presented. A discussion of both the practical and theoretical implications of both the descriptive and intervention research will follow. But first, some of the methodological issues relevant to developmental research need to be clarified.

METHODOLOGICAL ISSUES

The importance of methodological considerations can probably best be illustrated by the research on adult age differences in performance on psychometric intelligence tests. A number of different research designs have been employed to investigate age differences in this area, so the results obtained with different designs can be compared. The two designs traditionally used in developmental research are the cross-sectional and longitudinal designs. With cross-sectional designs individuals of different ages are all tested during the same testing period; thus, the performance of different individuals of different ages are compared. With longitudinal designs the same individuals are tested at all of the ages under investigation; thus, the performance of the same individual is compared at different ages and, therefore, at different testing periods. The use of these two designs has often given a somewhat different perspective on age differences in adult intelligence. Most of the cross-sectional studies have shown an increase in performance up until the early adult years and a decline thereafter (Droppelt & Wallace, 1955; Riegel, 1958; Schaie & Strother, 1968a; Wechsler, 1958). Longitudinal studies, on the other hand, have tended to show stability or slight increases in intelligence from early adulthood through most of the adult years with declines only during the later adult years (Bayley & Oden, 1955; Burns, 1966; Owens, 1953, 1966; Schaie & Strother, 1968a).

These discrepancies are at least partially a result of the fact that age changes and cohort differences are confounded in cross-sectional but not in longitudinal designs. With the cross-sectional design, the individuals of different ages are also members of different cohorts or generations. Thus, if members of different cohorts differ from each other, these differences will be confounded with actual age changes in cross-sectional studies. The drop in intelligence after early adulthood obtained with the cross-sectional studies may be a result of cohort differences rather than a result of actual age changes. The older cohorts may never have functioned as well as the younger cohorts, possibly because they never received as much education or never experienced as many cognitive demands as the younger cohorts. If this were the case, even if there were no real age changes, older individuals would perform less well and, as a consequence, age differences would be obtained.

With the longitudinal design, however, such cohort differences will not be confounded with age since only one cohort is sampled. The developmental curve obtained with the longitudinal studies would be indicative of actual age change. However, there are difficulties with longitudinal studies as well. The age-change function obtained for one cohort in a longitudinal study cannot be generalized to other cohorts; other cohorts could very well exhibit different age-change functions. In the longitudinal study age and time of measurement are confounded. If the circumstances occurring at one time of measurement actually have an effect on performance, this effect would be confounded with any age-change effects occurring at the same time. It is difficult to find an example of how a time of measurement effect might have an effect on adults' intellectual abilities. However, the importance of the confounding of time of measurement with age change in the longitudinal design can be illustrated with the following hypothetical example. Suppose a longitudinal study were done on the activity levels of individuals between the ages of 60 and 80. Suppose also that a new bus program was instituted about 10 years after the study was begun. The program provided buses to transport elderly individuals from their homes to wherever they wanted to go within the city at any time. The institution of the bus program might substantially increase the activity level of the elderly individuals so that an increase in activity would be observed after the tenth year of the study; yet that increase would not reflect a generalized age-change or maturational effect. Rather it would be a function of the time in which the measurement was taken. Thus, the investigator should not conclude that 70-year-olds are more active than 60-year-olds. It is important to realize that the age-change function obtained with one cohort may not generalize to other cohorts. The difficulties associated with longitudinal and cross-sectional designs have been discussed in detail by

Baltes (1968), Buss (1973), Riegel (1973b), Schaie (1965, 1970, 1974), and Wohlwill (1970).

Both Schaie (1965) and Baltes (1968) have proposed research designs that at least partially remedy some of the difficulties associated with the interpretation of the results obtained from cross-sectional and longitudinal designs. Schaie suggested that any analysis of developmental change should take into account three sources of variation: age, cohort, and time of measurement. These three components usually are confounded in developmental research. In cross-sectional designs age and cohort are confounded, as was shown earlier. Time of measurement is not confounded in these designs because only one time of measurement is included. Thus, with cross-sectional designs no estimate of the importance of time of measurement is obtained. In longitudinal designs age and time of measurement are confounded; no estimate of the importance of cohorts is obtained because only one cohort is measured.

Schaie (1965) proposed three new data-collection strategies or designs that might be used to at least partially separate the effects of these three components. The cross-sequential design involves the measurement of two or more cohorts at two or more times of measurement. The cohort-sequential method involves the measurement of two or more cohorts at two or more age levels. The time-sequential design would involve the measurement of two or more ages at two or more times of measurement. Two of the three components in each of these designs can be independently varied, but the third is always determined and confounded with the other two.

With the designs proposed by Schaie it is possible to separate the effects of two of the three components by using one of the proposed designs. Further, Schaie described how estimates of the variance contributed by all three of the components could be obtained by using more than one of the above designs. Although the designs proposed by Schaie are in many ways more informative than the traditional cross-sectional and longitudinal designs, they have not been employed in most of the studies presented in this chapter because of their recent development and difficulty of implementation. Because the more informative designs are not frequently employed, it is important to have a clear understanding of what the strengths and weaknesses of each of the designs commonly employed in developmental research are and what kinds of conclusions can be drawn from the results obtained with each of them.

With the cross-sectional design it is important to

keep in mind that any differences between age groups do not necessarily represent age changes. Further, it is important to remember that the age-change effect obtained in a longitudinal study might not represent a general age-change function. With these considerations in mind, we can proceed to the descriptive research on cognition.

DESCRIPTIVE RESEARCH

Psychometric Tradition

One of the major approaches to understanding cognition is the psychometric intelligence tradition, which is largely correlational. The emphasis has been on identifying the structure of intelligence by determining the interrelationships among different abilities thought to comprise intelligence (Cattell, 1971; Guilford, 1967; Horn, 1970; Thurstone, 1938). The main psychometric theorists with a strong developmental orientation are Cattell (1971) and Horn (1970). They attempted to reduce a number of the primary mental abilities obtained by factor analytic tests by factoring them. This procedure resulted in a small number of second-order factors. The two second-order factors that have received most attention in the area of adult intellectual changes were labeled *fluid* and *crystallized* intelligence. Fluid intelligence included such abilities as inductive reasoning, figural relations, and associative memory and was purported to be closely associated with the neurophysiologic state of the individual. Crystallized intelligence, on the other hand, included such abilities as vocabulary, verbal comprehension, and semantic relations and was purported to be largely determined by learning and acculturation. Horn and Cattell (1967) found that performance on measures of fluid intelligence decreased from adolescence on throughout the life span whereas performance on measures of crystallized intelligence increased throughout the entire life span.

Other researchers have also found that different intellectual abilities follow different developmental patterns over the life span. Nonverbal abilities such as abstract reasoning, perceptual–motor speed, and spatial abilities appear to decline from early adulthood through old age (Birren & Morrison, 1961; Eisdorfer, Busse, & Cohen, 1959; Eisdorfer & Wilkie, 1973; Foulds & Raven, 1948). Verbal abilities, on the other hand, appear to increase throughout most of the life span (Birren & Morrison, 1961; Rhudick & Gordon, 1973; Schaie & Strother, 1968a; Strother,

Schaie, & Horst, 1957), with the exception of a possible decline after the age of about 60 (Birren, 1968; Jarvik & Blum, 1971; Riegel & Riegel, 1972; Schaie & Labouvie-Vief, 1974). Thus, it appears that there are eventual declines in almost all of the abilities tested on standard intelligence tests. However, the research clearly indicates that the age at which such abilities begin to decline may vary considerably depending on the type of ability tested.

These conclusions regarding the development of intellectual abilities across the life span have been based upon traditional cross-sectional and longitudinal research designs as well as newer research designs suggested by Schaie (1965) and Baltes (1968). Thus, it is possible to conclude that there are some actual age changes in intellectual functioning. However, it is important to note that there are also substantial cohort differences in intellectual functioning (Nesselroade, Schaie, & Baltes, 1972; Schaie & Labouvie-Vief, 1974; Schaie, Labouvie-Vief, & Buech, 1973; Schaie & Strother, 1968b).

Piagetian Tradition

A second major approach to understanding cognition is based on Piagetian theory (Flavell, 1963). Piaget has developed a very comprehensive stage theory of cognitive development that includes development from birth through adolescence. The different stages result from changes in the cognitive structures of the child that take place as the child matures and interacts with the environment. Piaget used a wide variety of different tasks to assess cognitive functioning. Recent research on adult age differences in performance on such tasks indicates that elderly adults tend to perform less well than middle-aged adults. For example, elderly adults have been found to perform less well on a variety of different types of tasks that are purported to measure classification skills (Annett, 1959; Denney, 1974a; Denney & Cornelius, 1975; Denney & Lennon, 1972), animistic thinking (Dennis & Mallinger, 1949), egocentric thinking (Bielby & Papalia, 1975; Comalli, Wapner, & Werner, 1959; Looft & Charles, 1971; Rubin, 1974; Rubin, Attewell, Tierney, & Tumolo, 1973), and scientific thinking (Clayton, 1972; Tomlinson-Keasey, 1972).

While the results of these studies seem to indicate a lower level of performance by elderly individuals than by middle-aged individuals on Piagetian tasks, studies of conservation abilities are more equivocal. In tests of conservation, the subject is presented with two quantities of something that are equivalent with respect to a specific relevant dimension. Then the experimenter changes one of the two quantities in some way that does not change it with respect to the relevant dimension. The subject is then asked whether the two quantities are the same with-respect to the relevant dimension. For example, the experimenter might present the subject with two balls composed of the same amount of clay. After the subject has agreed that they are the same amounts of clay, the experimenter might change one of the balls into a flat, pancake-like shape. The experimenter might then ask the subject which ball has more clay. Of course, the correct answer would be that the two balls have the same amount of clay even though they look different. In several cross-sectional studies, elderly individuals have been found to conserve less than younger adults (Papalia, 1972; Rubin et al., 1973; Sanders, Laurendeau, & Bergeron, 1966), while in other studies such age differences have not been obtained (Rubin, 1976; Selzer & Denney, 1977). Thus, it appears that, while age differences were obtained on most Piagetian tasks, conservation may be an exception. The difference between conservation and some of the other Piagetian abilities may be that while most of the other abilities are not exercised much by elderly individuals, conservation abilities would be used by virtually all of the elderly population on almost a daily basis.

It is important to keep in mind that all of the Piagetian studies to date have been cross-sectional and, as a result, it is not possible to determine whether the age differences reflect age changes, cohort differences, or both.

Problem-solving Tradition

With a few exceptions (Smith, 1967; Wetherick, 1964), most of the studies involving performance on traditional problem-solving tasks have yielded age differences with elderly adults exhibiting poorer performance than younger adults. Such differences have been obtained with cross-sectional studies of performance on traditional concept-learning problems. With these problems the individual is presented with stimuli that vary on a number of dimensions and is told, with each presentation, whether the stimulus is a positive or negative instance of the concept. The individual's task is to figure out the concept. For example, the individual might be presented with stimuli that vary in shape, color, and size. If the concept were "red and square," the individual would be told that all stimuli that were both red and square were examples of the concept, while all stimuli that were not red *and* square were not examples of the concept. On the basis of this information the individual should eventually learn that the concept is red and square. Studies by Arenberg (1968), Brinley, Jovick, and McLaughlin (1974), and Carpenter (1971) have demonstrated that elderly adults perform less well than younger adults on such tasks.

Similar age differences have been found with cross-sectional studies of performance on a variety of "search" tasks, in which the individual is supposed to find the correct stimulus or stimulus arrangement from a variety of alternatives. In these tasks the subject selects stimulus alternatives and is told whether the correct stimulus or stimulus arrangement is included in the selected sample. The object is to find the correct solution in as few sample selections as possible. Elderly adults have been found to be less efficient on both nonverbal problems in which the subjects select their stimuli with and receive feedback from a mechanical apparatus (Arenberg, 1974; Jerome, 1962; Young, 1966, 1971) and verbal problems in which the subjects ask questions and receive verbal feedback from the experimenter (Denney & Denney, 1973; Rimoldi & Woude, 1971).

Elderly adults also seem to do more poorly than younger adults on tasks that require that they change the concept or strategy that they are using during the experimental session. In this type of task, the subjects learn to solve a problem or a set of problems with a certain strategy. Then the problem or problems are changed so that the original strategy is either no longer useful at all or is no longer the most efficient strategy. Both Heglin (1956) and Wetherick (1965) found that elderly individuals had more difficulty changing the concept they were using on such tasks than younger adults.

Cross-sectional age differences in verbal reasoning have also been obtained. Bromley (1957) reported that elderly adults performed less well on proverb interpretation tasks than younger adults. Friend and Zubek (1958) reported similar age differences in "critical thinking" on a test composed of a number of practical problems. On a test of logical reasoning, Morgan (1956) also found that elderly adults performed at a lower level than younger adults.

There have been at least two cross-sectional studies of the relationship between problem complexity and age differences. Both Clay (1954) and Kay (1954) found that as the complexity of the problem increased, the difference between the performance of middle-aged and elderly adults also increased.

Arenberg (1974) conducted a longitudinal study of the more traditional type of problem solving. He tested individuals between the ages of 24 and 87 on logical problem solving and then retested the same individuals 6 years later. His cross-sectional comparison showed an increase in errors with increasing age; the largest differences occurred between groups under 60 and groups over 60. On the other hand, his longitudinal trends revealed the decline only in individuals over the age of 70.

Summary

Generally, studies eminating from different theoretical and historical backgrounds indicate that there are age differences among adults in cognitive abilities. The cross-sectional studies typically yield larger differences starting at younger ages than the longitudinal studies primarily because age changes are confounded with cohort differences in the cross-sectional studies, but not in the longitudinal studies. Thus, it appears that the obtained age differences are a result of both age change (evidenced by the results of longitudinal studies) and cohort effects (evidenced by the fact that age differences are greater in cross-sectional studies than in longitudinal studies). Indeed, the issue of whether the obtained age differences are a result of age changes or cohort effects is an important one. Equally important, however, for both theoretical and practical reasons, is to know whether or not the performance of the elderly can be improved. The purpose of the remainder of this chapter will be to review research dealing with the issue of whether the cognitive abilities of elderly individuals can be changed and to discuss the theoretical and practical implications of both descriptive and intervention research.

INTERVENTION RESEARCH

A variety of intervention approaches have been used to facilitate the cognitive performance of elderly individuals. These approaches have been categorized into five basic groups, namely, modeling, direct instruction, feedback, practice, and noncognitive intervention techniques. This categorization system is somewhat simplistic but it does lend some organization to the diverse intervention approaches that have been employed. Each of these basic approaches and its effectiveness will be reviewed separately.

Modeling

A number of investigators have used modeling to facilitate various cognitive abilities in the elderly. In these studies the elderly adults usually view an adult model using cognitive strategies similar to those employed by younger adults. This intervention approach is typically a very effective means of modifying the performance of elderly individuals on cognitive tasks. Denney & Denney (1974) found that modeling improved the question-asking efficiency of older adults on a verbal search task. In another study, Denney (1974a) was able to facilitate the classification performance of elderly adults through modeling. Meichenbaum (1972), likewise, was able to facilitate the performance of elderly adults on concept-learning problems with a modeling procedure. Crovitz (1966) found that elderly individuals were better able to learn to sort a deck of cards according to the ''relevant'' dimension after having observed a model sort the cards three different times according to different dimensions.

In two additional studies, modeling techniques have been used to improve performance on inductive reasoning problems such as those typically included on intelligence tests. The results of these studies, however, do not provide clear evidence for the effectiveness of modeling. Labouvie-Vief and Gonda (1976) employed two modeling procedures, one to facilitate cognitive strategies and one to reduce anxiety. The authors reported that both procedures were effective in increasing inductive reasoning but they were no more effective than a control procedure that consisted only of practice with inductive reasoning problems. Panicucci (1975) also attempted to increase inductive reasoning by modeling the use of problem-solving strategies. Her modeling procedure was not effective in improving performance, although performance did improve in her control group, which received only practice on the problems without any training. Thus, these two studies indicate that inductive reasoning ability may be facilitated by practice, but they are less clear on the effects of modeling. However, with the exception of these two studies on inductive reasoning, the results of research indicate that modeling is a very effective method for improving the performance of elderly adults on cognitive tasks.

Direct Instruction

A second group of intervention procedures could be called direct instruction. These procedures are similar in many ways to modeling procedures. However, rather than being shown how to perform, the participants in these studies are told how to perform on the relevant task.

Heglin (1956) trained young, middle-aged, and elderly adults on a series of set-induction tasks. His training consisted of telling the subjects that their difficulty on some of the later problems was due to their continued use of methods that they had learned for solving some of the earlier problems. He also told the participants that they should try to avoid using only one way to solve the problems. Heglin reported that middle-aged individuals gained more from the training than did either the younger or older adults; the older adults gained the least. Heglin did not analyze pretraining versus posttraining differences within each age group, so it is not possible to determine whether significant increases were obtained for any of the age groups.

Young (1966) used a direct-instruction procedure to facilitate the performance of middle-age and elderly adults on a nonverbal search task. Her instructions were designed to impose order on the subjects' search strategy and to decrease the demands on short-term memory. She found that, even after training, the elderly adults still performed at a lower level than did the younger adults. However, since she did not include a control group of individuals who were not given such instructions, it is not possible to determine whether the instructions had a facilitating effect for either age group.

It is difficult to draw conclusions on the basis of the results of the direct-instruction studies because of the inadequate research designs and inadequate reporting of the results. In spite of their problems, these studies do suggest that elderly adults may benefit less from direct-instruction training than younger adults. This is somewhat surprising since elderly adults start out with a lower level of performance, thus leaving room for improvement. It also would be surprising if direct instruction were not effective when modeling is, because direct instruction involves just telling the subjects how to perform whereas modeling involves showing the subjects how to perform. However, it is possible that the verbal instructions may be too abstract for the elderly to comprehend as well as they comprehend the more concrete modeling instructions in which they are actually shown how to perform.

Feedback

A third type of intervention approach consists of providing the subjects with feedback regarding the correctness of their performance. Schutz and Hoyer (1976) investigated the effects of verbal feedback contingent on the correctness of elderly individuals' responses on a spatial egocentrism task. In addition to the verbal feedback, the elderly individuals in the training condition were shown how each pattern appeared from the experimenter's perspective by rotating the pattern 180°. On the posttest more correct responses were obtained in the feedback condition than in either the practice or the no-practice control conditions.

Sanders, Sterns, Smith, and Sanders (1975) assigned elderly adults in a concept-learning experiment to one of four experimental conditions: a reinforced training condition, a training condition, a practice condition, and a control condition. In the training condition, the participants were given verbal feedback after each response and, if necessary, they were also given "strategy hints" and "memory cue cards." In the reinforced training condition they were given tokens for correct responses in addition to the training. In the practice condition, if the participant failed a problem, the solution was given before he or she went on to the next problem, but no other feedback was given. In the control condition, the participants were given only the pretest and the posttest. Both the reinforced training and the training conditions resulted in better performance on the posttest than either the practice or the control conditions.

There is at least one study in which only feedback was given without any additional instruction. Hornblum and Overton (1976) attempted to train elderly people to conserve by providing them with feedback contingent on their responses to conservation problems. The control subjects received the same problems without feedback. Significantly, more conservation responses were obtained on the posttest in the feedback condition than in the control condition.

Since most of the investigations of the effectiveness of feedback have also included some instructions regarding strategy similar to those employed in the modeling and direct instruction procedures, it is difficult to assess the effects of feedback alone. However, since the feedback in the Hornblum and Overton study, which was not confounded with any other procedures, was effective, it suggests that feedback alone may actually have a beneficial effect on cognitive abilities.

Practice

Some investigators have suggested that elderly individuals may not perform as well as younger individuals on cognitive tasks because they are not frequently required to use the cognitive abilities tested in their everyday living (Denney & Denney, 1974; Selzer & Denney, 1977). If this were the case, then practice on identical or similar problems might facilitate performance. A number of the previously mentioned studies have included practice-only control groups. In at least two of these studies, practice by itself resulted in improved cognitive performance (Labouvie-Vief & Gonda, 1976; Panicucci, 1975). However, there are studies that show no significant practice effects (Hoyer, Hoyer, Treat, & Baltes, 1978–1979; Sanders et al., 1975; Schutz & Hoyer, 1976). Because of these conflicting results, the effects of practice on cognitive abilities in the elderly are difficult to assess. Practice may be more beneficial for some types of abilities than for others, or some practice procedures might be more conducive to facilitating performance than others.

Noncognitive Intervention

A number of investigators have suggested that elderly individuals' performance might be lower than the performance of younger individuals for reasons other than differential cognitive ability. They have suggested that elderly individuals may not perform as well as they are capable for reasons such as lack of motivation, general slowing of response speed, insufficient consideration of the tasks' demands, or lack of self-confidence regarding cognitive performance. Thus, a variety of noncognitive intervention techniques have been developed to try to change the characteristic that the researchers think might be responsible for the less-than-optimal performance of the elderly.

One intervention technique that has been used to change some characteristic of the subject other than cognitive ability itself is that of altering the elderly individuals' response speed. Hoyer, Labouvie, and Baltes (1973) hypothesized that the fact that elderly individuals tend to respond more slowly than younger adults might very well be a result of experience rather than a result of neurophysiologic deficits, as is usually assumed. They also hypothesized that their slower rate of responding might be responsible, at least in part, for their poorer performance on intellectual tests. They attempted to increase the response speed of elderly women on speeded perceptual-motor tasks in order to further determine whether the resulting increases in response speed would be reflected in performance on the intellectual tasks that contain a speeded component. Three treatment conditions included a reinforcement condition, in which the subjects were reinforced whenever they completed a trial in less time than in earlier trials, a practice condition, in which the subjects performed

all of the tasks but were not given feedback, and a control condition, in which the subjects were not presented with the training tasks. The results indicated that response speed increased as a function of practice but that the actual reinforcement procedure had little effect. Further, neither the training nor the practice had any effect on the intellectual task. In a second study, Hoyer et al. (1978–1979) increased the number of training sessions, but again no treatment-condition effects were found either in response time on the training tasks or in performance on the intelligence subtests. Thus, attempts to increase cognitive performance indirectly by reinforcing response speed on some unrelated task does not seem to be as effective as some of the more direct cognitive methods.

Denney (1978) conducted a series of studies to determine whether manipulating variables other than cognitive performance itself might directly influence cognitive performance on verbal search tasks. She hypothesized that elderly individuals might not perform efficiently on the 20-questions task, a verbal search task, because they are not motivated to try to perform well, because they lack confidence in their ability to perform well, or because they do not take enough time to consider the strategy they are going to use on the task. Thus, she manipulated each of these variables before presenting her elderly subjects with the task in order to see if these manipulations had an effect on performance. She attempted to increase motivation by setting up a system in which the elderly received more money as the number of questions required to solve the problem decreased. She found no difference between the performance of the subjects who were reinforced with money for efficient performance and those who were not reinforced.

Denney also tried to manipulate self-confidence by presenting the elderly adults with a series of problems on which they were told that they were doing extremely well before presenting them with the actual 20-questions task. Individuals in the control condition were given the same problems but no feedback. No difference was obtained between the training and the control groups.

Denney also suggested that the elderly might not perform as well on the 20-questions task as younger individuals because they might not take the time necessary to consider the demands of the task and think of the most appropriate strategy given these demands. Thus, in one study individuals in the experimental group were given a forced 3-minute delay between the time when the experimenter gave the instructions for the task and the time when the task was to be started. The control group was given no such delay. Again, no differences between the experimental and control groups were obtained.

The results of this series of studies certainly do not prove that the manipulation of variables such as motivation, self-confidence, and time to plan a strategy could not be effective. It is possible that better manipulation of these variables might be more effective or that manipulations of these variables might be effective for improving performance on other types of congitive tasks. It is also possible that the manipulation of other peripheral, noncognitive variables might be more promising than the manipulation of those studied by Denney. However, until more research is done in this area, we must conclude that it does not appear as if short-term manipulation of such peripheral variables is a very effective means for facilitating cognitive performance among the elderly.

Summary

In summary, both the modeling and feedback intervention techniques appear to be rather effective in changing cognitive performance among the elderly. Direct instruction may also be effective, although it is difficult to evaluate some of the direct-instruction studies because the research designs do not permit one to draw any clear conclusions regarding the effectiveness of training. The effect of practice on identical or similar problems also is unclear; in some studies practice alone resulted in improved performance while in others it did not.

On the other hand, none of the studies aimed at changing some noncognitive characteristics of elderly individuals resulted in improved cognitive performance. Thus, research so far indicates that any cognitive deficits exhibited by elderly individuals might best be remedied by cognitive rather than noncognitive intervention programs. Further, the results tend to suggest that the cognitive performance deficits result from actual cognitive deficits rather than from changes in noncognitive factors.

THEORETICAL IMPLICATIONS

The descriptive research indicates that in general elderly individuals perform less well on cognitive tasks than do younger adults. The results of the intervention research indicates that the cognitive performance of the elderly can often be facilitated

rather easily with very brief, short-term intervention techniques. Further, the intervention research indicates that the best way to facilitate cognitive performance among the elderly is to give them direct training on the abilities involved. These findings have both theoretical and practical implications.

Age Change versus Cohort Differences

The descriptive studies provide evidence relevant to the issue of whether the age differences that have been found in cognitive ability are a result of age-change effects or cohort-difference effects. The sequential and the longitudinal studies of intelligence and Arenberg's (1974) longitudinal study of logical problem solving indicate that there are actual age changes in cognitive performance during the adult years. However, these studies also indicate that there are cohort differences as well, evidenced by the fact that cross-sectional age differences are usually larger than longitudinal age differences and the fact that cohort effects are usually obtained in studies of intelligence. However, the longitudinal and sequential designs have been employed mainly with studies of psychometric intelligence. Thus, it is not clear that similar results would be obtained in other areas of cognitive functioning. More longitudinal and sequential research needs to be done in these other areas.

Antecedents of Age Changes and Cohort Differences

A second theoretical question involves the antecedents of age differences in cognition among adults. Cognitive deficits among the elderly have traditionally been thought to result from declines in neurophysiologic functioning that accompany aging (Dennis & Mallinger, 1949; Hooper, Fitzgerald, & Papalia, 1971; Horn, 1970; Rubin et al., 1973; Young, 1971). However, more recently some investigators have suggested that the age differences that have been found in cognitive ability may result, at least in part, from experiential differences. For example, some investigators have suggested that a decline in social interaction that occurs with aging may be responsible for changes in cognitive performance (Looft & Charles, 1971; Rubin et al., 1973). Others have suggested that decreases in educational and occupational demands that occur during the later adult years could be responsible for changes in cognitive performance. The intervention studies also indicate that, in addition to neurophysiologic changes with age, experiential factors contribute to age differences in cognitive abilities.

Although there has been much discussion and controversy regarding the environmental and/or biological determinants of age changes in cognitive ability, there has not been much investigation of the antecedents of cohort differences. Both the environmental and biologic variables that might be responsible for cohort differences need to be considered. The only variable that has received much attention as a possible cause of cohort differences to date is education. Education is one of the few variables that varies as a function of cohort and is easily measurable. The relationship between education and cognitive ability, however, is not clear. A number of investigators have reported significant relationships between education and cognitive performance (Kesler, Denney, & Whitely, 1976; Papalia, Kennedy, & Sheehan, 1973; Papalia, Salverson, & True, 1973; Selzer & Denney, 1977; Young, 1971), while others have reported that education was not significantly related to cognitive performance (Rubin, 1974; Rubin et al., 1973; Storck, Looft, & Hooper, 1972). Although not definitive, these results suggest that differences in education could be responsible for some of the cohort effects in cognitive abilities. Additionally, there are a number of other environmental variables that need to be investigated as potential contributors to cohort effects. In addition to environmental variables that might vary across cohort, biologic variables such as nutrition, physical exercise, physical illness, and drug consumption should also be investigated as possible contributors to cohort effects in cognition.

Schaie's Theory of Adult Cognition

Although the amount of empirical research in the area of cognitive development during adulthood has increased in recent years, there still has been very little theoretical work in the area. One theoretical attempt was made by Riegel (1973a) who proposed a fifth stage, that of dialectic operations, to supplement Piaget's theory of cognitive development in children. A more recent attempt was made by Schaie (1977–1978). Schaie reasoned that any stage theory of cognitive development that depicted the childhood years as those in which cognitive abilities are acquired and the adolescent or early adult years as those in which the abilities reach asymptote needs additional stages to adequately describe cognition during

the adult years. He suggested that if the purpose of the first part of life is to acquire those skills, then it is necessary to postulate further stages in which those acquired skills are employed in real life situations.

Schaie (1977–1978) proposed a theory of cognitive development involving five stages that cover the entire life span. These stages are illustrated in Figure 7–1. The first stage is characterized as the *acquisitive stage*. During this stage, the child acquires cognitive abilities while still functioning in a protected environment. The second stage, called the *achieving stage,* occurs in young adulthood when the individual is no longer functioning in a protected environment. During this stage individuals must accept responsibility for themselves and, as a consequence, the main goal is no longer the acquisition of cognitive abilities but rather the application of the cognitive skills already learned. Schaie referred to this process as the achievement of competence. During this stage, the individual must achieve independence and, as a consequence, must use the abilities acquired during the acquisition stage in a much more goal-directed manner. During this stage Schaie suggested that the individual will function cognitively in a much more efficient and effective manner with respect to tasks that have "role-related achievement potential."

The third stage, the *responsible stage,* occurs when the individual has established role competence and begins to take on responsibility for other individuals while establishing a family. The demands of this period in one's life, Schaie suggested, result in further changes in cognitive functioning. During this stage, the individual needs to integrate long-range goals as well as responsibilities for one's family in the solution of real-life problems. Schaie suggested that the demands during this period of one's life should result in increased performance on problem-solving tasks that are relevant to real-life situations, increases in cognitive flexibility, and decreases in field dependence, as well as a gain in crystallized intelligence and a loss in fluid intelligence. Schaie suggested that crystallized abilities will increase during this stage because they are relevant to the kinds of problems the individual has to deal with on a daily basis, while fluid abilities will decrease because they are not typically used on a daily basis.

For other individuals during this same period of life, the *executive stage* may be reached. This stage is reached by individuals who have to assume responsibility for societal systems rather than, or in addition to, responsibility for family units. This assumption of

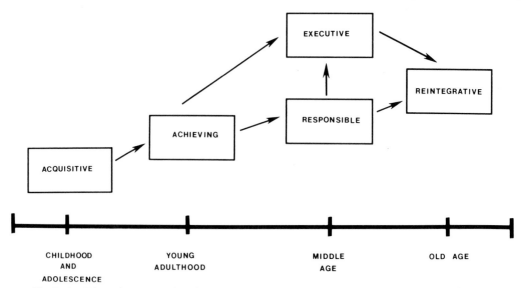

Fig. 7–1: Schematic representation of the five-stage life-span theory of cognitive development as proposed by Schaie. (Reprinted with permission from Schaie, K. W. Toward a theory of adult cognitive development. *Journal of Aging and Human Development*, 1977–1978, 8 (2), 129–138. © 1977, Baywood Publishing Co., Inc.)

responsibility demands the development of cognitive abilities for integrating complex and high-level hierarchical relationships. The assumption of such responsibility, Schaie contended, should result in increases in performance on tests of pattern recognition, inductive reasoning, and complex problem solving with corresponding decreases in the ability to deal with very specific problem-solving tasks and new bits of information.

Schaie suggested that standard intelligence tests are not really very good indicators of cognitive functioning during the responsible and executive stages. He added that the abilities measured by standard intelligence tests are those acquired during the acquisition and achieving stages but not those that are acquired when the individual takes on organizational, integrative, and interpretative roles. Schaie suggested that new measures of cognitive functioning may have to be developed to measure the abilities that are used most frequently during these later stages.

While the first four stages in Schaie's theory deal with cognitive abilities that are developed in response to the need for integration of learned intellectual skills at increasing levels of role complexity, the final stage in Schaie's theory deals with cognitive changes that occur during the last part of life when the degree of societal involvement and responsibility

decreases and when biologic changes may once again impose limits on cognitive functioning. Schaie referred to the final stage as the *reintegrative stage*. He suggested that the cognitive processes that are adaptive during this stage of one's life may be somewhat unrelated to the processes that are adaptive during the earlier stages. He further suggested that cognitive processes during this stage are probably much more heavily influenced by motivational and attitudinal variables than at any other stage. This stage occurs at a time when "the complexity of the adult cognitive structure has reached an overload stage, and consequently demands simplification, and where environmentally programmed role requirements are reduced due to occupational retirement, relinquishment of responsibilities for children and family, and other role restrictions" (Schaie, 1977–1978). As a result, the individual responds by being more selective in attending to cognitive demands that remain meaningful or attain new meaning. Thus, problem-solving behavior no longer occurs as a simple response to competence-motivational situations, but rather, occurs in situations that have meaning and purpose within the life situation of the individual. Schaie recommended that new types of measurement instruments must be devised to measure the cognitive functioning of elderly individuals. Such measurement will first require the analysis of criterion variables relevant to the life experiences and roles of elderly individuals.

PRACTICAL IMPLICATIONS

The intervention research reported previously was typically undertaken to determine whether some of the deficits that have been observed in the cognitive functioning of elderly individuals can be ameliorated and, if so, by what techniques. By determining what needs to be done in order to change cognitive performance, we presumably gain a better understanding of the antecedents of cognitive functioning. However, in a number of these studies, the underlying assumption was that it would be beneficial to change the cognitive functioning of elderly individuals if successful techniques could be found. Presumably no permanent changes would be effected with the brief, short-term training procedures used to date. However, the same procedures might possibly be expanded into long-term training programs to facilitate cognitive functioning in the elderly. Before such programs are instituted, however, it is extremely important that we first determine whether changing the cognitive functioning of elderly individuals would be beneficial.

It is possible, for example, that elderly individuals function in a very adaptive way, given their particular life situations. For example, Denney (1974b) has suggested that elderly individuals may classify stimuli in a way that is often considered to be less sophisticated but is actually more adaptive for them. The elderly often classify stimuli according to complementary criteria, that is, they put things together that show some complementary relationship, such as hammer and nail, rather than putting together things that are similar, such as hammer and axe. Denney suggested that both young children and elderly adults may classify according to complementary criteria because these criteria are the most natural and salient. That is, objects are grouped according to complementary criteria in the world and, therefore, in one's natural experience. She further suggested that the natural tendency to group according to complementary criteria may only be overcome when individuals are encouraged to classify in more abstract ways because of educational and/or occupational demands. If this hypothesis is correct, then there would be nothing to be gained by trying to change the way in which elderly adults classify.

It is possible that the ways in which elderly adults perform on other types of cognitive tasks also might represent more adaptive ways of interacting, given their life situations, than some of the ways in which younger adults approach the same problems. This possibility needs to be carefully considered. More harm than good might be done by the institution of long-term training procedures. At the very least, it might be a waste of time and effort for both the elderly individuals involved and the investigators.

REFERENCES

Annett, M. The classification of instances of four common class concepts by children and adults. *British Journal of Educational Psychology*, 1959, *29*, 223–236.

Arenberg, D. Concept problem solving in young and old adults. *Journal of Gerontology*, 1968, *23*, 297–282.

Arenberg, D. A longitudinal study of problem solving in adults. *Journal of Gerontology*, 1974, *29*, 650–658.

Baltes, P. B. Longitudinal and cross-sectional sequences in the study of age and generation effects. *Human Development*, 1968, *11*, 145–171.

Bayley, N., & Oden, M. H. The maintenance of intellectual ability in gifted adults. *Journal of Gerontology*, 1955, *10*, 91–107.

Bielby, D. D., & Papalia, D. E. Moral development and egocentrism: Their development and interrelationship across the life-span. *International Journal of Aging and Human Development*, 1975, *6*, 293–308.

Birren, J. E. & Morrison, D. F. Analysis of the WAIS subtests in relation to age and education. *Journal of Gerontology*, 1961, *16*, 363–369.

Birren. J. E. Increments and decrements in the intellectual status of the aged. *Psychiatric Research Reports*, 1968, *23*, 207–214.

Brinley, J. F., Jovick, T. J., & McLaughlin, L. M. Age, reasoning, and memory in adults. *Journal of Gerontology*, 1974, *29*, 182–189.

Bromley, D. B. Some effects of age on the quality of intellectual output. *Journal of Gerontology*, 1957, *12*, 318–323.

Burns, R. B. Age and mental ability: Re-testing with thirty-three years interval. *British Journal of Educational Psychology*, 1966, *36*, 116.

Buss, A. R. An extension of developmental models that separate ontogenetic change and cohort differences. *Psychological Bulletin*, 1973, *80*, 446–479.

Carpenter, W. L. The relationship between age and information processing capacity of adults. *Industrial Gerontology*, 1971, *8*, 55–57.

Cattell, R. B. *Abilities: Their structure, growth and action*. Boston: Houghton Mifflin, 1971.

Clay, H. M. Changes of performance with age on similar tasks of varying complexity. *British Journal of Psychology*, 1954, *45*, 7–13.

Clayton, V. The role of formal operational thought in the aging process. Unpublished manuscript, State University of New York at Buffalo, 1972.

Comalli, P. E., Wapner, S., & Werner, H. Perception of verticality in middle and old age. *Journal of Psychology*, 1959, *47*, 259–266.

Crovitz, E. Reversing a learning deficit in the aged. *Journal of Gerontology*, 1966, *21*, 236–238.

Denney, N. W. Classification abilities in the elderly. *Journal of Gerontology*, 1974, *29*, 309–314. (a)

Denney, N. W. Evidence for developmental change in categorization criteria for children and adults. *Human Development*, 1974, *17*, 41–53. (b)

Denney, N. W. The effect of the manipulation of peripheral variables on problem-solving performance among the elderly. Unpublished manuscript, University of Kansas, 1978.

Denney, N. W., & Cornelius, S. Class inclusion and multiple classification in middle and old age. *Developmental Psychology*, 1975, *11*, 521–522.

Denney, D. R., & Denney, N. W. The use of classification for problem solving: A comparison of middle and old age. *Developmental Psychology* 1973, *9*, 275–278.

Denney, N. W., & Denney, D. R. Modeling effects on the questioning strategies of the elderly. *Developmental Psychology*, 1974, *10*, 400–404.

Denney, N. W., & Lennon, M. L. Classification: A comparison of middle and old age. *Developmental Psychology*, 1972, *7*, 210–213.

Dennis, W., & Mallinger, B. Animism and related tendencies in senescence. *Journal of Gerontology*, 1949, *4*, 218–221.

Droppelt, J. E., & Wallace, W. L. Standardization of the Wechsler Adult Intelligence Scale for older persons. *Journal of Abnormal and Social Psychology*, 1955, *51*, 312–330.

Eisdorfer, C., Busse, E. W., & Cohen, L. D. The WAIS performance of an aged sample: The relationship between verbal and performance I.Q.'s *Journal of Gerontology*, 1959, *14*, 197–201.

Eisdorfer, C., & Wilkie, F. Intellectual changes with advancing age. In L. F. Garvik, C. Eisdorfer, & J. E. Blum (Eds.), *Intellectual functioning in adults*. New York: Springer Publishing Co., 1973.

Flavell, J. H. *The developmental psychology of Jean Piaget*. New York: D. Van Nostrand, 1963.

Flavell, J. H. Cognitive changes in adulthood. In L. B. Goulet & P. B. Baltes (Eds.), *Life-span developmental psychology: Research and theory*. New York: Academic Press, 1970.

Foulds, G. A., & Raven, J. C. Neural changes in mental abilities of adults as age advances. *Journal of Mental Science*, 1948, *94*, 133–142.

Friend, C. M., & Zubek, J. P. The effects of age on critical thinking ability. *Journal of Gerontology*, 1958, *13*, 407–413.

Guilford, J. P. *The nature of human intelligence*. New York: McGraw-Hill Book Co., 1967.

Heglin, H. J. Problem solving set in different age groups. *Journal of Gerontology*, 1956, *11*, 310–317.

Horn, J. L. Organization of data on life-span development of human abilities. In L. B. Goulet & P.

B. Baltes (Eds.), *Life-span developmental psychology: Research and theory.* New York: Academic Press, 1970.

Horn, J. L., & Cattell, R. B. Age differences in fluid and crystallized intelligence. *Acta Psychologica (Amsterdam),* 1967, *26,* 107−129.

Hooper, F., Fitzgerald, J., & Papalia, D. Piagetian theory and the aging process: Extensions and speculations. *Aging and Human Development,* 1971, *2,* 3−20.

Hornblum, J. N., & Overton, W. F. Area and volume conservation among the elderly: Assessment and training. *Developmental Psychology,* 1976, *12,* 68−74.

Hoyer, F. W., Hoyer, W. J., Treat, N. J., & Baltes, P. B. Training response speed in young and elderly women. *International Journal of Aging and Human Development,* 1978−1979, *9,* 247−253.

Hoyer, W., Labouvie, G., & Baltes, P. Modification of response speed and intellectual performance in the elderly. *Human Development,* 1973, *16,* 233−242.

Jarvik, L. F., & Blum, J. E. Cognitive declines as predictors of mortality in twin pairs: A twenty-year longitudinal study of aging. In E. Palamore & F. Jeffers (Eds.), *Prediction of lifespan.* Lexington: D. C. Heath & Co., 1971.

Jerome, E. A. Decay of heuristic processes in the aged. In C. Tibbitts & W. Donahue (Eds.), *Social and psychological aspects of aging.* New York: Columbia University Press, 1962.

Kay, H. The effects of position in a display upon problem solving. *Quarterly Journal of Experimental Psychology,* 1954, *6,* 155−169.

Kesler, M. S., Denney, N. W., & Whitely, S. E. Factors influencing problem solving in middle-aged and elderly adults. *Human Development,* 1976, *19,* 310−320.

Labouvie-Vief, G., & Gonda, J. N. Cognitive strategy training and intellectual performance in the elderly. *Journal of Gerontology,* 1976, *31,* 327−332.

Looft, W. R., & Charles, D. C. Egocentrism and social interaction in young and old adults. *International Journal of Aging and Human Development,* 1971, *2,* 21−28.

Meichenbaum, D. Training the aged in verbal control of behavior. Paper presented at the International Congress on Gerontology, Kiev, Russia, 1972.

Morgan, A. B. Differences in logical reasoning associated with age and higher education. *Psychological Reports,* 1956, *2,* 235−240.

Nesselroade, J. R., Schaie, K. W., & Baltes, P. B. Ontogenetic and generational components of structural and quantitative change in adult behavior. *Journal of Gerontology,* 1972, *27,* 222−228.

Owens, W. A. Age and mental abilities: A longitudinal study. *Genetic Psychology Monographs,* 1953, *48,* 3−54.

Owens, W. A. Age and mental ability: A second adult follow-up. *Journal of Educational Psychology,* 1966, *57,* 311−325.

Panicucci, C. L. The effect of training on inductive reasoning behavior in young and old adults. Paper presented at the 28th Annual Meeting of the American Gerontological Society, Louisville, Kentucky, October 1975.

Papalia, D. E. The status of several conservation abilities across the life-span. *Human Development,* 1972, *15,* 229−243.

Papalia, D., Kennedy, E., & Sheehan, N. Conservation of space in non-instutionalized old people. *Journal of Psychology,* 1973, *84,* 75−79.

Papalia, D. E., Salverson, S. M., & True, M. An evaluation of quantity conservation performance during old age. *International Journal of Aging and Human Development,* 1973, *4,* 103−109.

Rhudick, P. J., & Gordon, C. The age center of New England study. In L. F. Jarvik, C. Eisdorfer, & J. E. Blum (Eds.), *Intellectual functioning in adults.* New York: Springer Publishing Co., 1973.

Riegel, K. F. Ergebnisse und probleme der psychologischen alternsforschung. Teil I & II. *Vita Humana,* 1958, *1,* 52−64, 204−243.

Riegel, K. F. Dialectic operations: The final period of cognitive development. *Human Development,* 1973, *16,* 346−370. (a)

Riegel, K. F. Language and cognition: Some life-span developmental issues. *Gerontologist*, 1973, *13*, 478–482. (b)

Riegel, K. F., & Riegel, R. M. Development, drop, and death. *Developmental Psychology*, 1972, *6*, 306–319.

Rimoldi, H. G. A., & Woude, K. W. V. Aging and problem solving. *Industrial Gerontology*, 1971, *8*, 68–69.

Rubin, K. The relationship between spatial and communicative egocentrism in children and young and old adults. *Journal of Genetic Psychology*, 1974, *83*, 295–301.

Rubin, K. Extinction of conservation: A life-span investigation. *Developmental Psychology*, 1976, *12*, 51–56.

Rubin, K. H., Attewell, P., Tierney, M., & Tumolo, P. The development of spatial egocentrism and conservation across the life-span. *Developmental Psychology*, 1973, *9*, 432.

Sanders, S., Laurendeau, M., & Bergeron, J. Aging and the concept of space: The conservation of surfaces. *Journal of Gerontology*, 1966, *21*, 281–285.

Sanders, J. C., Sterns, H. L., Smith, M., & Sanders, R. E. Modification of concept identification performance in older adults. *Developmental Psychology*, 1975, *11*, 824–829.

Schaie, K. W. A general model for the study of developmental problems. *Psychological Bulletin*, 1965, *64*, 92–107.

Schaie, K. W. A reinterpretation of age related changes in cognitive structure and functioning. In L. R. Goulet & P. B. Baltes (Eds.), *Life-span developmental psychology: Research and development*. New York: Academic Press, 1970.

Schaie, K. W. Translations in gerontology—from lab to life: Intellectual functioning. *American Psychologist*, 1974, *29*, 802–807.

Schaie, K. W. Toward a stage theory of adult cognitive development. *Journal of Aging and Human Development*, 1977–1978, *8*, 129–138.

Schaie, K. W., & Labouvie-Vief, G. Generational versus ontogenetic components of change in adult cognitive behavior: A fourteen-year cross-sequential study. *Developmental Psychology*, 1974, *10*, 305–320.

Schaie, K. W., Labouvie-Vief, G. F., & Buech, B. U. Generational and cohort-specific differences in adult cognitive functioning: A fourteen-year study of independent samples. *Developmental Psychology*, 1973, *9*, 151–166.

Schaie, K. W., & Strother, C. R. A cross-sectional study of age changes in cognitive behavior. *Psychological Bulletin*, 1968, *70*, 671–680. (a)

Schaie, K. W., & Strother, C. R. The effects of time and cohort differences on the interpretation of age changes in cognitive behavior. *Multivariate Behavioral Research*, 1968, *3*, 259–294. (b).

Schutz, N. R., & Hoyer, W. J. Feedback effects on spatial egocentrism in old age. *Journal of Gerontology*, 1976, *31*, 72–75.

Selzer, S. C., & Denney, N. W. Conservation abilities among middle-aged and elderly adults. Paper presented at the Biennial meeting of the Society for Research in Child Development. New Orleans, March 1977.

Smith, D. K. The Einstellung effect in relation to the variables of age and training. *Dissertation Abstracts*, 1967, *27B*, 4115.

Storck, P. A., Looft, W. R., & Hooper, F. H. Interrelationships among Piagetian tasks and traditional measures of cognitive abilities in mature and aged adults. *Journal of Gerontology*, 1972, *27*, 461–465.

Strother, C. R., Schaie, K. W., & Horst, P. The relationship between advanced age and mental abilities. *Journal of Abnormal and Social Psychology*, 1957, *55*, 166–170.

Thurstone, L. L. Primary mental abilities. *Psychometric Monographs*, 1938, *1*.

Tomlinson-Keasey, C. Formal operations in females from eleven to fifty-six years of age. *Developmental Psychology*, 1972, *6*, 364.

Wetherick, N. E. A comparison of the problem-solving ability of young, middle-aged and old subjects. *Gerontologia*, 1964, *9*, 164–178.

Weatherick, N. E. Changing an established concept: A comparison of the ability of young, middle-aged and old subjects. *Gerontologia,* 1965, *11,* 82−95.

Wechsler, D. *The measurement and appraisal of adult intelligence* (4th ed.). Baltimore: Williams & Wilkins, 1958.

Wohlwill, J. F. Methodology and research strategy in the study of development change. In L. R. Goulet & P. B. Baltes (Eds.), *Life-span development psychology: Research and theory.* New York: Academic Press, 1970.

Young, M. L. Problem-solving performance in two age groups. *Journal of Gerontology,* 1966, *21,* 505−509.

Young, M. L. Age and sex differences in problem solving. *Journal of Gerontology,* 1971, *26,* 330−336.

Anderson D. Smith
Audrey M. Fullerton

8

Age Differences in Episodic and Semantic Memory: Implications for Language and Cognition

INTRODUCTION

The purpose of this chapter is to describe some of the experimental research currently being conducted on age-related differences in memory performance. Memory is the core of cognition and a necessary prerequisite to the understanding of the cognitive processing involved in language production and comprehension. Language use is characterized by the abilities to learn, that is, to encode information into memory; to store, that is, to retain information over both brief and long intervals of time; and to retrieve, that is, to decode information at the time speech is initiated. If older subjects are deficient in one or more of these mnemonic stages, a correlated change might occur in their ability to use language, either as a speaker or as a listener.

One popular view of memory, depicted in Figure 8−1, is the multistore model (Atkinson & Shiffrin, 1971; Waugh & Norman, 1965), which holds that memory can be divided into separate stores or types. After briefly being held in sensory-memory, information is attended to and stored in short-term memory. The information may then be encoded into

The preparation of this manuscript was supported in part by a National Institutes of Health research grant (No. AG-00445) from the Institute on Aging to Anderson D. Smith.

long-term memory where it can be retained for longer periods of time prior to retrieval and utilization.

Information in long-term memory can be considered to be either episodic or semantic (Tulving, 1972). Episodic memory is the internal diary, that is, memory traces organized by temporal context or experience. Semantic memory, on the other hand, is the internal dictionary, that is, memory traces organized by concept and semantic meaning. For episodic memory, temporal and/or contextual information about the original encoding is used for retrieval. Whereas these types of information form the basis for retrieval from episodic memory, they are not useful for retrieval from semantic memory. In other words, we know our names and that two plus two equals four and that a canary is a bird, but we do not remember the contextual information about when or how we learned these items from semantic memory. Concepts and facts form the structure of semantic memory, together with rules about the organization of concepts, the mental lexicon, and the rules of language. In contrast, questions such as "What did you have for breakfast this morning?" or "Who was the person you just met?" or "What were the items on the memory list you just saw?" involve episodic memory in that contextual or temporal cues about the information are used for retrieval.

In this chapter, we will review studies using the theoretical framework shown in Figure 8−1. While there are some conceptual problems with this formu-

139

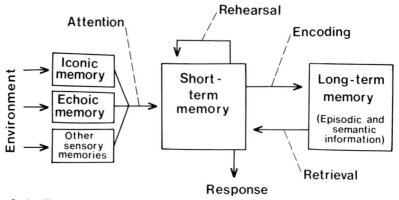

Fig. 8−1:   The multistore memory model used to organize the research discussed in this chapter.

lation (Craik & Lockhart, 1972; Postman, 1975), it serves as a useful framework to organize and discuss current research. First, we will discuss age differences in sensory and short-term memory, followed by consideration of age differences in long-term memory for both episodically and semantically stored information.

SENSORY MEMORY

As illustrated in Figure 8−1, information from the environment enters via the senses and is stored briefly in a raw, unanalyzed form between the time that it is received from the environment and the time when it is attended to. The information is not only preattentive, but decays rapidly with time.

Iconic Memory

Visual sensory memory, or iconic memory, has been estimated to last approximately ¼ to ½ second in young adults (Walsh & Thompson, 1978). While there is some evidence that the duration of visual sensory storage is shorter in older subjects, the significance of this finding for later information processing (i.e., short-term and long-term memory) is equivocal. In one experiment, for example, Walsh and Thompson (1978) measured age differences in the duration of iconic memory using the method of Haber and Standing (1969). Subjects were presented two visual stimuli separated by a variable interstimulus interval. The longest interstimulus interval for which subjects reported a single visual stimulus was then determined. This threshold value was found to be 41 msec shorter in the older age group. In other words, visual sensory memory duration was shorter in the older age group. Such a find-

ing is typical and has been reported by other investigators using different procedures to tap visual memory (Abel, 1972; Schonfield & Wenger, 1975).

The difference in interstimulus interval values between young and old subjects, however, is a small one, a difference of only 15 percent. It is not clear that such a small difference could account for the substantial deficits seen in later memory processing of older people. Further, short-term memory, the next step in the information-processing system, is relatively unaffected by age. The lack of an age deficit in short-term memory indicates that there is no general and ubiquitous deficit caused by early sensory memory problems. If a deficit in iconic memory is the cause of all memory deficits seen in older age groups, then effects should be seen at all stages in the memory system subsequent to iconic memory. It is unlikely, therefore, that the small deficit in iconic memory can account for later memory deficits in long-term memory. This is essentially the conclusion reached by Walsh and Thompson (1978).

Echoic Memory

There has been very little study of possible age differences in the auditory-sensory store, or echoic memory, but indirect evidence from dichotic-listening studies does suggest an age deficit. Age differences on dichotic-listening tasks are found for information assumed to be recalled from a preperceptual auditory store. In such experiments, subjects are presented two messages simultaneously, one message to each ear. At recall, subjects tend to recall the message from one ear followed by the message from the other. Recall of the message in the unattended ear could be accomplished by using the auditory-sensory store, but because such storage decays rapidly with time and because recall of the unattended message is delayed until the attended message is recalled, such recall is typically poor. Several studies have reported that age differences are found with such a task, but only in the "second half" of recall, the message recalled from the auditory-sensory store (Inglis & Caird, 1963; Mackay & Inglis, 1963). There are problems, however, with the interpretation that such findings are indicative of sensory-memory deficits. For one, thing, several investigators have found age deficits in both messages rather than in the recall only of the unattended message (Clark & Knowles, 1973; Craik, 1965). One possible interpretation of the results of the dichotic-listening studies is that the older group is at a disadvantage when selective attention is required. Craik (1977), for example, has suggested that older subjects are especially penalized when attention must be divided because this situation takes undue time that could be used to process the individual items. In summary, there is evidence to suggest that sensory-memory duration for older subjects is shorter, at least for visual information, although implications of this finding for later information processing are most likely negligible.

SHORT-TERM MEMORY

Once attended to, information moves from the modality-specific sensory memories into short-term memory. The multistore model of memory considers short-term memory to be the "working memory": it is where information processing takes place. For example, adequate short-term memory capacity is crucial for both the production and comprehension of speech. Because speech is continuous, early information in a sentence must be held briefly in memory in order for speech to be comprehended. Word meaning, for example, is often determined by the context of the surrounding sentence. Likewise, speech production must include some mechanism for briefly storing linguistic units prior to production.

It is well-known that short-term memory capacity is limited. In other words, short-term memory can process or retain only a small amount of information at any one time. Further, this information must be rehearsed in order to be maintained in short-term memory. If the information is not rehearsed, then it is quickly displaced by other incoming information either by attention to the sensory stores or by retrieval from long-term memory.

Most investigators agree that short-term memory is not changed with age, at least in terms of capacity. The immediate digit span, for example, is often used as a measure of the capacity of short-term

memory, and several studies have shown that digit span is unaffected by age (Botwinick & Storandt, 1974; Craik, 1968; Talland, 1968). Another indicant of short-term memory is the "recency" portion of the serial-position curve in free recall (i.e., the last few items presented in the list). Craik (1968) and Smith (1975) found that both young and old subjects recalled the recency items equally well, even though age differences were found for earlier serial positions (i.e., information assumed to be recalled from long-term memory).

While the capacity of short-term memory is the same in different age groups, there does seem to be evidence to suggest that older subjects take longer to search short-term memory at retrieval (Anders & Fozard, 1973; Waugh, Thomas, & Fozard, 1978). For example, in Waugh, Thomas, and Fozard's experiments, subjects were presented short lists of paired associates, and at some point into the list, the stimulus for the just-presented pair would be presented again for the subject to produce the response. The subject was aware that he or she would be recalling the second member of the latest pair seen, and also that the speed of response was important. The older the subject, the slower the response time on this task.

In summary, there seems to be no difference among age groups in short-term memory capacity but only in the time necessary to respond. Because short-term memory is the "working" memory where information processing occurs, the lack of significant age effects implies equal capacity to process ongoing information. The processing of language, for example, obviously involves the ability to temporarily store a small amount of information in order to process and comprehend the incoming message. A major function of the short-term memory system is to match information coming from the sensory store (e.g., speech through the auditory sensory store or text through the visual sensory store) with information stored in the more permanent long-term memory. Therefore, if short-term memory capacity is reduced with age, there should be serious problems in the older person's ability to engage in normal, everyday language processing. Differences in short-term memory capacity, however, are not found.

LONG-TERM EPISODIC MEMORY

Most laboratory memory tasks are tests of episodic memory; subjects are asked to reproduce or recognize lists of items presented in the experimental session. More often than not, subjects are familiar with the materials used so the task involves retrieving the items with the proper temporal context, that is, the context of the experimental session. As stated earlier, long-term memory can be considered a sequence of stages; information must be (1) encoded into memory at presentation, (2) retained over a retention interval, and (3) retrieved when memory is tested. We shall consider the three stages of encoding, storage, and retrieval in episodic memory separately.

Encoding

There are qualitatively different kinds of processing in which a subject can engage during learning, and what the subject does during presentation of the material determines the strength and quality of the memory trace. For example, if the subject forms a mental picture of a word as it is being presented, visual and spatial features will predominate in what is stored in long-term memory. We shall consider three different types of encoding processes in this section: (1) verbal elaboration, the degree to which each item is distinctively encoded; (2) visual elaboration, the use of imagery as a type of encoding; and (3) organization, the degree to which the items are related to each other during acquisition. If there are age differences in encoding, then they should become apparent later when memory is tested because the nature of encoding determines the nature of memory.

VERBAL ELABORATION

Verbal elaboration can be viewed as the "depth" or "breadth" of processing for each individual item during encoding (Craik & Lockhart, 1972; Craik & Tulving, 1975). This type of encoding is typically studied by giving the subject different tasks to perform during acquisition assumed to differ in the degree of elaborative processing required. For example, a word can be processed for some physical

characteristic (Does it rhyme with . . .?) or for meaning (Is it an animal?), depending on the task. These "orienting task" experiments with college-aged subjects have shown that the more elaborate the encoding, the better the later memory performance (Craik & Tulving, 1975; Schulman, 1971; Walsh & Jenkins, 1973). For example, memory performance is better if a subject looks at the word *rabbit* to decide if it is an animal name than if the subject has to decide whether the word rhymes with "habit." The rhyme question, in turn, leads to better memory performance than if the subject decides whether the word rabbit has double letters in it. These results suggest that memory performance is determined by the extent of verbal elaborative processing done at the time of encoding.

Eysenck (1974) examined elaborative processing in different age groups using this orienting-task methodology. Old and young subjects were tested by free recall after performing one of three orienting tasks differing in the degree of elaborative encoding necessary to perform the task. One group counted the number of letters in the word, for example, while another group had to write down a meaningful adjective modifier for the word. As shown in Table 8−1, Eysenck found no memory differences between the age groups after a nonsemantic orienting task like counting letters, but found significant differences after the semantic task of supplying adjectives. In other words, the greater the degree of elaborative processing required to perform the orienting task, the larger the age differences seen in later recall performance, a finding that has been replicated by other investigators (Mason, 1977; Perlmutter, 1978; White, as reported in Craik, 1977).

There are conflicting results, however, when recognition is used to test retention. In a recognition task, subjects pick the presented items from a test list composed of the test items as well as of distractors not presented at input. For recognition, the subject does not have to reproduce the items at test and so

Table 8−1
Age Differences in Recall as a Function of Elaborative Orienting Task

	Orienting task			
Age Group	Letter Counting	Rhyming	Adjective	Control
Young (18−30 years)	6.5	7.6	14.8	19.3
Old (55−65 years)	7.0	6.9	11.0	12.0

Derived, with permission, from Eysenck, M. W. Age differences in incidental learning. *Developmental Psychology,* 1974, *10,* 936−941.

retrieval is minimized. White (as reported in Craik, 1977) and Perlmutter (1978) found that the large age differences seen in recall after semantic orienting tasks were not observed when recognition tasks were used. Craik (1977) interpreted this finding to indicate that the difference in recall was a retrieval effect rather than purely an encoding effect because age differences were reduced when recognition, a task that is less senstitve to retrieval differences, was used. There are problems with this interpretation, however, which will be discussed in a later section on retrieval. In addition, Mason (1977) found age differences in both recall and recognition after semantic orienting tasks. Future research will have to clarify these conflicting results. Nevertheless, the recall results are clear. Older subjects show a deficit in recall performance when verbal elaboration is required during encoding.

VISUAL ELABORATION

A second type of encoding strategy is visual elaboration or imagery. Imagery is distinguished from verbal elaboration in that the subject encodes visual or spatial features of the to-be-remembered items, rather than verbal or linguistic features. Some investigators have concluded that older subjects are deficient in their use of visual imagery as an encoding strategy. In a classic experiment, Hulicka and Grossman (1967) investigated the use of imagery mediators in paired-associate learning in young and old subjects. The older subjects reported using imaginal mediators less often than did younger subjects (See Table 8−2). With imagery instruction, however, older subjects could improve their memory performance, relative to younger subjects. Hulicka and Grossman (1967) concluded that older subjects used

Table 8-2

Age Differences in Paired Associates Recall with and without Instructions to Use Mediators

	Instructions	
Age Group	No Mediators	Mediators
Young ($\bar{x}$ = 16.1)	63%	83%
Old ($\bar{x}$ = 74.1)	13%	65%

Derived, with permission, from Hulicka, I. M., & Grossman, J. L. Age-group comparisons for the use of mediators in paired-associate learning. *Journal of Gerontology*, 1967, 22, 46−51.

fewer imagery mediators than did younger subjects and instead used inappropriate verbal mediators if they used any at all. Canestrari (1968), however, found that older subjects not only used fewer visual mediators, but also fewer verbal mediators. Treat and Reese (1976) found that "self-generated" imagery mediators were more beneficial than "experimenter-provided" mediators, but that older subjects did not spontaneously develop and use such mediators without instruction.

One could conclude from these experiments that older subjects are deficient in the use of visual elaboration or imagery, but not because they could not perform such operations. With proper instructions and/or experimental conditions, older subjects can be "taught" to use imagery to improve recall (Poon, Fozard, & Sweeney, 1980). In other words, one could conclude that the deficit in imagery is only a "production deficit" (Flavell, 1970; Reese, 1976).

There are problems, however, with this conclusion. The paired-associate task used in all of these experiments confound encoding strategy controlled by instruction, such as visual imagery in the above studies, with the necessary organizational requirement of associating the stimulus to the response in order to perform the task. If imagery is used as a mediator, it might serve either or both of two functions. First, it could increase visual elaboration of the stimulus and response members of the pair, and second, it could increase organization by making it easier to relate the stimulus to the response. It is not clear, therefore, whether imagery improves performance on the paired-associate task because it causes better visual elaboration of the individual items or because it causes, through mediation, easier association. Theories of paired association have long recognized that these two separate stages of learning with such a task can be affected differently by manipulating variables (Underwood & Schulz, 1960).

There are relatively few experiments that separate imagery as an organizational cue from imagery as an elaborative cue. In one experiment, Mason and Smith (1977) looked at the effects of imagery versus standard instructions on free-call performance. The subjects were told to image or "picture" each word as it was presented. These instructions had no effect on a young group (20−39 years), but their performance was already high. The instructions did improve the recall of a middle-aged group (40−59 years) up to the level of the younger group. The oldest group (60−80 years) showed the lowest overall level of free recall and the imagery instructions had no effect on recall performance. The authors concluded that the young group used imagery spontaneously, while the older groups were less willing or less able to do so. A similar result was found in our laboratory in collaboration with Eugene Winograd and Elliott Simon (Winograd & Simon, 1980). In this experiment, a comparison was made between recall of pictures (line drawings) and words. In a previous experiment, Paivio and Csapo (1973) had found a picture superiority effect with young subjects, twice as many pictures as words being recalled, and suggested that the effect was due to the increased visual elaboration caused by the picture stimuli. We replicated Paivio and Csapo's findings with the young group, but found no such effect in an older group. In fact, there was a slight reversal in favor of words. These results are presented in Table 8−3. The outcome of this experiment supports the hypothesis that older people have difficulty with visual elaboration, especially in forming imaginal codes or in using such codes effectively at retrieval. Whether or not the imagry deficit can be overcome by instruction is clouded by the tendency of experimenters to confound imagery as an aid to visual elaboration with imagery as an aid to organization. This problem is discussed more fully by Winograd and Simon (1980).

ORGANIZATION

A third type of encoding strategy is organization, the process of grouping or relating items to each other at the time of encoding. Organization of the to-be-remembered information makes retrieval easier at the time memory is tested. Two different procedures have been used to study organization. The first method varies organization at the time of learning by manipulating either instructions, orienting tasks, or the experimental conditions. This is essentially the method used to study elaboration in the studies discussed so far. The second method is to measure directly the extent organization is used by examining the recall protocols of the subject. In the latter procedure, the tendency of the subject to recall consistently the same items together trial after trial is measured.

Table 8−3
Age Differences in the Recall of
Pictures and Words

Age Group	Pictures	Words
Young (18−22 years)	13.50	11.77
Old (60−80 years)	8.95	9.20

One problem with measuring organization directly, however, is that there are a variety of different measures that one could use. In an often-cited experiment, Laurence (1967) measured organization used by different age groups and found no differences. However, Laurence's measure of organization penalized the older group unduly for making fewer responses (Sternberg & Tulving, 1977). In recent studies using more appropriate measures, age differences in organization have been found (Hultsch, 1974; Smith, 1980), suggesting that older subjects do not spontaneously organize information as much as younger subjects.

While older subjects are deficient in spontaneous organization, recent studies suggest that with proper instructions, older subjects can and will organize appropriately. Hultsch (1974), for example, found that by requiring the subjects to organize material by sorting the to-be-remembered items prior to test, the recall performance of the older group improved relative to the younger group. Furthermore, older subjects performed more like the younger subjects on recall. In another experiment, Hultsch (1969) also was able to reduce age differences in recall by giving different instructions. Older subjects were given a specific means of organizing a list of words prior to the memory test and were instructed to make use of this organization at recall. Hultsch found that the age decrement in recall, observed in standard instruction conditions, was eliminated with this specific organizational plan. Hultch concluded that the older subjects were "compensated" by the organizational instructions (see Table 8−4).

SUMMARY

Research results to date suggest that there are qualitative differences in the use of encoding strategies between age groups. There is evidence to suggest that older subjects organize less, image less, and elaborate less than do younger subjects. If encoding differences exist, then it becomes difficult to interpret age differences in the remaining stages in the memory process. If different age groups process the items differently during acquisition, then qualitatively different memory traces are formed. The quality of these traces in turn would then determine the durability of the memory trace during the retention interval (i.e., storage) and the ease with which the traces can be found and used at the time of test (i.e., retrieval). This should be kept in mind as age differences in storage and retrieval are discussed.

Table 8–4

Mean Total Words Recalled in Sixteen Trials
as a Function of Age and Organizational Instructions

Age Group	Standard Instructions	General Organization Instructions	Specific Organization Instructions
Young (16–19 years)	252.8	268.3	269.2
Middle (30–39 years)	217.2	226.9	254.4
Old (45–54 years)	220.3	227.3	246.6

Derived, with permission, from Hultsch, D. F. Adult age differences in the organization of free recall. *Developmental Psychology,* 1969, *1,* 673–678.

Storage

Between encoding and retrieval, the information must be maintained or stored in memory during the retention interval. Other events occur during this interval and these events have been shown to interfere with storage (Postman & Underwood, 1973). One hypothesis of the age deficit in recall suggests that older subjects are more susceptible to interference from these intervening events (Kay, 1959; Welford, 1958). Recent research, however, has failed to support this hypothesis (Gladis & Braun, 1958; Smith, 1974, 1975).

In one series of experiments, Taub and his associates (Taub, 1968; Taub & Grieff, 1967; Taub & Walker, 1970) have found age differences in response interference, a particular kind of retroaction in which the previous act of responding interferes with later responding. In these experiments, larger age differences were seen in the recall from the second half of the recall sequence. Often, however, these investigations did not separate short-term memory from long-term memory in the analysis of recall responses. An interaction between age and position would be expected if short-term memory were not controlled. As noted earlier, there are no age differences in recall from short-term memory. By delaying recall until late in the recall sequence, the probability of recalling accurately from short-term memory is decreased and the probability of recalling accurately from long-term memory is increased. As the probability of long-term recall increases, age differences increase. The effect of response interference could be due, therefore, to age differenes in long-term memory at later recall positions in the sequence. This interpretation was supported by an experiment by Smith (1975) that revealed an interaction between age and position in the response sequence only for those items assumed

to be recalled from short-term memory, that is, the recency items from the presentation list.

In summary, there is little or no evidence to support the hypothesis that older persons are more susceptible than younger persons to retroactive interference.

Retrieval

One of the most popular explanations for the age deficit on most memory tasks has been the retrieval hypothesis, which suggests that older subjects have special problems in retrieving information at the time of test. The evidence most often cited to support this hypothesis comes from a classic experiment by Schonfield and Robertson (1966). A list of 24 words was presented to subjects from different age groups followed by a free recall task, and then followed by a recognition task. The results, shown in Table 8–5, indicate that differences were found between the age groups in the recall task, but no age differences were found with the recognition task. Schonfield and Robertson (1966) interpreted this finding in terms of the retrieval hypothesis in that recognition was assumed to be less sensitive to retrieval problems in the aged since the words were provided at the time of test. Other studies have replicated the recognition data (e.g., Craik, 1971) showing no age differences, and even though some investigators have found age differences in recognition (Erber, 1974; Botwinick & Storandt, 1974), these effects are typically much smaller than differences found with recall.

On the surface, the retrieval hypothesis gains support from these data. But an alternative hypothesis is possible based on the findings discussed in the earlier section on encoding. There is a great deal of evidence in the memory literature suggesting

Table 8—5
Age Differences in Recall and Recognition

Age Range	Recognition	Recall
20—29 years	20.01	13.78
30—39 years	19.48	12.30
40—49 years	19.53	10.01
50—59 years	19.90	9.57
60 + years	20.09	7.50

Reprinted with permission from Schonfield, D., & Robertson, B. A. Memory storage and aging. *Canadian Journal of Psychology,* 1966, *20,* 228—236.

that recall and recognition are differentially sensitive to different encoding strategies (Connor, 1977; Griffith, 1975; Tversky, 1973; Winograd & Smith, 1978). Griffith, for example, found that organizational processing during learning of a list of words was beneficial for a recall test, but not for recognition. It is likely that these differences in free recall between age groups are related to decreased organizational processing in older subjects. Organization is an appropriate strategy for recall tasks, and age differences occur because aged subjects engage in less organizational processing. This difference in processing strategy would not be seen on a recognition task, however, since recognition is not sensitive to organizational processing (Griffith). Retrieval differences are difficult to interpret, therefore, when there are reasons to believe that processing differences exist between age groups.

Other cited evidence for the retrieval hypothesis comes from studies by Hultsch (1975) and Laurence (1967), which also showed that age differences are reduced when cued recall is used rather than free recall. If age differences were due to retrieval, then providing retrieval cues or prompts at the time of test should improve the recall of the older group relative to the younger group. The results of an experiment by Drachman and Leavitt (1972), however, conflict with this hypothesis. The reason for the conflicting results of Drachman and Leavitt, however, is probably due to the type of cues they used in their study. Most cued-recall experiments use category labels (e.g., flowers) as retrieval cues and present category members (e.g., tulip, rose, carnation) in the to-be-remembered list. Drachman and Leavitt, on the other hand, used the initial letter of the word as the cue for retrieval. Smith (1977) found improvement in the older group only when category cues were used. Initial-letter cues failed to improve recall in any of the age groups.

Again, as with the recognition experiments, there are problems with the retrieval explanation of the cued-recall studies. First, in order for category cues to be effective, the items have to be organized conceptually during acquisition. The relatively greater improvement with the category cues in the older group could be due to the fact that pointing out the categorical nature of the word list in the cued-recall condition causes the older group to organize more during learning. Evidence for this interpretation is provided by the Smith (1977) experiment, which showed that the presence of the cues during learning was the important factor in improving the recall of the elderly group. No age differences in recall were observed when the category cues were provided at the time of list presentation. It was not just the presence of the cues at recall that helped the older group, however, but also the facilitated organizational encoding by the older group stimulated by the presence of the categories while learning the list.

The weight of the evidence in the literature suggests that age differences in episodic memory are best accounted for by the encoding hypothesis. Older subjects, for whatever reasons, fail to engage in the same encoding operations during acquisitions as do younger subjects. It may be that certain encoding strategies, such as organization, are reinforced in formal education, and as one grows older and becomes further and further removed from the educational setting, the reliance on these kinds of encoding strategies is gradually removed. Everyday remembering does not involve the active, strategic encoding emphasized for academic remembering. While this is only speculation, some evidence to this effect has been provided by a study by Hartley, Parker and Fisher (1976), who found no differences in the episodic recall of college students who differed widely in adult age. That is, a college student who was 60 years old recalled as well as did the typical college student of 20. While there are obvious sampling problems with such a comparison, it does provide a tentative basis on which to explain the strategic differences between age groups in encoding information into episodic long-term memory.

LONG-TERM SEMANTIC MEMORY

Many of the experiments in the area of semantic memory have attempted to map the organization or structure of information as it is stored in memory. Collins and Quillian (1969), for example, suggested that semantic information is stored hierarchically in terms of subsets and supersets of categories (i.e., a canary is a bird is an animal is a living being). Rips, Shoben, and Smith (1973), on the other hand, felt that the meaning of a word can be represented as a set of semantic features. Both theories assume that information in semantic memory is ordered in some way, and therefore that a search through semantic memory will take measurable time. Experiments in the area of semantic memory that have measured the time taken by a subject to answer semantic questions such as "Does a canary have wings?" have shown that semantic memory is highly organized.

Semantic memory theoretically involves the same stages of encoding, storage, and retrieval used with episodic memory, and like episodic memory, the division is somewhat artificial in that what is encoded obviously affects what is stored and retrieved. It does provide a convenient way to organize the results of a number of different experiments, however, and is used for this reason.

Encoding

Research on memory for sentences has concentrated on the question of what aspects of sentences are remembered. Bransford and Franks (1971) conducted a classic experiment that indicated that the grammatical aspects of sentences are less important than the propositional, semantic content of sentences. Results of their experiment suggested that when a sentence is encoded, it is broken down into basic ideas or "propositions," which can then be combined in a variety of ways. More specifically, subjects were presented with a series of related sentences, each containing one, two, or three main ideas. On a subsequent recognition task, the subjects were shown not only the original sentences, but also a number of "new" sentences not seen before. For example, if two of the original sentences were "The ants are red" and "The ants are on the table," then a new sentence on the recognition task might be "The red ants are on the table." It was found that subjects more often "recognized" never-presented sentences (new sentences) that combined several propositions, and with higher confidence, than they recognized actually presented sentences containing fewer propositions (old sentences). Bransford and Franks (1971) found that the semantic structure of language is more important as an encoding dimension than the syntactic structure of language, lending support to the theory that meaning is abstracted and assimilated into networks of linguistic information. In other words, the semantic content of the information is most important in semantic memory; it is what is said rather than how it is said that is stored. The syntactic format, however, is important as an aid to initial comprehension, which must precede the semantic encoding of the material.

Walsh and Baldwin (1977) used Bransford and Franks' (1971) paradigm of linguistic abstraction to investigate possible age differences in semantic memory encoding. As seen in Figure 8−2, no differences were found between young (mean age 18.7 years) and old (mean age 67.3 years) groups in the recognition of propositions, indicating that encoding into semantic memory is accomplished similarly across the adult age span. These data emphasize the importance of the distinction between episodic and semantic memory and further indicate that semantic memory may not show the decrements with age that are often shown by episodic memory.

The distinction between episodic and semantic encoding is also illustrated by an experiment by Nebes and Andrews-Kulis (1976), who investigated age differences in the the speed of sentence formation. Subjects were given pairs of nouns and asked to form sentences incorporating each pair. No age differences were found in speed of sentence formation or in the grammaticality of the generated sentences. When memory for the noun pairs was tested as a measure of episodic memory, however, the older subjects showed poorer recall than the younger subjects.

Encoding into semantic memory, however, is not totally constrained by the semantic content or "gist" of a sentence. Haviland and Clark (1974), for example, pointed out that all Bransford and Franks' (1971) sentences began with "the," a syntactic device that serves to connect sentences in a common context. In other words, "a red ant" and "an ant on the table" might not be taken to be the same ant as readily as the "the red ant" and "the ant on the table"

Another syntactic element important for encoding into semantic memory is redundancy, or the degree to which one linguistic element implies another. Offir (1973) and Clark and Clark (1977) suggested that users of a language learn to make the distinction between "given" and "new" information in language, one form of grammatical redundancy. These investigations further suggest that language users store the new information more consistently than the given information. Haviland and Clark (1974) pointed out that the given information may be used primarily as a method of access to relevant information already stored in memory. Once access is gained, then the given information is no longer needed and therefore is not stored again.

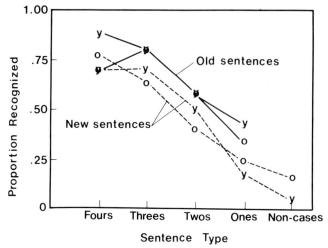

Fig. 8–2: Mean recognition rates on "old" and "new" sentences for young (Y) and old (O) subjects across sentence types in the Bransford and Franks (1971) paradigm. Number of propositions included in the last sentence determines sentence type. (Derived, with permission, from Walsh, D. A., & Baldwin, M. Age differences in integrated semantic memory. *Developmental Psychology*, 1977, *13*, 509–514.

A given–new sequence usually consists of several sentences (Hupet & Le Bouedec, 1977). A subject is introduced as new in one sentence and then is commented on in one or more following sentences. For example, the speaker might say, "Kate has a new car." This information might then be followed by "Kate's new car is a convertible." In the second sentence, the fact that Kate has a new car is now given information, whereas the fact that the car is a convertible is "new". Singer (1976) found that the effect can also occur when isolated sentences are presented that have certain syntactic forms conducive to division into given and new parts. Such sentences are said to contain "presuppositions," a form of grammatical redundancy. For example, the sentence "It was the king who led the troops" can be divided into given information, that someone led the troops, and new information, that it was the king who led them. Following presentation of such a sentence, Singer (1976) asked subjects whether they recognized both given and new nouns from the sentences. He found that the new nouns were recognized better than the given nouns. From the example above, subjects would be more likely to say that "king" had been presented than "troops".

Using Singer's (1976) paradigm, Fullerton (1978) replicated this result using different age groups. Although older subjects recognized relatively fewer words overall, they recognized more new nouns in comparison to given nouns than did the younger subjects (see Table 8–6). Age differences in the use of grammatical redundancy not only support the idea that syntactic elements of the language can have effects on semantic memory but also indicate that these syntactic elements may have differential effects due to age. The finding of a better memory for new items among older subjects, coupled with the decrement in overall recognition, supports the hypothesis that older subjects use learned rules of the language to compensate for memory deficits. Further support for this conclusion comes from Arenberg (1968), who found that older subjects are less likely to remember negative instances in a concept-attainment task when excessive demands are made on

Table 8–6

Mean Number of New and Given Words Recognized from Presuppositional Sentences as a Function of Age

Age Group	New	Given
Young (20–39 years)	9.4	8.7
Middle (40–59 years)	9.6	8.2
Old (60–80 years)	8.4	7.1

From Fullerton, A. M. Age-related differences in the use of presuppositional and phonological redundancy rules in semantic memory. Unpublished master's thesis, Georgia Institute of Technology, 1978.

memory. He suggested that negative instances are forgotten more quickly because they contain less information. Arenberg's results pertain directly to this experiment if the assumption that subjects are using learned rules of syntactic redundancy is correct, because, by definition, the given items contain less information than the new items.

Storage

The question of whether the manner in which information is stored in semantic memory changes with age has not been studied directly. Several studies, however, have dealt with vocabulary-size differences as estimates of the size of the mental dictionary across the adult age span. An increased vocabulary is an indication that the size of semantic memory may have also increased. Riegel (1958) found that vocabulary size increased, although at a decreasing rate, until the age of about 35, and then remained fairly stable.

An increase in vocabulary with age might also indicate a change in the structure of the semantic memory, that is, in how items are organized. Birren (1970) suggested that bits of information in semantic memory are reorganized into larger units or chunks, and thus an increased number of items can be stored in semantic memory. An indirect way of determining how items are stored is to analyze responses to a test of free associations. Riegel and Riegel (1964), using a 120-item free-association test, found that the proportion of the total number of responses represented by a few common associates decreased slightly with age. In other words, older subjects were more likely to give idiosyncratic responses than were younger subjects. This was particularly true for stimulus words of low and high frequency, whereas greater response variability was found for words in the middle-frequency range.

Riegel (1968) also noted the importance of considering both syntactic and semantic classes from which associative responses are drawn. A response from the same semantic class is called a paradigmatic response. For example, if the stimulus word is "knife," a paradigmatic response would be "fork," another eating utensil. If the response to "knife" were "cut," however, it would be a syntagmatic response, one which is based on the syntax of the stimulus word. In this case, a noun is being paired with a verb. Other possible syntagmatic pairings include nouns with adjectives, and verbs with adverbs. Riegel (1968) found that younger subjects preferred paradigmatic responses, whereas older subjects

tended to alternate between paradigmatic and syntagmatic responses. Specifically, older subjects used more verbs with concrete-noun stimuli, more concrete nouns with adjective stimuli, and more adjectives or abstract nouns with verb stimuli. These results suggest that the structure of semantic memory, at least the part that stores words from the language, may change with age. Riegel (1968) concluded that the tendency toward syntagmatic responses indicates a preference among older subjects for more meaningful functional relations, that is, a preference for concrete relations over abstract, conceptual relations.

As vocabulary size increases with age, verbal fluency, that is the speed of producing written or verbal associations to a word, seems to decrease (Riegel & Birren, 1966). In order to determine whether this effect is due to a general slowing of responses or to increased interference from a larger number of known words, Riegel and Birren (1966) asked subjects to give one word as a response to a two-, three-, or four-letter stimulus that was to be the first syllable of the response word. Although older subjects were slower than younger subjects in all conditions, they were relatively slowest when a four-letter stimulus was given, that is, when the response restriction was greatest. Riegel and Birren (1966) concluded that two speed factors are probably involved in such a task, namely, the time required for emergence of a response and the time needed to make a selection between alternative responses. The slower response of older subjects was apparently due to a decrease in emergence speed because older subjects were able to increase their response speed during the test to the level of younger subjects by learning to restrict their answers to the most common response.

A recent study by Stones (1978) also used word fluency as a means of investigating age differences in the structure of semantic memory. Unfortunately, only young ($\bar{x}$ = 17 years) and middle-aged ($\bar{x}$ = 49 years) subjects were used. All subjects in this experiment were matched in terms of education, in addition to the fact that the young subjects were all children of the old subjects. A synonym task was used to assess vocabulary size, followed by a word fluency task with both initial-consonant and conceptual-category cues. In general, the results of this study point to greater diversification in semantic memory by middle age, including increased intraindividual variability, and support the finding of more idiosyncratic responses in free association in older subjects (Riegel & Riegel, 1964).

In summary, these studies suggest that there may be changes in semantic memory due to increased verbal input over the life span. It is not clear, however, whether these changes are due to structural change, that is, to a change in the organization of information, or simply to increased amounts of information being held in semantic memory.

Retrieval

The investigation of retrieval from semantic memory necessarily interacts with investigation of the other two stages, as discussed earlier. The studies of verbal fluency and free association, for instance, not only provide information about how knowledge is organized but also about possible retrieval routes.

A paradigm that may provide some indication of the wide variety of information that can be retrieved from semantic memory is that of release from proactive interference. Proactive interference is interference with memory caused by previously learned responses. Wickens (1972) used this method to show that a particular attribute of a word has been encoded by the subject. On the first trial, the subject is presented with three words from the same category or class. This is followed by a rehearsal-preventing task and then by recall. The second and third trials follow the same pattern, and words are drawn from the same class as on the first trial. On the fourth trial, however, the three words presented to the experimental subjects are from a new category or class. Proactive interference produces a decline in recall over the first three trials. Thus, if recall recovers when a change is instituted on the fourth trial, the improvement is known as "release from proactive inhibition." When release occurs, it indicates that the subject is sensitive to a change in the category and, thus, to different attributes of the words presented.

The greatest release effects are typically found when semantic category shifts are made. Gardiner, Craik, and Birtwistle (1972) have suggested that the release occurs at the time of retrieval. When their subjects were given a shift from "garden flowers" to "wild flowers," for example, no release was found unless a category retrieval cue was presented at recall on the shift trial. In other words, subjects were able to use the category cue as a retrieval strategy. Whichever explanation is correct, that is, whether the release effect is due to encoding or to retrieval, the release-from-proactive-interference paradigm illustrates the richness of semantic memory by showing that any given word has a number of different attributes that can be used by the subject.

Using this paradigm, Elias and Hirasuna (1976) found that the relative amount of release from proactive interference with both semantic and phonological categories was similar in pattern for both young and old subjects. This finding has been replicated by Mistler-Lachman (1977) and suggests that loss of information or reduced access to information does not inevitably occur with age.

The question of age differences in speed of retrieval search from semantic memory has been investigated by Eysenck (1975). A young group (18−30 years) and an older group (35−65 years) were tested on recall using the category−letter task. In this procedure, the subject was presented with a category name followed by a single letter. The subject's task was to provide an example of the category that began with the letter presented. For example, given "fruit−A," the subject might respond "apple." Subjects were also tested on recognition using a category−word task. In this condition, subjects were required to tell whether or not a given word was a member of a given category (e.g., fruit−table). While there were no differences in speed of recall, older subjects performed significantly more slowly on the recognition task. Eysenck (1975) suggested that the time taken for recognition is mostly decision time and older subjects take more time to make the decision. Recall, however, involves both search and decision time, and older subjects may actually search semantic memory more quickly than younger subjects, even though they need more time to make decisions. He further suggested that the faster search time may be due to overlearning items in semantic memory as a function of age.

A common complaint of older people, however, is of difficulty in retrieving names of objects or people. In order to study retrieval, Thomas, Fozard, and Waugh (1977) designed an experiment to measure the time needed to retrieve names of common objects from semantic memory. In the first condition, the subject was simply required to name a picture of a common object. In the second condition, however, a word was presented just prior to the picture. Sometimes the presented word was the name for the picture and sometimes it was not. In either event, the subject was required to name the picture correctly. Naming time could thus be divided into a perceptual−motor component (i.e., the time necessary to make the motor response) and a search component (i.e., the time necessary to find the name in memory). Although age differences in speed were found, these were mainly attributable to the perceptual−motor component. Speed of search through semantic memory as a component of speech production did not change.

Because the Thomas, Fozard, and Waugh (1977) experiment suggested that search speed and strategy seem to be stable over age, Poon and Fozard (1978) conducted a second experiment to study the effect of familiarity on search speed. Pictures of objects were selected that were either contemporary or dated and either frequently used or unique. Contemporary, frequently used objects were named more rapidly by all age groups. However, older subjects named dated objects more rapidly than younger subjects, whereas younger subjects named contemporary, unique objects more rapidly. Poon and Fozard (1978) hypothesized that these results indicated that speed of retrieval was determined by the familiarity of the material rather than by age, thereby explaining older adults' difficulties in retrieving names of objects or people.

Further support for this hypothesis is provided by an experiment by Thomas, Waugh, and Fozard (1978) that required subjects to determine whether a single test letter was present in a short list. Two six-letter sequences were used, one familiar and one unfamiliar. When time simply to answer ''yes'' or ''no'' was subtracted from total time, no differences between age groups were found for search time in the ''familiar'' condition. In other words, age differences were due primarily to slowing in the perceptual–motor component rather than to differences in search speed through semantic memory. However, this was not the case when the ''unfamiliar'' sequence was presented. The search time in unfamiliar lists slowed with age, again indicating familiarity of the material was an important variable in retrieval from semantic memory for different age groups.

The importance of familiary in semantic memory has implications for the ability of older persons to adapt to their environment, that is, to get along in the world. As Fozard and Popkin (1978) point out, if a person is especially familiar with a particular environment, he will be well adapted to it in terms of being able to remember information about it and to make decisions concerning it. However, a possible consequence of familiarity is that abrupt changes in the environment may result in disruption of behavior.

The environment can be defined to include knowledge of language and its description of the relationships among items in the world. Adaptation to environment in this larger sense is, then, at least partly a function of age, because more time provides more exposure. Due to the greater experience provided by age, older people may be able to maintain effectiveness in their environment even though physical and perceptual slowing occurs. A study of age differences in the ability to use the world knowledge stored in semantic memory would seem to be one way to determine the effectiveness of adaptation.

Although little research has been done so far in this area, there are a few studies that indicate that memory decrements with age may not occur when semantic memory is studied, perhaps due to an adaptive change resulting from increased experience with the environment. As noted above, Fullerton (1978) found that older subjects were able to make better use of syntactic information in sentences to aid memory of text material. Also, Riegel (1968) found an increased preference among older subjects for syntagmatic, that is, functional responses. This latter finding has often been interpreted as a regression, since children also tend to prefer this kind of response. However, Riegel (1973) aptly concluded that paradigmatic responses are not necessarily adaptive for everyday living, but result from formal education and are adaptive primarily in that milieu. Syntagmatic responses, on the other hand, are adaptive, functional responses as they correspond to linguistic relationships. This conclusion is similar to the one reached earlier to explain strategic differences in episodic memory.

Lachman and Lachman (1980) suggested that there are three components involved in the successful use of knowledge stored in semantic memory to respond and deal with the environment. These components are retrieval, inference, and metamemory (memory control processes). Lachman and Lachman (1980) have conducted several experiment that attempt to isolate the ability of older people to use knowledge from their semantic memory. Subjects were asked a number of factual questions in order to obtain an estimate of their knowledge and of their ability to retrieve that knowledge. Questions covered a wide range of topics including the Bible, history, and sports. After each subject had an opportunity to recall the answers, they were given a recognition test. The estimate of retrieval efficiency was based on the number of answers correctly recognized compared to the number correctly recalled. In general, the results indicated that retrieval efficiency does not decline with age. A further study designed to test inferential ability by answering questions such as ''Which way does the Statue of Liberty face?'' also showed no decrements with age.

Much of this research seems to indicate that the changes seen in memory in older subjects are not detrimental and negative ones but are rather of an adaptive and positive nature. Even though older adults may have difficulty in performing laboratory tasks of episodic memory, they seem to be able to use the knowledge stored in semantic memory on a day-to-day basis as effectively as younger subjects. In addition, even the well-documented episodic-memory differences seem to be due to qualitative differences in processing strategy, and the choice of strategy could easily be considered an adaptive response to a changing environment. For these reasons, the picture of the interaction between memory and aging is probably not as bleak as it often has been painted.

SUMMARY AND CONCLUSIONS

There is no strong evidence to suggest that memory changes that occur with age are detrimental to the ability to use language effectively, because short-term memory capacity, which is of primary importance to speech comprehension and production, does not decrease with age. There are age differences in the ability to recall episodic information from long-term memory. These differences are most likely due to differing encoding strategies, that is, younger subjects use more active elaborative and organizational strategies than do older subjects. There is some evidence to suggest that active encoding strategies are emphasized by formal education and therefore that the apparent change in strategies with age may be due to the change from an academic to an everyday environment. This view supports the concept of an adaptive change rather than decreased cognitive ability.

Although there has been little research on age differences in semantic memory, the few experiments that have been performed do not show the age decrements found in studies of episodic memory. For example, no differences have been found between older and younger subjects in either the ability to abstract linguistic information into semantic memory or in the ability to generate grammatically correct sentences rapidly, both necessary components of language use. Furthermore, the ability to use syntactic components of language, such as redundancy, as an aid to the encoding of semantic information, may actually increase with age.

The size of semantic memory, that is, the number of items stored in the internal lexicon, may also increase with age, as indicated both by increased vocabulary size and increases in idiosyncratic responses on free-association tests. It is not clear whether the amount of information in semantic memory merely increases with age or whether the organization of that information also changes. In either case, the ability to use language would not be impaired.

Retrieval from semantic memory also does not appear to be adversely affected by age. This is an especially important finding because the ability to retrieve both information and specific words is essential to language performance. The problem of difficulty in retrieving a particular word or name, a problem of which older people often complain, may be an effect of the familiarity of the material rather than of age.

REFERENCES

Abel, M. The visual traces in relation to aging. Unpublished doctoral dissertation, Washington University, St. Louis, Mo., 1972.

Anders, T. R., & Fozard, J. L. Effects of age upon retrieval from primary and secondary memory. *Developmental Psychology,* 1973, *9,* 411−415.

Arenberg, D. Concept problem solving in young and old adults. *Journal of Gerontology,* 1968, *23,* 279−282.

Atkinson, R. C., & Shiffrin, R. M. The control of short-term memory. *Scientific American,* 1971, *224,* 82−90.

Birren, J. E. Toward an experimental psychology of aging. *American Psychologist,* 1970, *25,* 124−135.

Botwinick, J., & Storandt, M. *Memory, related functions and age.* Springfield, Ill.: Charles C Thomas Publisher, 1974.

Bransford, J. D., & Franks, J. J. The abstraction of linguistic ideas. *Cognitive Psychology,* 1971, *2,* 331−350.

Canestrari, R. E. Age changes in acquisition. In G. A. Talland (Ed.), *Human aging and behavior.* New York: Academic Press, 1968.

Clark, H. H., & Clark, E. V. *Psychology and language: An introduction to psycholinguistics.* New York: Harcourt Brace Jovanovich, 1977.

Clark, L., & Knowles, J. Age differences in dichotic listening performance. *Journal of Gerontology*, 1973, *28*, 173–178.

Collins, A. M., & Quillian, M. R. Retrieval time from semantic memory. *Journal of Verbal Learning and Verbal Behavior*, 1969, *8*, 240–248.

Connor, J. M. Effects of organization and expectancy on recall and recognition. *Memory and Cognition*, 1977, *5*, 315–318.

Craik, F. I. M. The nature of the age decrement in performance on dichotic listening tasks. *Quarterly Journal of Experimental Psychology*, 1965, *17*, 227–240.

Craik, F. I. M. Short-term memory and the aging process. In G. A. Talland (Ed.) *Human aging and behavior*. New York: Academic Press, 1968.

Craik, F. I. M. Age differences in recognition memory. *Journal of Experimental Psychology*, 1971, *23*, 216–223.

Craik, F. I. M. Age differences in human memory. In J. E. Birren & K. W. Schaie (Eds.) *Handbook of the psychology of aging*. New York: Van Nostrand Reinhold, 1977.

Craik, F. I. M., & Lockhart, R. S. Levels of processing: A framework for memory research. *Journal of Verbal Learning and Verbal Behavior*, 1972, *11*, 671–684.

Craik, F. I. M., & Tulving, E. Depth of processing and the retention of words in episodic memory. *Journal of Experimental Psychology: General*, 1975, *104*, 268–294.

Drachman, D., & Leavitt, J. Memory impairment in the aged: Storage versus retrieval deficit. *Journal of Experimental Psychology*, 1972, *93*, 302–308.

Elias, C. S., & Hirasuna, N. Age and semantic and phonological encoding. *Deveolopmental Psychology*, 1976, *12*, 497–503.

Erber, J. T. Age differences in recognition memory. *Journal of Gerontology*, 1974, *29*, 177–181.

Eysenck, M. W. Age differences in incidental learning. *Deveolopmental Psychology*, 1974, *10*, 936–941.

Eysenck, M. W. Retrieval from semantic memory as a function of age. *Journal of Gerontology*, 1975, *30*, 174–180.

Flavell, J. H. Cognitive changes in adulthood. In L. R. Goulet & P. J. Baltes (Eds.) *Life-span developmental psychology: Research and theory*. New York: Academic Press, 1970.

Fozard, J. L., & Popkin, S. J. *Optimizing adult development: Ends and means of an applied psychology of aging* Boston: Veterans Administration Outpatient Clinic, 1978. (Technical report No. 78–01)

Fullerton, A. M. Age-related differences in the use of presuppositional and phonological redundancy in semantic memory. Unpublished master's thesis, Georgia Institute of Technology, 1978.

Gardiner, J. M., Craik, F.I.M., & Birtwistle, J. Retrieval cues and release from proactive inhibition. *Journal of Verbal Learning and Verbal Behavior*, 1972, *11*, 778–783.

Gladis, M., & Braun, H. W. Age differences in transfer and retroaction as a function of intertask response similarity. *Journal of Experimental Psychology*, 1958, *55*, 25–30.

Griffith, D. Comparison of control processes for recognition and recall. *Journal of Experimental Psychology: Human Learning and Memory*, 1975, *1*, 223–228.

Haber, R. N., & Standing, L. G. Direct measures of short-term visual storage. *Quarterly Journal of Experimental Psychology*, 1969, *21*, 43–54.

Hartley, J. T., Parker, J. F., & Fisher, L. A. Free-recall learning in older and younger college students: The effect of list organization on performance. Paper presented to the meeting of the Southeastern Psychological Association, New Orleans, La., March 1976.

Haviland, S. E., & Clark, H. H. What's new? Acquiring new information as a process in comprehension. *Journal of Verbal Learning and Verbal Behavior*, 1974, *13*, 512–521.

Hulicka, I. M., & Grossman, J. L. Age group comparisons for the use of mediators in paired-associate learning. *Journal of Gerontology*, 1967, *22*, 46–51.

Hultsch, D. F. Adult age differences in the organization of free recall. *Developmental Psychology*, 1969, *1*, 673–678.

Hultsch, D. F. Learning to learn in adulthood. *Journal of Gerontology*, 1974, *29* 302–308.

Hultsch, D. F. Adult age differences in retrieval: Trace-dependent and cue-dependent forgetting. *Developmental Psychology*, 1975, *11*, 197–201.

Hupet, M., & Le Bouedec, B. The given-new contract and the constructive aspect of memory for ideas. *Journal of Verbal Learning and Verbal Behavior*, 1977, *16*, 69–75.

Inglis, J., & Caird, W. K. Age differences in successive responses to simultaneous stimulation. *Canadian Journal of Psychology*, 1963, *17*, 98–105.

Kay, H. Theories of learning and aging. In J. E. Birren (Ed.), *Handbook of aging and the individual*. Chicago: University of Chicago Press, 1959.

Lachman, J. L., & Lachman, R. Age and the actualization of world knowledge. In L. W. Poon, J. L. Fozard, L. Cermak, D. Arenberg, & L. Thompson (Eds.) *New directions in memory and aging: Proceedings of the George A. Talland Memorial Conference*. Hillsdale, N.J.: Lawrence Erlbaum Associates, 1980.

Laurence, M. W. Memory loss with age: A test of two strategies for its retardation. *Psychonomic Science*, 1967, *9*, 209–210.

Mackay, H. A., & Inglis, J. The effect of age on a short-term auditory storage process. *Gerontologia*, 1963, *8*, 193–200.

Mason, S. E. The effects of orienting tasks on the recall and recognition memory of subjects differing in age. Unpublished doctoral dissertation, Georgia Institute of Technology, 1977.

Mason, S. E., & Smith, A. D. Imagery in the aged. *Experimental Aging Research*, 1977, *3*, 17–32.

Mistler-Lachman, J. L. Spontaneous shift in encoding dimensions among elderly subjects. *Journal of Gerontology*, 1977, *32*, 68–72.

Nebes, R. D., & Andrews-Kulis, M. S. The effect of age on the speed of sentence formation and incidental learning. *Experimental Aging Research*, 1976, *2*, 315–331.

Offir, C. E. Recognition memory for presuppositions of relative clause sentences. *Journal of Verbal Learning and Verbal Behavior*, 1973, *12*, 636–643.

Paivio, A., & Csapo, K. Picture superiority in free recall: Imagery or dual coding? *Cognitive Psychology*, 1973, *5*, 176–206.

Perlmutter, M. What is memory aging the aging of? *Developmental Psychology*, 1978, *14*, 330–345.

Poon, L. W., Fozard, J. L., & Sweeney, L. W. Memory skill training for the elderly: Salient issues on the use of imagery mnemonics. In L. W. Poon, J. L. Fozard, L. Cermak, D. Arenberg, & L. Thompson (Eds.) *New directions in memory and aging: Proceedings of the George A. Talland Memorial Conference*. Hillsdale, N.J.: Lawrence Erlbaum Associates, 1980.

Poon, L. W., & Fozard, J. L. Speed of retrieval from long-term memory in relation to age, familiarity, and datedness of information. *Journal of Gerontology*, 1978, *5*, 711–717.

Postman, L. Verbal learning and memory. *Annual Review of Psychology*, 1975, *26*, 291–335.

Postman, L., & Underwood, B. .J. Critical issues in interference theory. *Memory and Cognition*, 1973, *1*, 19–40.

Reese, H. W. The development of memory: Life-span perspective. In H. W. Reese (Eds.) *Advances in child development and behavior*. New York: Academic Press, 1976.

Riegel, K. F. Ergebnisse und Probleme der psychologischen alternsforchung: Teil II. *Vita Humana*, 1958, *1*, 243–284.

Riegel, K. F. Changes in psycholinguistic performances with age. In G. A. Talland (Ed.), *Human aging and behavior*. New York: Academic Press, 1968.

Riegel, K. F. Dialectic operations: The final period of cognitive development. *Human Development*, 1973, *16*, 346–370.

Riegel, K. F., & Birren, J. S. Age differences in verbal associations. *Journal of Genetic Psychology*, 1966, *75*, 346–370.

Riegel, K. F., & Riegel, R. M. Changes in associative behavior during later years of life: A cross-sectional analysis. *Vita Humana*, 1964, *7*, 1–32.

Rips, L. J., Shoben, E. J., & Smith, E. E. Semantic distance and the verification of semantic relations. *Journal of Verbal Learning and Verbal Behavior*, 1973, *12*, 1–20.

Schoenfield, D., & Robertson, B. A. Memory storage and aging. *Canadian Journal of Psychology,* 1966, *20,* 228−236.

Schonfield, D., & Wenger, L. Age limitation of perceptual span. *Nature,* 1975, *253,* 377−378.

Schulman, A. I. Recognition memory for targets from a scanned word list. *British Journal of Psychology,* 1971, *62,* 335−346.

Singer, M. Thematic structure and the integration of linguistic information. *Journal of Verbal Learning and Verbal Behavior,* 1976, *15,* 549−558.

Smith, A. D. Response interference with organized recall in the aged. *Developmental Psychology,* 1974, *10,* 867−870.

Smith, A. D. Aging and interference with memory. *Journal of Gerontology,* 1975, *30,* 319−325.

Smith, A. D. Adult age differences in cued recall. *Developmental Psychology,* 1977, *13,* 326−331.

Smith, A. D. Age differences in encoding, storage, and retrieval. In L. W. Poon, J. L. Fozard, L. Cermak, D. Arenberg, & L. Thompson (Eds.) *New directions in memory and aging: Proceedings of the George A. Talland Memorial Conference.* Hillsdale, N.J.: Lawrence Erlbaum Associates, 1980.

Sternberg, R. J., & Tulving, E. The measurement of subjective organization in free recall. *Psychological Bulletin,* 1977, *84,* 539−553.

Stones, M. J. Aging and semantic memory: Structural age differences. *Experimental Aging Research,* 1978, *4,* 125−132.

Talland, G. A. Age and the span of immediate recall. In G. A. Talland (Ed.), *Human aging and behavior.* New York: Academic Press, 1968.

Taub, H. A. Aging and free recall. *Journal of Gerontology,* 1968, *23,* 466−468.

Taub, H. A., & Greiff, S. Effects of age on organization and recall two sets of stimuli. *Psychonomic Science,* 1967, *7,* 53−54.

Taub, H. A., & Walker, J. B. Short-term memory as a function of age and response interference. *Journal of Gerontology,* 1970, *25,* 177−183.

Thomas, J. C., Fozard, J. L., & Waugh, N. C. Age-related differences in naming latency. *American Journal of Psychology,* 1977, *90,* 499−509.

Thomas, J. C., Waugh, N. C., & Fozard, J. L. Age and familiarity in memory scanning. *Journal of Gerontology,* 1978, *33,* 528−533.

Treat, N., & Reese, H. W. Age, imagery and pacing in paired-associate learning. *Developmental Psychology,* 1976, *12,* 119−124.

Tulving, E. Episodic and semantic memory. In E. Tulving & W. Donaldson (Eds.), *Organization of memory.* New York: Academic Press, 1972.

Tversky, B. G. Encoding process in recognition and recall. *Cognitive Psychology,* 1973, *5,* 275−287.

Underwood, B. J., & Schulz, R. W. *Meaningfulness and verbal fluency.* Philadelphia: J. B. Lippincott, 1960.

Walsh, D. A., & Baldwin, M. Age differences in integrated semantic memory. *Developmental Psychology,* 1977, *13,* 509−514.

Walsh, D. A., & Jenkins, J. J. Effects of orienting tasks on free recall in incidental learning: "difficulty," "effort," and "process" explanations. *Journal of Verbal Learning and Verbal Behavior,* 1973, *12,* 481−488.

Walsh, D. A., & Thompson, L. W. Age differences in visual sensory memory. *Journal of Gerontology,* 1978, *33,* 383−387.

Waugh, N. C., & Norman, D. A. Primary memory. *Psychological Review,* 1965, *72,* 89−104.

Waugh, N. C., Thomas, J. C., & Fozard, J. L. Retrieval time from different memory stores. *Journal of Gerontology,* 1978, *5,* 718−724.

Welford, A. T. *Ageing and human skill.* London: Oxford University Press, 1958.

Wickens, D. D. Characteristics of word encoding. In A. W. Melton & E. Martin (Eds.), *Coding processes in human memory.* Washington, D.C.: V. H. Winston & Sons, 1972.

Winograd, E., & Simon, E. W. Visual memory and imagery in the aged. In L. W. Poon, J. L. Fozard, L. Cermak, D. Arenberg, & L. Thompson (Eds.), *New directions in memory and aging: Proceedings of the George A. Talland Memorial Conference.* Hillsdale, N.J.: Lawrence Erlbaum Associates, 1980.

Winograd, E., & Smith, A. D. When do semantic orienting tasks hinder recall? *Psychonomic Society Bulletin,* 1978, *11,* 165−167.

Section II

Speech and Language Pathology and the Aging Process

EDITORS' INTRODUCTION

In the first chapter of this book, Knox suggested that speech and hearing professionals can improve their understanding of communicative disorders and their ability to deliver meaningful services by being familiar with the influence of adult development and aging on communicative disorders. The purpose of the chapters in Section II is to illustrate his point relative to speech and language disorders. Therefore, the following five chapters cannot be characterized as overviews of expressive disorders that "old people" have, but, rather, are attempts to delineate relationships between the factor of age and the nature and treatment of these disorders. Since little research has been done in this regard, these chapters contain a healthy amount of instructive speculation designed to provide direction for needed research. The inquisitive reader can add to this speculation by relating the topics of this section to pertinent information on normal aging found in Section I.

Rosenbek and LaPointe (Chapter 9) discuss the motor speech disorders of dysarthria and apraxia of speech. The dysarthrias arise from a variety of neurologic conditions that are somewhat related to age in terms of onset. The authors point out several considerations that should be given to the diagnosis and treatment of these disorders when they occur in adulthood.

Though many adults have the problem of stuttering, very little is known about stuttering in adulthood except in the population of young adults attending college. Manning and Shirkey (Chapter 10) explore the question of what happens to stutterers after they leave school and provide a framework for the investigation of this question. Their hypotheses about stuttering in middle and late adulthood are based on investigations of articulatory, phonatory, and psychologic characteristics of this age group.

Meyerson and Shanks (Chapter 11) describe a variety of voice disorders of adults including laryngectomy and voice problems not related to organic pathology. Etiologies common among the elderly are specified. Functional disorders may be related to adjustments and anxieties that are common in the transition between stages of adult development. Treatment and prevention of voice disorders are discussed.

Aphasia is a language disorder that, during peacetime, is most frequently seen in middle-aged and older adults. Davis and Holland (Chapter 12) explain the reason for this and analyze investigations of the contribution of age to the type of aphasia, severity of aphasia, and recovery from aphasia. The theme in this chapter shifts to a topic that is applicable to rehabilitation of any of the communication disorders in adulthood. The authors consider the possible effect of attitudes toward aging on the treatment process, especially when the clinician is relatively young.

The communication disorder of any individual has an impact on immediate family and friends, and the integrity of the individual's support system affects his or her responsiveness to treatment. Webster and Newhoff (Chapter 13) provide a framework for the investigation of family problems related to communicative disorders and for intervention with these families. The authors address the disorders of adulthood specifically. The sudden communication disorder is examined as a life crisis much like other traumatic events that are common in an older population.

John C. Rosenbek
Leonard L. LaPointe

9
Motor Speech Disorders and the Aging Process

Man's incessant search for uniqueness has directed a good portion of effort to the task of cataloging features that separate him from other animals. The list is long and varied. Included are features such as characterisitc odor, thumbs that move in opposition to the fingers, the ability to use complex tools, a vocal tract positioned to permit easy choking on food, the power of reason and abstraction, a system of ethics, command of verbal and written language, and the ability to grasp the idea of aging and consequently fear it.

Two of these ideas, the verbal realization of language and the concept of aging, are within the domain of this chapter. Of necessity, we intend to consider a somewhat myopic and segmented relationship between the two, that is, how the process of aging relates to the breakdown of efficient motoric realization of language.

Just as we are blessed with the utility and beauty of speech, we are equally susceptible to its loss. Neuorogenic disorders of this singularly human trait have been traced periodically through the literature of several civilizations, from ancient Egyptian slaves and Greek fishermen to the slight dysarthria of a recent president of the United States. In the mid-1800s curiosity revolved around the peculiar and fascinating disturbances of speech, auditory comprehension, reading, and writing that came to be known as *aphasia*. But at this time, astute observers such as Hughlings Jackson (1878) began to realize that many output-transmissive disturbances of speech were not necessarily linked to symbolic impairment.

The communicative process is a unitary one

from a neurologic standpoint and every bit of communication a person undertakes is a product of his or her nervous system. Functionally, the entire speech production mechanism is a complex, interrelated system requiring synergy and precise coordination of its components. Consequently, neurologic abnormalities that disturb this delicate orchestration of sensory–neural–muscular events can and do affect the functions of the respiratory mechanism, the phonatory mechanism, and the resonatory–articulatory system.

Practical considerations dictate, though, that this integrated system be considered in more managable segments. Disturbances of voice and the linguistic–integrative process are treated in other chapters of this book. This chapter will focus on output-transmissive disorders that primarily but not exclusively fall within the realm of impaired phonology. These motor-speech disturbances include the dysarthrias and apraxia of speech.

DEFINITIONS OF MOTOR SPEECH DISORDERS

The Dysarthrias

Current usage of the term *dysarthria* is more comprehensive and precise than the traditional concept of dysarthria as imperfect articulation of speech caused by nervous system damage. Also, the idea of a unitary dysarthria is being refined to the more inclusive view of the *dysarthrias* (Darley, Aronson, &

159

Brown, 1975)—a *group* of related motor speech disorders resulting from disturbed muscular control over the speech mechanism.

A useful definition has grown from the work on motor speech disorders at the Mayo Clinic (Darley et al., 1975):

> The term will encompass coexisting motor disorders of respiration, phonation, articulation, resonance, and prosody. It will also comprise isolated single-process impairments, such as isolated articulation problem due to cranial nerve XII involvement, an isolated palatopharyngeal incompetence of neurogenic origin, or an isolated dysphonia due to unilateral vocal fold paralysis (p. 3).

Apraxia of Speech

The other communication impairment to be considered in this chapter, apraxia of speech, has been a fertile area of controversy for more than a century. Theoretic and interpretive arguments have abounded (Johns & LaPointe, 1976) but the term "apraxia of speech" seems to be gaining acceptance in the literature, despite the objections of some researchers (Martin, 1974).

We consider apraxia of speech to be a neurogenic phonologic disorder resulting from sensorimotor impairment of the capacity to program the positioning of the speech musculature and the sequencing of muscle movements for the volitional production of phonemes. Weakness, slowness, or incoordination in reflexive or automatic acts do not adequately explain the observed pattern of deviant articulation, and the movement disturbance is not attributable to deficient muscle groups. Prosodic alterations may be associated with the articulatory problem, both as a primary component of the condition and perhaps to a degree in compensation for it. From 10 to 15 behaviors have been cataloged as characteristic of the apraxic patient, but the hallmarks appear to be: (1) *initiation difficulty* characterized by stops, restarts, pauses, audible groups, nonaudible oral posturing, and phoneme, syllable, and/or whole word repetitions; (2) *more phonemic substitutions than distortions and omissions,* sometimes including additive substitutions of complex consonant clusters for singleton consonants; and (3) *change in production pattern on repeated trials* of the same stimulus target, including error change and performance that may vary on and off target.

ETIOLOGIES OF MOTOR SPEECH DISORDERS

A wide variety of congenital and acquired neuropathologies can affect the speech-production system. Damage can be located in cortical areas re-

sponsible for encoding the motor patterns of speech in the pyramidal system, extrapyramidal system, or in the peripheral nervous system composed of the cranial and spinal nerves and their associated ganglia. Both the quality and the severity of the speech impairment caused by neurologic damage not only depends on the site and extent of the offending lesion, but also when the insult occurs in the development of the individual. Figure 9–1 is a schematic illustration of the sections of the nervous system associated with motor speech disorders.

Conditions responsible for this damage represent an array of congenital injuries and anomalies as well as a variety of acquired conditions such as cerebral infections, toxic processes, space-occupying neoplasms, demyelinating diseases, neuromuscular diseases, closed-head and open-head trauma, and the multiple varieties of cerebrovascular disturbance. Wertz (1978) has presented a useful outline of these conditions and their effects on speech.

With a few exceptions, notably congenital malformations, cerebral palsy, and multiple sclerosis, most motor speech disorders are associated with the neuropathologies that accompany the aging process. The following section traces the relationship of these neuropathologies to age.

AGE-RELATED CONDITIONS

Cerebral Palsy

Cerebral palsy is not a specific disease or syndrome but a category of nervous system dysfunction that occurs in many forms. Perinatal neurologic damage creates the condition and impairs functioning of the motoric components of the speech-communication system. The condition often referred to as *cerebral palsied speech* is actually an example of one of the dysarthrias that occurs during childhood. Practically, cerebral palsy has been referred to as a microcosm of the whole world of neurologic disabilities (LaPointe, 1975). For many years it was known as Little's disease or spastic paralysis. This congenital neuromuscular condition may embody an array of associated defects such as impaired hearing, impaired vision, orthopedic abnormalities, epilepsy, perceptual problems, and retarded cognitive development.

In addition to these concomitants, the onset age of cerebral palsy assures that the condition will be a significant burden to normal social, emotional, and academic development. Of all the conditions treated in this chapter that cause motor speech disorders, this condition can have the most pervasive influence on subsequent developmental aspects of a person's life.

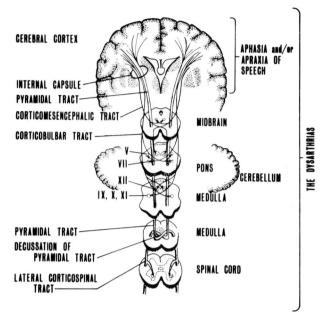

Fig. 9–1. Schematic illustration of the sections of the nervous system associated with motor speech disorders. (Adapted with permission from Wertz, R. T. Neuropathologies of speech and language: An introduction to patient management. In D. J. Johns (Ed.), *Clinical management of neurogenic communicative disorders.* Boston: Little, Brown, 1978.)

Clear correlations between cerebral palsy and speech dysfunction have been difficult because of the great variety of neuromuscular signs and symptoms that are included in this category. Cerebral palsy can include several diagnostic types, such as spastic paralysis, athetosis, ataxia, and rigidity. A wide range of severity within each type is possible as well as a blending of some of the characteristics of several types.

Multiple Sclerosis

Another neurologic impairment that can result in motor speech disturbance and that is related to a particular age is multiple sclerosis. Most typically, this disease has its onset in the second and third decades of life. As in cerebral palsy, the signs and symptoms that result encompass a good portion of the spectrum of the field of neurology. Though a great deal of research has focused on multiple sclerosis, its exact cause remains elusive. This demyelinating disease is gradually progressive in some people and affects a course of exacerbation and remission in others. Commonly reported symptoms include visual loss, ataxic gait, weakness and incoordination of the arms and legs, nystagmus, tremor, and dysarthria. Darley et al. (1975), however, have concluded that dysarthria is not a universal symptom of the disease. Many

subjects covering a fairly wide range of illness duration were judged in Mayo Clinic studies (Darley, Aronson, & Goldstein, 1972) to have adequate speech. When speech is affected, though, communication can be sorely reduced in intelligibility and present a bizarre impression. The most prominent speech deviations include impaired control of loudness and pitch, harshness, and imprecise articulation.

Amyotrophic Lateral Sclerosis

A number of progressive, degenerative diseases of the nervous system have their onset during adulthood. One of these is amyotrophic lateral sclerosis (ALS), a disease that appears in the fourth or fifth decade and results in widespread impairment of motor function by attacking both upper- and lower-motor-neuron systems (Darley et al., 1975). The course of the disease is not consistent from individual to individual, but for the most part the muscles of the upper extremities are affected first, followed by the lower extremities, and then those systems under control of bulbar structures. When the bulbar structures are invaded, the life-support systems of respiration or other vital functions may be compromised with resultant rapid degeneration and eventually death.

The degenerative progression of ALS is much

more rapid than in multiple sclerosis and the speech characteristics comprise a mixture of spastic and flaccid dysarthria traits. Since the degeneration does not necessarily proceed in an orderly or uniform fashion, the characteristics from either the damaged upper-motor-neuron or the lower-motor-neuron system can be the most outstanding at any given point in time. This multisystem impairment presents a devastation of speech that eventually leads to grossly impaired and unintelligible speech, laboriously slow rate, short phrases, extreme hypernasality, and marked hyperkinetic laryngeal valving, which in turn results in a harsh and strained−strangled voice quality (Darley et al., 1975).

Parkinsonism

Another condition that commonly has its onset later in life, usually after 50 years, is parkinsonism. This classic syndrome is characterized by hypokinesia, tremor at rest, muscular rigidity, and festination of movement. It is often associated with neurochemical degenerative changes in the basal ganglia, particularly the substantia nigra. A variety of less frequent causes has been suggested, however, including occasional association with encephalitis, slow virus infections, central arteriosclerosis, repeated head trauma (as in boxers), or toxic processes (such as manganese and carbon monoxide poisoning) (Darley et al., 1975). Drug-induced parkinsonism has been associated with the phenothiazides and tricyclic antidepressants commonly prescribed for elderly patients. This potential association was underscored in a recent experience of the second author in which severe hypokinetic dysarthria in a referred patient disappeared after discontinuation of the drug haloperidol. The effects of medication on control of the motor speech system is an area much in need of study.

Cerebrovascular Disorders

By far the greatest single cause of morbidity and disability in the elderly is the presence of arterial disease, and when this pervasive condition affects the cerebrovascular system, impaired control of the motor speech system can result (Locke & Galburda, 1978). Clearly, the acute incident referred to as a cerebrovascular accident (CVA) is not caused by a sudden structural change in the cerebral arterial system but is commonly present and insidiously progressive long before the insult to the brain.

Attempts at definitions of cerebrovascular accident have resulted in a good deal of variety. Implicit and common to all definitions is the concept of destruction of nervous tissue. The lay word *stroke* is appropriately chosen, for most often the patient is struck down, swiftly and suddenly. However, the onset may be gradual, stepwise, or transient, and these temporal differences in the nature of onset have accounted for the terms *completed* or *evolving* stroke, as well as *transient ischemic attack* (Locke & Galburda, 1978).

Infarction or tissue death due to the arrest of circulation in the supplying artery may be caused by thrombosis, embolism, stenosis, or hemorrhage. The term *thromboembolic* is being used with increasing frequency to refer to both stationary and moving obstructions.

According to Toole and Patel (1974), the adult cerebrovascular system strains a maximum of 20 percent of the total of circulatory blood, yet almost 50 percent of all symptom-producing arterial obstructions lodge in the brain. Consequently, neurologic impairment is often the first sign of multiple emboli to many parts of the body. Two reasons for the frequency of clinical signs of cerebral blockage have been proposed (Toole & Patel, 1974):

1. Much of the brain is extremely sensitive to obstruction of its flow. A 1-mm speck of material lodged in a brain stem artery can produce a disastrous neurologic deficit but will result in no symptoms if lodged in another organ or in the extremities.
2. The great vessels arise from the aortic arch in such a way that solid material expelled from the left ventricle tends to enter the left common carotid so that it travels to the brain instead of rounding the arch.

Also, the cerebral hemispheres seem to attract the majority of intracranial emboli because the amount of blood traversing the carotid system (more than 300 ml/min) is far greater than that carried by the vertebral artery (less than 100 ml/min). The middle cerebral artery, which nourishes many of the motor and associate areas that subserve speech and language, is a direct continuation of the internal carotid artery, and nearly 80 percent of the internal carotid blood supply is directed to the trunk and branches of the middle cerebral artery. Recurring emboli, therefore, have a tendency to lodge in the same cerebral artery, and unfortunately for the aging individual, cognitive, language, and motor speech functions are therefore vulnerable to and associated with vascular disease.

The most frequent source of cerebral emboli is the heart. Cardiac diseases form clots, and the continued movement of the beating heart throws them off into the circulatory system. Other relatively common sources of blood clot obstructions include the pulmonary veins and the veins of the legs, pelvic plexus, and the liver.

Though a blood clot is the most common cause of vascular obstruction, any solid, liquid, or gaseous foreign material can hinder the flow of blood through an artery and compromise the integrity of the nervous system. One such cause is the emboli composed of cholesterol crystals that are thrown off from plaques located in the carotid and cerebral–basilar arteries. Portions of these crystals may be cast off into the arterial stream by trauma to the arteries during compression, arteriography, or ligation (Toole & Patel, 1974).

Other cerebrovascular conditions that are less frequent than thromboembolic incidents include intracranial and subarachnoid hemorrhage, arterial aneurysms, and arteriovenous malformations.

EPIDEMIOLOGIC FACTORS

Epidemiology is the study of the frequency of diseases or conditions, including geographic distribution and the characteristics of the individual or environment that affect incidence or course (Kurtzke & Kurland, 1973). Information of this nature can be valuable in attempts to clarify the scope of a problem and put it into perspective. Estimates of the cost of a disease or handicapping condition can be used not only in terms of the number of affected persons and the expense of their care, but also in terms of the effect of the condition on the family, community, and future productivity of the individual. The scope of the problem of neurogenic motor speech disorders is difficult to assess from the literature either in clinical neurology or speech pathology.

Incidence of Motor Speech Disorders

No extensive study that addresses the question of either incidence or prevalence of the dysarthrias or apraxia of speech can be found in the literature at this time, and the scarcity of data prevents even an educated estimate. In one study of soldiers during World War II, Peacher (1945) suggested that 25.31 percent of all those with speech disorders were dysarthric.

The Veterans Administration has an active program in audiology and speech pathology throughout the United States, and an indication of the incidence of a variety of communication disorders can be appreciated from annual VA records. Even from these records, however, incidence of the motor speech dis-

orders is difficult to establish for a number of reasons. First, an individual may possess more than one communication disorder. The lesion that produces aphasia may also produce one of the dysarthrias or apraxia of speech, and the condition may be recorded as representative of only a single category. Second, since most VA programs enroll referred patients and do not conduct a screening of all hospitalized veterans, some selection bias may exist in the caseload. Staff and funding resources may not be sufficient to care for all those who in fact present a motor speech disorder. In a 1976 census of 87 speech pathology programs within the Veterans Administration, 15.9 percent of all patients exhibited speech disorders, but due to limited resources only one quarter of these were being treated for their communication impairment (Spuehler, 1978).

In fiscal year 1977, 87 speech pathology programs in the VA system reported seeing 8,215 patients with dysarthria for a total of 31,850 patient visits (Spuehler, 1978). These figures probably underestimate the number of veterans with motor speech problems because apraxia of speech is not used as a separate tally category, and perhaps a large percentage of the 44,910 patients categorized as aphasic presented a coexisting motor speech problem. Further, since only 87 of the nearly 200 VA medical centers are equipped to treat speech disorders, no doubt many persons who possess motor speech impairments go untreated and untallied. An accurate appreciation of the scope of the problem is elusive at this time. Studies of incidence and prevalence at hospitals throughout the country are sorely needed.

Incidence of Neurologic Disease

Though certainly not all neurologic conditions result in a motor speech disorder, some appreciation of the scope of the problem can be gained by consideration of the incidence and prevalence of nervous system disease in general. As Kurtzke and Kurland (1973) indicated, 1 in 70 of the general population has some form of neurologic disease. Further, each year about 1 in 130 of the general population is newly affected with a neuropathology. Translated into prevalence—the number of cases in a community at a given time—this means that over 3 million people in the United States have some sort of damage or anomaly of the nervous system.

GEOGRAPHIC FACTORS

The majority of these disorders appear with essentially equal frequency throughout the country. The disorders that do have large geographic dif-

ferences include congenital neurologic malformations and multiple sclerosis (Kurtzke & Kurland,
1973). Among congenital neurologic problems in the
United States, some concentration of incidence exists
on the eastern seaboard and there is a decline from
east to west. Multiple sclerosis shows a remarkable
geographic distribution and has been the subject of
extensive study for over 20 years. The disease is
much more common in the temperate zone than in the
tropics and subtropics. This unbalanced distribution
is apparent dramatically when prevalence rates from
the northern and southern tiers of the United States
are compared. Most studies indicate that persons who
migrate between regions, especially after the age of
15, retain the prevalence of their birthplace. Though
the condition becomes clinically apparent in the
twenties and thirties, these migration data suggest
that the pathologic onset probably occurs at an ap-
preciably younger age, perhaps the result of a
"slow" virus (Poser, 1975).

SEX AND RACE

Studies of the sex distribution of neurologic disease show few significant differences between males
and females, particularly for the conditions that result
in motor speech disorders, though a preponderance of
stroke incidence in males is still argued (Kurtzke &
Kurland, 1973).

Almost all epidemiologic data on race differences are from studies of death rates. Whites apparently have a higher incidence of malignant brain
tumor, multiple sclerosis, parkinsonism, dystonia,
amyotrophic lateral sclerosis, and muscular dys-
trophy as well as most congenital malformations of
the nervous system. Blacks seem to have higher rates
of cerebrovascular disease, epilepsy, and cerebral
palsy (Kurtzke & Kurland, 1973). These racial differences must be interpreted cautiously since race and
geography could be confounded, and variations in the
adequacy and availability of medical care could
further affect reported rates.

AGE

Age is related to a number of neurologic conditions and is particularly closely related to those conditions that are likely to create a motor speech disorder. Table 9–1 has been adapted from data presented by Kurtzke and Kurland (1973) to illustrate
the relationship of age to neurologic disease.

The most striking feature of these data and the
aspect that is most relevant to this chapter is the
geometric increase of cerebrovascular disease with
age. The average annual rate of strokes of all types

Table 9–1
Relationship of the Incidence of
Neurologic Disorders to Age

Maximal Incidence in Infancy
    Congenital malformations
    Cerebral palsy

Stable Incidence through Adulthood
    Subarachnoid hemorrhage
    Benign brain tumors
    Astrocytoma, grade I

Peak Incidence at Certain Ages
    Multiple sclerosis (20–40)
    Parkinsonism (75–80)
    Malignant brain tumors (55–65)
    Amyotrophic lateral sclerosis (57–61)

Geometric Incidence Increase with Age
    All cerebrovascular disease (rate doubles with
    each 5 years of age)

Adapted from Kurtzke, J., & Kurland, L. The
epidemiology of neurologic disease. In A. Baker (Ed.),
Clinical neurology. Hagarstown, Md.: Harper & Row,
1973.

was recently reported at 72 per 100,000 population
per year among persons 45 to 54 years old, and 1,786
per 100,000 population per year among those more
than 75 years of age (Whisnaut, 1974). Some progress has been made in reducing the risk factors associated with both cardiovascular and cerebrovascular mortality. Some have suggested that decreases in
cigarette smoking, cholesterol and saturated fat intake, and the sharpened American consciousness regarding physical fitness have accounted for this
trend. Whatever the cause, death rates from cerebrovascular disease were extremely stable from 1920
to 1951 and dropped 28.4 percent from 1951 to 1973
(Walker, 1976).

The trend of an aging American population is
clear, however. A well-publicized projection to the
year 2000 suggests that more than 30 million people,
or 12 percent of the population, will be 65 years of
age or over (Wilson, 1976). This growth, coupled
with the striking relationship between age and cerebrovascular disease, suggests that damage to the
brain will increase in importance as a major American health problem. When the delicate balance of the
nervous system is compromised we can expect a con-
sanguinity of disruptions in those motor systems that
allow efficient expression of our needs and whims.
Shattered verbal communication can be devastating

and dehumanizing. Attempts at restoration or compensation can and must be made, and that is the concern of the remainder of this chapter. The interaction of age with neuromotor control will be addressed throughout the discussions of evaluation, treatment, and prognosis of disturbances of motor speech.

NEUROMOTOR CONTROL OF SPEECH

Central or peripheral nervous system damage can produce a variety of motor symptoms such as paralysis, rigidity, uncontrolled and writhing movements, and incoordination. Usually the results of these motor deficits are obvious. The patient with multiple sclerosis is confined to bed because his legs no longer carry him; Lou Gehrig retired from baseball because amyotrophic lateral sclerosis robbed him of strength; the patient with parkinsonism shuffles along because he cannot take normal steps; the stroke patient drags one of his legs and is forced to change the hand with which he writes; the cerebral palsied child writhes in a wheel chair. The same motor abnormalities that cause such obvious changes in patients' ability to walk, work, and care for themselves may also cause a variety of speech deficits that have come to be called the motor speech disorders.

In order to better understand these speech disorders and the neuromuscular deficits that underlie them, various authors have hypothesized features of neuromotor performances on which normal speech depends. Darley et al. (1975) named six such features: strength, speed, range, accuracy, steadiness (of contraction), and tone. Netsell (1978) identified similar features but organized them differently. He posited that movement can be impaired in *range, velocity,* and *direction* because of abnormalities in muscle *strength, tone,* and *timing.* Like two recipes for ratatouille, the Darley et al. and Netsell schemes share some common ingredients but organize them somewhat differently.

Both systems have much to recommend them as guides to understanding the physiologic bases of the dysarthrias, that is, to understanding the relationships between clusters of speech symptoms and disturbances of neuromotor control and movement. Darley et al. (1975) based their hypotheses about such relationships on the statistical correlation of the perceptual (audible) symptoms of certain dysarthric speech types and the "known physiologic and neuromuscular elements" (p. 293) assumed to be characteristic of the disease causing those speech symptoms. For

example, they hypothesized that the speech symptoms of hypokinetic dysarthria in parkinsonism are caused by a reduced range of movement and rigidity. Netsell and his colleagues have taken a more physiologic approach by relying less on the ear and more on acoustic, aerodynamic, and cineradiographic measures (Kent & Netsell, 1975, 1978; Kent, Netsell, & Bauer, 1975; Netsell, Daniel, & Celesia, 1975; Netsell & Kent, 1976). They hypothesized, for example, that weakness and a tendency to accelerate are also important contributions to the symptoms of hypokinetic dysarthria (Netsell et al., 1975).

Besides normal strength, tone, and timing, human activity requires the contribution of cortical motor programmers. This level of motor function, sometimes called the psychomotor level, is hypothesized (DeJong, 1967) to involve the selection and ordering of movement sequences, which are then passed to the descending motor system and thence to the appropriate muscle groups. Motor programming for limb gestures is thought to reside in the parietal lobe and that for speech gestures in the frontal—parietal area, including Broca's area of the major hemisphere. When a programmer is disrupted apraxia results. A patient with limb apraxia may have trouble with the sequence of activities in lighting a cigarette or putting on his shirt. Disruption of the frontal—parietal motor programmer causes a characteristic pattern of articulatory and prosodic abnormalities called apraxia of speech or verbal apraxia.

As anyone who has tried to learn a new motor skill in middle age knows, age and neuromotor performance are related. Older persons become weaker and slower. These changes need not be seen as pathologic nor do they need to be treated. Their possible presence should be recalled, however, each time a clinician diagnoses a suspected motor speech disorder in an older patient, for such natural changes may masquerade as a mild motor speech disorder (Ryan & Burk, 1974). A similar complication may arise with children, for just as two normal children may differ in height and weight, so may they differ in strength and coordination. The best evidence for the presence of a motor speech disorder then is a child's consistent and significant failure to keep pace with his peers. Among the most difficult decisions to make about children is whether they are developing normal praxis or programmed movements. While it has not been demonstrated experimentally, at least to our knowledge, it might be hypothesized that the range of normal neuromotor control is greatest for the very old and the very young. This may explain, at least in part, our own clinical experience, which is that these two groups are the most challenging diagnostically.

DIAGNOSING MOTOR SPEECH DISORDERS

Taking a history of the patient's past and present status and making both informal and standardized observations of his speech and nonspeech oral performance are the beginnings of diagnosis. These data, when passed through a filter created by the clinician's training, professional reading, and clinical experience, allow decisions (or hypotheses) about (1) whether the patient's speech is normal or abnormal, (2) the type, distribution, and severity of symptoms, if the speech is abnormal, (3) the abnormalities of strength, timing, and tone that account for those symptoms, (4) the label(s) or classification(s) that best fit the patient's symptoms, (5) the appropriateness and type of treatment, and (6) the prognosis. Generally, these decisions need to be made regardless of the patient's birth date, but making them, as has been suggested, may be complicated in part by the patient's age.

Models to Direct the Diagnosis

The questions, like the testing that follows, need not be exhaustive, but neither should they be random or perfunctory. Focus for both can come from a model or scheme of motor speech activity that alerts the clinician about what to ask and look and listen for. One of the traditional models for this purpose divides speech into respiration, phonation, resonation, articulation, and prosody, and directs the clinician primarily to perceptual abnormalities such as inadequate loudness, hoarseness, hypernasality, consonant distortion, equal and even stress, and so on. Another model (Netsell, 1978) emphasizes the *functional components* of the speaking mechanism and the previously discussed neuromotor controls (strength, timing, and tone) and movement variables (range, velocity, and direction) responsible for normal speech.

Figure 9–2, taken from Netsell (1978), identifies the ten most important *functional components* by number. This model does not divert the clinician's attention from perceptual symptoms; the sound of patient's speech is still important. The model, however, does direct equal attention to the structures and portions of structures whose movements are primarily responsible for the perceptual symptoms. It also frees the clinician to consider each component's total contribution to the speech signal. The larynx, for example, has primary phonatory and articulatory functions but contributes as well to loudness, which is primarily a respiratory function.

The History

The history can be taken from the patient (unless age or illness prevents it) and confirmed by a family member. Many of the early questions about the medical and social history and about the developmental history (if the patient is a child) will be standard (Johnson, Darley, & Spriestersbach, 1963) regardless of whether or not the patient is suspected of having a motor speech disorder. In addition the interviewer will want the patient and family to highlight the patient's particular speech differences. Questions can be organized according to the logic provided by the ten functional components. Questions about the patient's loudness may reveal something about the respiratory structures because loudness is primarily a respiratory function. The answers to questions about voice quality may reveal something about laryngeal integrity, just as answers to questions about hypernasality will reveal something about the velopharynx. The answers to a host of questions may inform on the upper airway. Is articulation distorted? Is it slow? What of the patient's other deficits? Does he or she drool? Can he or she chew? Swallow? The history of any deficits also needs to be explored. When were difficulties first noticed? How have they changed? Does or did any other family member have a similar problem?

Formal Testing

After the history is complete, a patient thought to have a motor speech disorder can be taken through a series of speech and nonspeech tasks that evaluate each of the functional components alone and in various combinations. The patient's performance on these tasks can be evaluated perceptually and/or instrumentally. Perceptual evaluation is relatively quick and within the reach of most clinicians if they have been trained to listen and to identify dysarthric symptoms. Instrumental evaluation requires equipment and, like perceptual evaluation, specialized training. Much of the equipment is inexpensive, such as the manometer for measuring subglottal air pressure (Netsell & Hixon, 1978). A potential advantage of instrumental evaluation is improved precision. A

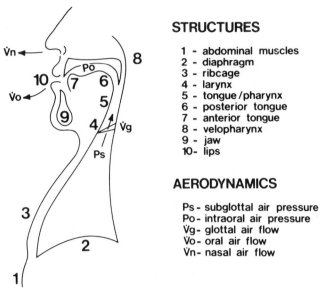

STRUCTURES

1 - abdominal muscles
2 - diaphragm
3 - ribcage
4 - larynx
5 - tongue/pharynx
6 - posterior tongue
7 - anterior tongue
8 - velopharynx
9 - jaw
10- lips

AERODYNAMICS

Ps- subglottal air pressure
Po- intraoral air pressure
Vg- glottal air flow
Vo- oral air flow
Vn- nasal air flow

Fig. 9–2. Schematic representation of ten functional components of the speaking mechanism and the air-pressure and air-flow characteristics generated by the activity of those components. (Adapted with permission from Netsell, R. Physiologic recordings in the evaluation and rehabilitation of dysarthria. *Communicative disorders: An audio journal for continuing education.* New York: Grune & Stratton, 1978.)

calibrated machine is less subject to educational bias, fatigue, and the need to prove a hypothesis than is a clinician. Increasingly, standard clinical practice is to use both perceptual and instrumental approaches.

Clinicians should begin with an evaluation of connected speech, if only because a patient, regardless of age, is likely to be put at ease by a greeting and on the defensive by a command to say /pʌpʌpʌ/ or to blow into a manometer. Also, the patient's attempts at connected speech will give the clinician a feeling about overall speech adequacy while providing clues to specific loci, frequency, and types of dysfunction. These clues can be followed up by progressively more controlled speech tasks such as are found in several standard speech samples (Darley et al., 1975) and in sentence and word articulation tests (Templin & Darley, 1960).

Even more discriminating speech and nonspeech tasks may be used to confirm global judgements and to expose deficits that may be camouflaged during other tasks. The unveiling of reduced respiratory support for speech can be accomplished instrumentally by measuring subglottal breath pressure. The inability to sniff, pant, or to make loudness changes during the prolonged production of /a/ may also unmask respiratory deficits (Hixon, 1975). Instrumental measures of oral and nasal air flow may permit evaluation of laryngeal and velopharyngeal integrity.

The ability to cough and to make rapid pitch changes on prolonged /a/ are among the perceptual tests of laryngeal function (Hixon, 1975). Resonance changes on prolonged /i/ when the patient's nostrils are occluded and when they are not, and resonance balance on such phrases as /pa pa maps/ are among the perceptual tests of velopharyngeal competence. The neurophysiologic integrity of lips and tongue can be inferred from intraoral air pressure measurements made during diadochokinetic tasks such as rapid repetition of /pʌ/ and /tʌ/ (Netsell, 1978). Perceptually, the lips can be tested by having the patient pucker, smile, and say /pʌ/ rapidly several times. Tongue protrusion and rapid production of /tʌ/ and /kʌ/ are among the perceptual tests of the tongue. To test the jaw's contribution of diadochokinetic performance, repetition of /pʌ/, /tʌ/, and /kʌ/ can be repeated while the patient clutches a bite block (Netsell, 1978) between his teeth, thus forcing the lips and tongue to move independently of the jaw.

Intelligibility measures are the last essential ingredient of a total motor speech evaluation. Individual patients may be easier or harder to understand than one would predict on the basis of all the special testing described previously. It is for this reason— and because a measure of how well a person is understood is one of the best indicators of a treatment's success—that intelligibility measures are mandatory.

Presently, the clinician can use Tikofsky's 50-word intelligibility list (1970), the more extensive measures of Yorkston and Beukelman (1978), or he or she can create individualized tests.

The motor speech mechanism does not work by itself; rather it is affected by linguistic, cognitive, and sensory systems. These, too, should be evaluated for each dysarthric and apraxic patient regardless of age. The danger in diagnosis, however, is a kind of clinical pleonasm. Redundancy is to be avoided unless the clinician is unsure of his observations.

Interpreting the Data

The data are not the diagnosis. Clinicians realize that motor speech disorders are not identified by a single test (regardless of the test's title), nor by a battery of tests, no matter how exhaustive; nor is the label to be found in a test score. The motor speech disorders are distinctive patterns of speech behavior. These patterns emerge when stimuli and instructions are attuned to the patient's age, experience, and knowledge and when responses are held up to a number of criteria. Perkins (1971) mentioned four such criteria: linguistic, cultural, developmental, and optimal production. The last refers to voice production and will not be discussed further. The other three are important to a discussion of age and motor speech disorders.

According to Perkins, "Linguistically, speech that violates grammatical rules or that is unintelligible is defective" (p. 343), because it fails to meet linguistic criteria. Similarly in a given society, men, women, and children sound different; and the man who sounds like a woman because of an inappropriate fundamental frequency is violating a cultural criterion. Obviously, both the linguistic and the cultural criteria interact with the developmental or age criteria. Abnormal articulation for an adult may well be normal for a 3-year-old, and what may be normal prosody for a child may be abnormal for an adult. Some responses, however, such as severe hoarseness and hypernasality, are abnormal in a person of any age. Nonetheless, the bulk of data from the motor speech evaluation are more likely to be interpreted correctly if the clinician knows the patient's age.

Persons in their fifth decade or older are of special interest because the effects of aging on motor speech performance are as yet uncertain. Whereas some studies have reported the deleterious effects of aging on speech (Ptacek, Saunder, Maloney, & Jackson, 1966), others have not (Blonsky, Logemann, Boshes, & Fisher, 1975), and Meyer-son's (1976) statement that ". . . speech differences in the aging are largely unsupported" (p. 33) is apparently most consistent with the data. We would hypothesize that a person's age will be discovered by future researchers to be less or no more important to motor speech performance than is his or her history of wellness. If the patient eschewed alcohol and tobacco, inherited a durable body, exercised, escaped obesity, and learned to manage stress, then the probability is great that respiratory, laryngeal, and articulatory differences noted at evaluation are indeed either dysarthria or dyspraxia, especially if the history confirms their onset concurrent with some traumatic event. If the history fails to establish a definite, causal relationship between symptoms and a traumatic event, then all conclusions, especially about mild differences, will be tentative because a patient's wellness clings to his voice. For example, smoking and emphysema may reduce respiratory support for speech, and smoking and alcohol can alter the larynx and vocal tract.

The final uses of the data are to determine the therapy's focus and the patient's prognosis. It is to treatment and prognosis that this chapter now turns.

TREATING MOTOR SPEECH DISORDERS

Chapter-length discussions can include only a few specifics about treatment, especially the treatment of motor speech disorders, because the symptoms and coexisting nonspeech deficits are so varied. The reader in search of specific methodology can consult Rosenbek and LaPointe (1978) and Rosenbek (1978). We will discuss selected management goals and procedures briefly, especially as they are governed by the general nature of motor speech disorders and by the patient's place in life, including his age.

Improving Physiologic Support for Speech

For us, improving physiologic support for speech means modifying the strength, timing, and tone on which normal speech seems to depend. Canter (1965) ventured that "therapeutic measures designed to improve physiological support for speech might be fruitful" (p. 48). While the data are only now being collected, our clinical experience tells us that Canter's "might be" can be replaced by "are often." A variety of traditional behavioral and biofeedback methods are often fruitful. Unlike Froeschels (1943), however, we do not recommend delaying speech training until physiologic support has been improved, unless strength and tone are so badly impaired that the patient is speechless. And even in this last case we would try to teach the patient an alternative mode of communication such as gesturing so that he could make his needs known while efforts to modify his strength and tone were ongoing. To delay teaching the patient to utter an intelligible *urinal* or to make some signal for it until days or weeks of muscle strengthening had been completed would make one unpopular with other members of the treatment team.

Age is but one of the criteria influencing a clinician's decision to attempt improved physiologic support. It may be, for example, that this goal will be appropriate to a greater number of younger patients than older ones. The reason, at least on the surface, is simple: Improving physiologic support such as strength is often a tedious and protracted process. It may be worth it only for the patient who is younger, who has a limited number of coexisting medical problems in addition to the one that caused the motor speech disorder, and who has varied and strong needs to communicate. Improving physiologic support is a legitimate goal also if (1) the patient's speech would otherwise be unintelligible, (2) the patient's speech intelligibility could be significantly improved by increased support, and (3) a change in control appears to be all that is necessary for a change in speech. And, lest we leave the impression that older patients are somehow less deserving than younger ones, let us emphatically summarize by saying that it is more important to plan treatment with a view to what patients have and what they have ahead of them rather than on the basis of how long they may have it.

Compensating for Reduced Physiologic Support

The patient can also be taught to compensate, to make the best use of whatever abilities remain. Luria, Naydin, Tsvetkova, & Vinarskaya (1969) said that such compensation results from the patient's learning to substitute one behavior for another and from his learning to perform a set of responses, such as talking, using a new set of neural controls. Examples of compensation include having the patient speak more slowly, with artificially increased effort (e.g., while bearing down against the arms of a wheel chair), at a higher fundamental frequency, or by accompanying speech with a rhythmical tapping of the hand on the desk top. Such compensatory methods can be emphasized with the severely involved patient, with the patient incapable of improved physiologic support, and with the patient whose environment makes minimal demands for intelligibility. Note that the emphasis is on environment—not age. The patients' symptoms and what they want or need are again more profound influences on treatment than when they were born.

No examples have yet been drawn from the treatment of apraxia of speech because the division between the two major goals—increasing support or compensating for reduced support—are blurred in apraxia. However the systematic, successful drill of articulatory movements so characteristic of apraxia of speech therapy probably improves physiologic support by reestablishing cortical movement patterns. Similarly, teaching the apraxic patient to slow down and to exaggerate stress and rhythm patterns may be just the compensation necessary for improved intelligibility.

Patient Cooperation

Improvement begins with cooperation. The burden of a motor speech disorder, regardless of severity, does not guarantee that a patient will seek out a speech pathologist or allow a physician to make the referral. Nor will a patient necessarily accept even the most gracious and competent of clinicians if someone does manage to get them together. A speech disorder is not always a speech handicap. For example, a cerebral palsied infant may not recognize his difference from other people; an adolescent may recognize but try to ignore the difference; a geriatric patient may disagree with the clinician about the gravity of symptoms. This last is not to perpetuate the stereotype of resignation in the elderly; it may be instead that the old have a keener sense of the natural (untreated and unbothered) course of things. Without cooperation, however, almost nothing enduring can be accomplished. Improved speech is not molded by the clinician working with inert materials; it is earned by clinician and patient struggling together. The child and even the adolescent will sometimes need to be beguiled by fluff and pageantry. The old can be won over—unless they are demented or adamant—by explanations and counseling. And explanations and counseling are, of course, the right of every patient regardless of age and regardless of how much or little he or she seems to want treatment.

In addition to counseling, explanations, and pageantry, one other influence on whether a patient is cooperative is the relevance of the clinician's materials, procedures, and goals. Relevance in such matters usually implies something about the patient's age, environment, interests, and future. Age may influence the number and type of therapeutic materials, the length and scheduling of sessions, the number of repetitions one tries to elicit, and the amount of time one spends helping the patient to see the value of treatment. But it influences little else. These variables of treatment are likely to be governed by the patient's health, environment, and future. Fatigue, for example, may be as disastrous to the young as to the old. Institutions can be callous regardless of their residents' ages; the future may be as compelling for the 70-year-old as for the 7-year-old. When selecting materials and planning sessions the clinician responds most to what the patients have and what they want to do about it, regardless of their proximity to the age of consent.

Team Cooperation

The neuropathologies, namely aphasia, apraxia of speech, and dysarthria, require that the speech pathologist be involved with other professionals. When a patient is treated, if at all, the amount, type, and outcome of the treatment depends on the availability, timing, and success of medical/surgical managements and the involvement of teachers, dietitians, physical and occupational therapists, the clergy, and the special educator. Hegemony has no place in the management of motor speech disorders. For example, the patient with a brainstem stroke and dysarthria will first be seen by a physician who will oversee his medication and stabilization. Speech treatment will often be delayed while respiratory therapy and nursing personnel attend to his respiration and nutrition and while physical therapy provides range of motion exercises at the bedside. Very often it is only after the patient is stable and after his primary functions have been attended to that other therapies such as speech and occupational join the effort. From that point on, all these professionals will serve the patient best if they cooperate with each other.

Other etiologies of the motor speech disorders, such as multiple sclerosis and amyotrophic lateral sclerosis, have different courses and demand different efforts of the team. The patient with amyotrophic lateral sclerosis often take a rapid downhill course. Medicine has no treatments, and the usual procedure is to make the patient comfortable as he dies. The patient with multiple sclerosis may experience periods of exacerbation followed by long periods of remission. Again medicine has no cure, but the patient's course makes it more likely that a number of therapies, including speech, will be involved, especially in helping the patient make the best use of the resources he or she has. Other etiologies, courses, and expectations of the team are discussed at length in Rosenbek and LaPointe (1978).

Selection and Sequence in Treatment

Before the clinician begins a specific treatment, he or she needs to decide about the order in which the functional components will be treated and about the stimuli to treat them. As a general rule, treatment is directed toward the component that is most disruptive to the total speech signal. If that component can be treated successfully, intelligibility will most likely improve. For example, if evaluation demonstrates that velopharyngeal inadequacy is contributing to consonant distortion, improved velar function (Schweiger, Netsell, & Sommerfeld, 1970) should result in better articulation and resonance. Reduced respiratory support may be contributing to short phrases, reduced loudness, monoloudness, and imprecise consonants. Improving respiration may change all these symptoms.

If life-sustaining activities such as chewing and swallowing are seriously impaired, the clinician, or someone on the treatment team, should attempt to improve them. If the patient is very young, such treatment takes precedence over speech treatments. If the patient is older, treatment of life-sustaining and speech activities can proceed simultaneously, because such deficits, as in swallowing, for example, often persist even after functional speech has appeared. Finally, if the underlying neuromotor condition(s) accounting for the speech symptoms can be determined, and if treatments are available, these conditions alone may be treated because influencing the underlying neuromotor pathology may influence the speech. Or the underlying neuromotor condition(s) and speech symptoms may be treated simultaneously.

The stimuli to be practiced are to be logically rather than capriciously organized. Clinical tradition suggests that therapy begin with stimuli that provide early success for the patient, and, like so many other ideas that have withstood the buffeting of time, this is a good one. Such stimuli may help a patient transfer to speech those gains made in treatment of the underlying neuromotor conditions. For example, a patient may have been able to improve his lip strength by use of a lip force transducer (Barlow & Abbs, 1979). This strength can be transferred to speech by having the patient begin speech training with the systematic, careful production of (pʌ/, /bʌ/, and /mʌ/. The successful practice at such levels of speech production will increase the likelihood of successful transfer to more complex speech production. This last statement, however, is a hypothesis subject to experimental investigation.

For a number of reasons, the selection and sequencing of targets and materials can only be decided on after each patient has been evaluated. Motor speech disorders, such as apraxia of speech, are not the same in adults and children (Yoss & Darley, 1974), especially if the child is born with a defective motor speech mechanism or acquires one before speech—language development is complete. Further, two patients with the same diagnosis, regardless of age, often differ, sometimes radically. Using general principles as a guide, the clinician should tailor the selection and sequencing of treatment procedures to the unique deficits and needs of each client. Once started, therapy proceeds in orderly steps. The nature of the steps in treating an adult who once had normal speech may differ from those used in treating a person who never experienced normal speech. The characteristics of these differences have yet to be specified.

PROGNOSIS

Prognosis refers to a projected outcome (with or without treatment) and an estimate of how long certain achievements will take. No one has yet undertaken a general statement about prognosis in the motor speech disorders because the group lacks homogeneity. Scattered in the literature, however, are prognostic statements about selected motor speech disorders. Luchsinger and Arnold (1965) observed that speech therapy for most parkinson patients may benefit their psyches but would have little effect on their speech. Allan (1972) warned that therapy, if it is done in groups, may continue for the patient's lifetime. On the other hand, Farmakides and Boone (1960) predicted significant improvement from speech therapy for the patient with multiple sclerosis if his intelligence is preserved. Apraxic patients probably make a better recovery than aphasic patients (Marks, Taylor, & Rusk, 1957; Mohr, Pessin, Finkelstein, Funkenstein, Duncan, & Davis, 1978), but their recovery has not been contrasted with groups of dysarthric patients. The prognosis is

abysmal for the patient whose motor speech disorders is caused by a rapidly progressive degenerative disease such as amyotrophic lateral sclerosis.

Age is the ubiquitous prognostic variable. Eisenson's (1949) mention of it echoes in the literature on every disorder. Probably it is true that the young nervous system's plasticity makes recovery from an acquired motor speech disorder somewhat more likely in the young than the old. One cannot help but feel, however, that a patient's age is but a minor influence on recovery in many cases. The patient's history of wellness, the severity of the deficit, the relative intactness of the intellectual and sensory processes, and the will and need to change are probably at least equally important. And even more to be trusted than any of these traditional signs is the patient's response to treatment. If he or she learns the treated material and if that learning generalizes, the prognosis is good whether the patient be infant or octogenarian.

UNANSWERED QUESTIONS

Perhaps the overriding research need in most areas related to health care is the necessity of gaining a genuine understanding of disease mechanisms. Research on questions about irreversibility of cerebral tissue damage is crucial. The prevention or cure of neurologic diseases that cause motor speech disorders, though, is probably generations away, and we must be satisfied with less lofty goals. These include discovery and refinement of the most efficient management of the people afflicted with these disorders. The last two decades have seen trends toward greater research attention to the evolution of systematic strategies of therapy (LaPointe, 1977), along with improved standardization of precise, behaviorally defined terminology. Equally promising to the evolution of treatment of motor speech disorders is the accelerated effort in the application of improved technology to the objective measurement of deviant speech parameters (Netsell, 1978).

Certainly, the contribution of computerized axial tomography to neurodiagnostics has been a significant development of the 1970s (DiChiro, 1975). Perhaps further refinement of this technique will allow more accurate association of the quality and severity of motor speech disturbance with specific lesion sites. Predicted advances in the diagnostic and therapeutic application of the emerging technologies of acoustic holography, pulsatile electrical impedance, and nuclear magnetic resonance also have been made (DiChiro, 1975). The potential exists for these tools to aid us in developing a clearer understanding of the nature, cause, and plasticity of neurogenic speech disruptions. It remains to be seen whether or not the potential will be realized.

The value of concentrated effort toward rehabilitation such as the use of stroke teams and stroke units has been documented (Sahs, 1975). Research is needed on means of making this approach more cost-effective so it is not regarded as a luxury that creates unnecessary expense for the hospitalized patient. In general terms, more support in both funding and understanding is needed to develop a medical and behavioral research thrust to improve prevention, early detection, treatment, and follow-up of these disorders. Until this knowledge becomes available, however, we must give the most enlightened attention to those who are afflicted with these disturbances. A highly valued component of the quality of life is the ability of people to interact with each other as efficiently as possible. Research that nurtures that objective in any way is laudable.

REFERENCES

Allan, C. M. Treatment of nonfluent speech resulting from neurological disease: Treatment of dysarthria. *British Journal of Disorders of Communication* 1972, *5*, 3−5.

Barlow, S. M., & Abbs, J. H. Transducers for evaluation of articulatory muscle strength in dysarthria. Paper presented at the American Speech and Hearing Association Convention, Atlanta, Georgia, 1979.

Blonsky, E. R., Logemann, J. A., Boshes, B., & Fisher, H. B. Comparison of speech and swallowing function in patients with tremor disorders and in normal geriatric patients: A cinefluorographic study. *Journal of Gerontology,* 1975, *30,* 229−303.

Canter, G. J. Speech characteristics of patients with Parkinson's disease: II. Physiological support for speech. *Journal of Speech and Hearing Disorders,* 1965, *30,* 44−49.

Darley, F., Aronson, A., & Brown, J. *Motor speech disorders.* Philadelphia: Saunders, 1975.

Darley, F., Aronson, A., & Goldstein, N. Dysarthria in multiple sclerosis. *Journal of Speech and Hearing Research,* 1972, *15,* 229−245.

DeJong, R. N. *The neurological examination: Incorporating the fundamentals of neuroanatomy and neurophysiolgoy* (3rd ed.). New York: Harper & Row Publishers, 1967.

DiChiro, G. Neuroradiology as a discipline. In D. Tower (Ed.), *The nervous system. (Vol. 2: The clinical neurosciences.* New York: Raven Press, 1975.

Eisenson, J. Prognostic factors related to language rehabilitation in aphasic patients. *Journal of Speech and Hearing Disorders,* 1949, *14,* 262−264.

Farmakides, M. N., & Boone, D. R. Speech problems of patients with multiple sclerosis. *Journal of Speech and Hearing Disorders,* 1960, *25,* 385−390.

Froeschels, E. A contribution to the pathology and therapy of dysarthria due to certain cerebral lesions. *Journal of Speech Disorders,* 1943, *8,* 301−321.

Hixon, T. J. Respiratory−larngeal evaluation. Paper presented at the Veterans Administration Workshop on Motor Speech Disorders, Madison, Wisconsin, 1975.

Jackson, H. On affections of speech from disease of the brain. *Brain,* 1878, *1,* 304−330.

Johns, D., & LaPointe, L. Neurogenic disorders of output processing: Apraxia of speech. In H. Whitaker & H. A. Whitaker (Eds.), *Studies in neurolinguistics* (Vol. 1). New York: Academic Press, 1976.

Johnson, W., Darley, F., & Spriestersbach, D. C. *Diagnostic methods in speech pathology.* New York: Harper & Row Publishers, 1963.

Kent, R., & Netsell, R. A case study of an ataxic dysarthric: Cineradiographic and spectrographic observations. *Journal of Speech and Hearing Research,* 1975, *40,* 115−134.

Kent, R., & Netsell, R. Articulatory abnormalities in athetoid cerebral palsy. *Journal of Speech and Hearing Research,* 1978, *43,* 353−373.

Kent, R., Netsell, R., & Bauer, L. L. Cineradiographic assessment of articulatory mobility in the dysarthrias. *Journal of Speech and Hearing Disorders,* 1975, *40,* 467−480.

Kurtzke, J., & Kurland, L. The epidemiology of neurologic disease. In A. Baker (Ed.), *Clinical neurology*. Hagarstown, Md.: Harper & Row Publishers, 1973.

LaPointe, L. Neurological abnormalities affecting speech. In D. Tower (Ed.), *The nervous system, (Vol. 3: Human communication and its disorders)*. New York: Raven, 1975.

LaPointe, L. Base-10 programmed stimulation: Task specification, scoring and plotting performance in aphasia therapy. *Journal of Speech and Hearing Research, 1977, 42,* 90–105.

Locke, S., & Galburda, A. Cerebrovascular disorders in later life. In W. Reichel (Ed.), *Clinical aspects of aging*. Baltimore: Williams and Wilkins, 1978.

Luchsinger, R., & Arnold, G. E. *Voice–Speech–Language*. Belmont, Calif.: Wadsworth Publishing Co., 1965.

Luria, A., Naydin, V., Tsvetkova, L., & Vinarskaya, E. Restoration of higher cortical function following local brain damage. In P. Vinken & D. Bruyn (Eds.), *Disorders of higher nervous activity*. Amsterdam: North Holland, 1969.

Marks, M., Taylor, M., & Rusk, H. A. Rehabilitation of the aphasic patient: A survey of three years' experience in a rehabilitation setting. *Archives of Physical Medicine and Rehabilitation, 1957, 38,* 219–226.

Martin, A. D. Some objections to the term apraxia of speech. *Journal of Speech and Hearing Disorders, 1974, 39,* 53–64.

Meyerson, M. D. The effects of aging on communication. *Journal of Gerontology, 1976, 31,* 29–38.

Mohr, J. P., Pessin, M. S., Finkelstein, S., Funkenstein, H. H., Duncan, G. W., & Davis, K. R. Broca aphasia: Pathologic and clinical. *Neurology, 1978, 28,* 311–324.

Netsell, R. Physiologic recordings in the evaluation and rehabilitation of dysarthria. *Communicative disorders: An audio journal for continuing education*. Grune & Stratton, 1978.

Netsell, R., Daniel, B., & Celesia, G. G. Acceleration and weakness in parkinsonian dysarthria. *Journal of Speech and Hearing Disorders, 1975, 40,* 170–178.

Netsell, R., & Hixon, T. A noninvasive method for clinically estimating subglottal air pressure. *Journal of Speech and Hearing Disorders, 1978, 43,* 326–330.

Netsell, R., & Kent, R. Paroxysmal ataxic dysarthria. *Journal of Speech and Hearing Disorders, 1976, 41,* 93–109.

Peacher, W. Speech disorders in World War II: III. Dysarthria. *Journal of Speech and Hearing Disorders, 1945, 10,* 287–291.

Perkins, W. H. *Speech pathology: An applied behavioral science*. St. Louis: C. V. Mosby, 1971.

Poser, C. Multiple sclerosis. In D. Tower (Ed.), *The nervous system (Vol. 2: The clinical neurosciences)*. New York: Raven Press, 1975.

Ptacek, P. H., Saunder, E. K., Maloney, W. H., & Jackson, C. C. R. Phonatory and related changes with advanced age. *Journal of Speech and Hearing Research, 1966, 9,* 353–360.

Rosenbek, J. Treating apraxia of speech. In D. Johns (Ed.), *Clinical management of neurogenic communicative disorders*. Boston: Little, Brown & Co., 1978.

Rosenbek, J., & LaPointe, L. The dysarthrias: Description, diagnosis, and treatment. In D. Johns (Ed.), *Clinical management of neurogenic communicative disorders*. Boston: Little, Brown & Co., 1978.

Ryan, W. J., & Burk, K. W. Perceptual and acoustic correlates of aging in the speech of males. *Journal of Communication Disorders, 1974, 7,* 181–192.

Sahs, A. Medical management of vascular diseases of the brain. In D. Tower (Ed.), *The nervous system (Vol. 2: The clinical neurosciences)*. New York: Raven Press, 1975.

Sarno, M. T. Speech impairment in Parkinson's disease. *Archives of Physical Medicine and Rehabilitation, 1968, 49,* 269–275.

Schweiger, J. W., Netsell, R., & Sommerfeld, R. M. Prosthetic management and speech improvement in individuals with dysarthria of the palate. *Journal of the American Dental Association, 1970, 80,* 1348–1353.

Spuehler, H. Personal communication, 1978.

Templin, M. C., & Darley, F. *The Templin–Darley tests of articulation*. Iowa City: Bureau of Educational Research and Service, Extension Division, State University of Iowa, 1960.

Tikofsky, R. S. A revised list for the estimation of dysarthric single word intelligibility. *Journal of Speech and Hearing Disorders*, 1970, *13*, 59–64.

Toole, J., & Patel, A. *Cerebrovascular Disorders*. New York: McGraw-Hill Book Co., 1974.

Walker, W. Success story: The program against major cardiovascular risk factors. *Geriatrics*, 1976, *31*, 97–104.

Wertz, R. Neuropathologies of speech and language: An introduction to patient management. In D. Johns (Ed.), *Clinical management of neurogenic communicative disorders*. Boston: Little, Brown & Co., 1978.

Whisnaut, J. Epidemiology of cerebral infarction: Current concepts of cerebrovascular disease. *Stroke*, 1974, *9*, 1–4.

Wilson, A. Aging and the Veterans Administration. In A. Wilson & W. Martin (Eds.), *Aging and total health*. St. Petersburg, Fla: Eckerd College, 1976.

Yoss, K. A., & Darley, E. L. Developmental apraxia of speech in children with defective articulation. *Journal of Speech and Hearing Research*, 1974, *17*, 399–416.

Yorkston, K. M. & Beukelman, D. R. A comparison of techniques for measuring intelligibility of dysarthric speech. *Journal of Communication Disorders*, 1978, *11*, 499–512.

Walter H. Manning
Edward A. Shirkey

10
Fluency and the Aging Process

STUTTERING AS LONG-TERM BEHAVIOR

The behavior called stuttering most often appears for the first time during early childhood, and from this perspective stuttering may be viewed as a disorder of childhood. However, the problem often persists, developing and maturing along with the individual through adolescence into adulthood. Considerable effort has gone into the study of the onset and development of stuttering in children. Due partly to the general availability of young adults who stutter, the majority of research has been conducted by academic and service centers with this population. Stutterers in their middle- and late-adult years, however, have received very little attention. This lack of interest in older stutterers is illustrated by an informal survey of the articles dealing with the nature or treatment of stuttering in the *Journal of Speech and Hearing Research,* the *Journal of Speech and Hearing Disorders,* and the *Journal of Fluency Disorders,* from 1969 through 1978. During this 10-year period only a total of 80 stutterers over the age of 40 were included as subjects in articles on the topic of stuttering. Of this number, 50 were age 40 or older, 21 individuals were age 50 or older, 8 were age 60 or older, and only 1 was age 70 or older. The lack of research with older stutterers is also true in foreign literature. While writing the *Nature of Stuttering,* Van Riper (1971) reviewed over 80 translations of foreign literature without finding a single article concerning the nature of stuttering in older individuals (Van Riper, 1978). He also reported that Dr. Henry Freund, an individual who knew the European literature well, did not know of any investigations dealing with older stutterers (Van Riper, 1978).

The apparent lack of interest and obvious lack of study concerning the nature of stuttering in older individuals is unfortunate. It would seem that in order to completely understand and modify a behavioral problem such as stuttering it would be essential to appreciate the development of the behavior throughout the life cycle. For example, the phenomenon of "spontaneous recovery" from stuttering, normally associated with stuttering during the early teenage years, may also occur during the middle- and late-adult years. In addition to a possible decrease in the number of individuals who stutter with increasing age, many older stutterers may experience a decrease in the severity of their stuttering. If this is true, even for some people, there may be principles of attitudinal and behavioral change that need to be understood. Perhaps such understanding would enable us to help individuals of any age who are continuing to struggle with their speech. Most important, current models of stuttering development, while they have proved useful in formulating intervention strategies, cannot be complete without at least some knowledge of the developmental changes of stuttering behavior that take place during the middle- and late-adult years.

In this chapter we will emphasize what is presently known about the nature of stuttering in the middle- and late-adult years of life. We shall ask questions that we hope will stimulate others to search for answers. In addition, we will formulate a model to help describe the occurrence of dysfluencies in older stuttering, as well as nonstuttering, speakers.

We begin our examination of stuttering in older adulthood by looking briefly at younger stutterers. We do this for two reasons. First, it seems important to place what little we do know about the nature of stuttering in older individuals into a developmental perspective. Second, it appears that there are several important features of the onset and development of stuttering in children, adolescents, and young adults that have importance for understanding the disorder in the later years of life.

We will also consider the nature of dysfluency in older nonstuttering individuals in our attempt to understand the nature of stuttering in older individuals. We do this because present knowledge concerning the articulatory, phonatory, psychologic, and fluency characteristics of older nonstutterers may provide some valuable insights for the understanding of stuttering in late adulthood.

THE BEGINNINGS OF STUTTERING

The consistency with which stuttering first appears in the early years of childhood is well documented, with the first occurrence of stuttering typically observed between ages 2 through 7. Although there are cases in which the onset and development of stuttering are rather abrupt, it is generally agreed that the development of stuttering is gradual. In fact, there has been considerable controversy concerning whether or not the first fluency breaks noted in the speech of a young, yet-to-be-confirmed stutterer are normal (Van Riper, 1971, 1973). Adding to the difficult task of distinguishing among normal and abnormal fluency breaks during the early phases of stuttering is the fact that most children show great variability in the occurrence of abnormal speech, swinging back and forth between periods of abnormal and normal fluency breaks, often without obvious cause (Van Riper, 1971). Once stuttering behaviors become more pronounced and less variable, the continued development of stuttering is characterized by an increase in the number of breaks in the flow of speech as well as the development of additional avoidance and escape behaviors. There is also a significant increase in the fear associated with

the stuttering moment, as well as the development of a self-concept that may be influenced by patterns of fear and avoidance related to speaking situations. As stuttering behavior develops there is less variation within the individual stutterer in terms of overt stuttering behavior. There is, however, considerable variation between stutterers with each stutterer demonstrating his own unique, and often creative, avoidance and escape behaviors (Bloodstein, 1960; Johnson & associates, 1959; Van Riper, 1971).

The issue of normal-versus-abnormal fluency breaks is an important concept for understanding the development of stuttering in young as well as in older individuals. While the distinction between normal and stuttered speech can be painfully obvious at times, in many instances the distinction is clouded by a child's production of a combination of both normal and abnormal fluency breaks. Several authors (Adams, 1977; Cooper, 1973; Johnson & associates, 1959; Van Riper, 1971) have described both behavioral and attitudinal features that provide some help in differentiating between normal and abnormal fluency breaks. Generally, fluency breaks are more likely to be perceived as stuttering when (1) the fluency breaks are frequent, (2) the fluency breaks occur between sounds or syllables, (3) tension or struggle behavior is present prior to or during the break, (4) cessation of voicing or airflow occurs, (5) the speaking rate increases during a repetition, and (6) the individual evidences fear or avoidance of speaking.

One view of normal and abnormal breaks in the speech of young children was proposed by Bloodstein (1974), who described a model of stuttering characterized by tension and fragmentation of speech. Tension tends to result in prolongations during the production of continuant sounds. During the production of stop consonants tension leads to a prolonged pause followed by an overaspirated plosive release. Fragmentation of speech results in repetitions. Bloodstein hypothesized that while stutterers who have been stuttering for some time tend to fragment words, the earliest phase of stuttering is characterized by fragmentation of larger syntactic structures such as sentences, coordinate and subordinate clauses, verb phrases, noun phrases, and prepositional phrases. Bloodstein viewed the loci of stuttering as following the rules of the "eccentric grammar of stuttering" (p. 383). These results are reflected in the child's early stuttering as he or she attempts the production of relatively larger syntactic units. Eventually, however, the child begins to show similar breaks during the production of progressively smaller syntactic units. The break in fluency typically occurs at the beginning of the syntactic structures and rarely, if ever, at the end of these structures. As the child begins to experience fluency failure on specific words and sounds, these units of speech become associated with the experience of stuttering. Thus, according to Bloodstein, the development of stuttering is reflected by a change of the loci of stuttering from the initial portion of larger linguistic units to the initial portions of progressively smaller units.

Van Riper (1971) proposed a model of stuttering that, in many respects, is similar to the model discussed by Bloodstein (1974). Van Riper's model, however, is not specifically addressed to the development of stuttering in young children. The basis of Van Riper's model is the concept of stability of motoric sequencing. He argued that motoric sequencing becomes more stable with practice, but more complex sequences tend to be less stable, and the stability of a sequence is apt to be disrupted by alterations in feedback. With these points in mind, Van Riper described a hierarchy of motor speech units from most to least stable, namely, phoneme, syllable, word, phrase, and sentence. Van Riper (1971) suggested that supramorphemic fluency breaks at the phrase or sentence level are common and may be thought of as formulative breaks. These formulative breaks in fluency are most typical in nonstuttered speech. Fluency breaks at the sound, syllable, or word levels, on the other hand, were viewed as failures of motoric integration. These coordinative or motoric breaks are more typical of stuttered speech.

Van Riper completed his model by discussing the selective effects of communicative and emotional stress on speech fluency. During moderately stressful speaking situations (communicative stress) speech is likely to be disrupted at the least stable levels of sequencing, resulting in fluency breaks at the phrase and sentence level. During more stressful speaking situations (emotional stress), speech is likely to be disrupted at the more stable levels of sequencing, resulting in fluency breaks occurring within sounds, syllables, and/or words. To quote Van Riper's proposition, "The greater the stress, the more likely it is that the sequencing of speech will be disrupted at a more basic level of integration" (p. 424). Because the act of speaking for a stutterer is likely to be associated with emotional as well as communicative stress, the fluency breaks of stuttered speech tend to take the form of motoric breaks with fragmented sounds, syllables, and words.

Both of these models provide a strategy that help describe and explain the developmental stages of stuttering in young children. These models may also provide insight into the fluency characteristics of older stutterers.

ADOLESCENCE AND YOUNG ADULTHOOD

The onset of stuttering rarely occurs during the preadult and early adult years. When it does, it is usually associated with a specific organic or psychogenic problem (Van Riper, 1971; Ingham, 1976; Rosenbek, Messert, Collins, & Wertz, 1978). More typical during these years is the continued development and refinement of the stutterer's avoidance and escape behaviors. According to Young (1975), the prevalence of stuttering in the general population is apparently maintained at approximately 0.7 percent from early school-age years through adulthood. On the other hand, Gillespie and Cooper (1973), who surveyed 5054 junior and senior high school students, found a prevalence of 2.1 percent. This relatively high prevalence rate was apparently due, at least in part, to an unusually high percentage of black stutterers (2.8 percent) compared to white stutterers (0.7 percent).

Spontaneous recovery has been observed to occur during the early adolescent years. Some authors have suggested that as many as 80 percent of all those who stuttered at one time in their lives were likely to recover without formal intervention (Andrews & Harris, 1964; Sheehan & Martyn, 1966, 1970), although this percentage has been disputed by other investigators (Cooper, 1972; Ingham, 1976; Young, 1975). For example, Cooper (1972) found recovery rates of 30 percent and 44 percent in his sample of 5054 junior and senior high school students, respectively.

Although the question of how many stutterers recover spontaneously from stuttering remains unanswered, the results of several independent studies suggest that some recovery does occur for a significant number of stutterers (Andrews & Harris, 1964; Cooper, 1972; Shearer & Williams, 1965; Sheehan & Martyn, 1966, 1970; Wingate, 1964). In summary, these studies indicate that most, but not all, of the stutterers recover during adolescence. The average age of recovery appears to be approximately 12 years but with a range from 9 to 40 years. There is little evidence to indicate that these "recovered" stutterers have *fully* recovered and are now truly normal speakers. Furthermore, there is no evidence to indicate if these recovered stutterers are likely to begin to stutter again later in life. There is general agreement that, whatever the degree of recovery, the change from stuttered to fluent speech is a gradual one, sometimes taking several years. The findings of these studies also indicated that recovered stutterers tend to attribute their recovery to a combination of change in self-concept and "speech practice." With increased age they begin to feel better about themselves as they develop skills and accomplish a variety of tasks. Whereas practice of speech can take many forms, assertive behavior (nonavoidance of words, situations, and people) is often associated with increased fluency. In addition, several of the former stutterers interviewed indicated that "speaking slower" was a helpful procedure for attaining fluency.

Before leaving our discussion of spontaneous recovery during the adolescent years, we need to point out a problem that prevents complete understanding of this phenomenon. As Young (1975) indicated, there cannot be prevalance rates of 0.7 percent for both school-age children and young adults *and* the occurrence of spontaneous recovery for as many as 80 percent of school-age stutterers. At least one of these figures, as Young suggests, must contain substantial error. That is, if 30 to 80 percent of all stutterers recover during adolescence, then the question arises as to why the prevalence figures for adolescent and young-adult stutterers are the same. Clearly, the issue of spontaneous recovery from stuttering is not well understood at this time.

Other individuals, of course, continue to stutter as severely as ever through their adolescent and early adult years. To some degree, at least, the fact that a person is a stutterer begins to affect the individual's social, educational, and vocational choices. During these years many of the stutterer's actions are dictated by fears of stuttering. As individual stutterers reach the early adult years, their ability to compensate for their stuttering varies greatly. Some stutterers, despite severe stuttering, choose occupations that require considerable speaking (i.e., ministers, secretaries, teachers). Other stutterers, of course, tend to withdraw from most speaking situations and choose occupations that require minimal verbal communication (Van Riper, 1971, 1979).

During the early adult years many stutterers refer themselves for therapy, regardless of whether or not they have received therapy previously. Earlier in their lives they may have been unwilling partners in the therapy process. When faced with some of life's major decisions during their early adult years, however, many stutterers see the necessity of making a commitment and possibly a concerted effort to change their speech behaviors. Both nonstutterers and stutterers are apt to pause and consider the available options once a major phase of their life is completed and they face the possibility of a change in roles. Such changes are likely to occur in conjunction with "timing events" (Kimmel, 1974, p. 55) such as termination of schooling, discharge from military duty, being fired or resigning from a job, and divorce. It seems to be during such periods in life that adult stutterers are more apt to make self-referrals for therapy and are most likely to make progress in therapy.

After the years of young adulthood, there appears to be a dramatic decrease in the number of stutterers seen for therapy. Part of the explanation for this decrease may be that school-age and college-age stutterers are more apt to find or be referred to clinical facilities, whereas older stutterers are not. In addition, older stutterers with career and family responsibilities may not be willing to take the time and effort required for therapy. Finally, some stutterers may have been successful in spite of their stuttering and simply do not feel the need for therapy.

MIDDLE AND LATE ADULTHOOD

The reasons for the lack of information on the nature of stuttering in older individuals are unclear. It may be, quite simply, that there are extremely few older individuals who stutter or, as Van Riper (1978) has suggested, older individuals who stutter typically lack the motivation to seek professional help. On the other hand, it may be that if we were more effective in communicating to older individuals the availability and possible value of clinical services, more older stutterers would seek such help.

For many years authorities in the area of stuttering have suggested that the prevalence of stuttering decreases in late adulthood. Travis (1978) often told his students that ". . . death and old age were sure cures for stuttering . . ." and that ". . . he never knew of an old man who stuttered." An attempt to investigate the prevalence of stuttering in older age groups was made by Shames and Beams (1956). Although there were procedural problems that hindered accurate samplings of stutterers, the results were interesting. Noting that their clinical records indicated an obvious lack of clinical contact with stuttering individuals over age 45, the authors attempted to test the hypothesis that the prevalence of stuttering was lower in the middle- and late-adult years. One hundred fifty clergymen were sent questionnaires that required them to tabulate the number of males and females in each congregation and the number of stutterers by age and sex. The clergymen were asked to identify stuttering in individuals "from first hand information" (p. 314). Only 50 questionnaires were returned and, of that number, only 22 were usable. The authors found a downward trend in the number of stutterers as age increased with a high of 0.9 percent during ages 3 to 5 and a low of 0.25 percent during ages 50 to 80. There appeared to be an obvious change in the prevalence of stuttering before and after age 50 with ten times more stutterers under 50. Shames and Beams suggested that the lowered prevalence of stuttering in the older age groups could have been the result of lowered church attendance by stutterers who would tend to shun social activities. This would not, however, explain the pronounced difference in prevalence before and after the age of 50. They also suggested that stutterers may be under more stress and, consequently, do not live as long as their nonstuttering counterparts. This possibility also has been suggested by Van Riper (1978):

I've come across many of them, but they've given up all hope of relief so they seek no services. They don't go to church or take part in social activities. They build little living spaces as free from hurt as possible. They get others to do their talking for them. I doubt that the prevalence of stuttering in the aged declines except for the attrition due to early death because of the stress under which they live constantly.

The only other reference concerning the prevalence of stuttering in older individuals was Jones (1948) and his report of an article by Treitel written in 1894. Treitel was an ear, nose, and throat specialist in Berlin who worked with stutterers. Drawing from his own experience and citing figures accumulated by a colleague named Denhardt (see Table 10−1), Treitel suggested that there was an obvious decrease in the number of older people seeking formal help for stuttering. While acknowledging that Denhardt's figures indicated only the number of individuals per age category seen by him for therapy, Treitel suggested that the prevalence of stuttering decreases after puberty. He reasoned that the ". . . calm and self-possession of maturity give the psychic influences less importance than the impressional spirit of adolescence" (p. 22).

With so little known concerning the prevalence of stuttering during the middle- and late-adult years, it is not surprising that even less is known about the characteristic forms of stuttering in this population. It appears that whereas several people who stuttered earlier in their lives "recover" after age 50, others continue to stutter but less severely. Whether older stutterers actually stop stuttering or are able to de-

Table 10−1

The Number of Stuttering Clients Seen by Denhardt for Therapy Grouped by Age.

Age Grouping	Number of Stutterers Seen for Therapy
6− 8	49
9−12	323
13−15	336
16−20	631
21−25	549
26−30	207
31−40	133
41−50	48
51−60	14
62−and older	1

Reprinted with permission from Jones, M. V. Leopold Treitel on stuttering. *Journal of Speech and Hearing Disorders*, 1948, *13*, 19−22.

crease their stuttering to a point at which it is less obvious and less handicapping is a question that needs to be studied. Murray (1978) reported that several notable individuals in the field of speech and language pathology who stuttered severely earlier in life showed an obvious improvement in fluency from their forties through their sixties. Murray described how one such adult stutterer had explained his increase in fluency from his thirties to fifties. First, he felt that not having to prove himself and sell himself to others as being capable or skillful facilitated fluency. Second, he felt that he had less energy with which to spend on all the struggle behavior typical of his early stuttering. Finally, he felt that his ability to keep his stuttering "streamlined" when it did occur resulted in increased fluency.

On the other hand, the relatively fluent stutterer may experience an increase in stuttering during the late-adult years. Van Riper (1978), for example, reported that his own stuttering increased markedly in frequency, though not in severity, after an initial heart attack at age 65. The "little sluggish prolongations," as he described them, mostly disappeared after his recovery. Later, following retirement, he again noticed an increase in the frequency and, occasionally, the severity of his stuttering, including more frequent and longer tremors along with some laryngeal blockings. In that these fluency breaks were surprising when they occurred, Van Riper speculated that his increase in stuttering was probably due to a lack of monitoring of his speech. Perhaps, he suggested, the hard work of "stuttering fluently" was no longer worth the effort.

A note of caution in interpreting the above comments is in order. "Recovered" stutterers in the field of speech and language pathology are knowledgeable concerning the nature and modification of stuttering behavior, and this knowledge may have contributed to changes in the fluency of these individuals. The generally improved fluency of these stutterers, of course, is not necessarily reflective of the speech of stutterers who have little or no knowledge of such information.

Older Nonstutterers

In order to understand the nature of fluent as well as dysfluent speech in older stutterers, it is necessary to consider the fluent and dysfluent speech characteristics of older nonstutterers. Yairi and Clifton (1972) analyzed the dysfluent speech behavior of preschool children, high school seniors, and geriatric individuals. Each group contained 15 subjects. The geriatric subjects included 7 women and 8 men ranging in age from approximately 69 to 88 years. The average age of this group was 78 years, and all but one of these subjects were above the age of 70. All subjects were white and came from various socioeconomic levels. Spontaneous speech samples from each subject were analyzed according to the dysfluency categories shown in Table 10−2. The children had 7.65 dysfluencies per 100 words, the high school students had 3.83 dysfluencies per 100 words, and the geriatric group 6.29 dysfluencies per 100 words. These differences were statistically significant, with the high school group having significantly fewer dysfluencies than the other two groups. The relative distributions of each dysfluency type (see Table 10−2) indicated that the category of "interjections" was the main factor differentiating the three groups. Although the preschool and geriatric groups did not differ significantly in the total number of dysfluencies, the geriatric subjects demonstrated nearly twice as many interjections as the preschool children. The high school subjects, although having less total dysfluencies than the geriatric subjects, had a similar proportion of interjections. The dysfluency types most often produced by the geriatric speakers were interjections (2.92 per 100 words) and revision−incomplete phrase (1.47 per 100 words). The dysfluency type least produced by the geriatric subjects was the "tense pause" (0.02 per 100 words).

Yairi and Clifton's findings support the notion of increased fluency with increased chronological age through the early adult years, a view held by several investigators (Branscom, Hughes, and Oxtoby, 1955; Davis, 1939, 1940; Fisher, 1934; Johnson, Brown, Curtis, Edney, & Keaster, 1948). The Yairi and Clifton study, however, provides additional data indicating that the number of fluency breaks increase during late adulthood. As Yairi and Clifton noted, these fluency breaks are not characteristic of the dysfluencies of stutterers. Rather, these fluency breaks (interjections and revision−incomplete phrases) are among the dysfluencies that other investigators (Boehmler, 1958; Johnson, 1961; Williams & Kent, 1958; Wingate, 1962) have shown to be characteristic of normal adult speakers. These findings, as Yairi and Clifton suggested, may be one reason why the onset of stuttering seldom occurs in the late-adult years. They reasoned that because nonfluency in the aged is both expected and acceptable, listeners are less likely to react adversely to the nonfluencies of an older person. Of course, nonfluencies also are characteristic of the speech of children. However, children may be more susceptible to adverse reactions to fluency failure and the internal stress created by new linguistic and articulatory tasks.

While Yairi and Clifton's findings might help explain why the onset of stuttering would be less likely to occur in older speakers, their findings do not suggest why those who do stutter would be likely to stutter less as they grow older. An analysis of the speech of older stutterers using Yairi and Clifton's approach would be one way to investigate this question. It may be, for example, that for older stutterers there is an increase in the number of normal fluency breaks (interjections, phrase repetitions, revision−incomplete phrases). But what is particularly intriguing is the possibility of a corresponding decrease in the fluency breaks characteristic of stuttering (part−word repetitions and tense pauses).

In a related study, Gordon, Hutchinson, and Allen (1976) analyzed the fluency characteristics of normal young-adult and geriatric speakers. Citing studies that suggested a decrease in brain weight and neuron cell densities with increasing age, the authors were searching for evidence of differences in expressive language between young and geriatric subjects. Ten older nonstuttering subjects (average age 80 years) were matched with ten younger nonstuttering subjects (average age 23 years) for visual acuity, hearing acuity, and educational level. The subjects were asked to make up a story from a series of pictures. Analysis was conducted on the general features of "uncertainty behavior," pause location, and utterance length, each of which had several subcategories.

Table 10–2
Percentage Distribution of Each of the Seven Disfluency Types
for Preschool Children, High School Seniors, and Geriatric Persons

Disfluency Type	Preschool Children*	High School Seniors*	Geriatric Persons*
Interjection	24.82 (1.90)	43.23 (1.66)	46.42 (2.92)
Part–word repetition	7.84 (0.60)	4.70 (0.18)	6.20 (0.39)
Word repetition	16.21 (1.24)	10.68 (0.41)	12.87 (0.81)
Phrase repetition	7.71 (0.59)	7.81 (0.30)	4.77 (0.30)
Revision–incomplete phrase	32.55 (2.49)	28.65 (1.10)	23.37 (1.47)
Disrhythmic phonation	9.67 (0.74)	3.91 (0.15)	6.04 (0.38)
Tense pause	1.18 (0.09)	1.04 (0.04)	0.33 (0.02)
Total	100.00	100.00	100.00

Reprinted with permission from Yairi, E., & Clifton Jr., N. F. Disfluent speech behavior of preschool children, high school seniors, and geriatric persons. *Journal of Speech and Hearing Research,* 1972, *15,* 714–719.

*Numbers in parentheses are the corresponding mean frequencies of dysfluencies per 100 words.

The results showed that the geriatric and young-adult subjects performed the same in terms of pause location and utterance length. The geriatric subjects, however, exhibited more uncertainty behavior than their younger counterparts. Post hoc analysis indicated a significant difference between the young-adult and geriatric subjects for one of the subcategories of uncertainty behavior, hesitant interjections and fillers. Gordon et al. suggested that the increase in uncertainty behavior in the older subjects indicated word-retrieval problems in the absence of apparent semantic–syntactic organizational deficits. Their interpretation of the results is supported by Birren, Riegel, and Robbin (1962) who found that geriatric subjects needed approximately 40 percent more time to make word associations.

In summary, preliminary research findngs suggest that normal speakers increase in dysfluency as they reach late adulthood, particularly in the forms of hesitant interjections and fillers. Whether a similar increase in such phenomena is the case with stutterers remains to be determined. The data, in any case, do not suggest a reason why stutterers are likely to decrease their stuttering during the later years of life. There are, however, several studies concerning articulatory, phonatory, and psychologic characteristics of older, nonstuttering speakers that may explain why individuals who have stuttered most of their lives would be likely to decrease in, or recover from, stuttering in their later years.

ARTICULATORY CHARACTERISTICS

Perhaps the change in the speaking ability of older individuals that would be most likely to facilitate a decrease in stuttering is the slowing of articula-

tion. Several investigators (Hartman & Danhauer, 1976; Mysak, 1959; Pierce, Burk, & Hoyer, 1978; Ptacek & Sander, 1966; Ptacek, Sander, Maloney, & Jackson, 1966; Ryan, 1972; Ryan & Burk, 1974) found that a slowed articulatory rate is associated with older age. Mysak (1954) suggested that changes in speaking rate were a function of a general slowing of neuromuscular activity with advancing age. Ryan (1972), in an investigation of the acoustic aspects of the aging voice, studied groups of 20 subjects each across decades of 40 to 49, 50 to 59, 60 to 69, and 70 to 79. He found a general decrease in words per minute as age increased. The only statistically significant difference in words per minute, however, was between the youngest and the oldest age groups. Ryan stated that "as age increases, rate of speaking becomes slower due to some factor other than lengthened pause time" (p. 268). Ryan suggested that as articulatory changes associated with aging take place, increased effort must be expended by the speaker in an attempt to maintain his habitual level of feedback. As a consequence, rate of speaking slows to accommodate the more pronounced movement of the jaw, tongue, and lips. Another possibility is that a reduction in the rate of articulation typically leads to a concomitant increase in syllable and voicing duration. In two related studies, Ryan and Burk (1974) and Hartman and Danhauer (1976) found that a slow articulatory rate was highly associated with the perception of the aging male voice. Ryan and Burk (1974) also reported the occurrence of imprecise consonant articulation in older individuals. Ptacek et al. (1966) found a reduced diadochokinetic rate for both male and female subjects over 65 years of age. Hutchinson, Robinson, and Nerbonne (1978) compared nasal and oral sound pressure levels of 60 normal subjects ranging in age from 50 to 80 and found data that indicated that older adults experience changes in the control of velopharyngeal function.

The articulatory changes of older speakers (slowed rate, an overall decrease in neuromuscular efficiency and accuracy, and imprecise consonant articulation) might help to explain the trend for increased fluency breaks in older normal-speaking persons. These age-related changes in articulatory function also may account for apparent decreases in the fluency breaks of older stutterers. Several of the articulatory conditions that appear to be typical of the speech of older individuals coincide with current views of stuttering intervention techniques. Rate-control and rhythmic-timing approaches, as discussed by Curlee and Perkins (1969), Ryan (1971), Webster (1973), and Schwartz and Webster (1977), employ techniques requiring a slowed speech rate, prolonged vowel production, and gradual transition from one articulatory position to another. Furthermore, the findings of Brayton and Conture (1978) indicate that decreases in stuttering are related to increases in vowel duration. Slower rates of speaking and associated increases in voicing and vowel duration may also facilitate fluency. If older stutterers begin to articulate in this fashion as part of the normal aging process, these changes may result in increased level of fluency.

PHONATORY CHARACTERISTICS

Studies of the aging male and female voice suggest several laryngeal or phonatory factors that may prove to be important in understanding the fluency characteristics of older stutterers. Mysak (1959) noted a progressive increase in the fundamental frequency of male subjects from age 50 through 85 years. Hollien and Shipp (1972) noted a slight decrease in the mean fundamental frequency from 20 to 50 years of age, but for subjects beyond age 50, their results were similar to those of Mysak. On the other hand, in a study of the aging female voice McGlone and Hollien (1963) indicated no significant change in the fundamental frequency with increasing age. They explained these differences by suggesting that anatomic changes during puberty are not as extensive in the female larynx as in the male larynx, and therefore degenerative changes may not be as profound in women in later life. Related to these findings are reports of a decrease in the range of fundamental frequency with increasing age (Endres, Baubach, & Flösser, 1971; Hutchinson & Beasley, 1976; Ryan & Burk, 1974), although the relationship of this decrease to sex has yet to be determined.

Ryan and Burk (1974) used a multiple-regression-analysis technique to study the variables contributing most to the perception of the aging male voice. They noted that there were six variables accounting for a multiple regression correlation of 0.96: (1) laryngeal air loss, (2) laryngeal tension, (3) voice tremor, (4) imprecise consonants, (5) slow articulation rate, and (6) increasing fundamental frequency. Of these, the three factors contributing most to this relationship (laryngeal air loss, laryngeal tension, and voice tremor) were related to laryngeal function. The authors suggested that aging may result in "an alteration in the fine motor control of vocal fold vibratory activity" (p. 90). Mysak (1959) found a decrease in what he termed phonation/time ratios (the percentage of total speaking time during which phonation is taking place) with increasing age. Ptacek et al. (1966) found reduced maximum performances on a number of physiologic variables for geriatric speakers including pitch range, oral diadochokinetic movements, maximum vowel intensity, vowel duration, maximum intraoral air pressure, and vital capacity. Just as change in the speed and accuracy of articulatory functioning may result in increased fluency breaks, these changes in the laryngeal function of older speakers also may contribute to the increase in fluency breaks that were reported by Yairi and Clifton (1972).

The recent findings concerning the laryngeal behavior of stutterers and the role of the larynx in the physiology of the stuttering moment also suggest that much of the increased fluency of older stutterers may be attributed to age-related laryngeal changes. Several investigators (Conture, McCall, & Brewer, 1977; Freeman & Ushijima, 1975, 1978; Hutchinson & Navarre, 1977) have observed high levels of vocal-fold tension and simultaneous contraction of abductor−adductor laryngeal musculature during the moment of stuttering. For example, Conture et al. (1977), while noting that there was no single pattern of laryngeal activity during stuttering, found that the majority of the part−word repetitions were characterized by a separation of the posterior aspects of the vocal folds. This separation was due to the simultaneous contraction of the abductor and adductor muscles. As Freeman and Ushijima (1978) have demonstrated, strong contraction of laryngeal antagonists is incompatible with normal phonation. Freeman and Ushijima found that the termination of such antagonistic contraction was nearly always followed by a fluent utterance. Huchinson and Navarre (1977) also discussed the onset of the stuttering moment as a function of vocal fold tension. Using the Halle and Stevens (1971) model of laryngeal functioning, they suggested that the level of vocal-fold tension was often so high in stutterers as to limit the functional ranges of supra- to subglottal pressure and glottal width, thus limiting the possibility of adequate phonation. Hutchinson and Navarre also suggested that even when speaking fluently stutterers may demonstrate vocal fold conditions that approximate cessation of vocal fold activity. On the other hand, they reasoned, any condition that would promote the relaxation or lessening of vocal fold tension prior to the onset of vocalization would facilitate fluency. It should be pointed out, however, that this research has been conducted with young adults, not children or older individuals.

Therapeutic procedures designed to promote vocal fold relaxation have frequently been advocated and similar suggestions are found in the clinical approaches described by Schwartz (1976) and Webster (1973). It may be that in older stutterers, the same effect is accomplished more naturally as these individuals begin to experience less precise vocal control resulting in laryngeal air loss (Ryan & Burk, 1974) and a relative decrease in the amount of time spent in phonated speech (Mysak, 1959). This possibility is contraindicated, however, by the findings of Ryan and Burk (1974), which suggest the presence of laryngeal tension and vocal tremor in older nonstuttering subjects. Certainly there is much to be discovered concerning the nature of articulatory and phonatory changes during late adulthood. Exactly how these changes may expend or diminish fluency is not known at present.

PSYCHOLOGIC CHARACTERISTICS

As researchers have begun to describe each stage of the life cycle in terms of psychologic growth, the period from the midforties through the fifties often is described as a time of relatively intense psychologic change and has been portrayed in terms of rebirth or renewal. For example, Neugarten (cited in Kimmel, 1974, p. 58) indicated that middle age was characterized by "self-awareness," "control of environment," "heightened introspection," and "restructuring of experience." According to Sheehy (1974), the events of this midlife phase are typically initiated by a reexamination process during which time the individual begins to question many of his views of himself and others. Individuals who are able to reassess their goals and values, typically in the decade of the fifties, gain a more objective and valid view of themselves and others. They are likely to demonstrate greater insight concerning their own behavior as well as the behavior of others. In addition, there is often the acquisition of a deeper concern for

others. And finally, the individual now is more likely to readjust old responses to lifelong problems (Levinson, 1978; Sheehy, 1974; Vaillant, 1977).

Objective introspection and personal growth have often been advocated as an important part of the therapy process for adult stutterers (Cooper, 1977). Certainly helping the stutterer to evaluate his self-concept as well as his attitudes and feelings concerning stuttering is only a part of the therapy process. But these objectives seem to be particularly important if long-term fluency is to be expected (Guitar & Bass, 1978). Similar changes in self-concept and attitude also are likely to occur for stutterers in their fifties or sixties. Such changes may result in less avoidance and struggle behavior, which, in turn, could result in increased fluency.

A Model of Fluency Change

The available information indicates that older nonstutterers have more fluency breaks during the decades of their sixties and seventies. In addition, much of what we have discussed suggests that older stutterers are likely to experience a decrease in stuttering behavior during these same years. This seems paradoxical. However, if fluency breaks are considered as either formulative or motoric breaks, this apparent paradox may be resolved. Figure 10−1 is an attempt to explain what may be occurring in the fluency of stutterers as well as nonstutterers during the life cycle.

Drawing from the work of Van Riper (1971) and Bloodstein (1974), the preliminary information on older speakers obtained by Yairi and Clifton (1972) and Gorden et al. (1976), as well as other investigations of the nature of fluency breaks in stutterers and nonstutterers (Blood & Hood, 1978; Branscom et al., 1955; Cecconi, Hood, & Tucker, 1977; Davis, 1939, 1940; Fisher, 1934; Haynes & Hood, 1977; Johnson, 1955; Johnson & associates, 1959; McClay & Osgood, 1959; McDearmon, 1968; Metraux, 1950; Soderberg, 1967; Williams & Kent, 1958), we have attempted to distinguish formulative from motoric fluency breaks. Certainly the research has indicated that these two general forms of fluency breaks are not mutually exclusive since, to some degree at least, both types of fluency breaks may be found in the speech of stutterers as well as nonstutterers. This seems to be especially true for word repetitions (Cecconi et al., 1977; Johnson and associates, 1959).

In the present model formulative fluency breaks are characterized by (1) breaks in fluency between whole words, phrases, and larger syntactic units (including whole-unit repetitions of these units), (2) lack of obvious tension during the breaks, and (3) interjections between the larger syntactic units. These breaks are essentially normal dysfluencies and are observed in the speech of nonstuttering children and adults. They are also present, however, in the speech of stutterers. Motoric fluency breaks, on the other hand, are characterized by (1) breaks in fluency between sounds or syllables, (2) obvious tension during the breaks, and (3) pauses with possible cessation of air flow and voicing between small linguistic units. These motoric breaks are not considered normal dysfluencies and are most obvious in the speech of young-adult stutterers. They are also present, but to a lesser extent, in the speech of nonstuttering children and adults.

The model in Figure 10–1 traces the relative occurrence of formulative and motoric fluency breaks for stutterers and nonstutterers across four general age categories including preschool childhood, young adulthood, middle adulthood, and late adulthood. The fluency level of young adult nonstutterers is used as a baseline because this group is considered to be performing at optimal speech fluency.

The fluency breaks of the nonstuttering preschool child are characterized by formulative fluency breaks typical of most young children. As Bloodstein (1974) described, these fluency breaks may be considered a function of early language learning. Motoric fluency breaks also occur but are relatively infrequent. Motoric fluency breaks are a result of the child's attempts to articulate the sounds of the language at a rate approximating that of the child's adult models. Both formulative and motoric fluency breaks decrease as the child acquires language and speech

skills, and by puberty the individual has reached the peak level of fluency typical of the young adult. By young adulthood, the nonstuttering individual should be performing at an optimal fluency level. Although some formulative and possibly motoric breaks may be present under conditions of communicative or emotional stress, these fluency breaks are infrequent. This pattern of fluency should continue throughout most or all of middle adulthood. During the late-adult years, nonstutterers may begin to experience an increase in the number of formulative fluency breaks. The increase in these forumlative breaks would take place gradually and would not be obvious nor considered abnormal. While there may also be an increase in the occurrence of motoric fluency breaks, these would be much less frequent.

The pattern of fluency breaks for the young stutterer would be similar to that of the nonstutterer at the onset of development with relatively more formulative than motoric fluency breaks. However, these formulative fluency breaks would eventually decrease as the number of motoric fluency breaks increased. This change would be due to a combination of increasing linguistic complexity of the child's speech and the child's reaction to communicative or emotional stress. Exactly how and why this change may take place is, of course, a basic question of stuttering development. The child's fluency during the later stages of development would be characterized by a gradual increase in the number of motoric fluency breaks versus the number of formulative breaks.

During the young-adult years, the speech of the stutterer would be characterized by a pronounced dif-

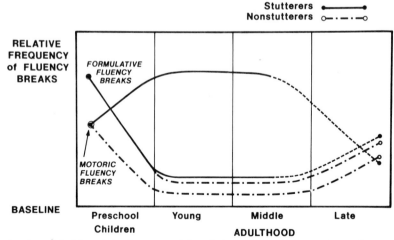

Fig. 10–1. A model of the relative frequency of formulative and motoric fluency breaks for stutterers and nonstutterers through four stages of life.

ference in the occurrence of motoric and formulative fluency breaks. This difference is one of the major speech characteristics that distinguishes the individual as a stutterer. The number and nature of motoric breaks vary of course, and would, along with other learned patterns of avoidance and escape behaviors, determine the severity of the stuttering. As with the nonstuttering adult, formulative breaks would be present. In addition, however, formulative breaks may occur in the absence of any real loss of formulative ability. That is, breaks in fluency that appeared to be formulative in nature would occur as a result of the stutterer's pattern of avoidance (postponement/substitution) behavior. For example, stutterers may choose to alter their choice of words or syntax in order to avoid or postpone feared sounds or words, giving the appearance of what we have described as formulative fluency breaks.

The description of the relative frequency of formulative and motoric fluency breaks through the first two stages of the model (preschool children and young adulthood) generally coincide with current research findings. The final two stages of the model, however, (middle and late adulthood) are predictive in nature and therefore represent hypotheses for future investigation. It is suggested that, at least with some stutterers, the physiologic changes that begin to take place in the decades of the forties through the sixties, combined with the beginnings of psychologic changes, may result in a decrease in frequency of motoric fluency breaks. There also may be, at least in the late-adult years, an increase in formulative fluency breaks in the same manner and for the same reasons that formulative breaks increase in nonstuttering individuals. Certainly the model we are proposing is far from complete. Based on what we do know, however, the model does appear to describe not only the fluency characteristics of stuttering onset and development but also the fluency characteristics and changes of nonstutterers during the aging process.

CLINICAL IMPLICATIONS

Much of what we need to know about the nature of fluency in older stutterers and nonstutterers has yet to be determined. What we do know suggests that nonstutterers tend to have more formulative breaks in fluency during later adulthood. What little we know about the nature of stuttering in older persons suggests that there may be a decrease in the number of people who stutter. There may also be a decrease in the severity of stuttering for those who continue to

stutter. Certainly not all stutterers stop stuttering during the final two or three decades of life. However, if further research substantiates recovery from stuttering during the later years of life, a reassessment of the concept of ''spontaneous recovery'' from stuttering would certainly be in order. It may be that stutterers are at least as likely to recover from stuttering during the last few decades of life as they were during the teenage years.

There are other important questions. Would recovering from stuttering in later life leave more residual effects in the form of avoidance and escape behaviors or inappropriate social relationships than recovery earlier in life? Would someone who recovered without the aid of formal intervention be more apt to experience a recurrence of stuttering during a period of emotional stress later in life? Would the lower prevalence of stuttering in females be reflected in the number of older female stutterers? Would the higher prevalence of stuttering in black populations as indicated by Gillespie and Cooper (1973) be reflected in the number of older black stutterers? These, of course, are only a few of the questions that need to be answered. Finding answers to some of these questions will be difficult without longitudinal studies. But we need to begin.

A more immediate task would be to determine whether therapy is effecive for older stutterers. Sheehan (1972) stated that the age of the stutterer is not a critical factor in predicting successful therapy. He suggested that emotional maturity was more important than age, and as one example, cited the case of a 78-year-old retired bandmaster who was able to successfully conquer his handicap through formal therapy procedures. However, the more typical view may be that of Makuen (1914), who stated that stutterers of ''somewhat advanced years soon grow weary of work and give it up'' (p. 385). Whereas older stutterers may well have the desire and potential to modify their speech, the daily requirement of speaking tasks necessary to effect change may not seem worth the effort. Anecdotal reports by Van Riper (1978) and Bloodstein (1978) indicated that the prognosis for a successful therapy outcome for older stutterers is rather poor. Van Riper (1978) further indicated that during his career he had seen six or seven stutterers in their seventies for diagnostic evaluations and only one of these people returned to begin therapy. The individual who did return for therapy died of a stroke a short time later.

To modify the behaviors and attitudes of stuttering takes considerable commitment and energy (Van Riper, 1973, 1978). Cooper (1977) uses the term "psychic energy" (p. 77) when discussing the effort that stutterers must continually employ to achieve and maintain fluency during, as well as after, formal intervention. Cooper also suggested that it is the speech and language pathologist's responsibility to assist the stutterer in evaluating just how much psychic energy he or she is able to expend on the shaping of fluency. Perhaps this would be especially important when a person is older and not enjoying the good health associated with earlier years of life. As Van Riper (1978) commented:

> It's hard work to stutter fluently and to maintain a certain amount of alertness and energy when you get older and more infirm. This energy level is very important; when it is high many little blockings can be overridden; when it is low, they appear. Without the energy necessary to operate the automatic controls which took care of the stuttering moments, the tiny lags in the transitions of speech become stuttering.

Stutterers who have undergone successful therapy earlier in life may be the most apt to experience a recurrence of stuttering if they also experience poor health or emotional stress. Part of the reason for the recurrence of stuttering could be a loss of the energy necessary to maintain the activities of monitoring and modification. Such energy levels also may be necessary to foster assertive behavior.

Without the desire and energy to work on modifying a long-standing behavioral problem such as stuttering the prognosis for improvement in older individuals would appear to be poor. However, if the individual experiences changes in self-concept and attitude during the middle- and late-adult years, he or she may be responsive to help provided by a speech and language pathologist. It also may be that information and techniques informally presented to older stutterers would facilitate increased fluency. Whether intervention should take the form of a rigorous and intensive program or a less direct, self-therapy program such as that suggested by Fraser (1978) is another question to be studied. Not only might we help these stutterers to become more fluent speakers but, by investigating stuttering during middle and late adulthood, we are likely to discover some important concepts that may contribute to the completion of the picture of the nature of stuttering throughout the life cycle.

REFERENCES

Adams, M. R. A clinical strategy for differentiating the normally nonfluent child and the incipient stutterer. *Journal of Fluency Disorders*, 1977, *2*, 141−148.

Andrews, G., & Harris, M. *The syndrome of stuttering*. London: Heinemann, 1964.

Birren, J. E., Riegel, K. F., & Robbin, J. S. Age differences in continuous word associations measured by speech recordings. *Journal of Gerontology*, 1962, *17*, 95−96.

Blood, W., & Hood, S. B. Elementary school-aged stutterers' disfluencies during oral reading and spontaneous speech. *Journal of Fluency Disorders*, 1978, *3*, 155−165.

Bloodstein, O. The development of stuttering: II. Developmental phases. *Journal of Speech and Hearing Disorders*, 1960, *25*, 366−376.

Bloodstein, O. The rules of early stuttering. *Journal of Speech and Hearing Disorders*, 1974, *39*, 379−394.

Bloodstein, O. Personal communication, 1978.

Boehmler, R. M. Listener responses to non-fluencies. *Journal of Speech and Hearing Research*, 1958, *1*, 132−141.

Branscom, M. E., Hughes, J., & Oxtoby, E. T. Studies of nonfluency in the speech of preschool children. In W. Johnson (Ed.), *Stuttering in children and adults*. Minneapolis: University of Minnesota Press, 1955.

Brayton, E. R., & Conture, E. G. Effects of noise and rhythmic stimulation on the speech of stutterers. *Journal of Speech and Hearing Research*, 1978, *21*, 285−294.

Cecconi, C. P., Hood, S. B., & Tucker, R. K. Influence of reading level difficulty on the disfluencies of normal children. *Journal of Speech and Hearing Research*. 1977, *20*, 475−484.

Conture, E. G., McCall, G. N., & Brewer, D. W. Laryngeal behavior during stuttering. *Journal of Speech and Hearing Research*, 1977, *20*, 661−668.

Cooper, E. B. Recovery from stuttering in a junior and senior high school population. *Journal of Speech and Hearing Research*, 1972, *15*, 632−638.

Cooper, E. B. The development of a stuttering chronicity prediction checklist: A preliminary report. *Journal of Speech and Hearing Disorders, 1973, 38,* 215–223.

Cooper, E. B. Controversies about stuttering therapy. *Journal of Fluency Disorders, 1977, 2,* 75–86.

Curlee, R. F., & Perkins, W. H. Conversational rate conrol therapy for stuttering. *Journal of Speech and Hearing Disorders, 1969, 34,* 245–250.

Davis, D. M. The relation of repetitions in the speech of young children to certain measures of language maturity and situtational factors: Part I. *Journal of Speech Disorders, 1939, 4,* 303–318.

Davis, D. M. The relation of repetitions in the speech of young children to certain measures of language maturity and situational factors: Parts II and III. *Journal of Speech Disorders, 1940, 5,* 235–246.

Endres, W., Bambach, W., & Flösser, G. Voice spectrograms as a function of age, voice disguise, and voice imitation. *Journal of the Acoustical Society of America, 1971, 49,* 1842–1848.

Fisher, M. S. Language patterns of preschool children. *Child Development Monographs, 1934, 15,* Columbia University.

Fraser, M. *Self-therapy for the stutterer: One approach.* Memphis: Speech Foundation of America, 1978.

Freeman, F., & Ushijima, T. The stuttering larynx: An EMG, fiberoptic study of laryngeal activity accompanying the moment of stuttering. *Haskins Laboratories Status Report on Speech Research,* 1975, SP-41. New Haven: Haskins Laboratories.

Freeman, F. J., & Ushijima, T. Laryngeal muscle activity during stuttering. *Journal of Speech and Hearing Research, 1978, 21,* 538–562.

Gillespie, S. K., & Cooper, E. B. Prevalence of speech problems in junior and senior high schools. *Journal of Speech and Hearing Research, 1973, 16,* 739–743.

Gordon, K. C., Hutchinson, J. M., & Allen, C. S. An evaluation of selected discourse characteristics in normal geriatric subjects. *Idaho State University Laboratory Research Reports, 1976, 1,* 11–21.

Guitar, B. E., & Bass, C. Stuttering therapy: The relation between attitude change and long-term outcome. *Journal of Speech and Hearing Disorders, 1978, 43,* 392–400.

Halle, M., & Stevens, K. N. A note on laryngeal features. *Haskins Laboratory Quarterly Report,* 1971, *101,* 198–213.

Hartman, D. E., & Danhauer, J. L. Perceptual features of speech for males in four perceived age decades. *Journal of the Acoustical Society of America, 1976, 59,* 713–715.

Haynes, W. O., & Hood, S. B. Language and disfluency variables in normal speaking children from discrete chronological age groups. *Journal of Fluency Disorders, 1977, 2,* 57–74.

Hollien, H., & Shipp, T. Speaking fundamental frequency and chronologic age in males. *Journal of Speech and Hearing Research, 1972, 15,* 155–159.

Hutchinson, J. M., & Beasley, D. S. Speech and language functioning among the aging. In H. J. Oyer & E. J. Oyer (Eds.), *Aging and communication.* Baltimore: University Park Press, 1976.

Hutchinson, J. M., & Navarre, B. The effect of metronome pacing on selected aerodynamic patterns of stuttered speech: Some preliminary observations and interpretations. *Journal of Fluency Disorders, 1977, 2,* 189–204.

Hutchinson, J. M., Robinson, K. L., & Nerbonne, M. A. Patterns of nasalance in a sample of normal gerontologic subjects. *Journal of Communication Disorders, 1978, 11,* 469–481.

Ingham, R. J. Letter to the editor. *Journal of Speech and Hearing Disorders, 1976, 41,* 280–281.

Johnson, W. A study of the onset and development of stuttering. In W. Johnson (Ed.), *Stuttering in children and adults.* Minneapolis: University of Minnesota Press, 1955.

Johnson, W. (Ed.). Measurements of oral reading and speaking rate and disfluency of adult male and female stutterers and nonstutterers. *Journal of Speech and Hearing Disorders Monograph Supplement,* 1961, *7,* 1–20.

Johnson, W. (and associates). *The onset of stuttering.* Minneapolis: University of Minnesota Press, 1959.

Johnson, W., Brown, S. F., Curtis, J. F., Edney, C. W., & Keaster, J. *Speech handicapped school children.* New York: Harper & Row, 1948.

Jones, M. V. Leopold Treitel on stuttering. *Journal of Speech and Hearing Disorders*, 1948, *13*, 19−22.

Kimmel, D. C. *Adulthood and aging*. New York: John Wiley & Sons, 1974.

Levinson, D. J. Becoming one's own man. *Esquire*, April 11, 1978, pp. 85−93.

Makuen, G. H. A study of 1000 cases of stammering, with special reference to the etiology and treatment of the affection. *Therapeutic Gazette*, 1914, *38*, 385−390.

McClay, H., & Osgood, C. I. The hesitation phenomena in spontaneous English speech. *Word*, 1959, *15*, 19−44.

McDearmon, J. R. Primary stuttering at the onset of stuttering: A reexamination of data. *Journal of Speech and Hearing Research*, 1968, *11*, 631−637.

McGlone, R. E., & Hollien, H. Vocal pitch characteristics of aged women. *Journal of Speech and Hearing Research*, 1963, *6*, 164−170.

Metraux, R. W. Speech profiles of the pre-school child 18 to 54 months. *Journal of Speech and Hearing Disorders*, 1950, *15*, 37−53.

Murray, F. P. Personal communication, 1978.

Mysak, E. D. Pitch and duration characteristics of older males. *Journal of Speech and Hearing Research*, 1959, *2*, 46−54.

Pierce, N. J., Burk, K. W., & Hoyer, E. A. Rate and duration characteristics of speech in the aging. Paper presented at the annual meeting of the American Speech and Hearing Association, San Francisco, November 1978.

Ptacek, P. H., & Sander, E. K. Age recognition from voice. *Journal of Speech and Hearing Research*, 1966, *9*, 273−277.

Ptacek, P. H., Sander, E. K., Maloney, W. H., & Roe Jackson, C.C. Phonatory and related changes with advanced age. *Journal of Speech and Hearing Research*, 1966, *9*, 353−360.

Rosenbek, J., Messert, B., Collins, M., & Wertz, R. Stuttering following brain damage. *Brain and Language*, 1978, *6*, 82−96.

Ryan, B. P. Operant procedures applied to stuttering therapy for children. *Journal of Speech and Hearing Disorders*, 1971, *36*, 264−280.

Ryan, W. J. Acoustic aspects of the aging voice. *Journal of Gerontology*, 1972, *27*, 265−268.

Ryan, W. J., & Burk, K. W. Perceptual and acoustic correlates of aging in the speech of males. *Journal of Communication Disorders*, 1974, *7*, 181−192.

Schwartz, D., & Webster, L. M. More on the efficacy of a protracted precision fluency shaping program. *Journal of Fluency Disorders*, 1977, *2*, 205−215.

Schwartz, M. F. *Stuttering solved*. New York: McGraw-Hill Book Co., 1976.

Shames, G. H., & Beams, H. L. Incidence of stuttering in older age groups. *Journal of Speech and Hearing Disorders*, 1956, *21*, 313−316.

Shearer, W. M., & Williams, J. D. Self-recovery from stuttering. *Journal of Speech and Hearing Disorders*, 1965, *30*, 288−290.

Sheehan, J. G. Message to a stutterer. In S. B. Hood (Ed.), *To the stutterer*. Memphis: Speech Foundation of America, 1972.

Sheehan, J. G., & Martyn, M. M. Spontaneous recovery from stuttering. *Journal of Speech and Hearing Research*, 1966, *9*, 121−135.

Sheehan, J. G., & Martyn, M. M. Stuttering and its disappearance. *Journal of Speech and Hearing Disorders*, 1970, *35*, 279−289.

Sheehy, G. *Passages: Predictable crises of adult life*. New York: Bantam Books, 1974.

Soderberg, G. A. Linguistic factors in stuttering. *Journal of Speech and Hearing Research*, 1967, *10*, 801−810.

Travis, L. E. Personal communication, 1978.

Vaillant, G. E. *Adaptation to life*. Boston: Little, Brown & Co., 1977.

Van Riper, C. G. *The nature of stuttering*. Englewood Cliffs, N.J.: Prentice-Hall, 1971.

Van Riper, C. G. *The treatment of stuttering*. Englewood Cliffs, N.J.: Prentice-Hall, 1973.

Van Riper, C. G. Personal communication, 1978.

Van Riper, C. G. *A career in speech pathology*. Englewood Cliffs, N.J.: Prentice-Hall, 1979.

Webster, R. L. Successive approximation to fluency: Operant response shaping procedures for use with stutterers. *Seventeenth International Congress of Applied Psychology*, 1971, Liege, Belgium. (Cited in R. J. Ingham & G. Andrews, Behavior therapy and stuttering: A review. *Journal of Speech and Hearing Disorders,* 1973, *38,* 405−441.)

Williams, D. E., & Kent, L. R. Listener evaluations of speech interruptions. *Journal of Speech and Hearing Research,* 1958, *1,* 124−131.

Wingate, M. E. Evaluation and stuttering: III. Identification of stuttering and the use of a label. *Journal of Speech and Hearing Disorders,* 1962, *27,* 368−377.

Wingate, M. E. Recovery from stuttering. *Journal of Speech and Hearing Disorders,* 1964, *29,* 312−321.

Yairi, E., & Clifton, Jr., N.F. Disfluent speech behavior of preschool children, high school seniors, and geriatric persons. *Journal of Speech and Hearing Research,* 1972, *15,* 714−719.

Young, M. A. Onset, prevalence, and recovery from stuttering. *Journal of Speech and Hearing Disorders,* 1975, *40,* 49−58.

Marion D. Meyerson
Susan J. Shanks

11

Voice Disorders in Adulthood

The study of voice disorders has been undergoing an aging process similar to that of the human body. The professional zygote containing the bases for the present state of vocal rehabilitation is found in early classic writings such as those of West, Kennedy and Carr (1937), Stinchfield (1928), Travis (1931), and others. Forces of knowledge, environmental stimuli, and social impact have provoked changes in the study of voice disorders as they do in the human organism. Moore (1977), in a retrospective review of the last 50 years of literature related to voice disorders, noted increasing governmental, scientific, and educational attention to the voice and voice disorders. Perhaps this can be viewed as evidence of the coming of age of voice science.

The purposes of this chapter are to develop a greater awareness of voice and aging processes and to introduce the specific vocal conditions that exist in the aged. The chapter will include an overview of maturation and aging of the voice, the incidence and descriptions of vocal disorders in adults, and rehabilitation and prevention of voice problems.

TERMINOLOGY

Michel and Wendahl (1971) observed that mutual understanding of terminology is an indicator of the stage of a science's advancement. In addition, a discussion of terminology is a requisite for the orientation of the reader of this chapter. The multitude of terms noted when perusing the literature reflects the complexity of voice problems and the lack of basic information about voice production (Moore, 1971a). The disparate nomenclature also appears to have a regressive influence on the further development of the field of voice disorders. Most authorities have agreed that pitch (frequency), loudness (intensity) and quality are three of the basic vocal parameters. Moncur and Brackett (1974) used the term *"paracode"* to denote speech phenomena not "directly related to the identification of the word" (p. 1). They added duration in time as a feature essential to the paracode. Cooper (1977) noted six vocal variables, including pitch, tone focus, quality, volume, breath support, and rate. He added that the person's vocal image, a unique learned concept of voice, depended on cultural and environmental experiences, and the training and direction of the voice. Perkins (1977) suggested that the behaviors to consider in producing an efficient voice are the traditional parameters of pitch and loudness plus voicing, constriction, mode (register), focus, effort, and smoothness. Perkins also listed three modes or registers including vocal fry or pulse, heavy (the mode used by most speakers), and falsetto. Hollien (1977) added a range of tones above loft (his term for falsetto) and called these flute, whistle, and pipe registers.

The above terminology is only a sample of what

can be found in the literature and suggests the multiplicity of psychologic, physical, social, and emotional perceptions to be considered when evaluating the voice. Although the terms define vocal parameters, they do not begin to describe the disorders of vocal behavior. Perkins (1977) cited five bases for laryngeal disorders: (1) those that disrupt synchrony and smooth approximation of the cords, (2) those that limit adduction or abduction, (3) those that alter the contractile ability of the vocal cords, (4) those in which endocrine imbalances alter anatomy and physiology, and (5) those in which essential tissue is destroyed. A host of terms resulting from the aforementioned anatomic and physiologic alterations varies from descriptions such as strident, harsh, breathy, thin, hoarse, and aphonic to action terms such as hyperfunction and spastic dysphonia. Further descriptors will be introduced in later sections of this chapter.

Normal human voice is dependent primarily upon the integrity of the laryngeal mechanism. The human body undergoes normal change throughout life and the vocal mechanism reflects the body alteration in its structure and function. Additionally, pathologic processes may intervene and further modify the quality.

MATURATION AND AGING OF THE VOICE: A DEVELOPMENTAL PROCESS

The human larynx is a remarkable example of millions of years of species-specific development. The genetic information that determines the anatomy and physiology of the larynx is present in the zygote at the moment of conception. Cells proliferate and allow for diversification of function in a manner that is surprisingly orderly and rarely in error. Nevertheless, differences are programmed into the genetic material and provide important prenatal influences on the structure of the larynx.

The male embryo, solely by virtue of the Y chromosome that heralds its maleness, is scheduled for increased laryngeal size and lower frequency of vocal-fold vibration in adulthood. The two X chromosomes marking the female embryo program a comparatively smaller larynx and higher fundamental frequency. Other genetic influences are determined at conception because voice is a hereditary trait, much the same as hair and eye color (Luchsinger & Arnold, 1965). Luchsinger and Arnold found that monozygotic twins with essentially identical genetic material

have similar voice qualities. Fraternal twins, on the other hand, do not demonstrate the same degree of similarity in voice patterns.

Beyond the range of normal hereditary variation, chromosomal or genetic malformations that affect the larynx and consequently the voice may occur sporadically or in accordance with Mendelian rules (Gorlin, Pindborg, & Cohen, 1976). Other genetic syndromes that may not alter laryngeal morphology but affect the central or peripheral nervous system or the endocrine system also may result in voice disorders.

Although prenatal factors exert significant control of postnatal behavior, phonatory performance in infancy through adulthood is subject to many other influences. All neonates cry, but their individual cries are as varied as will be their speaking voices. Greene (1972b) reported studies indicating variations in the crying patterns of newborns and the abilities of mothers to successfully identify their own babies' cries on tape. She concluded that the phonatory behavior of infants is quite idiosyncratic, based to some extent on genetic determinants, but also varying in quality and quantity according to external factors and particular personality traits.

In early childhood, vocal development becomes part of a coordinated totality utilizing the biologic systems that allow for the acquisition of language (Perkins, 1977). During childhood there is an absence of sex differences in laryngeal anatomy and vocal characteristics. In adolescence a change in the characteristics of the larynx occurs and is referred to as voice or laryngeal mutation. The nature of this mutation is different for boys and for girls. Boys undergo a more rapid growth of the larynx with more striking concomitant differences in voice quality. As the vocal folds increase in size and the natural frequency of vibration decreases, pitch and quality may fluctuate and produce voice breaks. Greene (1972b) cited a number of reports indicating that voice breaks and shifts occur in young children of both sexes and are a normal feature of juvenile laryngeal function. She further reported that "stormy mutations" in male adolescents are relatively uncommon and may not be pathologic.

In addition to the documented hormonal changes that account for normal mutation in puberty, both Moses (1954) and Greene (1972b) have made note of a myriad of sociocultural factors that begin to influence voice quality long before the endocrine changes take place. Certainly self-concept, peer pressure and vocal hygiene are parameters that affect our voices throughout our lives.

Aging is a process that begins at birth and continues through childhood and adulthood. Following the postpubertal stabilization of voice quality, subtle vocal changes continue throughout young adulthood and middle age and on to old age. The particular rate and pattern of aging and certainly the ultimate reality of aging and demise of the human organism are in large part genetically determined. Herndon (1976) noted two major genetic influences in aging: familial longevity and specific gene mutation that may alter the aging process by introducing a disease or disability.

The aged or senescent voice has been analyzed in relation to anatomic and physiologic changes (Hutchinson & Beasley, 1976; Meyerson, 1976; Schow, Christensen, Hutchinson, & Nerbonne; 1978; von Leden, 1977). Cartilages of the larynx ossify with age, muscles atrophy, joints stiffen, and hormonal responses decline, but contradictory findings leave direct relationships between anatomic changes and vocal behavior speculative (Meyerson, 1976). Although a number of reports have described the parameters of the aging voice (Luchsinger & Arnold, 1965; Meyerson, 1976; Ptacek & Sander, 1966; Ptacek, Sander, Maloney, & Jackson, 1966; Schow et al., 1978), there has been no consensus as to the actual vocal behaviors noted in older individuals. For example, rather than changes associated with aging laryngeal tissues, a mild neurologic slowdown may be responsible for what is recognized as the aging voice (Meyerson, 1976). In any event, ''normal'' aging variations with no pathologic component do not seem to seriously affect the ability of older individuals to communicate. Organic or functional voice disorders, however, might well interfere with easy communication.

INCIDENCE OF VOCAL DISORDERS

The incidence of voice disorders in children has been reported by Wilson (1979), White (1946), Luchsinger and Arnold (1965), and others. Curtis and Morris (1978) noted a higher incidence of voice disorders in children than in adults. The young population is relatively easy to study because of compulsory education and regular school attendance up to the age of 16 to 18 years. After the school years, however, there is no reliable method presently available for keeping track of the adult population to determine whether voice problems become more prevalent in certain age groups. Curtis and Morris postulated that the reduced incidence in adults was prob-

ably the result of the absence of child-related factors such as schoolyard screaming, growth and maturation, and frequent upper respiratory infections.

The vocal mechanism is durable and able to withstand prolonged use (Brodnitz, 1965). Nevertheless, consistent production under stressful conditions and in occupations such as teaching, preaching, acting, singing, and selling may increase the incidence of voice problems (Brodnitz, 1965). Additional factors influencing incidence figures in older individuals have been reported by Cooper (1970). He looked at the results of rehabilitation with 99 patients of 60 years of age and older. Cooper attributed their problems to inappropriate pitch because of fatigue or habit and varying emotional states such as grief, despair, and resignation.

The incidence of vocal disorders in adults is open to question because the figures are limited to those individuals who seek help from a physician or speech—language pathologist. Both Batza (1977) and Brodnitz (1965) published data on the number of individuals seen in their respective otolaryngological settings over a period of years. Batza listed 1000 cases examined over a 4-year period. A varied assortment of vocal problems including postoperative dysphonia, ventricular adduction, and spastic dysphonia were most prevalent during the middle years (the fifth and sixth decades). The abusive behaviors were probably of long standing, but the symptoms became more manifest with aging as the body failed to rebuild injured tisses (Batza, 1977). Of the 1000 cases reported by Batza, only 486 had actual laryngoscopic findings such as vocal nodules, contact ulcers, polyps, and bowed, edematous, or paralyzed folds. Of the 1404 patients with organic and functional voice problems reported by Brodnitz (1965), a large percentage was in the middle years.

Because of the lack of vocal screening in the adult population, it is difficult to make assumptions about the incidence and types of voice disorders that will appear in association with aging. For example, although Murphy (1964) indicated that vocal tremulousness is typical of old age, Brodnitz (1965) concluded that singers, especially males, retained their vocal abilities into senescence. Thus, it seems that patterns of aging are highly individualized.

Standards for determination of vocal deviation in adults have not been set to date. The presence of a disorder such as hoarseness may be less acceptable for a minister than for a rock star for whom it is an identifying feature. Certainly some transitory influences such as weight gain and loss, medication, and fatigue have not been adequately explored.

In summary, there is disparate terminology, a lack of evidence of actual widespread deterioration of the vocal mechanism in aging, questionable incidence figures of voice disorders in older individuals, and an absence of standards in judging the presence of voice disorders. Nevertheless, vocal problems do occur in adulthood and should be studied.

ORGANIC AND FUNCTIONAL VOICE DISORDERS

Voice disorders traditionally have been dichotomized causally as functional or organic. Because the precipitating factor suspected in many organic conditions such as vocal nodules and contact ulcers is misuse or abuse of the vocal mechanism, a number of authorities have questioned the appropriateness of this dichotomy (Boone, 1977; Moncur & Brackett, 1974; Murphy, 1964). For the purposes of this chapter, the functional and organic dichotomy will be used with full awareness of this overlap. Organic disorders will denote an alteration in the vocal mechanism that contributes to a voice problem. Functional voice disorders will refer to conditions in which the structures are unchanged but are malfunctioning for voice (Murphy, 1964). The term psychogenic will be used to refer to a functional disorder in which a psychologic disturbance is thought to be associated with a somatic disorder (Murphy, 1964).

Laryngectomy

The single most dramatic and critical organic voice problem associated with aging is removal of the larynx because of cancer. Approximately 2500 to 4000 individuals each year have laryngectomies and most of them are men over the age of 50 (Damste & Lerman, 1975). Cancer is suspected when persistent hoarsness is present for more than 6 weeks (Damste & Lerman). Therefore, immediate medical attention is necessary to determine the cause of the hoarseness. If cancer is present, medical treatment is imperative because the mortality rate is 100 percent if the cancer is not treated (Myerson, 1964) but is extremely low if proper care is received. Most laryngeal cancer is of the squamous cell carcinoma type (Myerson, 1964). The lesion may be localized or it may have metastasized, thereby requiring individual determinations as to the extent and type of surgery.

Removal of the larynx is the treatment most often preferred for those patients whose histologic analyses differentiate the disease from other conditions (Burns, Bryce, & van Nostrand, 1979; Myerson, 1964; Vaughan, Strong, & Jake, 1978). A conservative approach may involve a partial or hemilaryngectomy (Burns et al., 1979; Perkins, 1978) or a radical removal of the total larynx and adjacent tissues may be performed. Although Myerson (1964) stated that the results of surgery are not affected by age, he suggested greater care in the selection of cases over 70 years because of a less favorable cure rate in that group. Also radiation and chemotherapy and, more recently, cryosurgery (Hong, Silverstein, & Sadeghee, 1977) and laser therapy (Vaughan, et al., 1978) have been used as methods of treatment.

Discovery of laryngeal cancer and recommendation for surgery are disturbing facts that necessitate thoughtful preparation. Salmon (1977) described the need for counseling with the patient and his family concerning the physical, social, and emotional changes that follow laryngectomy. Loss of speech and methods of compensation such as esophageal speech and electrolarynx should be explained in a preoperative session (Sanchez-Salazar & Stark, 1972).

Postsurgical counseling should be both realistic and supportive. The patient must be told that he can no longer breathe through his nose and mouth and that the physical contours of his neck will be flattened (Levin, 1962). Levin (1962) noted that although swallowing usually remains normal, changes in pharyngeal morphology may make it effortful and accompanied by gurgling and gulping sounds. The patient must be aware that he will smell only strong odors, that his sense of taste will be altered, and that he no longer will sneeze but will cough through his tracheal stoma. Levin (1962) also reported the need to inform patients about the possibility of reduced range of shoulder movement with involvement of the spinal accessory nerve and of increased possibility of tracheobronchitis because of inadequate air filtration and warming through the stoma. Greene (1972b) further commented on the excessive dryness and crusting of the trachea, which may prevent easy breathing. If these physical conditions are understood and accepted as likely occurrences following laryngectomy, adjustment to the results of ablative surgery may be facilitated.

The individual recuperating from a laryngectomy knows that he has undergone a major operation for a serious problem that can recur. It is not surprising that fear is the main emotion that must be faced (Levin, 1962). Insomnia, suicidal feelings, euphoria, and depression are also found in the laryngectomee (Greene, 1972b). Supportive services including counseling must be maintained throughout the rehabilitative process.

The type of communication available after surgery will depend in part on the integrity of remaining structures. Immediate postsurgical frustrations may be alleviated with the use of a key chain containing plastic-disc key words as well as pencil and paper (Starmer, 1971). The method of long-term communication chosen by rehabilitative specialists depends on the extent of surgery and other factors. Currently, the preferred method is esophageal speech (Diedrich & Youngstrom, 1966; Hartman & Scott, 1974; King, Marshall, & Gunderson, 1971; Shanks, 1977), which involves the utilization of a portion of the esophagus as a pseudoglottis. Methods of teaching esophageal speech involve inhaling, sniffing, or injecting air through a new glottis, generally the cricopharyngeus sphincter (Boone, 1977; Damste, 1975; DiCarlo, Amster, & Herer, 1955; Diedrich & Youngstrom, 1966; Gardner, 1971; Gately, 1971; Gordon, 1971; Greene, 1972b; Rigrodsky, Lerman, & Morrison, 1971; Simmons & Shanks, 1971). Myerson (1964) described a study by Seeman of 342 laryngectomees from which he concluded that the type of surgical procedure had no influence on the quality of esophageal speech obtained or the amount of training necessary to obtain it. These findings are certainly open to question because a procedure that removes esophageal tissue or compromises its function would affect the attempt to achieve esophageal speech.

Snidecor (1971) gave several positive prognostic signs for determining the ease with which esophageal speech could be learned. These signs included the ability to eat a variety of foods and swallow normal-sized pieces, motivation to return to work, facility in talking in groups, relating well to family, and lack of embarrassment about stomach growls. Snidecor's additional inclusion of age younger than 62 and lack of fear of old age as positive prognosticators signified the possible negative influence of actual aging or perception of aging on success in rehabilitation of laryngectomees. Myerson (1964) described the person who learned esophageal speech quickly as aggressive, alert, and mechanically inclined rather than asthenic and retiring. Berlin (1963) added adequate hearing ability and general health, both of which may decline in aging, as important factors in rehabilitation.

When esophageal speech does not seem to be attainable, or if the quality of the speech is less than realistically desired, other methods have been used. Surgical techniques to build an internal pseudo-larynx have been reported by Asai (1972), Taub and Bergner (1973), Zwitman and Calcaterra (1973a), and others. Continued efforts to develop better surgical techniques for rebuilding a usable pseudoglottis may yield promising results in the future. In the meantime, mechanical devices may be necessary when surgical methods are unsuccessful or unadvisable. The electro-larynx is a noninvasive, mechanical device that is generally hand-held and has provoked controversy for a number of years. Our laryngectomized patients frequently state that they feel (or were told) that utilization of an electrolarynx is a "crutch" that precludes attaining good esophageal speech. Lauder (1968), Boone (1977), and others recommend using the mechanical device early as a supplement to esophageal speech therapy so that it is thought of as an adjunct rather than a failure device. Diedrich and Youngstrom (1966) reported a preference for esophageal speech over an electrolarynx among laryngectomees. Nevertheless, the electrolarynx has its place in the early postlaryngectomy period before esophageal speech is learned, in phone use where esophageal speech may not be successful, and at times of physical weakness when the physiologic effort necessary for esophageal speech may not be possible. Its use is most helpful for those for whom the amount of tissue removed was so extensive that development of a pseudoglottis is not possible.

Various other types of mechanical larynges have been described by Luchsinger and Arnold (1965), Boone (1977), and Greene (1972b). The wireless intraoral device reported by Zwitman, Knorr, and Sonderman (1978) offers promise because it frees both hands of the laryngectomee.

In summary, the combination of surgical intervention, voice therapy and mechanical assistance has resulted in communicative rehabilitation for most laryngectomees, and outstanding accomplishment for some. However, continued research is needed to improve surgical results, to develop better therapy methods, and to determine the effectiveness of rehabilitative procedures.

Vocal Fold Paralysis

Another organic voice disorder is the result of vocal-fold paralysis. Vocal fold paralysis may occur in older adults because of central or peripheral lesions and may be unilateral or bilateral.

Central lesions of bulbar origin can give rise to flaccid paralysis (Doyle, 1972) of the vocal mechanism. Some precipitating causes of bulbar paralysis include amyotrophic lateral sclerosis, central nervous system syphillis, and a variety of cerebrovascular accidents, all of which are encountered in greater frequency among older individuals.

Most causes of vocal fold paralysis, however, are peripheral in origin. The intrinsic laryngeal muscles that regulate the movement of the vocal folds are controlled by the superior and recurrent laryngeal branches of the Vagus nerve (Cranial nerve X). Brodnitz (1965) stated that the most frequent cause is damage to the nerve during thyroid surgery. Doyle (1972) noted a number of other etiologies including toxic neuritis, neoplasm, and cardiac pulmonary disease. Traumatic damage secondary to gunshot wounds or motor accidents may also result in vocal fold paralysis.

The symptoms of vocal fold paralysis run the gamut from none at all to total aphonia. In unilateral paralysis, the normal fold might well compensate in its movement patterns and voice quality may be perceived as normal. In bilateral vocal fold paralysis, the initial concern is an open airway, which may be compromised if the folds are fixed in the medial or closed position. If the folds are in the open position because of the paralysis or because they have been abducted permanently by surgery to aid breathing, the voice is likely to be breathy or aphonic.

Treatment procedures have included many attempts at nerve repair and nerve grafts (Doyle, 1972). Vocal fold injection with materials such as Teflon™ and silicone have also been reported (Brodnitz, 1965; Moore, 1971b). Brodnitz (1965) urged voice therapy prior to any decision for surgery because he felt that the majority of patients would respond well to this more conservative method. The efficacy of medical and voice therapy procedures needs to be documented in the aging population to assist in treatment decisions in the future.

Endocrine Dysfunction

Hormonal secretions, which are the significant end product in the endocrine system, may have significant effects on the structure and function of the larynx. In childhood, endocrine problems such as hypogenitalia, sexual precocity, pituitary malformation, and sexual ambiguity can change a number of vocal and other characteristics (Luchsinger & Arnold, 1965). Throughout life, gonadal functioning within the endocrine system can alter the quality of voice and the appropriateness of pitch level (Kirchner, 1970). As noted earlier, the normal mutational changes in adolescent males are brought about by

changing hormonal flow. Luchsinger and Arnold (1965), in fact, describe the voice as a secondary sex characterisic always subject to sex gland functioning. In older adults, changes in endocrine functioning are said to result in vocal involution, which is seen as regressive alterations in aging (Luchsinger & Arnold). Damste and Lerman (1975) reported vocal virilization with accompanying lowering of pitch in aging women because of postmenopausal drug therapy or ovarian neoplasm, both of which would alter the endocrine balance.

Pathologic changes in the endocrine system can affect hormones that are not generally associated with sexual functioning. For example, a decrease in thyroid hormone production can cause a condition known as myxedema and result in some degree of atrophy of the laryngeal muscles with accompanying vocal hoarseness (Luchsinger & Arnold, 1965). Excessive thyroid activity can result in a variety of voice problems including vocal fatigue and tremulo (Luchsinger & Arnold).

Abnormal functioning of the parathyroid, adrenal, and pituitary glands in adulthood results in generalized changes in body tissues that may include atrophy of laryngeal tissues. Among these problems is Addison's disease or hypoadrenalism, which is progressive and fatal and includes total aphonia as a prelude to death (Luchsinger & Arnold, 1965). Another disorder is acromegaly or hyperpituitarism, which is marked by laryngeal enlargement and a deep, rough voice quality (Kirchner, 1970).

Drugs may alleviate some endocrine-related voice disorders. Von Leden (1977) noted positive effects of sex hormones, steroids, potassium, and vitamins on the laryngeal mucosa. Medical intervention followed by voice therapy may provide relief from some of the vocal symptoms resulting from alterations in hormonal secretion. Accountability studies of these procedures to establish their usefulness would be valuable.

The Dysarthrias

Perkins (1977) described dysarthria as weakness, paralysis, or incoordination of the speech apparatus. Darley, Aronson, and Brown (1975) made frequent reference to the central or peripheral changes that would affect muscular control in phonation. Their list of dimensions that lead to the classification of several distinct types of dysarthrias contained many features dependent on laryngeal valve integrity. These included abnormalities in pitch and in loudness, in addition to quality differences such as harshness, hoarseness, breathiness, strained— strangled voice, aphonia, and tremor.

Many of these disease processes resulting in the reduction of laryngeal muscle control are more common among older individuals. Amyotrophic lateral sclerosis (ALS) generally develops in the fifth and sixth decades and is marked by progressive neuronal degeneration that leaves the patient extremely weak. Weaver (1976) noted that muscle fasciculations in the larynx may be an early sign of ALS. In pseudobulbar palsy secondary to multiple strokes, which are also common in older adults, Darley et al. (1975) described laryngeal hypertonicity in a majority of patients.

Parkinsonism is one of the most characteristic diseases of older individuals, striking 1 percent of the population over the age of 50 (Duvoisin, 1976). Its major feature is progressive hypokinesia. The reduced range of mobility that affects the entire body also makes for a lack of vigorous movement in the laryngeal mechanism (Darley et al., 1975). Logemann, Fisher, Boshes, & Blonsky (1978) reported laryngeal disorders in 89 percent of 200 patients with parkinsonism including significant reduction of variability resulting in monopitch and monoloudness and possible quality changes. Drug and speech therapy have yielded some reports of alleviated symptoms, although the progressive nature of parkinsonism precludes a cure. Sarno (1968), following speech (and voice) therapy with more than 300 patients, concluded that there was no real improvement in speaking ability. She did, however, allude to the benefit of therapy to the patient's self-image. Since communication is a multifaceted act involving more than simply the activity of the laryngeal or articulatory mechanisms, psychologic benefits associated with therapy are of value.

Spastic Dysphonia

Long assumed to be psychogenic in nature (Brodnitz, 1965), spastic dysphonia in adults has acquired new etiologic presumptions. Dedo, Townsend, and Izdebski (1978) have performed histologic analysis on the recurrent laryngeal nerves of patients with spastic dysphonia and have observed myelin abnormalities in 30 percent of the specimens. In addition, some patients demonstrated brain stem or basal ganglia disturbances with no manifest peripheral nerve problems. The authors postulated that spastic dysphonia may be the outcome of a number of organic and/or psychogenic pathologic conditions. Certainly, emotional stress appears to exacerbate a condition that may have an organic primary etiology. Barton (1979) felt spastic dysphonia was an involuntary hyperfunction syndrome that is often associated with compulsiveness or hostility over a period of many years.

Perkins (1977) described the hyperfunctional disorder of spastic dysphonia as a voice that "is a strained, squeezed, creaking, choking squawk" (p. 167). In his 1978 text he presented a detailed account of a public figure who had suffered from spastic dysphonia for 17 years. During that period, her status and prestige provided her with access to a plethora of diagnostic procedures and remedial techniques, none of which was deemed effective. Eventually, she underwent a surgical procedure involving recurrent laryngeal nerve resection (Barton, 1979; Dedo, 1976) and obtained excellent results. Her story was printed in many newspapers and scholarly journals following the surgery, thereby informing many professionals and adults with spastic dysphonia of a new remedial procedure for a heretofore debilitating communicative disorder.

Vocal Nodules and Contact Ulcers

Brodnitz (1965) noted two contrasting types of benign pathological changes in the vocal fold. One category includes papillomas and granulomas, which can result in voice disorders. The second type encompasses nodules, polyps, and ulcers that are the consequences of vocal misuse. Nodules in particular are relatively common occurrences in individuals who abuse their voices. Excessive shouting in childhood and vocal strain by teachers, singers, and actors result in bruises on the margin of one or both vocal folds that harden and become similar to calluses. In the "bruise" stage, vocal rest may result in prompt recovery (Luchsinger & Arnold, 1965). When nodes are long-standing, surgical removal with subsequent vocal rehabilitation may be prescribed.

Polyps are similar to nodules in origin and effect but may occur after just one episode of vocal abuse (Moore, 1971b). Luchsinger & Arnold (1965) noted that increased frustration with a changed position in life might facilitate the development of vocal nodules in aging persons and afford, along with possible endocrine changes, an explanation for voice changes. Additionally, continued use of alcohol and tobacco might irritate the vocal folds and necessitate excessive effort for maintaining phonation.

Contact ulcers are more common in adult males than females and are generally associated with tension and vocal abuse. Perkins (1977) described the ulcers as resulting from grinding, hammering contact of the vocal processes. Vocal rehabilitation and the avoidance of the irritants associated with drinking and smoking are the normal treatment procedures.

Additional pathologic conditions such as hyperkeratosis and leukoplakia are precipitated by vocal abuse and by excessive use of alcohol and tobacco (Bryce, 1974). Although in themselves benign, they may be premalignant. The cumulative effects of long-term poor vocal hygiene may make these inflammatory conditions increase in frequency with age.

Respiratory Problems

Changes in the adult respiratory mechanism may result in changes in breath support for voice. The ossification of rib cartilages in aging figures in the reduction of thoracic mobility and consequently in vital capacity. Luchsinger & Arnold (1965) mentioned the possibility of respiratory disorders emanating fron central nervous system lesions as might occur in extrapyramidal tract dysfunction. Perkins (1977) underscored the effect of bronchopulmonary disabilities on the maintenance of subglottal pressure necessary for phonation. Tuberculous laryngitis, a complication of pulmonary tuberculosis, was noted by Holinger (1976) to cause hoarseness, pain, and coughing.

Any respiratory problem that results in coughing could certainly precipitate a voice disorder. Peterson and Peterson (1960) reported that coughing is common among the aged, a behavior that Meyerson (1976) noted was likely to be the result of chronic or senile bronchitis. If excessive, the sphincteric valving in coughing can be abrasive to the vocal folds and cause temporary or permanent pathologic changes.

Functional Disorders

Laryngectomy, vocal fold paralysis, endocrine and respiratory problems, dysarthria, spastic dysphonia, vocal nodules and contact ulcers represent morphological changes in the phonatory apparatus. Some of these problems are precipitated by strain or misuse but all include organic components. Functional disorders are not manifested by structural changes. Most functional voice disorders are described as personality based (Greene, 1972a, 1972b; Irwin, 1960; Luchsinger & Arnold, 1965; Moses, 1954; Murphy, 1964). The voice, a product of glottal closure and breath flow, can mirror a person's emo-

tional state and can reflect adjustment problems (Moses, 1954). Rousey and Moriarty (1965), and Greene (1972b) wrote about the correlation between neuroses and the voice. Goldstein (1958) and later Block and Goldstein (1971) surveyed the literature and found little information on functional voice disorders. A few individual case studies and some contradictory investigations that did not use controls were noted. These authors concluded that because of the paucity of information and the ambiguous nature of personality as an etiological, consequential, or therapeutic factor, little was known about functional voice disorders.

Two recent investigations involving adult psychiatric patients have been reported. An objective attempt to evaluate the voice characteristics of six adults with depression following electroconvulsant therapy did not reveal any significant changes (Darby & Hollien, 1977). However, improved inflection and stress, more precise articulation, and increased vitality were noted in some patients. Another study, conducted by Chevrie-Muller, Seguier, Spira, & Dordain (1978), demonstrated that schizophrenics' personality traits can be perceived from their voices. Speech rate, pitch variation, and quality (timbre) were the vocal parameters judged by listeners to be associated with this syndrome. Generally, previous descriptions of the vocal parameters involved in functional disorders were found only in individualized case studies (Greene, 1972b; Moses, 1954; Strandberg, Griffith, & Hallowell, 1971).

Hysterical voice disorders and anxiety-based problems are categorized as psychogenic in origin by Greene (1972a, 1972b) and others. Hysterical aphonia or dysphonia is usually accompanied by conversion symptoms (Boone, 1977; Greene, 1972b). The aphonic person generally experiences a sudden loss of voice associated with a traumatic event such as marital stress, career dissatisfaction or financial reversal (Damste & Lerman, 1975; Murphy, 1964). Although speaking is affected, laughing and coughing are produced with normal vocalization (Greene, 1972b). Myerson (1964), Boone (1977), and others suggested explaining the nature of the problem to the client and convincing him or her that normal phonation is possible. As long as the person receives secondary gain from the condition, the prognosis is questionable (Boone, 1977; Damste & Lerman, 1975). For this reason referral for psychiatric services is often necessary (Greene, 1972b).

A generalized anxiety state may cause vocal weakness and/or hoarseness accompanied by feelings of pressure or choking from a lump in the throat or catarrh (Greene, 1972b). Like the hysterical condition, treatment should include supportive therapy combined with relaxation techniques and voice production activities (Greene, 1972a, 1972b).

Another vocal problem that may be organic or functional in origin is puberphonia, defined as lack of expected maturational voice change (Greene, 1972b) If functional, establishing a new pitch range by expanding the pitch range, by humming, by coughing, or by using digital pressure on the thyroid cartilage is recommended (Boone, 1977; Greene, 1972b). Exercises for persons exhibiting inappropriate use of falsetto or glottal fry are found in Moncur and Brackett (1974) and Boone (1977). Postoperative therapy for the adult transsexual individual who may desire stabilization of an appropriate habitual pitch level may also include many of these procedures.

Ventricular dysphonia, a functional disorder involving adduction of the false or ventricular folds, may unconsciously be employed to spare the true folds following infection (Boone, 1977; Myerson, 1964). However, ventricular phonation may be recommended in rare instances by a voice specialist following permanent and severe damage to the true vocal folds. When the true folds are healthy, normal phonation should be the goal. Phonating on inhalation and then shifting from exhalation to inhalation during phonation can assist in eliminating ventricular phonation and habituating true-fold phonation. Lowering the position of the larynx through means such as digital manipulation also may be used to achieve this goal (Boone, 1977).

The stress of a family illness, divorce, or bereavement, fear of cancer after losing a loved one with the disease, and arguments at work or at home are samples of behavior that can be accompanied by dysphonia, which is generally less severe than the complete aphonia previously described (Greene, 1972b). Myerson (1964) and Murphy (1964) linked the weak voice with depression in adults and adolescents. Macrophonia, the use of an excessively loud voice, is seldom seen in a clinic unless a hearing loss is present (Murphy, 1964). Improved vocal hygiene and training for better voice projection are recommended to prevent laryngeal abuse.

Pitch breaks and diplophonia may be functional problems when they occur in the voice of the adult whose profession demands clear voice production even when fatigued and/or under tension. Boone (1977) and Moncur and Brackett (1974) outlined methods of eliminating these problems, including the changing of pitch to a higher level.

Stage fright, although not considered a func-

tional voice disorder, was included in a text by Murphy (1964) as a phenomenon adults may experience. Attention to this problem may be necessary as more aging persons who lack public speaking experience attempt to achieve social and political change by expressing themselves in public and assuming leadership roles in society.

Breathiness, harshness with specific and/or general tension, shallow breathing, and hoarseness usually associated with organic voice problems can also result from abusive vocal patterns and become functional voice problems. Vocal nodules and contact ulcers are often referred to as functional in origin for this reason. Wilson (1979) reported that some children with the above vocal characteristics come from pathologic families where divorces, separation, and abnormal living conditions and family relationships were prevalent. Although not documented objectively, problems with adjustment during similar life crises or change of events may precipitate these voice disorders in adults, as suggested by case studies (Boone, 1977; Greene, 1972b; Murphy, 1964).

Wilson (1979) stated that deviant vocal behaviors can be learned through imitation. As an example, an adult who encounters people with excessively loud voices may emulate this undesirable vocal behavior. In such cases a program of vocal hygiene is recommended unless there are clinical indications of need for psychiatric referral.

Because psychologic problems are prevalent in persons with functional voice problems and because motivation and morale are important factors in vocal reeducation (Damste & Lerman, 1975), team management is recommended (Luchsinger & Arnold, 1965). Specialists who can use biofeedback (Boone, 1977), operant manipulation of vocal parameters (Moore & Holbrook, 1971), different types of relaxation therapies (Wolpe & Lazarus, 1966) and other technical procedures should work together to document their successes and/or failures with the aging population. The clinician should use all necessary resources available to give the adult the best service in an effort to remediate the funcational voice disorder.

REHABILITATION OF VOICE PROBLEMS IN OLDER ADULTS

Recognition and diagnosis of voice disorders constitute important preliminary steps in a total remedial process. The goal of the remaining steps should be ''the best adaptation for optimal phonation to the given anatomical situation'' (Damste & Lerman, 1975, p. 64). Rehabilitation must be a multidisciplinary, multidimensional effort involving physicians, other health professionals, counselors and social workers, clinicians and teachers, the patient and his peers and contacts. Fox and Blechman (1975) outlined the functions of such a team as identifying the problem, defining the objectives, initiating change, and stabilizing vocal patterns. These authors saw several rehabilitative options, including medical and surgical intervention in the treatment of cancer and other neoplasms, drugs in treating an endocrine system malfunction, and physical therapy techniques for neuromuscular disorders. In addition to these options, recent studies utilizing electromyographic biofeedback in treating hyperfunctional voice disorders (Prosek, Montgomery, Walden, & Schwartz, 1978) have demonstrated facilitation of vocal reeducation through the development of self-monitoring skills.

Fox and Blechman (1975), in addition to the medical category discussed above, described options including psychologic, behavioral, and environmental management. Psychologic therapy may be consigned to professionals with appropriate training and may be geared to motivation, socialization, and improved self-concept. Storandt (1976), Weiss (1971), and Bollinger (1974) have noted the advantages of group therapy in the development of empathy, support, and reinforcement of patients for each other.

Behavioral therapy as a means to change vocal behavior can include the myriad of direct therapeutic techniques that have been developed over the years of practice of voice science (Greene, 1972a, 1972b; Cooper & Cooper, 1977; Boone, 1977; Weiss & Beebe, 1951; Moncur & Brackett, 1974). Breath control, relaxation exercises, chewing therapy, auditory training, successive approximation, and many others are among these techniques. The particular combination of methods must be selected to suit the individual and to capitalize on his status as an adult and on his life experiences.

Older adults can be recipients of mature and meaningful clinical interactions. Weiss (1971) underscored the need to use stimulating materials and to avoid treating the aged as children. Leutenegger (1975), in describing therapy with parkinsonism patients, noted that explanation followed by demonstration worked well in reducing frustration and increasing cooperation of the patients. Certainly, there is a need to consider other problems common to older individuals such as hearing deficits, systemic ailments, and possible central nervous system changes

that may impinge on vocal behavior and the prognosis for remediation.

Environmental management, as described by Fox and Blechman (1975), might incorporate many strategies to prevent voice disorders and assist in encouraging the cooperation of family and friends in reinforcing habit changes and providing positive experiences for improved communication.

Interest in the geriatric patient is burgeoning (Oyer & Oyer, 1976; Schow, et al., 1978). Training programs dealing with specific problems and pleasures in remediation of all types of disorders found in the older adult remain few and far between. More courses such as graduate seminars and workshops in speech and hearing problems of the aged (Leutenegger & Stovall, 1971), as well as professional literature, have begun to provide the knowledge necessary for successful patient rehabilitation.

PREVENTION OF VOICE DISORDERS

Whereas a direct focus on identification and remediation of voice disorders is necessary, programs of prevention can encourage good vocal habits and undermine vocal abuse. Vocal abuse is responsible for many of the voice disorders discussed thus far and can also exacerbate disorders resulting from organic changes. During an individual's lifetime, vocal changes may occur from habitual behaviors that may or may not be considered detrimental in themselves. Reduction of these behaviors should result from a program of vocal hygiene, described by Luchsinger & Arnold (1965) as involving all factors necessary to maintain and promote the health of the vocal mechanism.

Vocal hygiene has been of major importance in the literature related to voice disorders in children (Anderson & Newby, 1973; Bryce, 1974; Cook, Palaski, & Hanson, 1979; Cooper, 1973; Fox & Blechman, 1975; Punt, 1974; Wilson, 1979). Clinicians normally would indicate that making changes in abusive vocal behavior in children requires herculean efforts and a large measure of luck. A program of vocal hygiene should be more amenable to use with adults. Cook et al. (1979) included information on the following topics in their program for children: the basic structure and functioning of the voice-producing mechanism, voice quality, hygienic use of the voice, vocal misuse, and voice disorders. A similar informational program including all subtopics could be geared to the older adult.

Brodnitz (1953), in an account of prerequisites

for good vocal hygiene, stressed attention to environmental factors such as weather, temperature control, and humidity in the home. Diet and posture also were noted as factors influencing vocal production. Cooper (1970) made note of the role of grief, despair, and resignation in precipitating a condition he called "vocal fatigue". Von Leden (1977) recommended the use of special amplifying equipment in the telephone or in the form of a microphone so as to avoid vocal fatigue. Voice conservation should be practiced in a noisy car, bus, or train, in a room with a radio or television set on, in large crowds and parties, and while mechanical devices such as lawnmowers or hairdryers are in operation. Loud laughing, shouting, coughing, and throat clearing, and speaking while engaged in strenuous physical exercise such as jogging also might be abusive to the laryngeal mechanism.

Excessive smoking and alcohol consumption, as well as fumes, dust, and smoke have been cited as detrimental to laryngeal tissues (Myerson, 1964; Wynder, Covey, Mabachi, & Mushinski, 1976; Ash, 1962). Some individuals appear to have allergic reacions to milk products (Wilson, 1979) and to certain drugs (Portnoy, 1975) that may affect the vocal folds by changing the mucosal surface. Greene (1972b) reported the possibility of dysphonia resulting from drugs given for mental depression.

The use of the silent cough described by Zwitman and Calcaterra (1973b) and other medically acceptable ways of lubricating the vocal folds such as drinking water may prevent harmful throat clearing and coughing. A reduction in talking time may be beneficial to persons who use their voices a great deal, especially during those times when there is fatigue or an upper respiratory infection. Speech should be accomplished without strain or tension. Increasing loudness without raising the pitch is a simple skill reflective of the independent operation of the two mechanisms. Individuals of all ages could use practice in this skill, which is basic to good vocal hygiene.

The learning centers incorporated into many day and residential senior citizen units are ideal settings for implementation of vocal hygiene programs. Older individuals in these units are encouraged to maximize communication through participation in activities requiring verbal expression of views and experiences with peers who are hard of hearing or have other communicative disorders. A program of vocal hygiene may include spontaneous counseling by a trained professional during all activities plus formal lectures on the prevention of voice disorders.

CONCLUSIONS

The field of voice disorders has increased in breadth and sophistication over the years but continues to grow and change. We have become aware of the maturation and the aging of the human voice. The physical and physiologic changes that transform the voice of a child into that of an adult are recognized but many of the specific aspects remain to be fully understood. We do know that voice disorders that are either organic or functional in nature can interfere with successful communication in adulthood. Some of these disorders, such as laryngectomy, the dysarthrias, and spastic dysphonia, are more common among older adults. Rehabilitation of voice problems involves an understanding of many parameters of human functioning—biologic, psychologic, sociologic, and environmental. Planning for prevention of voice disorders affords an opportunity for professionals to minimize patient problems and to provide for a fuller communicative life for older adults.

REFERENCES

Anderson, V. A., & Newby, H. A. *Improving the child's speech* (2nd ed.). New York: Oxford University Press, 1973.

Asai, R. Laryngoplasty after laryngectomy. *Archives of Otolaryngology,* 1972, *95,* 114–119.

Ash, J. E. Pathologic epithelial changes and tumors of the larynx. In N. M. Levin (Ed.), *Voice and speech disorders: Medical aspects.* Springfield, Ill. Charles C. Thomas Publisher, 1962.

Barton, R. T. Treatment of spastic dysphonia by recurrent laryngeal nerve section. *Laryngoscope,* 1979, *89,* 244–249.

Batza, E. M. Adventures in vocal rehabilitation. In M. Cooper & M. H. Cooper (Eds.), *Approaches to vocal rehabilitation.* Springfield, Ill. Charles C. Thomas: Publisher, 1977.

Berlin, C. I. Clinical measures of esophageal speech: I. Methodology and curves of acquisition. *Journal of Speech and Hearing Disorders,* 1963, *28,* 42–51.

Block, E. L., & Goldstein, L. D. Functional speech disorders and personality: A decade of research. *Journal of Speech and Hearing Disorders*, 1971, *36*, 295–314.

Bollinger, R. L. Geriatric speech pathology. *Gerontologist*, 1974, *14*, 217–220.

Boone, D. R. *The voice and voice therapy* (2nd ed.). Englewood Cliffs, N.J.: Prentice-Hall, 1977.

Brodnitz, F. S. *Keep your voice healthy*. New York: Harper & Row, 1953.

Brodnitz, F. S. *Vocal rehabilitation*. (3rd ed.). Rochester, N.Y.: American Academy of Ophthalmology and Otolaryngology, 1965.

Bryce, D. P. *Differential diagnosis and treatment of hoarseness*. Springfield, Ill.: Charles C. Thomas Publisher, 1974.

Burns, H., Bryce, D. P., & van Nostrand, P. Conservation surgery in laryngeal cancer and its role following failed radiotherapy. *Archives of Otolaryngology*, 1979, *105*, 234–239.

Chevrie-Muller, C., Seguier, N., Spira, A., & Dordain, M. Recognition of psychiatric disorders from voice quality. *Language and Speech*, 1978, *21*, 87–111.

Cook, J. V., Palaski, D. J., & Hanson, W. R. A vocal hygiene program for school age children. *Language, Speech, and Hearing Services in the Schools*, 1979, *10*, 21–26.

Cooper, M. Voice problems of the geriatric patient. *Geriatrics*, 1970, *25*, 107–110.

Cooper, M. *Modern techniques of vocal rehabilitation*. Springfield, Ill.: Charles C. Thomas Publisher, 1973.

Cooper, M. Direct vocal rehabilitation. In M. Cooper & M. H. Cooper (Eds.), *Approaches to vocal rehabilitation*. Springfield, Ill.: Charles C. Thomas Publisher, 1977.

Cooper, M., & Cooper, M. H. *Approaches to vocal rehabilitation*. Springfield, Ill.: Charles C. Thomas Publisher, 1977.

Curtis, J. F., & Morris, H. L. Disorders of voice. In J. F. Curtis (Ed.), *Processes and disorders of human communication*. New York: Harper & Row, 1978.

Damste, P. H. Methods of restoring the voice after laryngectomy. *Laryngoscope*, 1975, *85*, 649–655.

Damste, P. H., & Lerman, J. W. *An introduction to voice pathology*. Springfield, Ill.: Charles C. Thomas Publisher, 1975.

Darby, J. K., & Hollien, H. Vocal and speech patterns of depressive patients. *Folia Phoniatrica*, 1977, *29*, 279–291.

Darley, F. L., Aronson, A. E., & Brown, J. R. *Motor speech disorders*. Philadelphia: W. B. Saunders, 1975.

Dedo, H. H. Recurrent laryngeal nerve surgery for spastic dysphonia. *Annals of Otology, Rhinology and Laryngology*, 1976, *35*, 451–459.

Dedo, H. H., Townsend, J. J., & Izdebski, K. Current evidence for the organic etiology of spastic dysphonia. *Archives of Otology, Rhinology and Otolaryngology*, 1978, *86*, 875–880.

DiCarlo, L. M., Amster, W. W., & Herer, G. R. *Speech after laryngectomy*. Syracuse, N.Y.: Syracuse University Press, 1955.

Diedrich, W. M., & Youngstrom, K. A. *Alaryngeal speech* (2nd printing). Springfield, Ill.: Charles C. Thomas Publisher, 1966.

Doyle, P. J., *Vocal cord paralysis*. Rochester, N.Y.: American Academy of Ophthalmology and Otolaryngology, 1972.

Duvoisin, R. *Parkinsonism: Clinical symposia*. Summit, N.J.: CIBA Pharmaceutical Co., 1976.

Fox, D. R., & Blechman, M. *Clinical management of voice disorders*. Lincoln, Neb.: Cliff Notes, 1975.

Gardner, W. H. *Larngectomee speech and rehabilitation*. Springfield, Ill.: Charles C. Thomas Publisher, 1971.

Gately, G. A. A technique for teaching the laryngectomized to trap air for the production of esophageal speech. *Journal of Speech and Hearing Disorders*, 1971, *36*, 484–485.

Goldstein, L. D. Functional speech disorders and personality: A survey of the research. *Journal of Speech and Hearing Disorders*, 1958, *1*, 359–376.

Gordon, M. T. Speech therapy management following laryngectomy. *British Journal of Disorders of Communication*, 1971, *6*, 52–57.

Gorlin, R. J., Pindborg, J. J., & Cohen, M. M. *Syndromes of the head and neck.* New York: McGraw-Hill Book Co., 1976.

Greene, M. C. L. *Disorders of voice.* Indianapolis: Bobbs-Merrill, 1972(a).

Greene, M. C. L. *The voice and its disorders* (3rd ed.). Philadelphia: J. B. Lippincott, 1972(b).

Hartman, D. E., & Scott, D. A. Overt responses of listeners to alaryngeal speech. *Laryngoscope,* 1974, *84,* 410–416.

Herndon, C. N. Medical genetics. In F. V. Steinberg (Ed.), *Cowdry's The care of the geriatric patient.* St. Louis: C. V. Mosby, 1976.

Holinger, L. D. Inflammatory conditions of the larynx. In G. M. English (Ed.), *Otolaryngology.* New York: Harper & Row, 1976.

Hollien, H. The registers and ranges of the voice. In M. Cooper and M. H. Cooper (Eds.), *Approaches to vocal rehabilitation.* Springfield, Ill.: Charles C. Thomas Publisher, 1977.

Hong, S. W., Silverstein, H., & Sadeghee, S. The effects of cryosurgery on the canine and human larynx. *Laryngoscope,* 1977, *87,* 1079–1085.

Hutchinson, J. M., & Beasley, D. S. Speech and language functioning among the aging. In H. J. Oyer & E. J. Oyer (Eds.), *Aging and communication.* Baltimore: University Park Press, 1976.

Irwin, J. V. Psychological implications of voice and articulation disturbances. In D. A. Barbara (Ed.), *Psychological and psychiatric aspects of speech and hearing.* Springfield, Ill.: Charles C. Thomas Publisher, 1960.

King, P. S., Marshall, R. C., & Gunderson, H. E. Management of the older laryngectomee. *Geriatrics,* 1971, *26,* 147–157.

Kirchner, J. A. *Pressman and Kelemen's physiology of the larynx.* Rochester, N.Y.: American Academy of Ophthalmology and Otolaryngology, 1970.

Lauder, E. The laryngectomee and the artificial larynx. *Journal of Speech and Hearing Disorders,* 1968, *33,* 147–157.

Leutenegger, R. R. *Patient care and rehabilitation of communication-impaired adults.* Springfield, Ill.: Charles C. Thomas Publisher, 1975.

Leutenegger, R. R., & Stovall, J. D. A pilot graduate seminar concerning speech and hearing problems of the chronically ill and the aged. *ASHA: Journal of the American Speech and Hearing Association,* 1971, *13,* 61–66.

Levin, N. M. Esophageal Speech. In N. M. Levin (Ed.), *Voice and speech disorders: Medical aspects.* Springfield, Ill.: Charles C. Thomas Publisher, 1962.

Logemann, J. A., Fisher, H. B., Boshes, B., & Blonsky, E. R. Frequency and co-occurrence of vocal tract dysfunction in the speech of a large sample of Parkinson patients. *Journal of Speech and Hearing Disorders,* 1978, *43,* 47–57.

Luchsinger, R., & Arnold, G. E. *Voice-speech-language.* Belmont, Calif.: Wadsworth Publishing Co., 1965.

Meyerson, M. D. The effects of aging on communication. *Journal of Gerontology,* 1976, *31,* 29–38.

Michel, J., & Wendahl, R. Correlates of voice production. In L. Travis (Ed.), *Handbook of speech pathology and audiology.* New York: Appleton-Century-Crofts, 1971.

Moncur, J. P., & Brackett, I. P. *Modifying vocal behavior.* New York: Harper & Row, 1974.

Moore, G. P. *Organic voice disorders.* Englewood Cliffs, N.J.: Prentice-Hall, 1971(a).

Moore, G. P. Vocal disorders organically based. In L. Travis (Ed.), *Handbook of speech pathology and audiology.* New York: Appleton-Century-Crofts, 1971(b).

Moore, G. P. Have the major issues in voice disorders been answered by research in speech science? A 50-year retrospective. *Journal of Speech and Hearing Disorders,* 1977, *42,* 152–160.

Moore, J. C., & Holbrook, A. The operant manipulation of vocal pitch in normal speakers. *Journal of Speech and Hearing Research,* 1971, *14,* 283–290.

Moses, P. J. *The voice of neurosis.* New York: Grune & Stratton, 1954.

Murphy, A. T. *Functional voice disorders.* Englewood Cliffs, N.J.: Prentice-Hall, 1964.

Myerson, M. C. *The human larynx.* Springfield, Ill.: Charles C. Thomas Publisher, 1964.

Oyer, H. J., & Oyer, E. J. *Aging and communication.* Baltimore: University Park Press, 1976.

Perkins, W. H. *Speech pathology: An applied behavioral science* (2nd Ed.). St. Louis: C. V. Mosby, 1977.

Perkins, W. H. *Human perspectives in speech and language disorders*. St. Louis: C. V. Mosby, 1978.

Peterson, V. S., & Peterson, J. S. The health of the aging. In E. W. Burgess (Ed.), *Aging in western societies*. Chicago: University of Chicago Press, 1960.

Portnoy, R. A. Hyperkinetic dysarthria as an early indicator of impending tardive dyskinesia. *Journal of Speech and Hearing Disorders*, 1979, *44*, 214–219.

Prosek, R. A., Montgomery, A. A., Walden, B. E., & Schwartz, D. M. EMG biofeedback in the treatment of hyperfunctional voice disorders. *Journal of Speech and Hearing Disorders*, 1978, *43*, 282–294.

Ptacek, P. H., & Sander, E. K. Age recognition from voice. *Journal of Speech and Hearing Research*, 1966, *9*, 273–277.

Ptacek, P. H., Sander, E. K., Maloney, W. H., & Jackson, C. R. Phonatory and related changes with advanced age. *Journal of Speech and Hearing Research*, 1966, *9*, 353–360.

Punt, N. A. Lubrication of the vocal mechanism. *Folia Phoniatrica*, 1974, *26*, 287–288.

Rigrodsky, S., Lerman, J., & Morrison, E. *Therapy for the laryngectomized patient: A speech clinician's manual*. New York: Teachers College Press, Columbia University, 1971.

Rousey, C. L., & Moriarty, A. E. *Diagnostic implications of speech sounds*. Springfield, Ill.: Charles C. Thomas Publisher, 1965.

Salmon, S. J. Bridging communication gaps through interpersonal therapy with laryngectomized patients. In M. Cooper & M. H. Cooper (Eds.), *Approaches to Vocal Rehabilitation*. Springfield, Ill.: Charles C. Thomas Publisher, 1977.

Sanchez-Salazar, V. V., & Stark, A. The use of crises intervention in the rehabilitation of laryngectomees. *Journal of Speech and Hearing Disorders*, 1972, *37*, 323–328.

Sarno, M. T. Speech impairment in Parkinson's disease. *Archives of Physical Medicine and Rehabilitation*, 1968, *49*, 269–275.

Schow, R. L., Christensen, J. M., Hutchinson, J. M., & Nerbonne, M. A. *Communication disorders of the aged*. Baltimore: University Park Press, 1978.

Shanks, J. C. Variations on a vocal theme through interpersonal therapy with alaryngeal patients. In M. Cooper & M. H. Cooper (Eds.), *Approaches to vocal rehabilitation*. Springfield, Ill.: Charles C. Thomas Publisher, 1977.

Simmons, M. F., & Shanks, S. J. A comparative study of methods for teaching of post-laryngectomy speech. *British Journal of Disorders of Communication*, 1971, *6*, 58–62.

Snidecor, J. C. Presentation at Second Annual Post-laryngectomy Seminar, Los Angeles, October 15, 1971.

Starmer, G. Presentation at Second Annual Post-laryngectomy Seminar, Los Angeles, October 15, 1971.

Stinchfield, S. *Speech pathology*. Boston: Expression, 1928.

Storandt, M. Psychological aspects. In F. V. Steinberg (Ed.), *Cowdry's The care of the geriatric patient* (5th ed.). St. Louis: C. V. Mosby, 1976.

Strandberg, T. E., Griffith, J., & Hallowell, M. W. Case study of psychogenic hoarseness. *Journal of Speech and Hearing Disorders*, 1971, *36*, 281–286.

Taub, S., & Bergner, L. H. Air bypass voice prosthesis for vocal rehabilitation of laryngectomees. *American Journal of Surgery*, 1973, *125*, 748–756.

Travis, L. (Ed.). *Speech pathology*. New York: Appleton, 1931.

Vaughan, C. W., Strong, M. S., & Jake, G. J. Laryngeal carcinoma transoral treatment utilizing the CO_2 laser. *American Journal of Surgery*, 1978, *136*, 490–493.

von Leden, H. Speech and hearing problems in the geriatric patient. *American Geriatrics Society Journal*, 1977, *25*, 422–426.

Weaver, M. Neurological disorders of the larynx. In G. English (Ed.), *Otolaryngology*. New York: Harper & Row, 1976.

Weiss, C. E. Communicative needs of the geriatric population. *American Geriatrics Society Journal*, 1971, *19*, 640–645.

Weiss, D. A., & Beebe, H. H. (Eds.). *The chewing approach in speech and voice therapy*. New York: Karger, 1951.

West, R., Kennedy, L., & Carr, A. *The rehabilitation of speech*. New York: Harper & Brothers, 1937.

White, F. W. Some causes of hoarseness in children. *Annals of Otology, Rhinology and Laryngology*, 1946, *55*, 537–542.

Wilson, D. K. *Voice problems in children* (2nd ed.). Baltimore: William & Wilkins, 1979.

Wolpe, J., & Lazarus, A. A. *Behavior therapy techniques: A guide to the treatment of neurosis*. New York: Pergamon Press, 1966.

Wynder, E. L., Covey, L. S., Mabachi, K., & Mushinski, M. Environmental factors in cancer of the larynx. *Cancer*, 1976, *38*, 1591–1601.

Zwitman, D. H., & Calcaterra, T. C. Phonation using the tracho-esophageal shunt after total laryngectomy. *Journal of Speech and Hearing Disorders*, 1973, *38*, 369–373. (a)

Zwitman, D. H., & Calcaterra, T. C. The silent cough method for vocal hyperfunction. *Journal of Speech and Hearing Disorders*, 1973, *38*, 119–125. (b).

Zwitman, D. H., Knorr, S. G., & Sonderman, J. C. Development and testing of an intraoral electrolarynx for laryngectomy patients. *Journal of Speech and Hearing Disorders*, 1978, *43*, 263–269.

G. Albyn Davis
Audrey L. Holland

12
Age in Understanding and Treating Aphasia

A person is susceptible to brain injury resulting in aphasia at any age following language acquisition and well into the later years. Younger persons (i.e., those in their twenties and thirties) most commonly become aphasic as the result of traumatic head injury, whereas aphasias in persons over 50 most commonly occur as a result of a cerebrovascular accident (CVA), or stroke. As the arteriosclerotic processes of aging progressively weaken the cardiovascular system, the likelihood of suffering a stroke increases. Since about 50 percent of stroke cases survive and the proportion of elderly in our society is increasing, the demand for aphasia rehabilitation should remain substantial. Yet the physiologic changes and medical problems accompanying the aging process have led clinicians to believe that older patients have a poorer chance for recovery than do younger ones. The purpose of this chapter is to review and assess what is known about age relative to aphasia and to predicting recovery from it. The second part of this chapter shows why the clinician should understand adult development and aging in order to treat aphasic patients effectively.

UNDERSTANDING APHASIA

Understanding the nature of aphasia entails distinguishing this disorder from other pathologies related to cerebral dysfunction. Also, the clinician needs to understand the specific etiologies for aphasia while being sensitive to its different symptom complexes, severity levels, and factors pertaining to recovery. Chronological age, especially to the extent that it correlates with physiologic change, may be a factor in refining our understanding of these aspects of aphasia. After a brief introduction to the nature of aphasia, considerations of aging will be discussed relative to differential diagnosis, etiology, types of aphasia, severity of impairment, and recovery.

A Description of the Problem

Aphasia is a disruption of language caused by damage to certain areas of the brain (Goodglass & Geschwind, 1976). As a language disorder it differs from unimodal disorders such as hearing loss or dysarthria by involving not only speech and language production and comprehension but also reading, writing, and symbolic gesturing as well. The symptom complexes of individual patients vary as a function of the location and extent of brain damage, and these variations are evident in differing patterns and degrees of impairment in linguistic performance. Since the damage is to the so-called language areas of the cerebral cortex (usually the left hemisphere), aphasia differs from pathologies associated with damage to other cortical areas, the entire cortex, or certain subcortical structures. Some persons with aphasia have an accompanying right-sided paralysis or weakness of the muscles, but the major impact of this disorder lies in its frustration of communication through the speech modality. The aphasic person with damage restricted to the language areas of the left hemisphere is alert, responds to his environment relatively appropriately in nonverbal ways, and generally maintains a desire to communicate with others. He or she shows a knowledge of the rules of social discourse and communicates intentions and ideas in a restricted fashion through remaining linguistic and nonlinguistic means.

The varied impacts of aphasia on different people can be anticipated in part by considering when it may occur in the life cycle. Its consequences will depend on whether the victim has just begun building a family and career, has been involved in the activities of school-age children, has been adjusting to children leaving home, or has been planning for or adjusting to retirement. Aphasia requires adjustments to reduced abilities to carry out basic social roles that change throughout adulthood. Because of the unanticipated changes in roles of spouse and parent by the person with aphasia, other family members must adjust to fill in the newly created gaps. As a result, aphasia becomes a family problem as well as an individual problem.

Differential Diagnosis

The accurate identification of aphasic symptoms is an important first step in speech—language rehabilitation. This step typically leads the clinician to decide whether to try aphasia treatment or to refer to a more appropriate professional, whether some nonaphasic symptoms may impede attempts to treat aphasic symptoms, or whether treatment should be structured around parameters of language or speech. Such decisions about treatment can be made when the symptoms of aphasia are distinguished properly from behaviors characteristic of normal aging and from the symptoms of pathologies associated with the aging process.

Aphasia is superimposed on an individual who already possesses certain biologic and psychologic characteristics that continue to change and interact with the aphasic condition. Some of these conditions that intermingle with aphasia may be products of or associated with the normal aging process. This presents a differential diagnostic problem within an individual patient rather than between patients with different disorders. That is, the clinician must distinguish between behaviors due to aphasia and behaviors due to aging to the extent that this is possible.

The language problems of an elderly aphasic person need to be distinguished from the modality-specific sensory (Orchik and Burgess, 1977) and motor (Hutchinson, Robinson, & Nerbonne, 1978; Ptacek, Sander, Maloney, & Jackson, 1966) changes with normal aging. For example, the presence of presbycusis (Schuknect, 1964) in an elderly person with aphasia makes it necessary to estimate the relative effects of the hearing loss and aphasia on comprehension of speech, so that the appropriate treatment is chosen for each problem. Also, age-related changes in encoding strategies of episodic memory (Eysenck, 1974; Perlmutter, 1978) may interact with an aphasic person's performance on certain diagnostic and treatment tasks. Research is needed that will help the clinician determine whether behaviors related to aphasia and those related to aging are easily separable with regard to identification of symptoms.

Certain aspects of problem solving and word association by elderly persons risk being misinterpreted as being either abnormal in general or aphasic in particular. For example, elderly individuals use relatively unsophisticated methods of classifying stimuli that, as Denney (1974) suggested, are more adaptive to real-life situations than they are deficient. In studies of free word association, Riegel (1968) found that while young adults tended to give paradigmatic (in-class) responses, elderly subjects alternated between paradigmatic and syntagmatic (syntactically related) responses. Also, elderly subjects tended to give more atypical, idiosyncratic responses. Aphasic subjects were found to produce the same type of associations produced by normal controls (Sefer & Henrikson, 1966). However, clinicians must be careful not to apply standards relevant for young adults to response criteria for elderly aphasic patients when giving them word-association tasks.

Distinguishing between pathologic aging and normal aging in some elderly individuals may be difficult, and definitions of each are often circular (Bromley, 1974). The difference between aphasia and neuropathologies of old age is a common problem in institutionalized settings, such as nursing homes, and presents a differential diagnostic problem. The neuropathologies of older persons are included within the broad classification of chronic organic brain syndromes (Blazer, 1977) or generalized intellectual impairment (Halpern, 1971). The associated cognitive deficits or dementia are characterized by loss of memory for recent events, disorientation as to time and place, confusion of ideas, and faulty judgment (Blazer, 1977). Aphasia, on the other hand, usually involves loss of memory for words rather than events, while orientation is preserved. Confusion of ideas is minimal. In neuropsychologic examinations, patients with dementia show deficits equally in verbal and nonverbal measures, whereas patients with aphasia show more difficulty with verbal than with nonverbal measures (McFie, 1975). Aphasia differs from organic brain syndrome not only in the distinction between language and cognitive deficits but also in characteristics of etiology and onset. Chronic organic brain syndrome associated with aging processes is usually due to diffuse brain damage of insidious onset, whereas aphasia is due to focal brain insult of sudden onset (Wertz, 1978).

In a more thorough discussion of differential diagnosis and the different etiologies of dementia, Wertz (1978) considered generalized intellectual impairment to be a type of language disorder in accordance with an investigation by Halpern, Darley, and Brown (1973). They gave an adaptation of Schuell's (1957) short examination of aphasia to ten patients in this category and found mild reductions in most language categories. However, the qualitative aspects of the language behavior reflecting dementia were not clearly compared with aphasia.

In addition, certain psychopathologies are associated with aging, such as depression, hypochondriasis, and paranoid conditions (Blazer, 1977). The source of a general inertia and reticence in a person with aphasia and a prior history of chronic depression is sometimes difficult to determine. Depression is very common in old age (Butler, 1978), and it is a common reaction to aphasia (Eisenson, 1973). Further complicating the possibilities with aphasia in the elderly is that "many organic problems are first seen as psychiatric ones, and vice versa" (Butler, 1978, p. 7). Butler noted that depression may be an early sign of organic brain syndrome, so that the speech—language pathologist may be confronted with decisions about various combinations of aphasia and the neuropathologies and psychopathologies that are associated with aging.

The direct language treatment procedures employed with aphasic patients are frequently not appropriate for the language impairments of dementia (Wertz, 1978). Remediation is possible, however, for the symptoms of organic brain syndrome, and the speech—language clinician may have multifarious roles in this regard. The first question for the physician, however, is whether the patient's symptoms of dementia are due to reversible causes such as acute stress, anxiety, physical space reduction, malnutrition, alcoholism, pernicious anemia, fecal impac-

tions, and so on (Butler, 1975, 1978; Smith & Barker, 1972). Proper medical treatments and social adjustments can minimize forgetfulness, reduced concentration, and intellectual decline from these causes.

According to Wertz (1978), rehabilitation for cases of generalized intellectual impairment is directed toward "restitution of lost functions, reduction of the patient's need for functions that have been lost, and utilization of residual functions" (p. 59). Physical, occupational, and recreational therapies can maximize residual abilities and slow the progresion of dementia. Reality orientation is a method designed to minimize the effects of memory loss, confusion, and disorientation; classes usually are conducted by a nursing assistant, housekeeper, or other person having frequent contact with patients (Barnes, 1974; Barns, Sack, & Shore, 1973; Brook, Degun, & Mathes, 1975; Citrin & Dixon, 1977; Folsom, 1968). Other types of therapy for organic brain syndrome include resocialization, remotivation, attitude therapy, reinforcement therapy, milieu therapy, and so on (Barnes et al., 1973). Wertz (1978) described the speech—language pathologist's role in identifying treatable sensory and motor barriers to communication and in helping the hospital staff to improve communication with patients. Accurate recognition of symptoms as aphasia, normal or pathologic aspects of aging, or the unfortunate outgrowth of circumstances that can cluster at old age leads the clinician to decisions about the most appropriate treatment rather than simply to a decision about whether to treat at all.

Etiologies of Aphasia

The etiologies of aphasia are not equally likely to occur at any age. Because of the impact of this fact on research in aphasiology, it is important to consider the relationship among etiology, age, and aphasia in this report. The focal brain damage resulting in aphasia may be caused by a cerebrovascular accident (stroke), trauma (head injury), or neoplasm (tumor). The peak incidence of strokes is between 40 and 70 years of age (Chusid, 1976). The peak incidence of the most common primary brain tumor in adults, the malignant glioma or astrocytoma grades 3—4, is between 45 and 55 years of age (Weiss, 1978). Accidental head injury, of course, may occur at any age, although the literature on aphasia due to head injury is disproportionately centered on war injuries incurred by men in their twenties (Luria, 1970; Wepman, 1951). The ages of aphasic groups identified by etiology reflect the proportion of deaths from these three etiologies, with accidents being the major cause between 10 and about 35 years of age and cardiovascular diseases including stroke being the major cause after 45 years of age for men and 55 years of age for women (Kimmel, 1974). Much of our present lore concerning diagnostic methodology, classification, and treatment expectations in aphasiology is based on relatively large sample studies of the aphasic population that vary in etiological and age characteristics. The interaction of etiology and age complicates any attempt to establish general descriptions of aphasia because different etiologies produce different recovery patterns (Wertz, 1978) and increasing age produces changes in physical health and mental function.

The characteristics of large-sample studies of aphasia shown in Table 12–1 illustrate the relationship between etiology and age. These studies involved description, analysis, and classification of aphasic symptom patterns, as well as analyses of the extent of recovery from aphasia. Five of these studies reported standardization data on formal aphasia diagnostic batteries including those developed by Wepman and Jones (1961), Schuell (1965), Porch (1967), and Kertesz and Poole (1974). One of the authors (Holland, 1980), in standardizing a test for functional communicative abilities, controlled for age roughly in proportion to the normal frequency of occurrence of aphasia in the general population.

An examination of Table 12–1 reveals some substantial differences, as well as some similarities, among the studies. The studies of aphasia with predominantly traumatic etiologies involved young-adult samples with mean ages of 26 (Wepman, 1951) and 28 (Luria, 1970) and with 83 percent of another sample below age 45 (Butfield & Zangwill, 1946). Samples involving predominantly stroke victims are characterized by a broader age range, higher mean ages (49–62 years) with over half the subjects being 50 years of age and older. A gross estimate of these characteristics for a typical hospital clinical population was derived by averaging figures from studies not representing one etiology exclusively and by taking different sample sizes into consideration. We might predict, therefore, that 78 percent of aphasia cases would be due to stroke, making the average age of a clinical population with aphasia around 55 years. Variations from this frame of reference include the studies of effects of war injuries and, to a lesser degree, Porch's sample for standardizing his test battery with a relatively large proportion above 50 years. In another study of aphasia (Gosnave, 1977), not shown

in Table 12–1, 44 postsurgical cases had a mean age of around 40 years, which is somewhat younger than the more typical CVA-dominated groups.

At least in peacetime, stroke produces about 80 percent of our aphasia caseloads in the hospital setting. Thus, a closer look at this etiology relative to age is warranted. In a careful analysis of 16 studies of stroke done in a variety of communities in the United States, Sahs, Hartman, and Aronson (1976) estimated incidence (new cases per year) and prevalence (total cases in the community) of stroke for a hypothetical standard population of one million. These estimates are shown in Table 12–2. The estimated mean age of 55 for a clinical aphasia population with a broad age range begins to make sense when based on the data in Table 12–2, namely, that 93 percent of new cases and 82 percent of all cases of stroke occur at age 55 and older. In spite of the preponderance of stroke cases in clinical caseloads, clinical populations are younger than the average age of stroke victims in general partly because the mortality from stroke is greater for older victims (Millikan & Moersch, 1953). Furthermore, the proportion of people with strokes within each age group increases with chronological age. For example, it has been estimated that 9.5 percent of persons over 75 years of age have suffered a stroke (Sahs et al., 1976). We could get close to a prediction of the number of aphasics possibly needing treatment in this standard population by eliminating almost 50 percent of stroke victims who do not survive after 30 days and by guessing that roughly half of the survivors suffer left hemisphere lesions. (According to Sahs et al., 30-day survival rates are 20 percent for intracerebral hemorrhage, 50 percent for subarachnoid hemorrhage, and 60 percent for cerebral infarction.)

The increasing incidence and prevalence of stroke as people get older is probably a direct function of the physiologic aging process that occurs throughout the life span. This process is "the sum total of all changes that occur in a living organism with the passage of time and lead to functional impairment and death" (Timiras, 1978, p. 606). Changes in the cardiovascular system include the arteriosclerotic process commonly referred to as "hardening of the arteries." The effect of arteriosclerosis is to decrease cerebral blood circulation and increase blood pressure (Bromley, 1974). An abrupt onset of this process produces a stroke. Chusid (1976) cited a study of 1175 consecutive autopsies that points to the lifelong duration of the arteriosclerotic process. Vascular insufficiency resulting from stenotic vessels showed up as early as 30 to

Table 12–1

Age Means and Ranges for Large-Sample Studies of Aphasia

	N	Mean Age	Age Range	% of Sample Younger than 50	% of Sample Older than 50	% of Sample Older than 60	Major Etiology
Butfield & Zangwill (1946)	66			83			56% trauma
Weisenburg (1934)	60	44[1]	12 to 59				62% CVA
Wepman (1951)	68	26	19 to 38	100	0	0	97% trauma[2]
Brown & Simonson (1957)	100			33	67	42	68% CVA
Marks, Taylor, & Rusk (1957)	205			36	64	30	94% CVA[3]
Wepman & Jones (1961)	168	51	14 to 76	44	56[4]	36	77% CVA
Schuell et al. (1964)	152	52	19 to 72	38	62	50	83% CVA
Porch (1967)	150	61	18 to 90	18	82	57	89% CVA
Luria (1970)	267	28[5]	18 to 46[5]	100	0	0	All trauma
Smith (1971)	78	49	20 to 73	53[6]	47	14	All CVA
Kertesz & Poole (1974)	150	61					76% CVA
Duffy & Ulrich (1976)	44	62	22 to 88				77% CVA
Kertesz & McCabe (1977)	93	57	16 to 85				92% CVA
Obler et al. (1978)	167	56		27%	73%	32%	All CVA
Holland	130	59	20 to 82	(see Table 12–3)			90% CVA
Typical figures		55		34%	66%	38%	78% CVA

[1]Median.
[2]Based on initial 71 cases used in recovery study.
[3]Ninety-four percent cerebral "disease processes," primarily CVA.
[4]Over age 49.
[5]Based on 43 case studies reporting age.
[6]Under age 51.

Table 12-2

Estimated Incidence and Prevalence of Stroke in a Standard Population of One Million People

Age group	Standard million population	Estimated incidence per 1,000	Expected new cases per year	Estimated prevalence per 1,000	Expected total cases in community	Prevalence proportion per age group (in percent)
0 to 34	582,083	0.00*	0	0*	0	
35 to 44	113,561	0.25	28	0	0	
45 to 54	114,206	1.00	114	20	2,284	2.0
55 to 64	91,464	3.50	320	35	3,101	3.4
65 to 74	61,155	9.00	550	60	3,669	6.0
75 plus	37,531	30.00	1126	95	3,565	9.5
Total	1,000,000		2138		12,619	1.3

Reprinted from Sahs, A. L., Hartman, E. C., & Aronson, S. M. (Eds.). *Guidelines for stroke care* (DHEW Publication No. (HRA) 76-14017), Washington, D.C.: U.S. Government Printing Office, 1976.

*Frequency of stroke in the 0 to 34 age group is so low that estimated incidence and prevalence are considered 0 for the purposes of calculation.

212

40 years of age for 2 percent of his sample. This was true of 6 to 8 percent of the patients from age 60 to 70. Moreover, the location of narrowing in the Circle of Willis, a system of arteries at the base of the brain, differed between younger and older patients.

Type of Aphasia and Age

Both etiology and the resulting type of aphasia appear to vary as a function of age. For example, Jason Brown's (1977) theory of cerebral ontogenesis suggests that age itself may be a rough predictor of type of aphasia. The syndromes of aphasia to be considered in this section are those defined by Goodglass and Geschwind (1976) as being related to specific sites of lesion and include nonfluent aphasia (Broca's), the fluent aphasias (Wernicke's, conduction, anomic), and global aphasia.

Brown (1976, 1977) and Brown and Jaffe (1975) proposed that specialization of cerebral function is a lifelong process and that the point at which a brain lesion intercepts this process determines the resultant type of aphasia. In other words, the symptom patterns of aphasic patients may be determined by an interaction between site of lesion and the particular state of cerebral specialization at the time of onset. This theory not only offers a fresh way to predict the occurrence of aphasic syndromes but also may be useful in helping to resolve occasional disputes between unidimensional and multidimensional explanations of aphasia (Darley, 1977). The theory was supported in part by certain clinical observations pertaining to the effects of lesions in particular cortical areas at particular ages. For example, Brown and Jaffe (1975) cited three cases of patients age 31 or younger in which the surgical removal of Broca's area did not result in expressive aphasia. Specialization for speech programming in Broca's area therefore may not occur until later in life. From other cases, they concluded that lesions to Wernicke's area in the posterior temporal lobe may produce mutism or agrammatism in the young child, anomia or symptoms of conduction aphasia in adolescence and middle age, and jargon aphasia or Wernicke's aphasia later in life. Brown concluded that auditory comprehension may be represented diffusely in the brain in childhood with subsequent gradual focusing of this function in the left temporal lobe.

Brown and Jaffe predicted that anatomic correlation with aphasic syndromes would become more predictable with increasing age, that one would expect to find an age specificity of different aphasic syndromes, and that Wernicke's aphasia would be more common in older patients. In a review of records of 348 aphasic patients that addressed the second and third predictions, Obler, Albert, Goodglass, & Benson (1978) selected 167 patients in the five categories mentioned earlier to compare relative to their age characteristics. The ages of conduction, anomic, and global aphasics clustered around the group median of 55.8. However, Broca's aphasics were younger statistically at 51 years, and Wernicke's aphasics were older statistically at 63 years. The number of Wernicke's patients in each decade from the thirties to the seventies increased linearly, while the other four types of aphasia displayed a normal distribution peaking between ages 52 and 57. A further analysis of their data showed that Broca's patients accounted for 50 percent of the aphasic patients in their forties, dropping to 14 percent of the group in their seventies. On the other hand, Wernicke's patients accounted for 11 percent of the group in their forties and increased to 36 percent of the group in their seventies. These data suggest that there may be a rough age specificity for Broca's and Wernicke's aphasia and that Wernicke's aphasia indeed is more common among older persons with aphasia.

In standardizing her new test of functional communication, one of the authors (Holland, 1980) provided another substantiation of the Brown–Jaffe hypothesis. Because the large sample was controlled to replicate the aging characteristics of the aphasic population, type of aphasia, which was not controlled, could be examined as a function of age. Table 12–3 summarizes the results. Broca's aphasics dominated the youngest group. Wernicke's aphasics were absent from the youngest group, appearing in the next age group and increasing in frequency as group age increased. In fact, all varieties of aphasia observed occurred only in the upper two age ranges but with decreasing proportions of the milder posterior anomic and anterior Broca's aphasias. A one-way analysis of variance, testing the relationship of age to type of aphasia, corroborated Obler et al.'s (1978) finding that Wernicke's aphasics were significantly older than were Broca's and anomic aphasics. The mean-age difference between Broca's and Wernicke's aphasics was 13 years, comparable to the 12-year difference found by Obler et al. Contrary to the previous results, Holland's global aphasics tended to be older than Broca's and anomic aphasics.

Severity of Aphasia

In spite of a paucity of clear evidence, it is commonly believed that as age increases the severity of aphasic impairment increases. For example, Porch (1967) correlated PICA (Porch Index of Communica-

Table 12—3
Anterior, Mixed, and Posterior Types of Aphasia Related to Age

	Age Groups									
	46		*46 to 55*		*56 to 65*		*65*		*Total Sample*	
	N	%	N	%	N	%	N	%	N	%
Broca	14	70	13	43	10	25	10	25	47	36
global	1	5	3	10	8	20	8	20	20	15
mixed	1	20	6	20	12	30	7	17.5	26	20
Wernicke	—	—	1	3.5	5	12.5	11	27.5	17	13
transcortical										
sensory	—	—	—	—	1	2.5	1	2.5	2	2
anomic	4	20	6	20	2	5	2	5	14	11
conduction	—	—	1	3.5	2	5	1	2.5	4	3
Total	20		30		40		40		30	

Adapted from Holland, A. L. *Communicative abilities in daily living.* Baltimore: University Park Press, 1980, p. 20.

tive Ability) test scores with a variety of patient variables and found only a "slight tendency" (p. 24) for younger subjects to score higher than older subjects. Yet the awareness of physiologic changes with aging sometimes stirs some disbelief of the data. Porch added the following comment: "Although this negative correlation between age and test scores is not strong enough to preclude the possibility of a sampling error, it seems reasonable to expect the older patient, with an ageing cerebral vascular system, to function less well under test conditions than the younger patient" (p. 24).

Smith (1971) suggested that age is a variable positively correlated to severity of aphasia. He examined 78 patients who had suffered cerebrovascular accidents (Smith, 1971). Following Schuell's (1965) unidimensional concept of aphasia and using her aphasia test battery to measure severity, Smith did not differentiate among types of aphasia and examined levels of severity of aphasic disturbance within the four modalities of language use. To determine the relationship between age and severity, he divided his subjects into three groups: 9 subjects 20 to 35 years of age, 32 subjects 36 to 50 years of age, and 37 subjects over 50 years of age. The interval between onset of aphasia and testing ranged from 1 month to 10 years, and it is not clear whether the ages reported by Smith represented age at onset or age at the time of measurement. Smith found that the incidence of severe deficits in auditory comprehension, speech, and writing increased with advancing age. This trend was most pronounced in the speech modality, especially between the ages 36 to 50 and in the

over-50 group. Using a test of sentence production, Gosnave (1977) found a significant correlation between age and test performance, the older brain-injured subjects doing more poorly. Smith (1971), however, noted that conclusions from his study must be qualified since the youngest group consisted of only nine subjects.

Further indications of a relationship between age and severity come from observations of the most severe forms of aphasia, often referred to as global aphasia. Sarno's studies of treatment (Sarno, Silverman, & Sands, 1970) and spontaneous recovery (Sarno & Levita, 1971) with severe aphasia reported a mean age of 64 and a median age of 67 respectively. Schuell's (Schuell, Jenkins, & Jimenez-Pabon, 1964) most severely impaired groups also were much older than the less-impaired groups. For example, Group I (simple aphasia) had a mean age of 38 years and Group V (irreversible aphasia) had a mean age of 59.6 years. In studies of aphasia types, global and Wernicke's aphasias are usually the most severe disorders. Kertesz and Poole's (1974) global aphasics averaged 65 years, their Wernicke's aphasics averaged 60 years, and their Broca's aphasics averaged 57 years. These data differ from Obler et al.'s (1978) finding that global aphasics clustered around the median age of 56 while Wernicke's aphasics were much older. The differences may be due, in part, to variations in assigning patients to groups.

Holland (1980) also found significant age differences relative to severity of aphasia on her measure of functional communication. Her two younger age groups had a significantly higher mean test score than did those over age 65. However, because behaviors often attributed to aging can be attributed instead to other factors (Butler, 1978), an interaction was found within the two older groups implicating factors other than age as a basis for the observed difference in severity. For the two older age groups, equal numbers of patients were institutionalized and living at home, and subjects in both groups were almost equally divided by sex. Among the findings was that older persons with aphasia living at home had significantly higher test scores than those of the same age living in an institution. Thus, although simple aging may contribute to severity of aphasia, this relationship is complicated by living environment, possibly by male–female differences, and certainly by the interaction between age and whether the patient is living in an institution or at home.

Another variable that possibly interacts with age and affects aphasic persons' test performance is amount of formal education. As standards of education have increased dramatically during the present century, younger people have had more education than older people, as Porch (1967) found in his sample population used for standardizing his test battery. Porch suggested, therefore, that test scores that were correlated positively with education, such as writing skill, should correlate negatively with age. As expected, he found a negative correlation between age and writing ability displayed by his aphasic subjects. Again, it is suggested that factors correlated with aging, but not aging per se, may affect the level of aphasic performance.

Recovery from Aphasia

Predicting recovery from aphasia is a complex matter involving several endogenous variables such as etiology, type of aphasia, and initial severity and at least one exogenous variable, namely, speech–language treatment. Though each of these variables has been shown to affect the course of recovery, isolating any single variable by controlling for the others has been a difficult task for investigators. Furthermore, these variables may have differential effects on recovery relative to its extent, amount, rate, and pattern. Since Eisenson's (1949) early clinical observations, age has been considered to be another variable related to recovery and to the effectiveness of treatment (Darley, 1972; LaPointe, 1978a). The experimental evidence relating age to recovery is equivocal partly because age interacts with etiology, type of aphasia, and severity. However, the conclusion that old age has a negative impact on recovery makes sense because of age-related changes in neurophysiology, cognition, and susceptibility to disease as well as changes pertaining to living environment that often accompany aging. Most studies of recovery from aphasia have included subjects who had received treatment of various kinds during all or part of the time periods studied. In the ensuing review of such studies, recovery periods in which subjects did not receive treatment or received minimal treatment are distinguished from recovery periods that included speech–language treatment.

SPONTANEOUS RECOVERY

Since the clinical study of aphasia began, persons with aphasia have been observed to recover language functions to varying degrees in the few months after onset. The slope of the spontaneous recovery curve appears to be negatively accelerated, with most recovery occurring within the first month post onset (Culton, 1969; Sarno & Levita, 1971) until the process is completed, usually no more than six months post onset. In response to Smith's (1971) suggestion that Culton's (1969) data might be related to age, Culton (1971) noted that his five oldest subjects recovered to a greater degree than his five youngest subjects. Sarno and Levita compared age only to initial test scores and found no correlation. While studies of spontaneous recovery of language function have provided little evidence to suggest that age is correlated with amount or rate of recovery, Smith (1972) continued to promote age as a negative factor in predicting recovery by pointing to findings regarding diaschisis.

Diaschisis is defined as the temporary suspension of functions of intact ipsilateral and contralateral hemispheres remote from the focal lesion (Smith, 1972). The physiologic mechanism underlying this phenomenon appears to be a bilateral reduction of hemispheric blood flow following unilateral cerebral infarction. This reduction of blood flow was found to disappear in the healthy hemisphere within 2 or 3 weeks after onset (Meyer, Shinohara, Kanda, Fukuuchi, Ericsson, & Kok, 1970). Meyer, Kanda, Fukuuchi, Shimazu, Dennis, & Ericsson (1971) compared 17 subjects younger than 59 years of age to 27 subjects over age 60 and found that the effects of diaschisis were prolonged with the older subjects. They concluded that "during the acute stage of cerebral infarction the young individual has considerably more capacity for recovery from the remote effects of stroke than the older patient" (p. 393), defined as over age 60. However, diaschisis does not account for recovery from impairments attributed to the site of permanent infarction, and the role of age in the spontaneous recovery from these impairments has not been determined.

In a study of recovery rate measured with the Western Aphasia Battery (Kertesz & Poole, 1974), Kertesz and McCabe (1977) found a nonsignificant negative correlation between age at onset and amount of recovery during a 3-month interval. Only 5 of the 36 patients studied had received speech–language treatment during the 3-month interval. Amounts of recovery were measured at two successive 3-month intervals and at a third interval of 6 to 12 months or more with initial testing within 45 days after onset of aphasia. Age was correlated with amount of recovery during the first 3-month interval. Kertesz and McCabe qualified the nonsignificant correlation by suggesting that it would have been significant if four of the subjects had been removed from the analysis. One of these four exceptions, however, a 72-year-old global aphasic, made his "remarkable" recovery during the third interval instead of the interval used in the analysis. Furthermore, this older patient made his large improvement during the only interval in which he was treated. Two of these four subjects, both much younger global aphasics who made little improvement, were not treated. Therefore, the attempt to suggest a possible correlation between age and recovery is questionable, because the four exceptions were drawn, in one case, from data not included in the statistical analysis and from the presence of treatment in the older case and the absence of treatment in the younger cases.

Finally, Obler and Albert (1977) examined age relative to the sequence in which different languages are recovered by multilingual aphasic patients. They surveyed 106 cases from the literature and 3 cases of their own. Recovery of the most recently learned language occurred above chance level for aphasics under 60 years of age. Whether first or second language recovered most was not evident for older subjects. Obler and Albert concluded that age may be one determinant of recovery patterns in this respect.

In conclusion, the studies reviewed do not provide evidence that spontaneous recovery varies as a function of age. Culton's (1969) data actually suggest the unexpected conclusion that more older persons with aphasia recover than younger aphasics. However, the number of subjects in this study was small. The study of diaschisis (Meyer et al., 1971), in which the prognosis for younger subjects was more favorable than for older subjects, is not related to recovery from aphasia. Kertesz and McCabe (1977) found no correlation between age and amount of recovery.

None of these studies was created to answer the question about age and recovery from aphasia, and analyses pertaining to this question in Culton's and Kertesz's studies were post hoc in nature. A study designed to answer this question may still find a relationship between age and recovery, and this relationship may vary depending on whether the investigator considers the extent, amount, rate, or pattern of recovery.

SPEECH–LANGUAGE TREATMENT DURING RECOVERY

The relative contributions of age and etiology to treatment effectiveness have not been clearly established in the aphasia literature. Based on a review of 21 cases, Eisenson (1949) suggested that advancing age may reduce the benefits of treatment for aphasia. He also noted that traumatic cases improved more rapidly than vascular cases but that the former were younger than the latter. In addition, investigations of a potential interaction between age and treatment have been difficult to carry out, as evidenced by Vignolo's (1964) study of treatment effectiveness in which age and treatment variables could only be analyzed separately. He found that 72 percent of subjects aged 60 and younger improved in communicative abilities, whereas only 22 percent of subjects over age 60 improved. However, only 9 subjects were over age 60 while 60 subjects were under age 60, so that any conclusion regarding age and recovery during treatment was tentative. At a later stage of the same project with 281 treated and untreated subjects, Basso, Capitani, and Vignolo (1979) found that age was not significantly related to the recovery of all subjects and that age did not make a difference whether the subjects were treated or untreated.

A comparison of early studies of recovery in treated patients could lead to the conclusion that younger patients benefit more from treatment than older patients. Butfield and Zangwill (1946) and Wepman (1951) evaluated the amount of recovery by aphasic patients who were younger than 50 years of age, while Marks, Taylor and Rusk (1957) and Godfrey and Douglass (1959) evaluated amount of recovery by much older patients. In the Marks et al. study, 64 percent of the patients were over age 50, and Godfrey and Douglass studied a group with a mean age of 60. In these studies, amount of improvement was rated in different ways, such as with categories of much improved, improved, and unchanged (Butfield & Zangwill, 1946) or excellent, good, fair, and poor (Marks et al., 1957). A comparison of these different rating procedures is facilitated by collapsing levels of "improvement" into one category. In the studies of younger patients by Butfield and Zangwill (1946) and Wepman (1951), 81 percent and 87 percent respectively improved in varying amounts. In the studies of older patients, only 50 percent (Marks et al., 1957) and 37 percent (Godfrey & Douglass, 1959) showed improvement of language function to varying degrees. However, most of the younger subjects in the studies showing a high percentage of improvement had suffered traumatic injury as the cause of aphasia, while most of the older subjects in the studies showing less improvement had suffered strokes. Therefore, etiology may have contributed to this difference in recovery, and the relative contribution of age and etiology to recovery during treatment has continued to be obscure.

Two additional studies offer conflicting conclusions regarding the impact of age on recovery during treatment. Sands, Sarno, and Shankweiler (1969) concluded that age was the "most potent variable" (p. 205) influencing recovery in 30 stroke patients who received treatment for aphasia. The treatment ranged from 2 weeks to 2 years and 8 months in duration. All patients were followed from 4 months to a year after treatment was terminated. Their conclusion regarding age was based on a comparison between five patients who made the largest gains and five who made the least gains. The mean age of the former group was 47, and the mean age of the latter group was 61. On the other hand, Keenan and Brassell (1974), who rated recovery by reviewing 39 patients' files, found no difference in extent of recovery among six age groups from the twenties through seventies. Interpretation of this result is difficult, because etiology was not specified by the investigators. Like Keenan and Brassell's study, other retrospective searches through case records found that age was not a prognostic indicator for recovery (Messerli, Tissot, & Rodriguez, 1976; Rose, Boby, & Capildeo, 1976). These latter conclusions regarding age must be evaluated relative to the methodological weaknesses of retrospective studies, which include lack of control over confounding variables and indirect observation using subjective ratings.

The difficulties in constructing valid and reliable studies to examine the role of any single variable in recovery have certainly prevented us from making any definitive conclusion regarding age as a prognostic sign. Rating scales have been vague and inconsistent in their number and definition of scale points. However, formal test measures may provide their own difficulties. For example, Whitbourne (1976) found that elderly normal subjects exhibited more test anxiety for a cognitive task than did young-adult subjects. Younger patients therefore may be more toler-

ant of a test situation than elderly patients, creating another confounding variable. Other problems include balancing the number of subjects among age groups, controlling for the potential interaction of other variables such as etiology and initial severity, and examining all parameters of recovery including amount and rate.

TREATMENT AND ATTITUDES TOWARD AGING

The extent to which clinicians understand adult development and aging may have a subtle but important impact on the ability to treat older clients most effectively. Treatment of aphasia is facilitated by clinician attributes of unconditional positive regard and empathy toward the client, attributes which apply to the treatment of any communication disorder. A lack of understanding of aging and of one's own feelings about aging can inhibit the development of these attributes, affecting treatment through the clinician's attitudes and apprehensions about old age. In the rest of this chapter, we discuss the value of empathy and unconditional positive regard and suggest the possible impact of negative attitudes toward aging on the treatment of aphasia. Finally, we propose some ways to modify attitudes and, therefore, to maximize empathic understanding and unconditional positive regard for aphasic patients. In this discussion, we show how the patient's age is, in fact, suggestive of specific strategies of stimulus selection for treatment activities.

Unconditional Positive Regard and Empathy

Carl Rogers, who has had considerable influence on speech pathology (Van Riper, 1973), suggested that two conditions for successful psychotherapy are unconditional positive regard and empathic understanding on the part of the clinician for the client (Rogers, 1961). He defined unconditional positive regard as "an outgoing positive feeling without reservations, without evaluations" (p. 62). Rogers added that change is facilitated when the clinician experiences a warm, positive, and accepting attitude toward the client. Therefore, to be most effective in treating aphasic persons, the speech clinician must be accepting of a generally older person along with and in spite of his or her aphasia. The notion of an accepting atmosphere in the clinic should not be misconstrued to mean that "anything goes," that there are no boundaries within which the patient must function to achieve the goals of language treatment. It does mean, however, that the patient's depression, frustration, or anger is allowed in the clinical setting without reservation or evaluation by the clinician.

Empathy is the capacity to sense the feelings and personal meanings that the client is experiencing at each moment (Rogers, 1961). In their study of students in speech therapy interactions, Kaplan and Dreyer (1974) suggested that empathy was characterized by social support, encouragement, and positive facial and gestural responses. Haynes and Oratio (1978) surveyed clients in speech clinics around the country regarding clinician attributes that these clients found to have been most helpful in their treatment. Of six factors emerging in an analysis of 162 questionnaires, qualities reflecting "empathetic–genuineness" ranked second in importance to technical skill. In writing about the diagnosis of aphasia, Emerick and Hatten (1974) emphasized the value of understanding the person and what has happened to him or her as completely as possible. They added the following:

> It is dreadfully easy to be seduced by a particular diagnostic tool to the point that we come to see aphasia and the aphasic solely through a test. . . . it is worth at least as much time to appreciate the impact of aphasia upon an individual's humanity (p. 240).

Appreciating this impact of aphasia involves recognizing that aphasia is a devastating change event within the context of a continually developing adult.

Another comment regarding empathic understanding provides a reference point for subsequent discussions. Rogers (1951) advised that "it is the counselor's function to assume, in so far as he is able, the internal frame of reference of the client, . . . to lay aside all perceptions from the external frame of reference while doing so, and to communicate something of this empathetic understanding to the client" (p. 29). In the treatment of aphasia, this external frame of reference to be put aside may include the attitudes and beliefs about aging and old age that have been found in American society and, more specifically, within related health professions.

Attitudes about Aging and Old Age

Age has been found to be one of the important factors in determining the ways people behave toward each other in all societies (Neugarten & Moore, 1968). From their surveys of middle-class American men and women, Neugarten, Moore, and Lowe (1968) concluded that an elaborate and pervasive system of norms or expectations regarding age-appropriate behavior forms a "prescriptive time-table for the ordering of major life events" (p. 22). In one of their surveys, most men and women between ages 40 and 70 agreed that the best age for a man to marry is 20 to 25, that most people should be ready to retire between 60 and 65, that a good-looking woman is 20 to 35 years old, and that an old man is 65 to 75 and an old woman 60 to 75. In subsequent research, the actual ages at which certain milestones occurred corresponded to the expectations found previously (Neugarten, 1974). In another survey, three age groups showed a clear perception of expectations held by society regarding the most appropriate age for several behaviors, such as a woman's wearing a two-piece bathing suit, a man's living with his parents, or a couple's doing the "twist." Age norms operate in self-evaluations such as being "early," "late" or "on time" with regard to family and occupational milestones or in judgments of others such as "He's too old to do this" or "She's too young to wear that" (Neugarten et al., 1968). This age-consciousness includes attitudes directed specifically to old age.

Common attitudes toward the elderly have served to categorize them as a homogeneous group that is senile, rigid, unproductive, dependent, and untreatable, with problems solely due to irreversible physiologic aging (Blau & Berezin, 1975; Butler, 1975; Collette-Pratt, 1976). Ageism (Butler, 1969; Palmore & Manton, 1973) has been viewed as a pervasive prejudice; Butler (1975) defined it as "the process of systematically stereotyping and discriminating against people because they are old" (p. 894). Butler (1969) stated that it "reflects a deep seated uneasiness on the part of the young and middle-aged—a personal revulsion to and distaste for growing old, disease, disability; and a fear of powerlessness, 'uselessness,' and death" (p. 243). Studies have shown that negative attitudes toward the elderly develop early in childhood (Seefeldt, Jantz, Galper, & Serock, 1977; Thomas and Yamamoto, 1975), but adolescents have been found to have more positive than negative attitudes toward the elderly (Ivester & King, 1977).

Data reflecting ageism among adults was found in a survey of more than 4000 Americans conducted by Louis Harris and Associates and reported by Beverly (1975). She compared younger persons (age 18 to 64) with the elderly (over 65) regarding their perceptions about old age. In this study, the young (age 18 to 39) had the lowest image of old age, with far better images of the aged occurring for persons between 40 to 64 years of age and then declining again among the elderly themselves. In many respects, the self-image of the elderly was similar to the poor image of old age held by the youngest group. As exceptions to this general agreement, the young persons' ratings of open-mindedness and adaptability were much lower than the oldest group's view of themselves. Conversely, the youngest group thought more positively of the friendliness and wisdom of the elderly than did the elderly themselves. The general public's view of old age did not coincide with the elderly's self-image in some other respects as well. Whereas the total group felt that the major problems of old age were loneliness, not feeling needed, and lack of job opportunities, the elderly group did not feel these were significant problems compared to poor health and fear of crime. Finally, the elderly reported spending much less time watching TV, sitting and thinking, sleeping, and doing nothing than the general public thought they did. This data is especially suggestive that the younger public's stereotype of old age is inaccurate in many respects.

Butler (1975, 1978) stated that many psychiatrists and other mental-health specialists share society's negative attitudes toward older people. Biases of medical students were revealed in a study in which they made choices as to saving the life of one of two patients distinguished on the basis of race, sex, or age (Spence, Feigenbaum, Fitzgerald, & Roth, 1968). When race was a criterion, about 50 percent refused to make a choice; when sex was a criterion, 25 percent refused to make a choice; and when age was a factor, 3 percent refused to make a choice. These students thus showed a prejudice against age that was stronger than their prejudice against race and sex. Geiger (1978) found that medical students have certain misperceptions about the elderly, such as overestimating the percentage of the population that is over age 65 and the percentage of the elderly in extended-care facilities.

Many psychiatrists hold the view that the elderly are untreatable or resistant to change (Mutschler, 1971). Butler (1975, 1978), however, noted that only a third of those who die after age 80 have signs of senile brain disease and that many older people with acute brain syndromes can be helped with prompt and skillful diagnosis and treatment. He attributed psychiatrists' negative feelings toward the elderly to their apprehensiveness about their own old age, conflicts about their personal relationships with their own parents, and feelings of helplessness (Butler, 1975). Opinions held by nursing-home staff regarding the rehabilitation potential of the institutionalized elderly were found to vary depending on the role of the staff member (Kosberg & Gorman, 1975). Nurses, social workers, the board of directors, and secretarial staff held relatively positive views; housekeepers, nonprofessional nursing staff, and the residents themselves held negative views.

Strong preferences for working with younger patients were found in surveys of undergraduate occupational therapy students (Mills, 1972) and doctoral candidates in clinical psychology (Wilensky & Barmack, 1966). Most of the psychology students, for example, preferred to work with 19- to 24-year-old clients. Geiger (1978) found that 88 percent of the medical students studied would consider working with old people only as a last resort. Finally, Garfinkel (1975) used an attitude scale to determine if a 1964 reference to "the reluctant therapist" still applied to a group of psychologists, psychiatrists, and social workers. Though he found a generally more positive attitude toward old people, 34 of 38 agreed that "old people usually don't talk much," which he concluded was a new excuse for therapists, who rely on verbal interaction, to avoid elderly clients.

In summary, we reviewed how age is used as a criterion for evaluating and governing behavior, the negative attitudes of the general public and certain health professionals and students toward the elderly, and the preference shown by some health professionals for younger clients. Studies of attitudes toward aging held by speech−language pathologists are not found in the literature. However, speech−language pathologists and students in speech pathology might be expected to share similar attitudes and preferences regarding age and the elderly. These negative attitudes and sometimes inaccurate beliefs may interfere with treatment of aphasia.

Clinician−Client Age Differences

Jones and Seagull (1977) indicated that the qualities of unconditional positive regard, empathy, and trust correlate positively with perceived similarities between the clinician and the client. They discussed the potential impact of one clinician−client difference, that of race, on the relationship between a white therapist and black client in which the therapist may perceive the client in terms of a stereotype or as someone else familiar to the therapist. Ageism, like racism, has vast potential for creating a negative climate for therapeutic change. Clinicians, supplanting a relationship to the individual patient they are attempting to help with their stereotypes of the elderly or their attitudes toward their parents, can frequently be unaware of this tendency and its influences on the therapeutic process.

The clinician can more easily assume the client's internal frame of reference when the clinician and client are similar according to such features as race, sex, and age. For this reason, it is not surprising that the doctoral candidates in clinical psychology mentioned previously preferred to have clients of the same age as themselves. However, in graduate training programs in speech pathology, clinicians working with aphasic persons are usually much younger than their clients. Though a clinician of any age may hold negative attitudes and inaccurate beliefs about old age, this frequent age difference serves to emphasize the need to consider the potential influence of these attitudes and beliefs.

Negative attitudes and tendencies to stereotype that characterize ageism can interfere with developing unreserved positive feelings toward an older client and with assuming the client's internal frame of reference. Jones and Seagull (1977) suggested likely outcomes of guilt over racist attitudes that we believe are applicable to ageism as well. These outcomes included attempts to be too sympathetic and ingratiating toward the client due to a fear of realistic confrontation, communicating one's own anxiety to the client, and unrealistic approaches to the client's real-life problems. Jones and Seagull further pointed out that the therapist can become an overzealous "helper," becoming angry if the client does not respond. For example, Mutschler (1971) cited an observation by Myerson that "medical residents reacted to elderly patients as they might their own parents and became irritated if the expected gratitude was not forthcoming" (p. 233). The senior author knew one speech pathologist working in a hospital who openly expressed anxiety over treating elderly clients, fearing that they might die during therapy. Graduate students in speech pathology often comment on the difficulty of "switching roles" with an aphasic client, the young adult advising and directing an elderly adult. This concern indicates that age influences some clinicians' perceptions of roles in clinical interaction.

Solutions to the Problem

Some differences between clinicians and their clients are anticipated by speech pathology training programs. For example, with respect to disorders of childhood, the impact of the clinician–client age difference is reduced by substantial course requirements in child psychology and development. Training programs also frequently provide frameworks for experiencing what it "feels like" to stutter and to be communicatively impaired by disorders such as deafness and aphasia. Present course work on aphasia enables the clinician to communicate empathic understanding relative to the disorder with statements like "I know, you know what you want to say but can't say it." In outlining components of an ideal training program for clinical aphasiologists, Leutenegger (1975) wondered why a course on adulthood and aging could not be required, as are courses about children, particularly for students interested in treating the older brain-damaged population. Such a course should improve the clinician's understanding of older people and enhance awareness of his or her own attitudes and beliefs about old age. Though direct experience with older clients may enhance the ability to empathize with older patients, dealing with this issue during graduate training may affect students' preferences for working with certain clientele as well as speed the process of understanding.

The first step, however, in reducing the interference of an external frame of reference is to identify and acknowledge one's own attitudes, beliefs, or feelings about older people. This self-awareness facilitates being able to separate this external frame of reference from perceiving and understanding the elderly patient as an individual. Self-awareness training in general has been shown to increase the amount of social support, positive facial and gestural responses, attentiveness, and nonrestrictive behavior by students engaged in speech and language treatment (Kaplan & Dreyer, 1974).

Exposing trainees to information about the elderly has been shown to change attitudes toward old age. Smith and Barker (1972) measured such attitudes of physicians, nurses, social workers, occupational therapists, and graduate students in gerontology before and after they had participated in a five-day reality-orientation training program. These trainees made positive changes on an attitude scale that were significantly different and in the opposite direction from a control group that had not been exposed to the training program. Furthermore, the favorable attitude shift of the trainees was maintained on a second retest 6 months later.

Another solution is to require volunteer work in programs for the normally aging and visits to nursing homes, just as students observe and interact with normally developing children in their homes and in nursery schools. Contact with the aging and with their problems, pleasures, and life styles in natural context is as useful to understanding the aging aphasic person as the related experiences with normal children are to understanding the language-disordered child. The kind of contact may also influence attitudes toward the elderly. For example, medical students assigned to be companions to ambulatory, relatively healthy old people were found to have more positive attitudes toward the elderly than medical students assigned to wards for the chronically ill aged (Holtzman, Beck, & Coggan, 1978).

In order to maximize graduate students' understanding of their aphasic clients relative to stages of adulthood, a unique method for recording information about personal history has been used at Memphis State University. The personal history of each adult patient is recorded on a *life-cycle* form and a *historical time-line* form. These forms are based on Kimmel's (1974) discussion of the interaction between a person's life cycle or time of birth and the historical period in which the person goes through the typical stages of adulthood. This interaction is the source of cohort effects in research on aging (Kimmel, 1974; Knox, 1977).

The life-cycle form (see Fig. 12–1) contains a center column in which common milestones and stages of adult development are shown relative to the ages at which they usually occur. Milestones include birth, starting school and occupation, marriage, first child, children leaving home, and retirement. Stages of development are incorporated with the milestones, such as adolescence, early adulthood, middle adulthood (Bromley, 1974), and the stages of intimacy, generativity, and integrity described by Erikson (1963). To the left of this column, the student clinicians record the age and date at which each of these milestones and stages occurred for the patient, as well as the onset of aphasia relative to the life cycle. To the right of this column, detailed notes are recorded such as place of birth and names of children. A sense for the patient's history relative to standard stages of adulthood and for the stage of development at which aphasia has occurred may be obtained when personal history is recorded in this way.

Information from the life-cycle form is transferred to the historical time-line form (Fig 12–2). Selected "event cues" are listed on the right side of this second form. These cues include milestones and well-known events from recent American history since 1917 and are listed chronologically to the right of their respective dates at roughly 4-year intervals. These milestones and events include the start of presidents' terms of office, wars, famous achievements, and references to prominant figures in sports and entertainment at particular periods in the last 50 years.

To the left of these dates and event cues, the clinician records ages and milestones of the adult patient next to the corresponding period of historical time. The young clinician, who might not be readily familiar with periods of American life over the last 50 years, can obtain quickly and easily at least a superficial sense for the period in which the patient was attending high school, raising young children, or advancing in his or her occupation. For example, the clinician can note from Figure 12–2 that this patient's first vote was cast in the first election of Franklin Roosevelt as president. Different historical periods may influence different common stages of the life cycle in different ways, especially for the patient of 45 as opposed to the patient of 65. The historical milestones and events are suggestive of possible topics for individual or group discussion, and they cue patients into more personal recollections from different periods of their lives.

The historical time line illustrates the wealth of information available in each adult patient's personal history that can be used as content in treatment procedures for stimulating comprehension and expression. Holland (1978) recommended that stimuli be meaningful to the individual patient with reference to his or her daily activities. That is, if reading is to be exercised, then the patient should practice reading the mail and the phone directory. In another vein, stimulus material can be meaningful with reference to the patient's history; and, in a sense, the older the patient, the more information there is available to use in treatment. Valuable sources of cues to personal history, which were used to develop the historical time line, include a standard almanac and a collection of news photographs taken during the previous 50 years.

It is possible that stimulus content derived from personal history will improve linguistic performance because of the emotionalism or arousal that may be attached to it. For example, Boller, Cole, Vrtunski, Patterson, & Kim (1979) found that severely impaired aphasic patients were more responsive to "high emotional" questions and instructions than to neutral stimuli. They also noted the "common clinical experience that in emotionally loaded circumstances aphasics sometimes speak better than ordinarily" (p. 170). If the clinician is able to tap into the patient's personal experiences, he may be able to stimulate and channel arousal in ways that improve the patient's linguistic performance. The effectiveness of emotionally loaded stimuli could be investigated with single-case experimental designs by alternating phases of emotional and neutral materials (Davis, 1978) or by applying emotionally loaded

Name T. P.   Age   68   Onset   11/18/75

Date/Age	Milestones/Stages	Individual Notes
5/24/09	0: Birth	Little Rock, Arkansas
	6: Begin school	Moved to Memphis
	12: Puberty	Mother died
	Adolescence	
High school (16)	Identity	Central High School (Memphis)
	18: Begin occupation (or college)	University of South
	Intimacy	(Sewanee, TN)
	20: Early Adulthood	
1931 (22)	Marriage	Wife: Martha
	Parenthood	
1932 (23)	Vote	1933—First child William
	Generativity	Enters Navy
	25: Middle Adulthood	1937—Second Child Eleanor
	Family	
	Occupation	
	30: (Generation Gap)	
	40: Late Adulthood	
	"Middle Age"	
(42)	Children leave home	First grandchild
		Retires from Navy
		Becomes frozen food broker
	48: Death of parents	
	Menopause/male	
(53)	climatic	Father died
54	Grandparenthood	Retires
	60: Preretirement	
	65: Retirement	
11/18/75 (66)	Integrity	Stroke (thrombosis); onset
	Death of Spouse	of aphasia
	70: Old Age	
	Great-grandparenthood	

Fig. 12-1. Individual life-cycle form used for recording information about aphasic clients' personal history.

stimuli to one behavior but not to another behavior (LaPointe, 1978b).

Finally, an awareness of the literautre on cognitive processing relative to aging may provide the clinician with additional considerations for planning treatment of aphasia. For example, Poon and Fozard (1978) found that whether pictures of objects were contemporary or dated had an effect on speed of picture naming by normal adults. Dated objects, such as a churn, hand pump, wash board, and wringer, were named more rapidly by older subjects (60 to 70 years) than by younger subjects (18 to 22 years) whereas older subjects took longer to name contemporary objects. The dated and contemporary objects were selected from Sears-Roebuck and Montgomery Ward catalogues of 1910 and 1974. These results indicate

that a historical, and therefore age-related, dimension of stimulus content may have an impact on word-retrieval efficiency of adults with aphasia. An understanding of adulthood and of the individual patient's past experiences may have an effect not only on the young clinician's ability to establish empathy and unconditional positive regard toward older clients but also on the clinician's planning of typical treatment activities.

RESEARCH IMPLICATIONS

Two major challenges face investigators who are interested in determining the relationship between aging and aphasia. The first involves whether the

Name   T. P.   Age   68   DOB 5/24/09

Patient Age and Milestones	Year	Event Cues
8: In Memphis	1917	Wilson President
		World War I
		(1920) Prohibition in effect
12: Mother died	1921	Harding President
		First radio world series
		Schick: First electric shaver
16: High school	1925	Coolidge President
		Scopes trial in Tennessee
		H. Ford: Cars not just black
		(1926) H. Ford: 8-hr day, 5-day week
18: College		(1927) Dempsey–Tunney long count
		Babe Ruth's 60th home run
		Disney: First M. Mouse cartoon
		Lindberg's *Spirit of St. Louis*
		(1928) Amelia Earhart
	1929	Hoover President
		Southern textile strikes
		St. Valentine's Day Massacre
		DEPRESSION
22: Married		(1931) Charlie Chaplin in *City Lights*
First Vote	1933	FDR President-New Deal
		Prohibition repealed
Enters Navy		Dillinger shot
24: First child (boy)		(1935) Huey Long assassinated
		Joe Louis beats Max Baer
		(1936) Jesse Owens, Olympics in Germany
		Lou Gehrig retires
28: Second child	1937	FDR defeats Alf Landon
(girl)		Hindenberg disaster
		Spencer Tracy, Best Actor
		(1938) Bette Davis, Best Actress
		Disney's *Snow White*
		"Wrong Way Corrigan"
		(1939) Germany invades Poland
		Gone with the Wind
	1941	FDR defeats Wilkie
		Pearl Harbor—World War II
		Cary Grant, Best Actor

Fig. 12-2.   Individual historical time line relating milestones in adult patient's life to corresponding period of historical time. (Based on discussion of interaction between a person's life cycle or time of birth and the historical period in which the person goes through the typical stages of adulthood in Kimmel, DC: *Adulthood and Aging*. New York, John Wiley, 1974.)

clinician can distinguish reliably between cognitive changes associated with normal aging and the symptoms associated with aphasia. A clear distinction may not be possible within a single patient. Since both types of change result from changes in the central nervous system, one type gradual and the other sudden, a subtle interaction between the two processes is more likely, perhaps, producing certain forms of aphasia. For example, is the change in the central auditory system that increases rapidly after age 60 (Konkle, Beasley, & Bess, 1977) related to the finding that persons with Wernicke's aphasia tend to be older? In addition, if signs of aging are identifiable in aphasic persons, are these signs treatable with the methods employed by speech–language pathologists? Also, in what way might age-related changes interfere with the aphasia treatment process? Age-related changes in language use may represent adaptive strategies rather than deficits and may not be appropriate for treatment of any kind.

The second challenge involves clearly establishing the relationships between age and recovery from aphasia and between age and the benefits of treatment for aphasia. Though the belief is strong that increasing age reduces the amount and rate of recovery, experimental verification of this relationship is lacking. However, there is evidence to suggest that age is related to type of aphasia and its severity, both of which may be more directly related to recovery. The nature of the relationship between age and severity of aphasia requires further study since a variety of psychological and environmental factors accompany the aging process. As stated earlier in this chapter, difficulties in establishing control over variables in the study of age and recovery are derived from the general problem of isolating any single variable in the study of aphasia and from the specific problem of equating adequate sample sizes among different age groups.

Understanding these relationships may contribute to the clinician's ability to provide appropriate treatment of adults in an empathic manner. The attitudes that a young clinician, especially, may bring to treatment interactions should be examined further. An assumption was made in this chapter that the attitudes of relatively inexperienced speech–language clinicians may reflect the attitudes of society in general and of those found in related professions. However, the actual attitudes of clinicians at various levels of experience have not been determined. Such an investigation may lead to increased awareness of the possible impact of attitudes and beliefs about aging and "old age" on the clinical process in speech–language pathology.

REFERENCES

Barnes, J. A. Effects of reality orientation classroom on memory loss, confusion, and disorientation in geriatric patients. *Gerontologist,* 1974, *14,* 138–142.

Barns, E. K., Sac, A., & Shore, H. Guidelines to treatment approaches: Modalities and methods for use with the aged. *Gerontologist,* 1973, *13,* 513–527.

Basso, A., Capitani, E., & Vignolo, L. A. Influence of rehabilitation on language skills in aphasic patients. *Archives of Neurology,* 1979, *36,* 190–196.

Beverly, E. V. The beginning of wisdom about aging. *Geriatrics,* 1975, *30,* 117–119, 122–123.

Blau, D., & Berezin, M. A. Neuroses and character disorders. In J. G. Howell (Ed.), *Modern perspectives in the psychiatry of old age,* New York: Brunner/Mazel, 1975.

Blazer, D. G. *Psychopathology of aging.* Kansas City, Mo.: American Academy of Family Physicians, 1977.

Boller, F., Cole, M., Vrtunski, B., Patterson, M., & Kim, Y. Paralinguistic aspects of auditory comprehension in aphasia. *Brain and Language,* 1979, *7,* 164–174.

Bromley, D. B. *The psychology of human ageing.* Baltimore: Penguin Books, 1974.

Brook, P., Degun, G., & Mathes, M. Reality orientation, a therapy for psychogeriatric patients: A controlled study. *British Journal of Psychiatry,* 1975, *127,* 42–45.

Brown, J. R., & Simonson, J. A clinical study of 100 asphasic patients. *Neurology,* 1957, *7,* 777–783.

Brown, J. W. The neural organization of language: Aphasia and lateralization. *Brain and Language,* 1976, *3,* 482–494.

Brown, J. W. *Mind, brain, and consciousness: The neuropsychology of cognition.* New York: Academic Press, 1977.

Brown, J. W., & Jaffe, J. Hypothesis on cerebral dominance. *Neuropsychologia,* 1975, *13,* 107–110.

Butfield, E., & Zangwill, O. L. Reeducation in aphasia: A review of 70 cases. *Journal of Neurology, Neurosurgery and Psychiatry,* 1946, *9,* 75–79.

Butler, R. N. Age-ism: Another form of bigotry. *Gerontologist,* 1969, *9,* 243–246.

Butler, R. N. Psychiatry and the elderly: An overview. *American Journal of Psychiatry,* 1975, *132,* 893–900.

Butler, R. N. Overview on aging. In G. Usdin & C. K. Hofling (Eds.), *Aging: The process and the people.* New York: Brunner/Mazel, 1978.

Chusid, J. G. *Correlative neuroanatomy and functional neurology.* Los Altos, Calif.: Lange Medical Publications, 1976.

Citrin, R. S., & Dixon, D. N. Reality orientation: A milieu therapy used in an institution for the aged. *Gerontologist,* 1977, *17,* 39−43.

Collette-Pratt, C. Attitudinal predictors of devaluation of old age in a multigenerational sample. *Journal of Gerontology,* 1976, *31,* 193−197.

Culton, G. L. Spontaneous recovery from aphasia. *Journal of Speech and Hearing Research,* 1969, *12,* 825−833.

Culton, G. L. Reaction to age as a factor in chronic aphasia in stroke patients. *Journal of Speech and Hearing Disorders,* 1971, *36,* 563−564.

Darley, F. L. The efficacy of language rehabilitation in aphasia. *Journal of Speech and Hearing Disorders,* 1972, *37,* 3−21.

Darley, F. L. A retrospective view: Aphasia. *Journal of Speech and Hearing Disorders,* 1977, *42,* 161−169.

Davis, G. A. The clinical application of withdrawal, single-case research designs. In R. H. Brookshire (Ed.), *Clinical aphasiology conference proceedings.* Minneapolis: BRK Publishers, 1978.

Denney, N. W. Evidence for developmental change in categorization criteria for children and adults. *Human Development,* 1974, *17,* 41−53.

Duffy, R. J., & Ulrich, S. R. A comparison of impairments in verbal comprehension, speech, reading, and writing in adult aphasics. *Journal of Speech and Hearing Disorders,* 1976, *41,* 110−119.

Eisenson, J. Prognostic factors related to language rehabilitation in aphasic patients. *Journal of Speech and Hearing Disorders,* 1949, *14,* 262−264.

Eisenson, J. *Adult aphasia: Assessment and treatment.* New York: Appleton-Century-Crofts, 1973.

Emerick, L. L., & Hatten, J. T. *Diagnosis and evaluation in speech pathology.* Englewood Cliffs, N. J.: Prentice-Hall, 1974.

Erikson, E. H. *Childhood and society.* New York: W. W. Norton, 1963.

Eysenck, M. W. Age differences in incidental learning. *Developmental Psychology,* 1974, *10,* 936−941.

Folsom, J. C. Reality orientation for the elderly mental patient. *Journal of Geriatric Psychiatry,* 1968, *1,* 291−307.

Garfinkel, R. The reluctant therapist 1975. *Gerontologist,* 1975, *15,* 136−137.

Geiger, D. L. How future professionals view the elderly: A comparative analysis of social work, law, and medical students' perceptions. *Gerontologist,* 1978, *18,* 591−594.

Godfrey, C. M., & Douglass, E. The recovery process in aphasia. *Canadian Medical Association Journal,* 1959, *80,* 618−624.

Goodglass, H., & Geschwind, N. Language disorders (aphasia). In E. C. Carterette & M. P. Friedman (Eds.), *Handbook of perception* (Vol. 7): *Language and speech.* New York: Academic Press, 1976.

Gosnave, G. Sentence production test in sensory aphasic patients. In S. Rosenberg (Ed.), *Sentence production: Developments in research and theory.* Hillsdale, N. J.: Lawrence Erlbaum Associates, 1977.

Halpern, H. The differential diagnosis of language in the brain-injured adult. *Journal of Communication Disorders,* 1971, *4,* 176−183.

Halpern, H., Darley, F. L., & Brown, J. R. Differential language and neurological characteristics in cerebral involvement. *Journal of Speech and Hearing Disorders,* 1973, *38,* 162−173.

Haynes, W. O., & Oratio, A. R. A study of clients' perceptions of therapeutic effectiveness. *Journal of Speech and Hearing Disorders,* 1978, *43,* 21−33.

Heglin, H. J. Problem solving set in different age groups. *Journal of Gerontology,* 1956, *11,* 310−317.

Holland, A. L. Functional communication in the treatment of aphasia. In L. J. Bradford (Ed.), *Communicative disorders: An audio journal for continuing education.* New York: Grune & Stratton, 1978.

Holland, A. L. *Communicative abilities in daily living.* Baltimore: University Park Press, 1980.

Holtzman, J. M., Beck J. D., & Coggan, P. G. Geriatrics program for medical students. II. Impact of two educational experiences on student attitudes. *Journal of the American Geriatrics Society* 1978, *26*, 355−359.

Hutchinson, J. M., Robinson, K. L., & Nerbonne, M. Patterns of nasalance in a sample of normal gerontologic subjects. *Journal of Communication Disorders*, 1978, *11*, 469−481.

Ivester, C., & King, K. Attitudes of adolescents toward the aged. *Gerontologist*, 1977, *17*, 85−89.

Jones, A., & Seagull, A. A. Dimensions of the relationship between the black client and the white therapist. *American Psychologist*, 1977, *32*, 850−855.

Kaplan, N. R., & Dreyer, D. E. The effect of self-awareness training on student speech pathologist−client relationships. *Journal of Communication Disorders*, 1974, *7*, 329−342.

Keenan, J. S., & Brassell, E. G. A study of factors related to prognosis for individual aphasic patients. *Journal of Speech and Hearing Disorders*, 1974, *39*, 257−269.

Kertesz, A., & McCabe, P. Recovery patterns and prognosis in aphasia. *Brain*, 1977, *100*, 1−18.

Kertesz, A., & Poole, E. The aphasia quotient: The taxonomic approach to measurement of aphasic disability. *Le Journal Canadien Des Sciences Neurologiques*, 1974, *1*, 1−17.

Kimmel, D. C. *Adulthood and aging*. New York: John Wiley & Sons, 1974.

Knox, A. B. *Adult development and learning*. San Francisco: Jossey-Bass, 1977.

Konkle, D., Beasley, D., & Bess, F. Intelligibility of time-altered speech in relation to chronological aging. *Journal of Speech and Hearing Research*, 1977, *20*, 108−115.

Kosberg, J. I., & Gorman, J. F. Perceptions toward the rehabilitation potential of institutionalized aged. *Gerontologist*, 1975, *15*, 398−403.

LaPointe, L. L. Aphasia therapy: Some principles and strategies for treatment. In D. F. Johns (Ed.), *Clinical management of neurogenic communicative disorders*. Boston: Little, Brown & Co., 1978.(a)

LaPointe, L. L. Multiple baseline designs. In R. H. Brookshire (Ed.), *Clinical aphasiology conference proceedings*. Minneapolis: BRK Publishers, 1978.(b)

Leutenegger, R. R. Training of aphasiologists. In R. H. Brookshire (Ed.), *Clinical aphasiology conference proceedings*. Minneapolis: BRK Publishers, 1975.

Luria, A. R. *Traumatic aphasia*. The Hague, Paris: Mouton, 1970.

Marks, M. M., Taylor, M., & Rusk, H. A. Rehabilitation of the aphasic patient: A survey of three years' experience in a rehabilitation setting. *Neurology*, 1957, *7*, 837−843.

McFie, J. *Assessment of organic intellectual impairment*. New York: Academic Press, 1975.

Messerli, P., Tissot, A., & Rodriguez, J. Recovery from aphasia: Some factors of prognosis. In Y. Lebrun & R. Hoops (Eds.), *Recovery in aphasics*. Amsterdam: Swets & Zeitlinger, 1976.

Meyer, J. S., Kanda, T., Fukuuchi, Y., Shimazu, K., Dennis, E. W., & Ericsson, A. D. Clinical prognosis correlated with hemispheric blood flow in cerebral infarction. *Stroke*, 1971, *2*, 383−394.

Meyer, J. S., Shinohara, Y., Kanda, T., Fukuuchi, Y., Ericsson, A. D., & Kok, N. K. Diaschisis resulting from acute unilateral cerebral infarction. *Archives of Neurology*, 1970, *23*, 241−247.

Millikan, C. H., & Moersch, F. P. Factors that influence prognosis in acute focal cerebrovascular lesions. *Archives of Neurology and Psychiatry*, 1953, *70*, 558−562.

Mills, J. Attitudes of undergraduate students concerning geriatric patients. *American Journal of Occupational Therapy*, 1972, *26*, 200−203.

Mutschler, P. Factors affecting choice of and perseveration in social work with the aged. *Gerontologist*, 1971, *11*, 231−241.

Neugarten, B. L. Age norms. In M. L. Huyck (Ed.), *Growing older*. Englewood Cliffs, N. J.: Prentice-Hall, 1974.

Neugarten, B. L., & Moore, J. W. The changing age-status system. In B. L. Neugarten (Ed.), *Middle age and aging*. Chicago: University of Chicago Press, 1968.

Neugarten, B. L., Moore, J. W., & Lowe, J. C. Age norms, age constraints, and adult socialization. In B. L. Neugarten (Ed.), *Middle age and aging*. Chicago: University of Chicago Press, 1968.

Obler, L. K., & Albert, M. L. Influence of aging on recovery from aphasia in polyglots. *Brain and Language*, 1977, *4*, 460−463.

Obler, L. K., Albert, M. L., Goodglass, H., & Benson, D. F. Aging and aphasia type. *Brain and Language,* 1978, *6,* 318–322.

Orchik, D., & Burgess, J. Synthetic sentence identification as a function of age of the listener. *Journal of the American Audiology Society,* 1977, *3,* 42–46.

Palmore, E., & Manton, K. Agism compared to racism and sexism. *Journal of Gerontology,* 1973, *28,* 363–369.

Perlmutter, M. What is memory aging the aging of? *Developmental Psychology,* 1978, *14,* 330–345.

Poon, L. W., & Fozard, J. L. Speed of retrieval from long-term memory in relation to age, familiarity, and datedness of information. *Journal of Gerontology,* 1978, *33,* 711–717.

Porch, B. E. *Porch index of communicative ability.* Palo Alto, Calif.: Consulting Psychologists Press, 1967.

Ptacek, P. H., Sander, E. K., Maloney, W. H., & Jackson, C. C. R. Phonatory and related changes with advanced age. *Journal of Speech and Hearing Research,* 1966, *9,* 353–360.

Riegel, K. F. Changes in psycholinguistic performances with age. In G. A. Talland (Ed.), *Human aging and behavior.* New York: Academic Press, 1968.

Rogers, C. R. *Client-centered therapy.* Boston: Houghton Mifflin, 1951.

Rogers, C. R. *On becoming a person.* Boston: Houghton Mifflin, 1961.

Rose, C., Boby, V., & Capildeo, R. A retrospective survey of speech disorders following stroke, with particular reference to the value of speech therapy. In Y. Lebrun & R. Hoops (Eds.), *Recovery in aphasics.* Amsterdam: Swets & Zeitlinger, 1976.

Sahs, A. L., Hartman, E. C., & Aronson, S. M. (Eds.). *Guidelines for stroke care* (DHEW Publication No. [HRA] 76–14017). Washington, D.C.: U.S. Government Printing Office, 1976.

Sands, E., Sarno, M., & Shankweiler, D. Long-term assessment of language function in aphasia due to stroke. *Archives of Physical Medicine and Rehabilitation,* 1969, *50,* 202–207.

Sarno, M. T., & Levita, E. Natural course of recovery in severe aphasia. *Archives of Physical Medicine and Rehabilitation,* 1971, *52,* 175–179.

Sarno, M. T., Silverman, M., & Sands, E. Speech therapy and language recovery in severe aphasia. *Journal of Speech and Hearing Research,* 1970, *13,* 607–623.

Schuell, H. A short examination for aphasia. *Neurology,* 1957, *7,* 625–634.

Schuell, H. *The Minnesota test for differential diagnosis of aphasia.* Minneapolis: University of Minnesota Press, 1965.

Schuell, H., Jenkins, J. J., & Jimenez-Pabon, E. *Aphasia in adults.* New York: Harper & Row, 1964.

Schuknecht, H. F. Further observations on the pathology of presbycusis. *Archives of Otolaryngology,* 1964, *80,* 369–382.

Seefeldt, C., Jantz, R. K., Galper, A., & Serock, K. Using pictures to explore children's attitudes toward the elderly. *Gerontologist,* 1977, *17,* 506–512.

Sefer, J. W., & Henrikson, E. H. The relationship between word association and grammatical classes in aphasia. *Journal of Speech and Hearing Research,* 1966, *9,* 529–541.

Smith, A. Objective indices of severity of chronic aphasia in stroke patients. *Journal of Speech and Hearing Disorders,* 1971, *36,* 167–207.

Smith, A. Replies to two comments on "Objective indices of severity of chronic aphasia in stroke patients." *Journal of Speech and Hearing Disorders,* 1972, *37,* 274–278.

Smith, B. J., & Barker, H. R. Influence of a reality orientation training program on the attitudes of trainees toward the elderly. *Gerontologist,* 1972, *12,* 262–264.

Spence, D. L., Feigenbaum, E. M., Fitzgerald, F., & Roth, J. Medical student attitudes toward the geriatric patient. *Journal of the American Geriatrics Society* 1968, *16,* 976–983.

Thomas, E. C., & Yamamoto, K. Attitudes toward age: An exploration of school-age children. *International Journal of Aging and Human Development,* 1975, *6,* 117–129.

Timiras, P. S. Biological perspective on aging. *American Scientist,* 1978, *66,* 605–613.

Van Riper, C. *The treatment of stuttering.* Englewood Cliffs, N. J.: Prentice-Hall, 1973.

Vignolo, L. A. Evolution of aphasia and language rehabilitation: A retrospective exploratory study. *Cortex*, 1964, *1*, 344−367.

Weisenburg, T. H. A study of aphasia. *Archives of Neurology and Psychiatry*, 1934, *31*, 1−33.

Weiss, H. D. Neoplasms. In M. A. Samuels (Ed.), *Manual of neurologic therapeutics*. Boston: Little, Brown & Co., 1978.

Wepman, J. M. *Recovery from aphasia*. New York: Ronald Press, 1951.

Wepman, J. M., & Jones, L. V. *Studies in aphasia: An approach to testing*. Chicago: University of Chicago Education−Industry Service, 1961.

Wertz, R. T. Neuropathologies of speech and language: An introduction to patient management. In D. F. Johns (Ed.), *Clinical management of neurogenic communicative disorders*. Boston: Little, Brown & Co., 1978.

Wetherick, N. E. Changing an established concept: A comparison of the ability of young, middle-aged and old subjects. *Gerontologia*, 1965, *11*, 82−95.

Whitbourne, S. K. Test anxiety in elderly and young adults. *International Journal of Aging and Human Development*, 1976, *7*, 201−210.

Wilensky, H., & Barmack, J. Interests of doctoral students in clinical psychology in work with older adults. *Journal of Gerontology*, 1966, *21*, 410−414.

Elizabeth J. Webster
Marilyn Newhoff

13

Intervention with Families of Communicatively Impaired Adults

Rehabilitation specialists have recognized that the onset of a communication impairment in adulthood constitutes a crisis not only for the affected person but also for his or her family. Björn-Hansen (1957), Locke (1966), Farrell (1969), and Braconier (1974) pointed out numerous ways in which family life simply is not the same as it was prior to the traumatic event. In the postonset period all members of a family must cope with altered life styles. The amount and type of subsequent family disorganization will vary, of course, but some disruption is inevitable. Further, a client's family members are able to promote or seriously impede client progress. For example, Wepman (1951) cited contrasting cases of deleterious interference and of helpful cooperation of families of aphasic patients.

Because communicative impairments affect entire families and family members in turn influence rehabilitation efforts, family intervention should be an integral part of therapy for all adult clients. In this chapter a rationale is presented for viewing all communication impairments acquired in adulthood as family problems. Communication disorders specialists who have been trained to deal with family communication problems have employed various family intervention models, and several of these will be reviewed. Finally, we shall suggest directions for needed research in the area of family intervention.

THE FAMILY UNIT AND FAMILY HOMEOSTASIS

Family size, of course, varies from the single-parent unit to the extended family. Many families are what Rosow (1965) called "intergenerational" ones; that is, they are comprised of two or more generations who live in the same household or in close proximity. Today in the United States the number of intergenerational families may be increasing at a faster rate than at any time during the present century. There are two reasons for this: (1) the high rate of divorce, and (2) the fact that people are living longer. When a couple is divorced, it is common for one of the former partners to return to his or her original family, often accompanied by children. Further, as people age, they tend to want to live with or near their children (Butler, 1978; Schow, Christiansen, Hutchinson, & Nerbonne, 1978). Thus a family unit often includes members of more than one generation.

Whatever its size and composition, a family must be understood to function as a unique, cohesive, and delicately balanced unit. Each family member learns to fulfill a role that is constructed to complement the roles of other family members (Satir, 1967). In this way the entire unit is balanced and stable. Satir viewed a family's sense of being in balance as analogous to the physiologic state of homeostasis and thus used the term "family homeostasis" to refer to such stability. Every part of the unit is dependent on every other part, and this mutual dependence means that anything that changes one segment changes the whole unit. Consequently, the entire family is affected by changes that accompany the aging process.

As in the physiologic state, a family's homeostasis is transient; it can easily be disrupted. All types of events, even those that appear minor to the outer world, can seriously undermine a family's sense of well being. Satir noted that when family homeostasis is threatened, family members experience great anxiety. They then may try in ways that seem unproductive to regain their sense of well being. For example, a man in his midforties established his own retail business. Whereas his former employment had permitted him to arrive home in time for dinner each evening, his new responsibilities prevented his keeping regular hours and for a period of time he seldom spent an evening with his wife. During this period the wife developed severe and debilitating headaches. Her condition so frightened the husband that he began to close his store early in order to spend evenings with her. His business suffered, but his wife's headaches disappeared. Assuming that this woman's headaches were related to disruption of her sense of family homeostasis, it must also be assumed that neither she nor her husband were necessarily aware of this relationship.

The roles that are necessary to maintain a family's stability may be openly stated and understood by those who fulfill them, or such roles may only be inferred from the way family members behave. For example, in one family the grandfather is referred to as "the one who knows about history," whereas in another family he is not so labeled but he emerges as the one who is asked the questions about history. Satir (1967) noted that often one is unaware of the role one fulfills, as exemplified by the grandfather in the latter situation. Satir also suggested that once a person's familial role has been defined, he or she tends to be perceived in that light by all other family members and to behave accordingly. However, it is likely that a person's role is viewed differently by different family members. For example, a mother may be perceived in one way by her daughter and in another way by her husband.

A family-assigned role may have the desired effect of insuring family stability while at the same time having negative consequences for the person fulfilling the role (Meissner, 1964). The reader may think of numerous examples of stultifying role

assignments: young adults who are in college because their families want them to be, or older adults who pursue careers they no longer like and would not choose to continue except for their families' needs and expectations.

However negative the consequences of family-role assignment may be, family stability is threatened when a member tries to change his or her role. For example, when a woman who has stayed at home as a housewife and mother decides to work outside the home, it can temporarily disrupt other family members until they learn to adjust to the woman's new role. Likewise when the child who has been defiant and troublesome becomes helpful and considerate, the shift may be viewed with suspicion because no one is prepared for it. In either case the family's immediate wish is to return to the familiar, safe patterns.

As an extreme example of negative consequences of family-role assignment, Satir described families in which one member with a problem or disability was labeled as the "identified patient," that is, the sick or disabled family member. Similarly, Haspiel, Clement, and Haspiel (1972) and Taylor (1976) commented on the tendency in families to use their communicatively impaired members as scapegoats. This identified patient or scapegoat gives others a place to project family stress and/or blame for many of the family's failures. When the role of scapegoat or identified patient is essential to a unit's homeostasis, it may be impossible for other family members to participate in helping the impaired person to improve.

Fortunately not all families will need to identify one member as patient or scapegoat. All family members will have assigned roles, however, and these will influence the clinician's choices in both treatment for the patient and type of intervention for others within the family. This is the case because each family member communicates from the standpoint of his or her role. These previously learned roles, and the communication patterns that arise from them, provided security for the family in the past and thus were well rehearsed long before the communication disorder began. For example, if a husband who felt comfortable in the role of the relatively uncommunicative but stable provider for his family underwent the dramatic role change required when he suddenly became incapacitated, the shift would produce great anxiety in him and in members of his family, who also had adjusted to his former role (Rogers, 1972; Raymond, Slaby & Lieb, 1975).

In order to maintain stability, families develop rigid rules governing intrafamily communication: One does not shout after father comes home, one always speaks respectfully to one's elders, or one does not tell mother what to do. It is important that communication disorders specialists try to understand the unique communication rules of each adult client's family because these rules were in effect prior to the onset of a disability and are the ones with which a family feels most comfortable. Rehabilitation activities must be in accord with the family's communicative limits if such activities are to be continued at home.

THE CHANGING NATURE OF FAMILY COMMUNICATION

Within the constraints imposed by a family's need for stability, its communication patterns are likely to change as family members age (Riley & Foner, 1968). Change in family personnel due to births, deaths, and family mobility often result in at least temporary lack of homeostasis. Roles may have to be shifted somewhat and patterns of communication modified before the family can return to a stable state (Deutscher, 1964; Rollins & Feldman, 1970).

The aging process in family members is an extremely important variable in altering familial communication. Aging people are less likely to be caught up in establishing careers or planning for the future than they were earlier (Kuhlen, 1964; Kuhlen & Johnson, 1952). Therefore they become less inclined to talk at length about future aspirations. Likewise older people may more often talk about the past (Butler, 1978).

Jung (1971) thought that as people age they become more introspective and thus feel more concern about the meanings of events. In keeping with their more introspective pattern they may arrive at conclusions or suggest solutions more slowly than do younger people. Introspection is not abnormal behavior, but rather, as Jung noted, it signals a shift in attitudes about what the older person considers important. Such attitudinal change will be reflected in communication and must be accommodated within families (Spark & Brody, 1972). For example, an older family member may be more interested in discussing a situation at length than is a less reflective younger member.

Many older people report that they have a smaller circle of close friends than they did when they were younger, that they value their family and close friends more, and that they are less interested in trying to make new friends than they once were (Schow et al., 1978). Kuhlen (1964) and Kimmel (1974) noted that any such contraction in one's life-style will influence one's conversation. For example, older persons within a family may view the family both as their chief communicative outlet and as their chief topic of conversation.

Erickson (1950; 1968) postulated three stages in adult psychosocial development that influence how people adjust to and communicate with their families. Erickson thought that a crucial choice must be made within each of these stages of adulthood and that how well one chooses determines how well one will be equipped to deal with the next stage. In young adulthood the task is to develop intimacy as opposed to isolation. The ability to develop intimacy can lead to ability to adapt in later life (Lowenthal & Haven, 1968). In the middle years the choice is between what Erickson called generativity, that is, meaningful and productive activity, and its opposite, termed stagnation. A symptom of stagnation may be, for example, the persistent feeling that one is working hard at a task that is meaningless in the long term. Erickson believed that in the final stage of life the task is to develop a greater feeling of integrity and thus diminish the feelings of despair and disgust that Neugarten (1964) noted as fairly prevalent in later life.

It seems reasonable to assume that as a family ages some of its members may experience identity crises such as Erickson postulated. The period of life will certainly influence how older family members communicate. For example, Maddox (1978) thought that during these periods of crisis, aging people may communicate primarily in terms of their confusion, loss, and anger. On the other hand, Maddox cited evidence that older people who feel satisfied with their earlier social relationships and work are likely to report greater satisfaction in later life than do people who found their earlier lives less nourishing. Further, Butler (1978) stated that people who have experienced such earlier satisfactions are less subject to the depression that may accompany aging.

However, the differences in interests, concerns, and points of view between younger and older family members may strain intrafamily communication. Thus a family may experience problems in its communication prior to the onset of a communicative impairment in one of its members. Whether or not severe communication difficulties have existed, no two families will have identical communicative patterns. Communication in a household made up of older adults will be different from that of one populated by younger members, and both will differ from an intergenerational family.

CONSIDERATIONS FOR INTERVENTION

Effective family intervention depends in part on determining, as well as possible, (1) the nature of a family's longstanding communicative interaction, and (2) the nature of its communication immediately prior to the onset of the communicative impairment. In the absence of longitudinal studies of familial communication prior to the onset of an impairment, specialists involved in rehabilitation now assess these variables as best they can by administering questionnaires to key family members and by interviewing them (Hatzenbuehler & Webster, 1977). Individual interviews with several family members (Linebaugh & Young-Charles, 1978; Newhoff & Davis, 1978) in which each is asked to describe how people in the family communicated prior to the time one of them acquired an impairment is one way to reveal some of the intrafamily communication patterns (Satir, 1967). Satir further observed that within a group meeting family members quickly revealed their major communication problems.

It is essential for several reasons that communication disorders specialists assess intrafamily communication prior to planning any intervention procedures with clients. First, some of the drills used in speech rehabilitation may be meaningless in terms of a client's communication at home, and more meaningful activities might be substituted if the family's patterns were known. Further, communication-disorders specialists are prone to ask significant members of a patient's family to carry out speech and language activities at home. In some cases when the designated trainer tries to condut such activities, it so changes the family role structure that family stability is threatened. Such stress is counterproductive. Other types of tasks given to a family member can create stress if the person does not view such activities as consistent with his or her role. For example, during a group counseling session the wife of an aphasic man asked for suggestions for ways to make it easier to bathe him. She was given several suggestions that she systematically rejected as unworkable. Later she undoubtedly stated her primary problem with bath time when she said angrily, "Wives aren't supposed to have to bathe their husbands anyhow!" Wepman

(1951) stated that perhaps the most important item in a patient's case history is information about his or her role in the family. We are convinced that attempting to understand communication patterns that are essential to a family's stability will assist clinicians both in determining which family members to include in programs of family intervention and what type of intervention to provide.

The fact that individuals are reluctant to modify communication patterns that have seemed to insure family stability limits the amount and type of change that can result from the family intervention programs conducted by communication-disorders specialists. Nevertheless, there is a great deal that these professionals can do for the family faced with a communicatively impaired member.

FAMILY HOMEOSTASIS POSTONSET

Probably every family's communicative patterns undergo several of the aforementioned changes associated with aging. As part of the changing picture, therefore, most people in the family group may adjust very well to the gradual onset of one member's communicative impairment. Family members may, for example, learn to adjust their speech patterns to grandfather's deteriorating ability to hear. Often people do not realize that they have been compensating for some time for such a slowly developing impairment. In these cases, family stability remains intact.

Such adjustment is impossible with the sudden onset of a disability. The dramatic acquisition of an impairment will inevitably disrupt a family's communicative relationships and thus its homeostatic balance. Family distress is particularly acute if the communicative disability is acquired within the context of a life-threatening condition. It is traumatizing to know that a loved one must undergo removal of the larynx because of carcinoma or to witness the life and death struggle of one who has a stroke. McBride (1969) and Buck (1968) have provided personal accounts of the crisis induced by a person's stroke. Such accounts reveal agonizing emotional turmoil both to the affected individuals and to their families. Similar experiences of crisis were reported through the interviews with wives of stroke victims conducted by Malone (1969). Clinicians who understand that the sudden onset of a communication impairment produces severe family strain and disruption will not be surprised when both clients and their families exhibit reactions long after the acute crisis has passed.

STAGES IN THE REACTION TO CRISIS

Shontz (1965) postulated that when one experiences a major crisis one's reaction to it proceeds through various stages that can be described as shock, realization, retreat, and acknowledgment. Some people experience all four stages, others may go through the first two and seem to become fixed in retreat, while others seem to skip the retreat phase and move directly into acknowledgment. Although these phases are only postulated and can only be inferred, they suggest behaviors that communication-disorders specialists often see in families of adult clients.

The first stage in the reaction to crisis is shock. It is characterized by numbness, bewilderment, confusion, and a feeling of disbelief. Another symptom is the inability to think clearly. While in the period of shock, family members may be unable to attend to those who provide information and thus may appear later to be uninformed. Studies by Helmick, Watamori, and Palmer (1976) and Linebaugh and Young-Charles (1978) indicated that very frequently spouses of aphasic patients lacked information and failed to understand the severity of their spouses' disabilities. One can speculate that perhaps much of the misunderstood information was supplied during their shock phase when they were least able to make use of it. Haspiel et al. (1972) contended that clinicians cannot expect family members to utilize information given to them in this early period because family members' own needs for support are paramount. Likewise, interview information obtained by Hatzenbuehler and Webster (1977, p. 4) from wives of aphasic men support this contention. One woman reported, "I was told a lot of things I later understood; but early on, it was like the words only came at my face, not into my ears."

The shock period also is a poor time for helping professionals to seek as much cooperation from family members as will be necessary later in the rehabilitation process. Specialists who have developed listening skills, however, can serve family members well during this period by listening to and understanding their messages of distress. As an illustration, the wife of a man who had been struck by lightning said, "First I just wanted someone to sit with me while I cried and wondered how life would go on now that

my handsome husband had lost all his hair, had scars all over his face, and was deaf to boot." The wife of a stroke victim also told of her own needs when she described one of her early experiences:

I think I was a little crazy. Somebody came into Tim's hospital room while he was still unconscious and said she was a speech therapist. I remember telling her I'd forgotten how to talk and she said she'd sit with me instead. I'd like to thank her for that hour when I knew someone was there, but if I ever seen her again I probably won't recognize her.

Men also suffer. A husband reported,

Right after Nancy (his wife) had her stroke I started having horrible dreams. They were so bad I was afraid to go to sleep at night. My kids tried to cheer me up by telling me to forget them. One night when I was dreading leaving the hospital, this young intern came in to check on Nancy. All of a sudden I heard myself telling him about my awful dreams. Believe me, I didn't plan that conversation, but I guess I needed to tell somebody.

In the period of shock family members may thus exhibit symptoms of anxiety, disorientation, and disbelief that this crisis is really happening. To the extent that helping professionals can intervene early to offer support, a family member is more likely to trust them and to cooperate with them more fully in later rehabilitation.

Shock is followed by the period of realization. Whereas there has previously been shock, there is now recognition of the enormity of the problem. Such awareness produces great anxiety. In the case of families of communicatively impaired adults, the future may loom bleak and frightening because stability-insuring family roles are no longer applicable. In this stage of panic the desire is to regain equilibrium. A family therefore may shop frantically for a cure that will return the individual, and thus the family, to the former unimpaired state.

Realization often leads to retreat. In the retreat phase the situation is seen as overwhelming. Here again anxiety creates a desire to escape. One's tendency now is to want others to take over the case so that one need not further change one's lifestyle. For example, a wife's stance may be that she can do nothing to help her husband communicate more adequately and she may view the speech clinician as the only one able to effect such change. In this phase there may again be denial of the severity of an impairment. Shontz (1965) postulated that retreat is a normal reaction to realization; that is, faced with overwhelming future tasks, the desire is to run away. Communication-disorders specialists need to be aware that this is a frequently occurring stage in familial reaction to crisis. In the retreat stage family members will not be able to carry out home-training activities. At this time specialists can help family members by encouraging their involvement in selected aspects of the impaired person's program and by reinforcing even limited participation. As family members begin to feel they are helping, they can move through the retreat phase (Simmons-Martin, 1976).

The final stage of reaction is what Shontz (1965) termed acknowledgment. The person now has adjusted to the reality of the situation well enough to participate cooperatively in the rehabilitation process. Shontz's term "acknowledgment" recognizes that a person can become reconciled to having a communicatively impaired family member without welcoming the situation. Family members may still feel grief, or what Simmons-Martin termed "mourning," for the person who once was. However, a person at this stage can be counted on to carry out home speech and language activities, to carefully follow professionals' instructions, and to participate productively in rehabilitation.

Professionals cannot predict how long it will take members of a family to recover from the crisis of the sudden onset of a communication impairment, and probably individuals do so at different rates. According to Shontz's postulates, however, prior to family members' arrival at the stage of acknowledgment, they will need so much support for themselves that they cannot cooperate fully in rehabilitation programs. As family members become more adjusted to their new lifestyles they also become more active members of rehabilitation teams.

Figure 13-1 is based on Schontz's postulates, presenting them in relation to family members' reactions to the sudden onset of a relative's disability. It is hypothesized that such feelings as anxiety and helplessness would be overwhelming during certain phases and more within normal limits during other periods. A marked increase or decrease in these emotions is likely to have an impact on behavior. Figure 13-1 thus suggests that there will be variability in such behaviors as denial of the disorder's severity, understanding and use of information, and participation in rehabilitation activities.

MODELS OF FAMILY INTERVENTION

The primary goal of intervention programs should be that of helping families to regain stability in their functioning. There are many routes to this goal, and several of these are discussed in this section. Although a family's posttrauma homeostatic state will not be the same as that experienced prior to the communicative impairment, a new sense of stability and equilibrium can be acquired. Factors to be considered in helping families regain balance have emerged from research. For example, Helmick et al. (1976) and Linebaugh and Young-Charles (1978) highlighted families' needs for information, and Gardner (1966) and Malone (1969) showed that families may need to talk about attitudes and emotions arising from their relatives' disabilities.

Webster (1977) suggested that there are four functions to be served by those who intervene with families. These are (1) to receive the information that family members wish to share, (2) to give information to family members, (3) to help individuals clarify their ideas, attitudes and emotions, and (4) to provide them with options for changing their behaviors and/or the behaviors of the impaired persons. Some of these functions can also be served by lay people. Close friends can be supportive, and a family may benefit by visits from those who have recovered sufficiently from the same disability to lead productive lives (Gardner, 1966). Such visits, whether by professional or lay persons, are usually informal and unstructured. There are also various social-educational groups, such as a Stroke Club or a Lost Chord Club, with which impaired adults and their families can affiliate. Membership in such groups is to be encouraged. As valuable as they are, however, these affiliations cannot completely substitute for carefully planned and structured family-intervention programs under the auspices of professional practitioners.

Such intervention programs traditionally have included individual conferences with one or more members of a client's family. Programs that have evolved more recently have added group work to supplement individual conferences. Both types of conferencing can be used in family intervention programs because they serve somewhat different purposes.

Individual Counseling

Individual conferences are necessary because the specific needs and symptoms exhibited by each communicatively impaired person are unique. Through individual contacts professionals can both obtain and provide information that is pertinent to a particular family. These conferences also enable professionals to discuss specific treatment plans and give

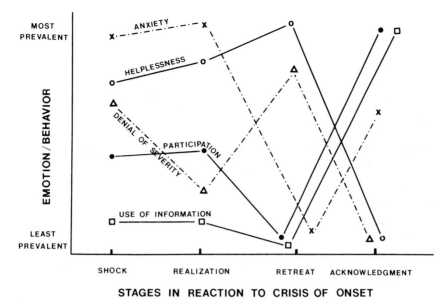

Fig. 13–1. Hypothesized emotions and reactions in relation to sudden onset of a communication impairment in an adult family member, based on Shontz, F. Reactions to crisis. *Volta Review,* 1965, *67,* 364–370.

progress reports (Duffy, 1975). Frequently individual counseling is used with family members prior to involving them in group counseling. For example, Haspiel et al. (1972) noted the need for individual counseling with hearing-impaired adults and their spouses prior to their involvement in group counseling. Individual sessions may also be the most beneficial for family members who are experiencing initial reactions to crisis (Schuell, Jenkins, & Jiminez-Pabón, 1964) because this format gives clinicians the opportunity to listen to one family's signals of distress, frustration, confusion or anger. Through such meetings family members may become increasingly ready to receive pertinent information and a feeling of trust may develop. Following such an initial period of individual counseling it is possible that family members may benefit from shared experiences within a group setting.

Group Counseling

The counselor functions outlined previously also are served as family members participate in sessions that include members of other families. Moreover, there are several advantages for those who participate in group meetings. For example, group sessions can give people an opportunity to question and discuss information that has been given to them. They can also obtain new information from other family members who have experienced similar problems. As an

illustration, one elderly woman who had caretaking responsibilities for her aphasic/hemiparetic sister commented to another group member during one session, "I've read and read and asked a lot of people, but I never found a successful way to help Anna with her bath until you explained how you handled that problem with your husband." In another meeting a man whose hemiplegic wife had just completed a driver-training course provided information about the course to other group members, several of whom had physically handicapped spouses but were unaware that such help was available. Later in the same meeting the married daughter of an aphasic woman spoke of the guilt she would feel if she did not invite her aphasic mother, a widow, to spend each evening with her and her family. Other group members helped her recognize that invitations prompted by guilt rather than by the desire to see her mother would only serve to strain their relationship. At the next group meeting the daughter was jubilant. She reported that only once during the week had she invited her mother for dinner and on that occasion had really enjoyed their interaction. She added that her mother also seemed relieved to have some evenings to herself. The daughter thanked other members of the group for helping her change a pattern that had been extremely troublesome to her.

The authors' experiences with groups of family members of communicatively impaired adults suggest that such group interactions have the potential for helping people to share needed information, to clarify their ideas, attitudes, and emotions, and to explore and experiment with ways to improve communication within their own famlies. Puts-Zwartjes (1973) also noted similar benefits of group experience for family members who face long-term adjustment of their intrafamily communication patterns.

The benefits of including group counseling, however, are not all on the side of families. As professional people observe group interactions they receive information and come to know each family better. Group sessions provide avenues to greater understanding of a family's pretrauma communicative patterns, thus enabling the specialist to better advise the family regarding their posttrauma communication adjustments. Since the time that Turnblom and Myers (1952) described a program that included discussion groups, many clinicians have used various formats to achieve one or more of the aforementioned benefits.

Derman and Manaster (1967) described a counseling program for relatives of aphasics. Housed in a rehabilitation hospital, it was conducted by a speech pathologist and a social worker. Group meetings enabled these professionals to provide information about the hospital and its programs as well as to obtain information about patients and their families. Group members were also able to discuss family problems and receive help with these problems. Derman and Manaster regarded this program as successful not only in giving help to families but also in improving hospital–community relations.

The group conducted by Porter and Dabul (1977) also met in a hospital setting and involved the disciplines of social work and speech pathology. Group members were wives of aphasic patients. Porter and Dabul designed group meetings for therapeutic purposes and centered discussions around the principles of transactional analysis (Harris, 1967). From analysis of themes discussed by a wife, the clinicians pointed out instances when either she or her husband had played parent, adult, or child roles. The authors reported that these sessions enabled wives to recognize these roles, to help their husbands function more consistently in the adult state, and to give their spouses cues that led them to use more propositional speech.

In a different vein, Goodkin, Diller, and Shah (1973) trained spouses of aphasic patients to serve as supplemental speech clinicians. Goodkin et al. devised a system for analyzing, from a conversational sample, the speech of both the aphasic member and the spouse. Target verbal behaviors were subsequently determined from the sample. Spouses were then taught basic principles of behavior modification and instructed to use these with their spouses at home. Results indicated significant gains in the functional communication of the aphasic partners. Goodkin et al. noted that a secondary but important advantage of their program was that the partners spent more time together during the training period.

The family counseling program discussed by Newhoff and Davis (1978) was based on the intervention model discussed by Webster (1977). The group leader was a speech pathologist experienced in counseling techniques. The group held six consecutive weekly sessions of 1 hour each during each semester that aphasic adults were enrolled for therapy in a university speech and hearing clinic. The family member who interacted most regularly with the patient was encouraged to attend all six sessions. The majority of the participants were patients' spouses, but adult children or other relatives were included in many groups.

Participants offered suggestions and support that may have helped others adjust to their aphasic relatives. They also had opportunities to express their emotions. Likewise these meetings provided the leader with a vehicle for transmitting information to family members and for assessing their understanding of such information. The leader also helped participants sort out and understand their ideas and attitudes about aphasia and the particular symptoms evidenced by their family members. Finally, the group meetings were used to help participants experiment with ways of changing their own behavior and/or that of the aphasic.

Based on their research with members of this group, Newhoff and Davis (1978) reported that although family members needed basic information regarding the causes and characteristics of cerebrovascular accidents and aphasia, this need was not primary. Family members expressed a greater desire to relate with caring professionals who would listen to them, understand their feelings, and give them support. As one spouse put it, "I don't care *how* he got that way or *why*, I want someone to understand how lost I feel now" (Newhoff & Davis, 1978, p. 324). The findings of Linebaugh and Young-Charles (1978) support those findings of Newhoff and Davis. Specifically, Linebaugh and Young-Charles reported that most of the family members with whom they worked did not find reading materials concerning stroke and aphasia to be adequate as support mechanisms. More importantly, once family members indicated they had a sufficient knowledge of aphasia, the majority reported a continued need for counseling. It appears, therefore, that knowledge about a patient's condition and the problems associated with it is not sufficient to aid family members in coping with their many problems. Rather, family members need continued support and guidance in clarifying their attitudes and feelings regarding their present life situation. As Newhoff and Davis (1978) pointed out, the need for exchanging information may be met early in the counseling experience. As counseling progresses the needs of the group seem to dictate that group discussions will focus on clarification of ideas, attitudes, and emotions and on suggestions for changing behavior. Thus, although a group such as that described by Newhoff and Davis is not designed to be primarily a psychotherapeutic one, it is thought to have psychotherapeutic benefits.

Haspiel et al. (1972) reported on their program of involving hearing impaired adults and their spouses in an intensive counseling experience. Counseling sessions were held for two or three consecutive days and occurred several times a year. The group met within the Veterans Administration Hospital where the hearing impaired spouse had been diagnosed and, when appropriate, fitted with a hearing aid and oriented to its use. All new patients were recommended for enrollment. Couples who had attended previous sessions were invited to return as space permitted, and Haspiel et al. reported that many of them returned quite regularly.

In this program group sessions were conducted by two audiologists trained in Satir's (1967) principles of family counseling. Under their leadership, discussions were centered around issues in intrapartner communication. For example, the authors noted that very often a spouse tended to blame the partner who had recently acquired a hearing impairment for all the difficulties between them or for longstanding and persistent communication problems. Such attitudes and behaviors were confronted by the leaders and explored by members of the group.

In summary, this review of intervention programs shows that they vary in purpose, scope, and intensity. Some programs are primarily geared toward the exchange of information whereas others seek to effect behavior change as well as to inform. Evidence (Puts-Zwartjes, 1973; Newhoff and Davis, 1978) is beginning to suggest that the latter type have more potential benefits for families. Methods used within a program vary with the orientation and training of professionals responsible for formulating and maintaining it, because clinicians of course choose intervention techniques that are consistent with their previous training and with their assumptions about

the needs of families. Other factors that contribute to a clinician's choice of method include availability of family members, nature of the particular setting, and operating procedures of the clinic in which the family intervention program is housed.

DIRECTIONS FOR FURTHER RESEARCH

There are a multitude of unanswered questions about intervention with families of communicatively impaired adults. These questions are researchable, and we suggest three major areas in which studies are needed.

Needs for Intervention

Previous research has established that communication disorders specialists need to intervene with families in which there is a communicatively impaired adult. In planning intervention programs, it would be helpful to know how to differentiate the families most in need of immediate assistance from those for whom it is less crucial (Hatzenbuehler & Webster, 1977). A related question concerns the amount of assistance that may be required by a particular family. Theoretically, all families should not need the same amount of professional help. It is not yet known how to distinguish the families needing long-term support from those which regain stability with very little help. Likewise it is unclear what variables determine when individual counseling should precede group work. Further, it would be important to know which factors govern the decision to move a family member from individual to group counseling.

Intervention Methods

Future research may show that one or several of the methodologies used by speech, hearing, and language clinicians are superior to others in terms of long-term benefits to families. Or perhaps it will be found that any method must be adapted to accommodate differences in the populations to be served. For example, older family members may respond better than younger ones to certain procedures, or the length of time since onset may be more important than age. Because of role differences that may exist, an adult child or sibling of a communicatively impaired adult may have needs quite unlike those of the client's spouse. As we learn more about specific benefits of different methods of intervention, there will be a great need for further study of how best to train clinicians to use these methods.

Outcomes of Intervention

Before methods can be assessed, clinicians must delineate their goals for family intervention. If the desire is to help family members adjust and clarify their attitudes, instruments should be devised to assess changes during and after intervention, such as those described by Newhoff and Davis (1978). If, however, clinicians wish to help family members modify their behavior, target behaviors must be identified and behavioral measures used to assess change.

In either case it is essential to develop methods for describing the communication between aphasic adults and their family members. This descriptive information will enable both the planning of appropriate intervention strategies and assessment of the effects of various types of intervention. In a preliminary investigation that explored such a descriptive method, Smith (1979) examined communicative interactions of family members meeting in a series of videotaped group discussions conducted by a communication-disorders specialist. Smith classified such variables as types of questions family members asked, types of statements they made, and the relative frequency with which they requested information, provided information, and made suggestions to each other. Harrell (1979) employed the same videotaped source of data to study questions, statements, and suggestions in the communication of the leader of these discussion groups. Both Smith and Harrell reported interjudge agreement ranging from 95 to 100 percent on classifying the aspects of verbal behavior that they studied. Therefore this means for describing communicative interaction is being further developed to study variables observed in both the nonverbal and verbal interaction between aphasic adults and their spouses. Specifically, these authors are comparing videotaped pre- and postintervention interactions between patient and spouse. Comparisons are made on such dimensions as a spouse's initiation of open-ended questions, statements of understanding, and voluntary repetition to assure that the partner understands a verbally expressed item. These projects represent those that must be undertaken in order to determine the value of family intervention programs.

Clinicians who have spearheaded programs in the area of family intervention have not only attempted to serve troubled people but have also pointed the way for a great deal of further study. Communication disorders specialists are in a uniquely favorable position both to intervene with families and to conduct research with them. Clinicians understand that they must retrain impaired adults to communicate within their families. They also know that what happens to other family members during the posttrauma periods will influence every rehabilitation effort. Finally, clinicians are trained to use the method of science in their therapeutic endeavors; that is, they are trained to observe, to describe, to make inferences, and to evaluate. Such training makes the clinician an ideal candidate for conducting the types of clinical research we have outlined.

The task of those who train communication disorders specialists is to include family intervention as an integral part of professional training. Professional specialists who work with communicatively impaired adults will have to interact with their clients' families. Thus they must be taught both how to study the needs of these people and how to meet these needs more adequately.

REFERENCES

Björn-Hansen, V. Social and emotional aspects of aphasia. *Journal of Speech and Hearing Disorders,* 1957, *22,* 53–59.

Buck, M. *Dysphasia: Professional guidance for family and patient.* Englewood Cliffs, N.J.: Prentice-Hall, 1968.

Butler, R. D. Overview on aging. In G. Usdin & C. J. Hofling (Eds.), *Aging: The process and the people.* New York: Brunner/Mazel, 1978.

De Branconier, L. Emotional problems in the aphasic and his environment. *Logopaedie en Foniatrie,* 1972, *44,* 237–242 (Disorders of Speech and Hearing Abstracts, 1974, *614,* 15–16).

Derman, S., & Manaster, H. Family counseling with relatives of aphasic patients at Schwab Rehabilitation Hospital. *ASHA: Journal of the American Speech and Hearing Association,* 1967, *9,* 175–177.

Deutscher, I. The quality of postparental life. *Journal of Marriage and the Family,* 1964, *26,* 263–268.

Duffy, B. J. Medical care of the elderly. In M. G. Spencer & C. J. Door (Eds.), *Understanding aging: A multidisciplinary approach.* New York: Appleton-Century-Crofts, 1975.

Erickson, E. H. *Childhood and society.* New York: W. W. Norton & Co., 1950.

Erickson, E. H. *Identity: Youth and crisis.* New York: W. W. Norton & Co., 1968.

Farrell, B. *Pat and Roald.* New York: Random House, 1969.

Gardner, W. H. Adjustment problems of laryngectomized women. *Archives of Otolaryngology,* 1966, *1,* 57–68.

Goodkin, R., Diller, L., & Shah, N. Training spouses to improve the functional speech of aphasic patients. In B. B. Lahey (Ed.), *The modification of language behaviors.* Springfield, Ill.: Charles C. Thomas Publisher, 1973.

Harrell, R. D. A clinician's communicative behavior with family members of aphasic adults. Unpublished Master's thesis, Memphis State University, 1979.

Harris, T. A. *I'm O.K.—You're O.K.* New York: Harper & Row, 1967.

Haspiel, M., Clement, J. R., & Haspiel, G. S. Aural rehabilitation for hard of hearing adults. San Francisco Veterans Administration Hospital, unpublished manuscript prepared for distribution, 1972.

Hatzenbuehler, R., & Webster, E. Helpful hints for speech pathologists from family members of aphasics. Paper presented at Tennessee Speech and Hearing Association Meeting, Chattanooga, 1977.

Helmick, J. W., Watamori, T. S., & Palmer, J. M. Spouses understanding of the communication disabilities of aphasic patients. *Journal of Speech and Hearing Disorders,* 1976, *41,* 238–243.

Jung, C. G. The stages of life. In J. Campbell (Ed.), *The portable Jung.* New York: Viking Press, 1971.

Kimmel, D. C. *Adulthood and aging.* New York: John Wiley & Sons, 1974.

Kuhlen, R. G., & Johnson, G. H. Change in goals with increasing adult age. *Journal of Consulting Psychology,* 1952, *16,* 1–4.

Kuhlen, R. G. Developmental changes in motivation during the adult years. In J. E. Birner (Ed.), *Relations of development and aging.* Springfield, Ill.: Charles C. Thomas Publisher, 1964.

Larkins, P. G., & Webster, E. J. An analysis of the communicative behavior of aphasic adults and their spouses. Memphis: Memphis State University, in progress.

Linebaugh, C. W., & Young-Charles, H. Y. The counseling needs of the families of aphasic patients. In R. K. Brookshire (Ed.), *Clinical Aphasiology Conference proceedings.* Minneapolis: BRK Publishers, 1978.

Locke, B. Psychology of the laryngectomee. *Military Medicine,* 1966, 593–599.

Lowenthal, M. F., & Haven, C. Interaction and adaptation. Intimacy as a critical variable. *American Sociological Review,* 1968, *33,* 20–30.

Maddox, G. L. The social and cultural context of aging. In G. Usdin & C. J. Hofling (Eds.), *Aging: The process and the people.* New York: Brunner/Mazel, 1978.

Malone, R. L. Expressed attitudes of families of aphasics. *Journal of Speech and Hearing Disorders,* 1969, *34,* 140–150.

McBride, C. *Silent victory.* Chicago: Nebon-Hall, 1969.

Meissner, W. W. Thinking about the family—Psychiatric aspects. *Family Process,* 1964, *3,* 1–40.

Neugarten, B. L., & Associates (Eds.), *Personality in middle and later life.* New York: Atherton, 1964.

Newhoff, M. N., & Davis, G. A. A spouse intervention program: Planning, implementation and problems of evaluation. In R. H. Brookshire (Ed.), *Clinical Aphasiology Conference proceedings.* Minneapolis: BRK Publishers, 1978.

Porter, J. L., & Dabul, B. The application of transactional analysis to therapy with wives of adult aphasic patients. *ASHA: Journal of the American Speech and Hearing Association,* 1977, *19,* 244–248.

Puts-Zwartjes, R. A. Group therapy with the husbands or wives of aphasics. *Logopaedie en Foniatrie,* 1973, *45,* 93–97.

Raymond, M., Slaby, A., & Lieb, J. *The Healing Alliance.* New York: W. W. Norton & Co., 1975.

Riley, N. W., & Foner, A. *Aging and society. Vol. I: An inventory of research findings*. New York: Russell Sage Foundation, 1968.

Rollins, B. C., & Feldman, H. Marital satisfaction over the family life cycle. *Journal of Marriage and the Family, 1970, 32,* 20—28.

Rogers, C. R. *Becoming partners: Marriage and its alternatives*. New York: Delacorte Press, 1972.

Rosow, L. Intergenerational relationships: Problems and proposals. In E. Shancs & G. F. Strieb (Eds.), *Social structure and the family: Generational relations*. Englewood Cliffs, N.J.: Prentice-Hall, 1965.

Satir, V. *Conjoint family therapy*. Palo Alto, Calif.: Science and Behavior Books, 1967.

Schow, R. L., Christiansen, I., Hutchinson, J. M., & Nerbonne, M. A. *Communication disorders of the aged*. Baltimore: University Park Press, 1978.

Schuell, H., Jenkins, J. J., & Jimenez-Pabón, E. *Aphasia in adults: Diagnosis, prognosis and treatment*. New York: Harper & Row, 1964.

Shontz, F. Reactions to crisis. *Volta Review, 1965, 67,* 364—370.

Simmons-Martin, A. A home demonstration approach with hearing impaired children. In E. J. Webster (Ed.), *Professional approaches with parents of handicapped children*. Springfield, Ill.: Charles C. Thomas Publisher, 1976.

Smith, C. L. Families of communicatively impaired adults. Unpublished Master's thesis, Memphis State University, 1979.

Spark, G. M., & Brody, E. M. The aged are family members. In C. J. Sager and H. S. Kaplan (Eds.), *Progress in group and family counseling*. New York: Brunner/Mazel, 1972.

Taylor, F. C. Project cope. In E. J. Webster (Ed.), *Professional approaches with parents of handicapped children*. Springfield, Ill.: Charles C. Thomas Publisher, 1976.

Turnblom, M., & Myers, J. S. A group discussion program with families of aphasic patients. *Journal of Speech and Hearing Disorders, 1952, 17,* 393—396.

Webster, E. J. *Counseling with parents of handicapped children: Guidelines for improving communication*. New York: Grune & Stratton, 1977.

Wepman, J. *Recovery from aphasia*. New York: The Ronald Press, 1951.

Section III

Audiology and the Aging Process

EDITORS' INTRODUCTION

As we age, "normal" changes are to be expected in the human sensory systems. Significant among these changes is that of human hearing. Nadol (Chapter 4) provided a vivid explanation of these expected changes in audition, which collectively have been referred to as "presbycusis," but he cautioned that perhaps our use of the concept of presbycusis heretofore has been far too simplistic, given that we are only now beginning to search adequately for the causes of changes in audition with age.

The first two chapters in Section III reflect the growing commitment by audiologists to achieve a better clinical understanding of changes in audition with age. Orchik (Chapter 14) provides statistical data that emphasize the significant interaction between peripheral hearing loss and age. After a review of the concept of "presbycusis," Orchik discusses audiologic manifestations of the amount and rate of change in audition with age as reflected in data from standard audiometric measurement as well as various special tests, some of which have been developed only within the past few years. Throughout his chapter, Orchik uses research to challenge generalized application of accepted concepts, such as the all-too-common practice of explaining reduced speech discrimination by simply using the term "phonemic regression," which only describes a clinical behavioral pattern observed in a restricted population of

patients. The emphasis, then, by Orchik is that of approaching each older adult as a unique study that, at least based on current data, is not likely to fit into a neat diagnostic package.

Hayes (Chapter 15) carries this theme beyond the peripheral hearing mechanism to the auditory pathways of the central nervous system. Early in the chapter she follows the lead of Denney (Chapter 7) and discusses the research methodologies used in this field of study, and she provides results from investigations using the various methodologies. She reviews newer developments in understanding the changes in the central auditory system with age, such as use of the "peripheral/central ratio," a measure that has led to some clarification of the role of factors other than peripheral hearing loss in accounting for age-related changes in auditory processing.

Both Orchik and Hayes refer to the importance of considering diagnostic results in view of necessary rehabilitation needs. Garstecki (Chapter 16) continues this theme by discussing aural rehabilitation for older adults, an area that, until recently, has received relatively little attention. A particularly unique aspect of this chapter is Garstecki's description of several scales that have been reported to be useful in the aural rehabilitation process. This discussion provides the reader with the opportunity to contrast and compare these various scales, which are likely to become significant measures of progress in aural rehabilitation in the future.

Freeman and Sinclair (Chapter 17) provide an overview of the most popular but likely the least understood rehabilitation area—that of hearing aids. They review certain controversies that have been prominent in recent years in this area, and then provide a discussion of types of aids and the need to fit an aid to the individual, taking into consideration not only the hearing loss per se, but also the patient's socioeconomic status, personal and familial interactions and obligations, and related concerns that were emphasized by Webster and Newhoff (Chapter 13). They emphasize not only the positive aspects of hearing amplification devices but also highlight the problems to be encountered in the evaluation and use of such devices.

Daniel J. Orchik

14

Peripheral Auditory Problems and the Aging Process

The most recent data on the incidence of hearing loss in the United States suggests that approximately 8 million Americans suffer some degree of significant hearing loss, of which approximately 6 million present a bilateral hearing loss (U.S. Public Health Service, 1967). A close examination of the incidence statistics with respect to age reveals some interesting facts. For example, the incidence of hearing loss in individuals 17 years of age or younger is approximately 3.5 per 1000 persons. However, for those 65 years of age and above, the incidence increases to 133 per 1000 persons (U.S. Public Health Service, 1967). Viewed from another perspective, of the 6 million individuals with significant bilateral hearing loss, slightly more than 6 percent are school-age children. In contrast, 80 percent are over the age of 45 years and 55 percent are over 65 years of age (U.S. Public Health Service, 1967). Clearly the majority of hearing-impaired persons are represented by the senior citizen population.

The most common cause of hearing loss in the adult population is presbycusis, or the loss of hearing due to the aging process (Sataloff, 1966). Presbycusis originally was felt to manifest changes primarily in the cochlea, but more recent thinking has suggested that the entire auditory system undergoes a variety of significant changes through the aging process (Schuknecht, 1955).

The high incidence of presbycusis coupled with increased longevity suggests that the magnitude of the problem is likely to increase. It should be clear, then, that an understanding of the auditory problems related to aging is of importance to anyone interested in the diagnosis and rehabilitation of communicative disorders in this population. In this chapter, the focus shall be upon the peripheral auditory problems that result from the aging process. In that the manifestations of peripheral auditory problems cannot be fully appreciated without some understanding of the pathophysiology of presbycusis, a brief review of the degenerative process of the peripheral auditory mechanism will be presented. Some of the unique aspects of the speech discrimination problems of the elderly cannot be appreciated without a discussion of the central auditory deficits presented by this population.

Finally, the ramifications of a hearing loss cannot be isolated from the complicating factors of physical illness, as well as emotional and social problems of aging. In addition to a decline in hearing sensitivity, the elderly person is faced with a number of stressful changes in life including the death of loved ones, increased crime, and economic setbacks (Butler & Lewis, 1973). Certainly the professional interested in the communication problems of the elderly must have an appreciation of the other factors that influence the everyday life-style of the aging client. Economic and social factors may exert significant influence on the degree of hearing handicap as well as the eventual outcome of rehabilitative efforts.

PATHOPHYSIOLOGY

Schuknecht (1955) described two types of changes in the peripheral auditory mechanism related to the aging process. The first is represented by epithelial atrophy, which involves the membranous labyrinth and is similar to the degenerative processes affecting supportive tissues elsewhere in the body. Included are both afferent and efferent fibers along the organ of Corti, observed first at the basal end and spreading toward the apex with advancing age. Schuknecht suggested the onset of sensory presbycusis occurs during middle age and is characterized by a relatively slow progression.

The second degenerative change involves the auditory neurons and is manifested by a descrease in the number of neurons in the eighth nerve as well as reduced second-, third-, and fourth-order neurons in the higher auditory pathway. This neural atrophy is superimposed on the epithelial changes and shows its effects on hearing sensitivity somewhat later (Schuknecht, 1955). However, it has been hypothesized that the neural atrophy accounts for the inordinately reduced speech discrimination to be discussed later. That is, a significant reduction in first-order neurons is required to affect threshold sensitivity, whereas a relatively slight reduction in neurons can influence perception of the complex speech signal (Schuknecht & Woellner, 1955).

Additional changes that have been observed in the auditory system as a function of aging include vascular alterations in the cochlea (Hansen & Riske-Nielsen, 1965) and calcification of the basilar membrane (Hinchcliffe, 1962). Further, the structural changes in the peripheral auditory system tend to be bilaterally symmetrical, although some ear asymmetry has been observed (Hansen & Riske-Nielsen, 1965).

In 1964, Schuknecht expanded on his earlier conceptualization (Schuknecht, 1955) of presbycusic changes in the peripheral auditory system, with the addition of the clinical entities of metabolic and mechanical presbycusis. Metabolic presbycusis, according to Schuknecht (1964), is the result of deficiencies in both the physical and the chemical aspects of energy production, particularly involvement of the stria vascularis, which is important to the maintenance of biochemical and bioelectrical properties of endolymph. Atrophy of the stria vascularis adversely affects these processes and results in a relatively flat hearing-sensitivity loss across all frequencies.

Mechanical presbycusis, on the other hand, is the result of increased stiffness in the basilar membrane, particularly toward the basal end. Consequently, cochlear motion mechanics are disrupted and a gradually sloping high-frequency hearing loss is in evidence. This mechanical change coupled with more recent evidence of spiral-ligament atrophy (Wright & Schuknecht, 1972) has been used to support the concept of an inner ear conductive hearing loss. An air–bone gap may not be present, but the sensitivity loss in mechanical presbycusis is in excess of that to be expected on the basis of hair cell reduction along the organ of Corti.

For an in-depth discussion of the peripheral anatomic changes in the hearing mechanism, the reader is referred to Chapter 4 of this text. From the preceding discussion, however, it should be clear that the effects of age on the auditory system are rather generalized. As will be observed in the following sections of this chapter, the physiologic changes are manifested in a number of ways in the peripheral audiologic test battery.

AUDIOLOGIC MANIFESTATIONS

Characteristically the hearing loss associated with aging, known as presbycusis, has been viewed as a gradually progressive, sensorineural hearing loss. Another unique characteristic of presbycusis has been an excessive reduction in speech discrimination ability in terms of the degree of sensitivity loss. Also considerable variability on the peripheral site-of-lesion auditory test battery has been observed, although less frequently. The manifestations are consistent with the position that the aging process affects each segment of the peripheral auditory system in varying degrees.

Hearing Sensitivity

AMOUNT AND RATE OF CHANGE

A change in hearing sensitivity, as reflected by the pure-tone audiogram, is probably the best known alteration in auditory function associated with the aging process. Bunch (1929, 1931), an early investigator who studied these changes, described a gradually progressive reduction in sensitivity beginning at about age 30. The hearing loss primarily affected frequencies above 1000 Hz and was shown to progress systematically through and beyond age 60. Bunch's original impression has been well documented (Corso, 1963a, 1963b; Glorig & Nixon,

1960; Goetzinger, Proud, Dirks, & Embrey, 1961; Sataloff & Menduke, 1957) and subsequently refined to reflect unique characteristics of the threshold changes (Carhart, 1958; Glorig & Davis, 1961; Rosen, Bergman, Plester, El-Mofty, & Salti, 1962; Rosen, Plester, El-Mofty, & Rosen, 1964).

Sataloff and Menduke (1957) observed little increase in hearing loss in men or women from age 65 through age 90. The hearing loss tended to be bilaterally symmetrical, as only 10 percent of the subjects had an ear difference of 10 dB or more. Sataloff and Menduke speculated that the low correlation between age and degree of hearing loss suggested that the presbycusic process may proceed at a reduced rate of change beyond age 65. A similar observation was made by Melrose, Welsh, and Luterman (1963) in a select group of 62 men between the ages of 74 and 89 years. As a group, these subjects exhibited a gradually sloping, bilaterally symmetrical, sensorineural hearing loss with greater loss in the high frequencies. However, no correlation was found between age and degree of hearing loss. Considerable variability in the form of standard deviations of 15 dB or greater at all frequencies also was observed.

The age-related hearing sensitivity loss has been shown to differ between men and women (Corso, 1963a, 1963b; Glorig & Nixon, 1960; Goetzinger et al., 1961). Using a sample of over 900 subjects, age 18 to 65 years, with relatively negative otologic and noise-exposure histories, Corso (1963a, 1963b) found that a reduction in hearing sensitivity developed in males between the ages of 26 and 32 years and in females at about the age of 37. Although the onset was seen to be more gradual in women, the rate of progression was greater in females, such that by age 51 to 57 years, women exhibited poorer low-frequency hearing than men. At this age the hearing-loss curves for men and women were shown to intersect such that men showed better hearing for the low frequencies whereas women exhibited better high-frequency hearing (see Fig. 14–1).

Sex differences in hearing sensitivity have been further demonstrated for subjects aged 60 through 90 years by Goetzinger and his associates (1961), who examined the hearing sensitivity of 90 men and women equally divided among three age decades (60 to 70, 70 to 80, 80 to 90). The women showed consistently better hearing in the high frequencies whereas the men showed more sensitive hearing in the low frequencies. Further, when thresholds were averaged across test frequencies, right-ear sensitivity was somewhat better than left-ear sensitivity.

Two more recent studies (Milne, 1977a; Milne & Lauder, 1975) have confirmed the impression of earlier investigators regarding the age and sex differences in presbycusis. Milne and Lauder (1975) examined the pure-tone sensitivity of nearly 500 persons between 62 and 90 years of age. Women demonstrated a greater hearing loss at 1000 Hz and below, whereas men exhibited a greater loss at 2000 Hz and above. In a subsequent study (Milne, 1977a), longitudinal data were provided for over 250 of the original subjects of Milne and Lauder (1975) tested at 1-year and 5-year intervals following the initial data collection. Their report represents one of very few documentations of changes in hearing sensitivity over time in the same group of elderly subjects. As a group, these subjects demonstrated increased hearing loss over the 5-year period, including the 70- to 90-year age group. There was an interaction, however, between initial hearing loss and change in threshold over the 5-year period; that is, the greater the initial hearing loss, the less the change in hearing sensitivity over the 5-year period. These data suggest a plateauing effect in the sensitivity change due to aging and indicate that a point may be reached beyond which further hearing loss does not occur.

AIR AND BONE CONDUCTION COMPONENTS

Although the hearing loss related to aging is generally reported to be sensorineural in nature, singular changes in the bone conduction response have been reported and related to the aging process (Carhart, 1958; Melrose et al. 1963). Further, in at least one investigation an age-related conductive component has been reported (Glorig & Davis, 1961).

Carhart (1958) described the Bernero effect, which is manifested by a greater loss by bone conduction than air conduction at 500 Hz. He interpreted this peculiar change in responsivity as a central perceptual disturbance. According to Carhart, the Bernero phenomenon is a condition whereby cortical differentiation of two trains of neural impulses (bone conduction) is more difficult than the differentiation of a single (air conduction) train. Such a condition could only exist at 500 Hz, according to Carhart, and therefore the reduced bone-conduction response at 500 Hz is more likely a reflection of central auditory dysfunction. Less sensitive bone-conduction responses were observed in 20 percent of the cases examined by Melrose and his associates (Melrose et al., 1963). However, the change in bone-conduction sensitivity was hypothesized as being related to alterations in impedance of the skull.

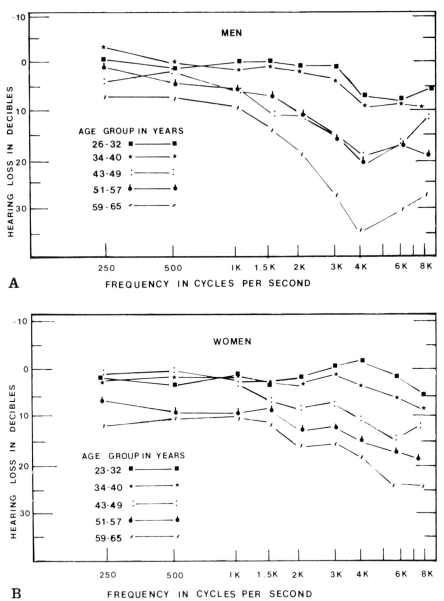

Fig. 14–1. (A) Mean hearing loss for men and women as a function of age. Thresholds are presented in decibels relative to those for the 18- to 24-year-old group. (B) Mean hearing thresholds for women as a function of age. Thresholds are presented in decibels relative to those for the 18- to 24-year-old group. (Reprinted, with permission, from Corso, J. Age and sex differences in pure-tone thresholds. *Archives of Otolaryngology,* 1963, 77, 385–405. Copyright 1963, American Medical Association.)

Glorig and Davis (1961) described a high-frequency air–bone gap that they ascribed to an age-related increase in stiffness of the cochlear partition. The air–bone gap was in evidence at 4000 Hz and increased from 10 dB at 50 years of age to 40 dB by 80 years of age. It was suggested that the age-related air–bone gap might be applied in the identification of noise-induced hearing loss and allow for meaningful correction of compensable hearing losses. Other investigators have demonstrated degenerative changes in the middle ear related to the aging process, although the changes have not been linked specifically to an age-related conductive hearing loss (Belal & Stewart, 1974; Enholm & Belal, 1974).

Nixon, Glorig, and High (1962) also described a high-frequency air−bone gap in 124 men without significant history of noise exposure. The air−bone gap was again in evidence at 4000 Hz. These authors, however, suggested that the conductive component was related to pathologic changes in the connective tissues of the middle ear.

In an examination of approximately 500 men and women, aged 62 to 90 years (Milne, 1977b), air and bone conduction thresholds were compared at 1000 and 4000 Hz. At 1000 Hz, 16 percent of the men and 18 percent of the women demonstrated an air−bone gap greater than 10 dB, whereas at 4000 Hz, 58 percent of the men and 34 percent of the women exhibited a similar air−bone gap. There was no significant correlation between age and the size of the air−bone gap. Milne related the high-frequency air−bone gap to a loss in mechanical activity in the ossicular joints causing a dissipation of primarily high-frequency energy, as previously described by Nixon et al. (1962). Of further interest was the finding that the air−bone gap increased with increasing hearing loss.

The aforementioned age-related changes in hearing sensitivity have been related to a number of factors. Perhaps the most provocative observation was that made by Rosen and his associates (Rosen et al., 1962, 1964) in their examination of hearing in the primitive Mabaan tribe of the Sudan. When compared to the 1954 Wisconsin State Fair data (Glorig, Wheeler, Quiggle, Gungi, & Summerfield, 1957), these men continued to show hearing through their seventies as sensitive as that exhibited by American males in their teens. Based on his findings in the Mabaan tribesmen, Rosen et al. (1962) suggested that the presbycusic changes were related to genetic factors, vascular reactions, and differences in metabolism and nutrition. In addition, Rosen contended that the increased stress and environmental noise associated with modern civilization play a role in the age-related changes in hearing sensitivity.

Speech Discrimination

The reduction in speech discrimination ability related to the aging process has received considerable attention. In fact, next to the changes in hearing sensitivity, the deterioration in speech discrimination is the most commonly recognized characteristic of age-related changes in auditory function.

Gaeth (1948) is generally credited with bringing to light the inordinate reduction in speech discrimination that characterizes the auditory problems manifested by the aging client. Gaeth coined the term *phonemic regression* to describe this clinical phenomenon and the concept has since been expanded on by a number of investigators. Originally, Gaeth suggested that phonemic regression existed concomitantly with sensorineural hearing loss and was more noticeable in individuals with moderate-to-severe hearing loss.

The concept of phonemic regression was supported by the research of Pestalozza and Shore (1955), who studied speech discrimination in a group of subjects over 60 years of age. They demonstrated a reduction in speech discrimination that could not be related to degree of hearing loss or slope of the audiometric configuration. In some subjects speech discrimination was so poor as to affect the intelligibility of spondee words, which in turn resulted in poor pure-tone and speech reception threshold agreement. No correlation was found between the speech discrimination score and the presence or absence of recruitment. Pestalozza and Shore suggested, therefore, that the reduced speech discrimination was related to degenerative changes involving the spiral ganglion cells and fibers of the eighth cranial nerve.

Goetzinger and his associates (1961), using subjects ranging in age from 60 to 90 years, demonstrated a significant age and ear effect for discrimination scores obtained using the CID W-22 word lists. The reduced speech discrimination scores were even more apparent using the more difficult Rush Hughes recording of the PB-50 word lists. This suggested to the authors that the speech discrimination problems in aging were the result of a composite of changes in the auditory system and were not related to degeneration at any single level.

Reduction in speech discrimination scores has been related to the degree of sensorineural hearing loss rather than age by some researchers (Harbert, Young, & Menduke, 1966; Kasden, 1970). Harbert et al. (1966) examined 50 individuals over the age of 60 years who had negative otologic histories and pure sensorineural hearing losses. Although these subjects showed reduced speech discrimination scores for the W-22 word lists, the discrimination scores were more strongly related to degree of hearing loss than to the subject's age.

Kasden (1970) also has questioned the concept of phonemic regression. He suggested that previous studies may have failed to adequately control for the degree of peripheral hearing loss. Using two groups of subjects matched in terms of degree of hearing loss and differing in age, Kasden failed to demonstrate an age-related reduction in speech discrimination.

Rintelmann and Schumaier (1974), however, demonstrated a significant age-related reduction in speech discrimination in subjects over 60 years of age matched in terms of degree of hearing loss with younger hearing-impaired individuals. The results clearly demonstrated a reduction in speech discrimination for the older listeners that could only be explained on the basis of age. Rintelmann suggested that the failure of some researchers to demonstrate similar differences might be related to the speech discrimination test employed. Rintelmann used the Northwestern University Auditory Test No. 6 (NU−6) (Tillman & Carhart, 1966) in contrast to previous investigators, who had used the Central Institute for the Deaf W−22 word lists. Thus Rintelmann contended, as previously suggested by Carhart (1965), that the W−22s do not represent a sufficiently difficult task for separating normal from pathological ears.

An age effect on speech discrimination scores was also demonstrated by Bess and Townsend (1977) using the NU−6. Their data, however, suggested an interaction between age and degree of hearing loss. The speech discrimination scores obtained on 772 ears presenting sensorineural hearing loss were examined with respect to the degree of hearing loss and age of the listener. As shown in Fig. 14−2, subjects with pure-tone averages better than 40 dB (ANSI−69) did not demonstrate any apparent age-related reduction in speech discrimination. However, the age effect became readily apparent for individuals exhibiting a sensorineural hearing loss in excess of 40 dB. Moreover, the age effect apparently increased with the degree of hearing loss; that is, subjects as young as 31 to 50 years with a hearing loss between 60 and 69 dB showed an apparent reduction in speech discrimination ability when compared to the youngest age group with similar hearing loss.

The reduction in speech discrimination associated with the aging process, however, cannot be considered a purely peripheral auditory problem. Sufficient data exist to support the contention that the speech discrimination difficulty is related to a generalized degenerative change in the auditory system including the central auditory nervous system (Bergman, 1971; Jerger & Hayes, 1977; Konkle, Beasley, & Bess, 1977; Orchik & Burgess, 1977).

Bergman (1971) examined the speech discrimination ability of normal hearing adults between the ages of 20 and 79 years using a variety of altered speech tasks. Bergman demonstrated a significant reduction in discrimination ability in the absence of any peripheral sensitivity loss. Konkle et al. (1977)

reached a similar conclusion regarding the age-related change in speech-discrimination ability. Using a time-compressed speech discrimination task, these researchers demonstrated differential effects for age and time compression. Specifically, time-compressed speech discrimination scores showed a consistent decline with increasing age. Moreover, the greater the amount of time compression, the greater was the demonstrated age effect.

The implication of a central auditory aging effect is further supported by the report of Orchik and Burgess (1977), who examined synthetic sentence identification (SSI−ICM) as a function of the age of the listener. Four age groups were examined and all subjects had normal peripheral hearing sensitivity. Listeners in the two oldest age groups (40 to 49 years and 60 years and over) showed a significant reduction in discrimination when the synthetic sentences were presented against a competing message of continuous discourse mixed in the same ear (SSI−ICM). Further, speech discrimination became poorer as the message-to-competition ratio (MCR) became more difficult. This interaction between age and listening condition (MCR) suggested that the common complaint of difficult hearing in noisy environments, which often is made by adult hearing-impaired persons, may represent an interaction between the peripheral hearing loss and a central auditory deficit related to aging.

Jerger and Hayes (1977) have suggested that this central aging effect may be of prognostic value in assessing the possible benefits of amplification and other aspects of aural rehabilitation. They evaluated the peripheral component using performance−intensity (PI) functions generated for phonetically balanced (PB) words and described a possible central component using a performance−intensity function generated for synthetic sentences in the SSI−ICM condition utilizing a 0-dB MCR. Typically the maximum scores of the SSI−ICM function and the PB function are equivalent. What is often found in the aged client, however, is a reduced SSI−ICM maximum in the presence of a normal or near normal PB max. According to the authors, the magnitude of the difference between the SSI−ICM max and the PB max may be useful in helping generate accountable aural rehabilitative recommendations.

The point to be made is that reduced speech discrimination is a pivotal auditory problem associated with aging. Moreover, this well-documented reduction in speech discrimination undoubtedly represents an interaction between changes in the peripheral and central auditory systems.

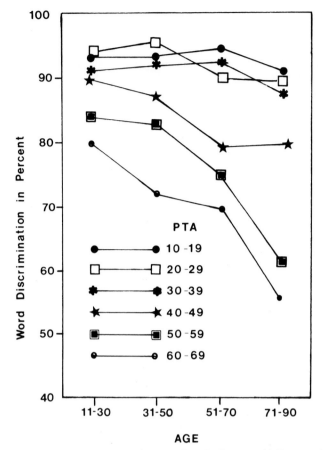

Fig. 14–2. Word discrimination as a function of age for listeners with flat sensorineural hearing loss. (Reprinted, with permission, from Bess, F., & Townsend, T. Word discrimination for listeners with flat sensorineural hearing losses. *Journal of Speech and Hearing Disorders,* 1977, *42,* 232–237.)

Special Auditory Tests

In this section the effects of aging on auditory function as they relate to the so-called special tests of peripheral auditory function shall be reviewed. As suggested by Pestalozza and Shore (1955), perhaps the most apparent indication is that "the usual relationships between auditory tests do not hold true for presbycusics" (p. 1161). Indeed it will become apparent that the presbycusic population exhibits wide variability on most measures designed to identify a site of lesion in the peripheral auditory mechanism. This variability simply reflects the generalized deterioration that characterizes the aging of the auditory system.

Despite the variability, it is felt that a review of the literature will provide at least two valuable insights. First, an understanding of the effects of age on

the special test battery should enable a more informed interpretation of special auditory test results in differential diagnosis. Second, and perhaps more important, the reader will hopefully arrive at the conclusion that more thorough evaluation of the aging client may yield greater understanding of the unique auditory problems confronted by the elderly individual.

In the discussion to follow, measures commonly employed in the peripheral special test battery will be treated individually. In each instance, the pattern of response found in the presbycusic population will be presented as available.

SHORT INCREMENT SENSITIVITY
INDEX (SISI)

The SISI test grew out of the earlier studies of the difference limen (DL) for intensity change (Jerger, 1955). In their original description of the

SISI test, Jerger, Shed and Harford (1959) described presbycusis as a clinical entity in which the SISI score was quite unpredictable. In a group of 34 elderly subjects SISI scores at 1000 Hz and 4000 Hz ranged from 0 percent (consistent with retrocochlear involvement) to 100 percent (consistent with a cochlear disorder). Thus, in presbycusis any level of performance on the SISI test might be expected.

LOUDNESS BALANCING

Recruitment, or an abnormal growth in the loudness function, is a clinical manifestation generally associated with cochlear pathology involving the hair cells. Tests of recruitment generally involve some form of pure-tone loudness-balancing procedure on the part of the subject. The presence of recruitment is generally indicative of cochlear pathology whereas the absence of recruitment is more consistent with neural involvement (Feldman, 1976).

Pestalozza and Shore (1955) evaluated the performance of 24 subjects over the age of 60 years who had sensorineural hearing losses, using the alternate binaural and monaural loudness-balance test. The results indicated considerable variability in performance on the part of the presbycusic subjects with no apparent correlation between the presence of recruitment and the speech discrimination score. On the other hand, Goetzinger et al. (1961) examined the performance of 90 subjects between the ages of 60 and 90 years using a variety of auditory tests including the alternate binaural and monaural loudness-balance tests. Only 27 of 80 men (35 percent) and 7 of 40 women (17 percent) demonstrated complete recruitment.

Harbert et al. (1966) used two monaural loudness-balance tests to assess the incidence of recruitment in 50 subjects over the age of 60 years. Recruitment was found in less than 30 percent of the subjects. The absence of recruitment was often associated with an elevated aural overload threshold, suggesting, according to Harbert, that the cochlear dysfunction in aging may be, at least in part, a mechanical disturbance such as increased stiffness of the basilar membrane.

Thus it can be seen that recruitment is not always manifested in the sensorineural hearing loss associated with aging. The absence of recruitment may be one indicator of a change in cochlear mechanics (Harbert et al., 1966) and is consistent with the changes in the cochlear-stiffness gradient reported by Schuknecht (1964).

AUDITORY ADAPTATION

Auditory adaptation is typically measured in two ways clinically, namely, through tone-decay testing and Bekesy audiometry. The presence of excessive auditory adaptation is generally regarded as a sign of acoustic nerve involvement. Tone decay tests may be of the threshold variety (Carhart, 1957) or may involve a suprathreshold stimulus (Olsen and Noffsinger, 1974; Jerger and Jerger, 1975).

Conventional Békésy audiometry is a patient-controlled threshold task (Jerger, 1960). However, recent modifications of Békésy audiometry use a suprathreshold procedure as well in assessing auditory adaptation (Jerger & Jerger, 1974; Orchik, Dunckel, & Culbertson, 1977).

Goetzinger et al. (1961) used a threshold tone decay procedure in evaluating the performance of subjects between the ages of 60 and 90 years. No significant tone decay was found at any age level. In those few subjects who demonstrated any degree of tone decay, it tended to occur at 2000 Hz. Further, the presence of tone decay appeared to be unrelated to speech discrimination performance in these subjects. Using a suprathreshold task, however, Jerger and Jerger (1975) demonstrated significant tone decay at 4000 Hz in ten patients with presumed cochlear hearing loss. The authors suspected a possible age effect in that six of the ten subjects were over 60 years of age, and the remaining four were between 43 and 59 years of age.

In his classic description of the application of Békésy audiometry in differential diagnosis, Jerger (1960) evaluated the results of 454 clinical cases. One subgroup consisted of 44 presbycusics who typically did not demonstrate significant auditory adaptation. Consistent with the variability found in this population, however, abnormal adaptation was found in isolated cases.

The above findings were supported in a subsequent investigation with older hearing-impaired subjects (Harbert et al., 1966). Using a conventional threshold Békésy procedure, Harbert et al. found abnormal adaptation in very few cases. When it was evident, adaptation tended to increase with increasing frequency. Thus, although not a typical finding, significant auditory adaptation may be evident in presbycusis, particularly in the high frequencies.

PI–PB FUNCTIONS

Jerger and Jerger (1971) have described the clinical utility of PB word functions in diagnostic audiometry, that is, the assessment of speech discrimination as a function of increasing intensity. In differentiating cochlear from eighth-nerve involvement, the phenomenon of *rollover* was of particular significance. Rollover implies a significant reduction in speech discrimination ability at high-intensity levels and is consistent with eighth-nerve dysfunction. The Jergers suggested that significant rollover is rarely found in cases other than eighth-nerve lesions, except in the elderly patient. Interestingly, only 9 of the 741 cases they examined (other than eighth nerve cases) demonstrated significant rollover. Of these 9 subjects, 8 were over 50 years of age, 7 were over 60 years of age, and 6 were over 70 years of age.

Gang (1976) examined the PB functions of 32 men over the age of 60 years who had sensorineural hearing losses. Gang found a strong relationship ($r = 0.83$) between the age of the listener and the amount of rollover, suggesting that the likelihood of eighth-nerve involvement increases with age. Further, because subjects failed to demonstrate any tone decay using a threshold test procedure, it may be contended that identifying eighth-nerve involvement in the elderly subject may be facilitated using a suprathreshold task.

IMPEDANCE AUDIOMETRY

Impedance audiometry has become a standard part of the audiologic battery. Its clinical utility includes applications in identification audiometry as well as differential diagnosis. The standard impedance battery typically includes three measures: tympanometry, static compliance, and acoustic reflex assessment.

Tympanometry represents an assessment of the change in efficiency of the middle ear system as air pressure is varied in the external auditory meatus (Jerger, 1975). The results of tympanometry are plotted graphically and referred to as a tympanogram and can be very useful in assessing middle ear function. Little is known concerning changes in tympanograms that might be related to the aging process. The changes that have been observed appear to interact with changes in the types of middle ear disorder that affect various age groups. That is, in children, a relatively high percentage of tympanograms associated with otitis media are observed, whereas the adult population shows a relatively small incidence of these tympanometric types. In contrast, an increased incidence of tympanogram types associated with ossicular abnormalities (i.e., stapes fixation) is observed with advancing age (Jerger, 1970).

Static compliance involves the measurement of the compliance of the middle ear in its resting or static state by determining the volume of air that has a compliance equivalent to that of the middle ear system (Jerger, 1975). A systematic decline in static compliance with advancing age has been demonstrated (Jerger, Jerger, & Mauldin, 1972). The effect was particularly evident in men, who showed a peak in compliance in the 30- to 39-year age group. In addition, women showed consistently lower static compliance at each age level. Hall (1979) generally confirmed the impression of age and sex differences in static compliance. In a well controlled investigation, Hall found the sex difference in static compliance to be most pronounced between 30 and 60 years of age. Both men and women showed a systematic decline in static compliance beyond age 30, which Hall attributed to changes in middle ear tissue, muscles, and ossicles.

The acoustic reflex threshold is the lowest sound intensity that will elicit a detectable contraction of the stapedius muscle (Jerger et al., 1972). In the normal-hearing population, approximately 95 percent of the acoustic reflex thresholds fall between 70 and 100 dB hearing level (HL) with a mean of approximately 85 dB HL (ANSI−69). A systematic decline in the acoustic reflex threshold with advancing age has been demonstrated (Jepsen, 1963; Jerger et al. 1972). No sex difference has been observed, however, and the age effect is of lesser magnitude than that observed in the static compliance data. Although the shift in acoustic reflex threshold is slight, the clinical impact is considerable.

Jerger, Hayes, and Anthony (1978) have demonstrated that the accuracy of predicting hearing sensitivity using acoustic reflex thresholds for pure tones and white noise is severely reduced in elderly patients. The effect of age upon the acoustic reflex threshold was more closely examined by Jerger et al. (1978). The decline in acoustic reflex threshold was found to be consistent across frequencies for pure-tone stimuli. However, for broad-band noise, the age effect was virtually nonexistent. Jerger et al. hypothesized that the differential effects were produced by increased cochlear distortion products due to aging and evident only in response to high intensity signals.

SUMMARY AND IMPLICATIONS

The effects of the aging process on the peripheral auditory system are considerable. Structural alterations involve both the sensory and neural components of the hearing mechanism and these widespread changes are characterized by a variety of effects on measures of auditory function.

The most apparent peripheral change is a gradually progressive sensorineural hearing loss with high-frequency sensitivity being affected first. The onset typically is during the fourth decade of life (Corso, 1963a, 1963b; Glorig & Davis, 1961) and there is some evidence that the process may be attenuated beyond age 65 (Melrose et al., 1963; Sataloff & Menduke, 1957). The peripheral sensitivity loss differs for men and women in terms of age of onset, rate of progression, and audiometric configuration. More specifically, the age of onset appears to be earlier in men, but the rate of progression appears to be somewhat more rapid in women. In addition, men show a greater hearing loss in the high frequencies, whereas women show a greater low-frequency hearing loss than men (Corso, 1963a, 1963b; Glorig & Nixon, 1960).

An inordinate reduction in speech discrimination is another characteristic audiologic finding. Although generally present regardless of the degree of hearing loss, there appears to be an interaction between age and degree of hearing loss in determining the extent of the speech discrimination loss (Bess & Townsend, 1977). Although the reduction in speech discrimination is at least in part related to central auditory dysfunction, the role of peripheral auditory changes cannot be discounted.

The results of the peripheral special auditory test battery are characterized by considerable variability in the presbycusic population. In measures designed to differentiate cochlear from retrocochlear pathology, findings suggestive of both sites of lesion are likely to be encountered in any group of older subjects. The variability simply reflects the widespread changes that occur within the auditory system as a result of the aging process.

The peripheral auditory changes have implications for diagnostic and rehabilitative audiology. In diagnostic audiology, the variability in test results found in the prebycusic population might be misconstrued as an indication of poor test validity or reliability. This misconception arises, however, from a lack of understanding as to the role of the special auditory test battery. As suggested by Jerger and Jerger (1976), the auditory test battery is designed to be specific as to site of lesion, not type of lesion. In other words, reduced speech discrimination and abnormal adaptation are as consistent with the atrophy found in neural presbycusis as with the presence of an acoustic neuroma. The insightful clinician should view the aged client as one who is likely to present a picture of multiple auditory dysfunction. Thus each presbycusic subject should be approached as a diagnostic challenge to delineate the extent of auditory pathology as it relates to that individual.

Moreover, the application of a differential diagnostic battery should represent more than a mere academic exercise. As suggested by McCandless (1977), the identification of the relative involvement of various parts of the auditory system should have far-reaching implications for aural rehabilitation. It seems reasonable to assume that the prognosis for successful rehabilitation, including but not limited to use of amplification, is in some way related to the relative involvement at various levels of the auditory system. Indeed, Jerger and Hayes (1977) have demonstrated a central aging effect that seems to influence the benefit derived from hearing aid use. Through continued research it should be possible to generate data-based recommendations regarding the aural rehabilitation of the patient with an age-related hearing loss. We can reach this level of competence only through a thorough understanding of the individual audiologic profile of the aging client both in terms of peripheral and central auditory function.

REFERENCES

Belal, A., & Stewart, T. Pathological changes in the middle ear joints. *Annals of Otology, Rhinology, and Laryngology*, 1974, *83*, 159–167.

Bergman, M. Hearing and aging. *Audiology*, 1971, *10*, 169–171.

Bess, F., & Townsend, T. Word discrimination for listeners with flat sensorineural hearing losses. *Journal of Speech and Hearing Disorders*, 1977, *42*, 232–237.

Bunch, C. C. Age variations in auditory acuity. *Archives of Otolaryngology*, 1929, *9*, 625–636.

Bunch, C. C. Further observations on age variations in auditory acuity. *Archives of Otolaryngology*, 1931, *13*, 170–180.

Butler, R., & Lewis, M. *Aging and mental health: Positive psychological approaches*. St. Louis: C. V. Mosby, 1973.

Carhart, R. Clinical determination of abnormal auditory adaptation. *Archives of Otolaryngology*, 1957, *65*, 32−39.

Carhart, R. Peculiarities of auditory function found in conjunction with presbycusis. *Laryngoscope*, 1958, *68*, 253−277.

Carhart, R. Problems in the measurement of speech discrimination. *Archives of Otolaryngology*, 1965, *82*, 253−260.

Corso, J. Age and sex differences in pure-tone thresholds. *Archives of Otolaryngology*, 1963, *77*, 385−405. (a)

Corso, J. Aging and auditory thresholds in men and women. *Archives of Environmental Health*, 1963, *6*, 350−356. (b)

Enholm, B., & Belal, A. Senile changes in the middle ear joints. *Annals of Otology, Rhinology and Laryngology*, 1974, *83*, 49−54.

Feldman, A. Diagnostic audiology. In J. Northern (Ed.), *Hearing disorders*. Boston: Little Brown & Co., 1976.

Gaeth, J. A study of phonemic regression associated with hearing loss. Unpublished doctoral dissertation, Northwestern University, 1948.

Gang, R. The effects of age on the diagnostic utility of the rollover phenomenon. *Journal of Speech and Hearing Disorders*, 1976, *41*, 63−69.

Glorig, A., & Davis, H. Age, noise and hearing loss. *Annals of Otology, Rhinology, and Laryngology*, 1961, *70*, 556−571.

Glorig, A., & Nixon, J. Distribution of hearing loss in various populations. *Annals of Otology, Rhinology, and Laryngology*, 1960, *60*, 407−516.

Glorig, A., Wheeler, R., Quiggle, R., Gungi, W., & Summerfield, A. 1954 Wisconsin State Fair Hearing Survey. *Monograph of the American Academy of Opthalmology and Otolaryngology*, 1957.

Goetzinger, C., Proud, G., Dirks, D., & Embrey, J. Study of hearing in advanced age. *Archives of Otolaryngology*, 1961, *73*, 622−674.

Hall, J. Effects of age and sex on static compliance. *Archives of Otolaryngology*, 1979, *105*, 153−156.

Hansen, C., & Riske-Nielsen, E. Pathological studies in presbycusis. *Archives of Otolaryngology*, 1965, *82*, 115−132.

Harbert, F., Young, I., & Menduke, H. Audiologic findings in presbycusis. *Journal of Auditory Research*, 1966, *6*, 279−312.

Hinchcliffe, R. The anatomical locus of presbycusis. *Journal of Speech and Hearing Disorders*, 1962, *27*, 301−310.

Jepsen, O. Middle-ear muscle reflexes in man. In J. Jerger (Ed.), *Modern developments in audiology*. New York: Academic Press, 1963.

Jerger, J. Differential intensity sensitivity in the ear with loudness recruitment. *Journal of Speech and Hearing Disorders*, 1955, *20*, 183−191.

Jerger, J. Békésy audiometry in the analysis of auditory disorders. *Journal of Speech and Hearing Research*, 1960, *3*, 275−287.

Jerger, J. Clinical experience with impedance audiometry. *Archives of Otolaryngology*, 1970, *92*, 311−324.

Jerger, J. *Handbook of clinical impedance audiometry*. Dobbs Ferry, N.Y.: American Electromedics, 1975.

Jerger, J., & Hayes, D. Diagnostic speech audiometry. *Archives of Otolaryngology*, 1977, *103*, 216−222.

Jerger, J., Hayes, D., & Anthony, L. Effect of age on prediction of sensorineural hearing level from the acoustic reflex. *Archives of Otolaryngology*, 1978, *104*, 393−394.

Jerger, J., Hayes, D., Anthony, L., & Mauldin, L. Factors influencing prediction of hearing level from the acoustic reflex. *Maico Audiological Monograph Series,* 1979, *1.*

Jerger, J., & Jerger, S. Diagnostic significance of PB word functions. *Archives of Otolaryngology,* 1971, *93,* 573−580.

Jerger, J., & Jerger, S. Diagnostic value of Békésy comfortable loudness tracings. *Archives of Otolaryngology,* 1974, *99,* 351−360.

Jerger, J., & Jerger, S. A simplified tone decay test. *Archives of Otolaryngology,* 1975, *101,* 403−407.

Jerger, J., & Jerger, S. Comment on ''The effects of age on the diagnostic utility of the rollover phenomenon.'' *Journal of Speech and Hearing Disorders,* 1976, *41,* 556−557.

Jerger, J., Jerger, S., & Mauldin, L. Impedance audiometry: normal and sensorineural ears. *Archives of Otolaryngology,* 1972, *96,* 513−523.

Jerger, J., Shedd, J., & Harford, E. On the detection of extremely small changes in sound intensity. *Archives of Otolaryngology,* 1959, *69,* 200−211.

Kasden, S. Speech discrimination in two age groups matched for hearing loss. *Journal of Auditory Research,* 1970, *10,* 210−212.

Konkle, D., Beasley, D., & Bess, F. Intelligibility of time-altered speech in relation to chronological age. *Journal of Speech and Hearing Research,* 1977, *20,* 108−115.

McCandless, G. Hearing aids and aging. *Hearing Aid Journal,* 1977, *6,* 44−45.

Melrose, J., Welsh, O., & Luterman, D. Auditory responses in elderly men. *Journal of Gerontology,* 1963, *18,* 267−270.

Milne, J. A longitudinal study of hearing loss in older people. *British Journal of Audiology,* 1977, *11,* 7−18. (a)

Milne, J. The air-bone gap in older people. *British Journal of Audiology,* 1977, *11,* 1−6. (b)

Milne, J., & Lauder, I. Pure tone audiometry in older people. *British Journal of Audiology,* 1975, *9,* 50−58.

Nixon, J., Glorig, A., & High, W. Changes in air and bone conduction thresholds as a function of age. *Journal of Laryngology and Otology,* 1962, *76,* 288−298.

Olsen, W., & Noffsinger, D. Comparison of one new and three old tests of auditory adaptation. *Archives of Otolaryngology,* 1974, *99,* 94−99.

Orchik, D., & Burgess, J. Synthetic sentence identification as a function of the age of the listener. *Journal of the American Audiology Society,* 1977, *3,* 42−46.

Orchik, D., Dunckel, D., & Culbertson, M. Békésy comfortable loudness: supportive case studies. *Journal of Speech and Hearing Disorders,* 1977, *42,* 126−129.

Pestalozza, G., & Shore, I. Clinical evaluation of presbycusis on the basis of different tests of auditory function. *Laryngoscope,* 1955, *65,* 1136−1163.

Rintelmann, W., & Schumaier, D. Five experiments on speech discrimination utilizing CNC monosyllables (N.U. Auditory Test No. 6). Experiment III: Factors affecting speech discrimination in a clinical setting: List equivalence, hearing loss, and phonemic regression. *Journal of Auditory Research,* 1974, *Supplement 2,* 12−15.

Rosen, S., Bergman, M., Plester, D., El-Mofty, A., & Salti, M. Presbycusis: Study of a relatively noise free population in the Sudan. *Annals of Otology, Rhinology and Laryngology,* 1962, *71,* 727−743.

Rosen, S., Plester, D., El-Mofty, A., & Rosen, H. High frequency audiometry in presbycusis. *Archives of Otolaryngology,* 1964, *79,* 18−32.

Sataloff, J. *Hearing loss.* Philadelphia: J. B. Lippincott, 1966.

Sataloff, J., & Menduke, H. Presbycusis. *Archives of Otolaryngology,* 1957, *66,* 271−274.

Schuknecht, H. Presbycusis. *Laryngoscope,* 1955, *65,* 202−210.

Schuknecht, H. Further observations on the pathology of presbycusis. *Archives of Otolaryngology,* 1964, *80,* 369−382.

Schuknecht, H., & Woellner, R. An experimental and clinical study of deafness from lesions of the cochlear nerve. *Journal of Laryngology and Otology,* 1955, *69,* 75−97.

Tillman, T., & Carhart, R. An expanded test for speech discrimination utilizing CNC monosyllables (N.U. Auditory Test No. 6). *Technical Report SAM-Tr-66-65,* USAF School of Aerospace Medicine, Brooks Air Force Base, Texas, 1966.

United States Public Health Service, National Center for Health Statistics. Characteristics of persons with impaired hearing in the United States. *Vital and Health Statistics,* 1967.

Wright, J., & Schuknecht, H. Atrophy of the spiral ligament. *Archives of Otolaryngology,* 1972, *96,* 16−21.

Deborah Hayes

15

Central Auditory Problems and the Aging Process

The hearing problems of elderly patients are exceedingly complex. In addition to loss in peripheral sensitivity, there may also be a handicap caused by central auditory aging. The principle effect of peripheral sensitivity loss is a decrease in the ability to hear speech; the usual effect of central auditory aging is a loss in the ability to understand speech, especially in difficult listening situations. Peripheral effects reduce overall speech intensity but central effects restrict overall speech understanding. It is not surprising, then, that the auditory complaint of many elderly patients is "Young people don't talk plainly" or "My grandchildren mumble too much."

In this chapter, techniques for the study of the progression and effects of central auditory aging will be discussed.

STUDY OF CENTRAL AUDITORY AGING

Traditionally, central auditory disorders and their resultant effects have been studied with test batteries designed to evaluate central auditory function at a specific level of performance (Jerger, 1960, 1973b; Jerger & Jerger, 1975; Lynn & Gilroy, 1977). A typical best battery might include measures of neural transmission in the brain-stem pathways, such as auditory brain-stem response (ABR) audiometry (Duane, 1977; Jerger, Mauldin, & Anthony, 1978;

Starr & Achor, 1975), and tests of temporal lobe speech processing, such as a dichotic (simultaneous, noncoherent) listening task (Calearo, 1957; Katz, Basil, & Smith, 1963). While these tests may work well with the young-adult patients on whom they were developed, their usefulness in evaluating central effects resulting from the aging process may be complicated by several factors.

First, central aging effects are diffuse and rarely site-specific. Histopathologic studies have shown age-related changes in both the brain stem and temporal lobe (Bondareff, 1977; Brody, 1955, 1973; Hansen & Reske-Nielsen, 1965; Kirikae, Sato, & Shitara, 1964). These changes affect the central auditory system at various rates and degrees. Traditional tests of central auditory function may be relatively insensitive to this diffuse, non-specific involvement.

Second, the peripheral sensitivity loss accompanying the aging process complicates the administration and interpretation of central auditory tests. Many tests designed to evaluate the central auditory system presume normal sensitivity because central auditory disorders do not produce sensitivity loss per se (Jerger, 1973b). The use of these tests in elderly patients with peripheral hearing loss may be inappropriate (Lynn & Gilroy, 1977).

Finally, it is often difficult to separate purely auditory effects from more general, nonauditory impairments. Aging in the central nervous system may affect intelligence, memory, recall, and learning

257

quite independently of central auditory involvement. Central auditory tests of complex, "sensitized" speech materials may be to a greater or lesser degree contaminated by these age-related, nonauditory effects.

These facts limit the usefulness of traditional central auditory test batteries in the evaluation of central aging effects. Investigators have employed a variety of other research techniques, therefore, for studying the central auditory aging process. Four methods of investigation have proved especially useful for aging research.

One method is histopathologic study of human and animal brains. Investigators may compare specimens from young and old individuals and infer age-related changes, or they may correlate postmortem physical findings with premortem behavioral results. Both methods have been employed in auditory aging research. Kirikae et al. (1964) and Hansen and Reske-Nielsen (1965), for example, demonstrated age-related changes throughout the central auditory system by histopathologic techniques. Hansen and Reske-Nielsen (1965) further correlated results of these studies with premorten audiograms of individual subjects. Investigations of this nature often provide important documentation of anatomic changes related to aging.

A second technique for evaluating age-related effects on central auditory function is cross-sectional analysis. By this technique, the performance of individual subjects of different age-groups is evaluated and age-group comparisons are made. This technique is frequently employed for investigations of the effect of age on speech understanding ability (Bergman, 1971; Bergman, Blumfield, Cascardo, Dash, Levitt, & Marguiles, 1976; Gaeth, 1948; Goetzinger, Proud, Dirks, & Embrey, 1961; Jerger, 1973a; Jerger & Hayes, 1977; Konig, 1969; Konkle, Beasley, & Bess, 1977; Orchik & Burgess, 1977; Pestalozza & Shore, 1955). The early work of Gaeth (1948), Pestalozza and Shore (1955), and Bergman (1971) provided important evidence of a decrease in speech understanding ability with increase in age by this technique. Cross-sectional analysis, then, is a useful research tool for revealing *differences* in auditory performance related to age.

The third technique, longitudinal study, is useful for revealing *changes* in auditory performance related to age. The performance of the same individuals is evaluated at two or more periods in time usually separated by an interval of several years or decades. The same methods and materials of investi-

gation are employed, and changes in performance over time are presumed to reflect aging effects. Longitudinal studies are necessarily more technically difficult than cross-sectional techniques. Both subject and experimenter availability over long periods of time can be troublesome. Nonetheless, these studies often provide information not readily available by other techniques. Bergman et al. (1976), for example, showed that the effect of age on ability to understand speech was only slight in subjects age 30 to 59 years, but considerably more pronounced in subjects age 60 years and older. Bergman and his colleagues tested the same individuals at two different periods in time with an intervening interval of approximately 7 years. Performance of subjects age 59 years and younger did not show a consistent change over time; performance decreased on some tasks but improved on others. Performance of subjects age 60 years and older, however, did show a systematic trend. On all tests, average performance decreased over time. By this longitudinal technique, Bergman et al. showed how the apparent rate of central aging changed (i.e., accelerated) in the seventh decade of life.

A fourth method for studying age-related effects on auditory behavior is to determine in individual subjects that portion of the hearing disorder that can be attributed to peripheral effects and that portion that can be attributed to central effects. Thus, subjects may be classified by their "peripheral/central ratio" rather than by their chronological age. This technique enjoys the theoretical advantage of examining effects on the basis of individual rates of aging rather than assuming consistent and uniform aging effects in similarly aged individuals. Hayes and Jerger (1979a; 1979b) have employed this technique to investigate the effect of central auditory aging on both pure-tone sensitivity and performance with a hearing aid. The peripheral/central ratio technique minimizes variability due to differences in rate of aging by classifying subjects by certain performance indices rather than by chronological age. It allows examination of subtle central effects frequently not revealed by cross-sectional or longitudinal analysis.

These four experimental techniques, histopathologic analysis, cross-sectional and longitudinal study, and the peripheral/central ratio procedure, are all useful in auditory-aging research. The selection of any particular method or procedure must necessarily depend on the underlying research question, the strengths and weaknesses of each procedure in approaching that question, and the resources available to the investigator. In the sections that follow, the contribution of each one of these procedures to the audiologic study of aging will become evident.

PROGRESSION OF CENTRAL AUDITORY AGING

Presence of central auditory aging effects is usually not predictable by chronological age. It is entirely possible to see an 80-year-old patient with no remarkable central aging effects and a 60-year-old patient with a severe central aging handicap. In a very general fashion, however, it is possible to predict the appearance and progression of central auditory aging.

Both histopathologic and behavioral studies suggest that age-related changes in the central auditory system occur as early as the fourth decade of life (Bergman, 1971; Bergman et al., 1976; Bondareff, 1977; Brody, 1955). Histopathologically observed changes include loss in neuronal population and accumulation of lipofuscin, a cytoplasmic material, throughout the central auditory system. Brody (1955), for example, reported a reduction of more than one half in the cells of the superior temporal gyrus (the primary auditory area) over the age range from 20 years to 75 years. Accumulation of lipofuscin in the brain-stem auditory nuclei begins in early middle age. Although its pathologic significance is unknown, it appears to be a reliable index of age-related central nervous system alterability (Bondareff, 1977).

Behavioral studies of "sensitized" (i.e., distorted) speech materials also suggest that central auditory aging begins in the age-decade 40 to 49 years. Using cross-sectional techniques, Bergman (1971) and Orchik and Burgess (1977) found performance decrements for complex speech listening tasks in subjects as young as age 40 years. Bergman (1971) evaluated the performance of subjects ranging in age from 20 to 80 years for a variety of speech materials including unaltered speech, reverberated speech, overlapping speech, and interrupted speech. Performance for all forms of distorted speech started to decrease in the age-decade 40 to 49 years. Performance for unaltered speech did not show substantial decrements until age-decade 70 to 79 years. Orchik and Burgess (1977) demonstrated a similar effect for undistorted sentence materials presented in the presence of speech competition. Three adult age-groups were evaluated; 20 to 25 years, 40 to 49 years, and 60 years and older. For the relatively easier listening

conditions, when the primary sentences were as loud as or louder than the secondary competition, performance of all three age-groups was about the same. As the listening condition became more difficult, performance of the oldest age-group (60 years and older) decreased relative to performance of the two younger age-groups (20 to 25 years, 40 to 49 years). Finally, in the most difficult listening condition, when the secondary competition was considerably louder than the primary sentences, performance of subjects age 40 to 49 years decreased relative to performance of subjects 20 to 25 years. As the listening task became progressively more difficult, performance decrements emerged at younger age-decades. The results of these studies and several other investigations (Gaeth, 1948; Goetzinger et al., 1961; Jerger, 1973a; Jerger & Hayes, 1977; Konig, 1969; Konkle et al., 1977; Pestalozza & Shore, 1955) suggest that central aging effects may be observed in subjects as young as 40 to 49 years if the listening condition is sufficiently difficult. However, the effect of central auditory aging on speech understanding in easy listening conditions is usually not evident until age-decade 60 to 69 years.

The rate of central auditory aging has been demonstrated by both cross-sectional and longitudinal techniques. Konkle et al. (1977) found a difference in performance for time-compressed, monosyllabic words of over 20 percent between subjects whose average age was 57 years and those whose average age was 78 years. The difference in performance between 57-year-old subjects and 21-year-old subjects, however, was less than 20 percent. In other words, performance changed less in the 36-year span from age 21 to 57 years than in the 20-year span from age 57 to 78 years. The longitudinal study of Bergman et al. (1976) also revealed acceleration of central aging effects in subjects age 60 years and older.

Histopathologic and cross-sectional behavioral studies, then, suggest that central auditory aging begins at about age 40 to 49 years. By behavioral techniques, the results are usually observed only by performance decrements for "sensitized" or distorted speech materials. In later age-decades, the effect may be observed on performance for easier, undistorted speech tests. Cross-sectional and longitudinal techniques suggest that central auditory aging progresses slowly until about age 60 years and then increases much more rapidly. In general, it is during the rapidly accelerating period of central auditory aging that its effect on everyday communication becomes apparent. Individual subjects age 60 years and older typically report more difficulty understanding speech, especially in difficult listening conditions, than younger subjects, irrespective of the presence or degree of peripheral sensitivity loss.

EFFECTS OF CENTRAL AUDITORY AGING

The effects of central auditory aging may be observed in all aspects of auditory behavior, from sensitivity to pure-tone signals to success of auditory rehabilitation. The principle effect, however, is loss in the ability to understand speech. Because of the importance of the loss in speech understanding ability and its implications for auditory rehabilitation, investigators have examined this aspect of central auditory aging in considerable detail.

Speech Understanding Ability

UNALTERED SPEECH MATERIALS

The effect of age on the ability to understand speech was first described over 30 years ago. Gaeth (1948) observed a disproportionate loss in intelligibility for "common" words in hearing-impaired subjects age 60 and older. He noted that the phenomenon was most prevalent in subjects with moderate-to-severe hearing losses, but that it was also associated with age. Gaeth's initial, controlled observations of the effect of age on speech understanding ability represent a pioneering contribution to the audiologic study of aging.

In the years immediately following Gaeth's observations, other investigators confirmed and extended his findings (Goetzinger et al., 1961; Konig, 1969; Pestalozza & Shore, 1955). Results of the study by Pestalozza and Shore, for example, showed that performance for monosyllabic phonemically balanced (PB) words for subjects age 60 years and older was 20 percent to 40 percent poorer than performance of subjects age 50 years and younger, in spite of control for degree of sensitivity loss. Pestalozza and Shore concluded that this phenomenon first described by Gaeth and more fully examined in their own investigation was best explained on a "non-peripheral" (i.e., central) basis.

The effects of central aging on speech understanding ability can also be observed with materials other than single words. Jerger and Hayes (1977) compared performance for PB words and for a sentence identification task in the presence of speech competition in 204 patients by age-decade. Figure 15–1 shows the result of this study for the left ear. Although average performance for both sets of materials decreases with increasing age, performance for sentences decreased to a much greater extent than performance for words. In addition, performance for sentences began to decrease slowly at about age 30 to 39 years and much more rapidly at about age 60 to 69 years. In contrast, performance for words did not show systematic decrement until about age 50 to 59 years. Apparently, undistorted PB words were not sufficiently stressful to reveal the effect of central aging until its influence was fairly pronounced. Jerger and Hayes attributed the discrepancy in performance for words and performance for sentences to the "central aging effect." They noted that the effect was similar in both magnitude and direction (performance for sentences poorer than performance for words by 20 percent or more) to the effect observed in younger subjects with documented central auditory lesions. In addition, they observed that no configuration of peripheral hearing loss resulted in the same pattern of speech understanding ability; performance for sentences poorer than performance for words was a uniquely central effect.

It is apparent that the decrease in speech understanding ability with age is not the result of peripheral hearing loss. Researchers have shown that, in spite of rigorous control for sensitivity loss, elderly subjects continue to exhibit a disporportionate loss in speech intelligibility. Jerger (1973a), for example, examined single-word intelligibility as a function of age with hearing loss held constant in over 2000 patients ranging in age from 6 to 89 years. He found that at virtually any level of sensitivity loss, there was a systematic decrease in performance for PB words with increase in age.

Furthermore, the speech intelligibility loss associated with the aging process can be observed irrespective of signal level or speech intensity (Jerger & Hayes, 1977; Konkle et al., 1977). If peripheral sensitivity loss were to alter speech understanding ability substantially by decreasing overall signal level, then speech amplification should overcome this effect. This is not the case, however. Amplifying the speech signal usually does not improve speech understanding ability of the elderly. In fact, in some cases, speech amplification appears to decrease performance. Gang (1976) reported that in some elderly subjects (age 60 years and older) performance for undistorted PB words paradoxically decreased as speech level increased. This phenomenon, termed "rollover," is often observed in younger subjects with eighth nerve or brain-stem auditory dysfunction.

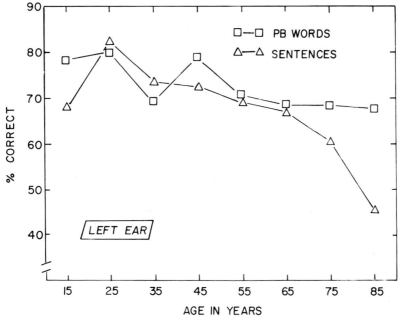

Fig. 15–1. Average performance for PB words and for a sentence identification task by age decade. Although performance for both sets of materials decreases with increasing age, performance for sentences decreases to a much greater extent than performance for words. (Reprinted, with permission, from Jerger, J., & Hayes, D. Diagnostic speech audiometry. *Archives of Otolaryngology*, 1977, *103*, p. 220. Copyright 1977, American Medical Association.)

Similar to the word–sentence discrepancy, then, the performance of elderly subjects for "amplified" speech is often quite similar to the performance of younger subjects with documented central auditory lesions.

Studies of performance for undistorted speech materials effectively rule out a peripheral basis for the speech understanding problems of the elderly. In addition, investigations have confirmed the progression of central auditory aging. For relatively difficult speech materials (sentences in competition) performance decrements appear in the fourth decade of life, increase slowly through the seventh decade, then accelerate much more rapidly. For easier speech materials (words in quiet) performance is not affected until about age 60 to 69 years. Nonetheless, performance for both speech materials is eventually affected by the central aging process, which emphasizes the importance of the effect.

DISTORTED SPEECH MATERIALS

Researchers also have investigated the performance of elderly subjects with distorted or sensitized speech materials. Early work by several Italian investigators (Antonelli, 1970; Calearo, 1957; Calearo &

Lazzaroni, 1957) revealed the effectiveness of distorted speech materials for evaluating central auditory dysfunction. Distorted speech tests, then, are used to investigate in finer detail the central auditory problems of the elderly. Among the most useful materials are temporally degraded speech items, especially interrupted and time-compressed words and sentences.

Calearo and Lazzaroni (1957) were among the first to report that altering speech rate severely affected speech understanding ability in the elderly. They presented simple sentences at approximately two and one half times faster than the normal rate. Young subjects showed no performance decrements in this condition, but elderly subjects exhibited a dramatic decrease in performance.

Bergman (1971) also found deterioration of performance for temporally distorted speech materials in subjects aged 40 to 49 years and older. He studied performance for a number of speech materials, including unaltered, overlapping, and interrupted words and sentences. Performance for all materials decreased as a function of age, but decrements were greatest for interrupted speech. Bergman concluded that the effect of age on speech understanding ability is similar to that of temporal interruption or reduction of speech on-time. As age increases, "time-sampling" of speech by the central auditory system effectively decreases, resulting in dramatic performance breakdowns.

Studies employing temporal distortion other than interruption also reveal severe performance deficits in the elderly. Both Sticht and Gray (1969) and Konkle et al. (1977) have shown this effect on time-compressed, monosyllabic words. In a series of carefully controlled investigations, Konkle and his colleagues observed that intelligibility for time-compressed, monosyllabic words decreased as a function of increasing time compression and age and decreasing sensation level. In spite of strict control for degree of sensitivity loss, the performance of subjects age 54 to 84 years systematically decreased as age increased. These investigators concluded that, "Changes in speech intelligibility associated with the aging process appear to be closely allied to changes in the temporal resolving power of the central auditory processing system." (p. 108).

Studies of performance for distorted speech materials, then, improve definition of the central age effect, more accurately reveal its rate and progression, and even suggest its underlying cause. Further studies of this nature in both young and elderly individuals should yield patterns of speech understanding performance diagnostic of the presence and magnitude of the central aging effect. Indeed, more refined techniques for the evaluation of the speech understanding problems of the elderly are among the most important research frontiers in audiology.

Pure-Tone Sensitivity

In contrast to the dramatic effects of central aging on speech understanding ability, central effects on pure-tone sensitivity are considerably more subtle. Bordley and Haskins (1955) were among the first to describe a central aging effect on pure-tone sensitivity. They assessed sensitivity in "older" subjects by two techniques, conventional behavioral measurement and electrodermal response (EDR) audiometry. In subjects who had been unsuccessful hearing aid users, the EDR audiogram showed substantially better pure-tone sensitivity than did the behavioral audiogram. Bordley and Haskins attributed this discrepancy to "damage to the cerebrum, probably to the cerebral cortex" (p. 382). Shortly thereafter, in an extensive review of literature dealing with the anatomic locus of presbycusis, Hinchcliffe (1962b) concluded that "degenerative changes in the end-

organ are not responsible for threshold shifts in presbycusis" (p. 304). He noted that all sensory systems undergo exponential deterioration with age and that the structure common to all sensory systems is the brain (Hinchcliffe, 1962a).

Hansen and Reske-Nielsen (1965) provided histopathologic support for a centrally based locus of pure-tone sensitivity loss. They reported the histopathologic and behavioral findings in 12 human subjects ranging in age from 60 to 91 years. The audiograms of all 12 subjects showed some degree of high-frequency hearing loss, but considerable variability in the degree of low-frequency hearing loss. In two subjects with substantial low-frequency hearing loss, no degenerative changes of the ganglion cells in the middle and apical coils of the cochlea could be observed. Degeneration throughout the central auditory system, however, was evident.

More recently, Hayes and Jerger (1979a) systematically studied the relationship of central auditory aging to pure-tone sensitivity. They divided elderly subjects (age 60 years and older) into three groups on the basis of their peripheral/central ratio. Figure 15−2 shows the average audiograms of three groups. Above 1000 Hz, all three groups demonstrated equivalent sensitivity loss. Below 1000 Hz, however, group C (central effect) showed considerably poorer low-frequency sensitivity than either group A (peripheral effect) or group B (intermediate effect). In other words, elderly subjects with substantial central effects show considerably poorer low-frequency sensitivity than elderly subjects with peripheral but no measurable central difficulties. Hayes and Jerger could not account for this difference in sensitivity on the basis of middle ear effects. Furthermore, purely peripheral hearing loss did not result in the same "central" speech understanding pattern originally employed to classify the subjects. The investigators concluded that low-frequency sensitivity loss is yet another sign of the central age effect as previously suggested by independent, histopathologic findings (Hansen & Reske-Nielsen, 1965).

Considerable research evidence, then, suggests that central auditory aging can influence pure-tone sensitivity. Although the majority of the well-documented (Pestalozza and Shore, 1955; Goetzinger, et al., 1961; Konig, 1969) sensitivity loss in the aged is the result of peripheral−sensory effects, central influences also are present.

It is important to recognize that the pure-tone audiogram of some elderly subjects may not reflect the true level of peripheral sensitivity. Hearing level

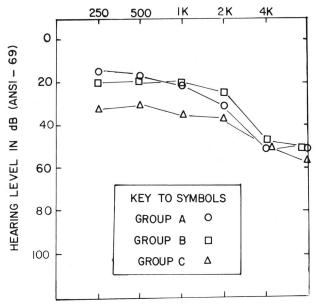

Fig. 15–2. Average audiograms for three groups of elderly subjects categorized by "central aging effect." Elderly subjects with substantial central effects (Group C) show poorer low-frequency sensitivity than elderly subjects with peripheral effects (Group A) or intermediate peripheral–central effects (Group B). (Reprinted, with permission, from Hayes, D., & Jerger, J. Low-frequency hearing loss in presbycusis: A central interpretation. *Archives of Otolaryngology,* 1979, *105,* p. 11. Copyright 1979, American Medical Association.)

may be substantially better than the pure-tone audiogram suggests. It is not surprising that auditory rehabilitation and hearing aid prescription based on pure-tone signals alone have been largely unsuccessful. Indeed, such techniques will predictably lead to overfitting and unsatisfactory hearing aid use by the elderly.

Auditory Rehabilitation

In no single aspect of auditory behavior is the influence of central factors more important than in the auditory rehabilitation of the elderly. The discrepancy between apparent potential and actual benefit from hearing aid use is usually attributed to central effects (Niemeyer, 1968; Jerger & Hayes, 1976). Unfortunately, however, relatively few research investigations have examined thoroughly the influence of central aging on auditory rehabilitation, and our knowledge of its effects is largely intuitive. Recently, however, two reports have appeared that suggest that the central effect in the auditory rehabilitation of the elderly is even more pervasive and deleterious than originally suspected.

Hayes and Jerger (1979b) performed a retrospective study of hearing aid performance in subjects age 60 years and older. They divided these subjects into three groups based on their peripheral/central ratio. They then examined aided speech understanding performance in the three groups. Aided performance was evaluated in the sound field with sentences in the presence of speech competition. Listening conditions ranged from "very easy" (sentences considerably louder than competition) to "very difficult" (competition considerably louder than sentences) (Jerger & Hayes, 1976).

Figure 15–3 summarizes the average aided performance of the three groups plotted relative to the expected performance of young adults with unaided normal hearing (shaded area). In the very easy listening condition, all three groups did quite well. As the listening task became more difficult, however, the three groups diverged. In the "difficult" listening condition, the average score of group A (peripheral effect) was 65 percent; group B (intermediate effect), 50 percent; and group C (central effect), 36 percent. As the central component (as measured by word–sentence discrepancy) increased, performance with a hearing aid systematically decreased.

Hayes and Jerger then studied the relationship

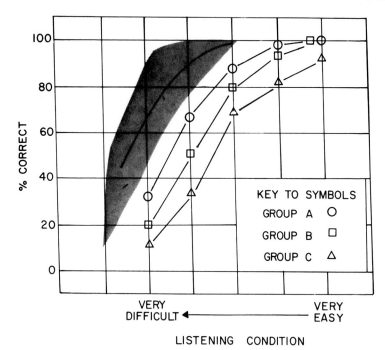

Fig. 15–3. Average aided performance for three groups of elderly subjects divided on the basis of central aging effect. As difficulty of the listening task and central component increase, aided performance decreases.

between the degree of sensitivity loss, the presence of a central component, and aided performance. This comparison resulted in the finding that elderly subjects with central aging effects and only mild sensitivity losses perform substantially more poorly with amplification than elderly subjects with moderate sensitivity losses but no central component. In other words, the presence of central auditory effects limits performance with a hearing aid to a greater extent than the degree of sensitivity loss.

The second study, by McCandless and Parkin (1978), entailed an examination of the relationship between successful hearing aid use and site of lesion. They found that as the site of lesion moved from peripheral to central, successful use of a hearing aid declined. In subjects with conductive hearing loss, success was as high as 94 percent. In subjects with a central site of lesion, the success rate was only 6 percent. Obviously, the successful use of a hearing aid is closely related to the site of the auditory lesion.

To every practicing audiologist, the results of these studies are hardly surprising. What is unexpected is the degree to which central effects limit performance with a hearing aid. The studies by both Hayes and Jerger (1979b) and McCandless and Parkin (1978) suggested that whereas the presence of a

central auditory disorder may not preclude the use of a hearing aid entirely, it will certainly limit expected benefits.

The findings have profound implications on the auditory rehabilitation of the elderly. The traditional formulae for predicting success with a hearing aid, based on degree of sensitivity loss and PB word understanding score, are probably inappropriate. Techniques yielding some measures of central auditory function may provide better prediction of potential for hearing aid use than aided PB word performance scores. Whatever the case, it is evident that successful auditory rehabilitation of the elderly is considerably more complex than simple hearing aid fitting.

COMMENT

Central auditory aging is one of the most serious communication problems of the elderly. It affects all aspects of auditory behavior, from sensitivity to pure-tone signals to performance with a hearing aid. Basically, and most importantly, however, central auditory aging affects the ability to communicate in everyday listening situations.

The recognition and understanding of central age-related effects has increased considerably in the past 30 years. Research efforts utilizing histopathologic study and the peripheral/central ratio as well as the more traditional methodology of cross-sectional and longitudinal analysis have shown the emergence, progression, and effect of central aging on a variety of auditory tasks. Recent studies utilizing sensitized speech materials are especially promising for suggesting possible underlying causes of the phenomenon.

The future for investigations in this area is certainly exciting. Among important research goals are (1) the refinement of methods for determining the relative contribution of both peripheral and central effects to auditory dysfunction in the aged, and (2) the development of techniques of auditory rehabilitation specifically designed for the complex hearing problems of the elderly. The list of potential research projects is virtually endless and represents one of the most challenging research frontiers of audiology.

REFERENCES

Antonelli, A. Sensitized speech tests in aged people. In C. Rojskjaer (Ed.), *Speech audiometry.* Second Danavox Symposium, Odense, Denmark: Danavox, 1970.

Bergman, M. Hearing and aging. *Audiology,* 1971, *10,* 164–171.

Bergman, M., Blumfield, V., Cascardo, D., Dash, B., Levitt, H., & Marguiles, M. Age-related decrement in hearing for speech: Sampling and longitudinal studies. *Journal of Gerontology,* 1976, *31,* 533–538.

Bondareff, W. The neural basis of aging. In J. Birren & K. Schaie (Eds.), *Handbook of the psychology of aging.* New York: Van Nostrand Reinhold Co., 1977.

Bordley, J., & Haskins, H. The role of the cerebrum in hearing. *Annals of Otology, Rhinology and Laryngology,* 1955, *64,* 370–383.

Brody, H. Organization of the cerebral cortex, III: A study of aging in human crebral cortex. *Journal of Comparative Neurology,* 1955, *102,* 511–556.

Brody, H. Aging of the vertebrate brain. In M. Rockstein (Ed.), *Development and aging in the nervous system.* New York: Academic Press, 1973.

Calearo, C. Binaural summation in lesions of the temporal lobe. *Acta Oto-Laryngologica,* 1957, *47,* 392–395.

Calearo, C., & Lazzaroni, A. Speech intelligibility in relation to the speed of the message. *Laryngoscope,* 1957, *67,* 410–419.

Duane, D. A neurologic perspective of central auditory dysfunction. In R. Keith (Ed.), *Central auditory dysfunction.* New York: Grune & Stratton, 1977.

Gaeth, J. A study of phonemic regression in relation to hearing loss. Doctoral dissertation, Northwestern University, 1948.

Gang, R. The effects of age on the diagnostic utility of the rollover phenomenon. *Journal of Speech and Hearing Disorders,* 1976, *41,* 63–69.

Goetzinger, C., Proud, G., Dirks, D., & Embrey, J. A study of hearing in advanced age. *Archives of Otolaryngology,* 1961, *73,* 662–667.

Hansen, C. & Reske-Nielsen, E. Pathological studies in presbycusis: Cochlear and central findings in 12 aged patients. *Archives of Otolaryngology,* 1965, *82,* 115–132.

Hayes, D., & Jerger, J. Low-frequency hearing loss in presbycusis: A central interpretation. *Archives of Otolaryngology,* 1979, *105,* 9–12. (a)

Hayes, D., & Jerger, J. Aging and the use of hearing aids. *Scandinavian Audiology,* 1979, *8,* 33–40. (b)

Hinchcliffe, R. Aging and sensory thresholds. *Journal of Gerontology,* 1962, *17,* 45–50. (a)

Hinchcliffe, R. The anatomical locus of presbycusis. *Journal of Speech and Hearing Disorders,* 1962, *27,* 301–310. (b)

Jerger, J. Observations on auditory behavior in lesions of the central auditory pathways. *Archives of Otolaryngology,* 1960, *71,* 797–806.

Jerger, J. Audiological findings in aging. *Advances in Oto-Rhino-Laryngology,* 1973, *20,* 115–124. (a)

Jerger, J. Diagnostic audiometry. In J. Jerger (Ed.), *Modern developments in audiology* (Vol. 2). New York: Academic Press, 1973. (b)

Jerger, J., & Hayes, D. Hearing aid evaluation: Clinical experience with a new philosophy. *Archives of Otolaryngology,* 1976, *102,* 214−225.

Jerger, J., & Hayes, D. Diagnostic speech audiometry. *Archives of Otolaryngology,* 1977, *103,* 216−222.

Jerger, J., & Jerger, S. Clinical validity of central auditory tests. *Scandinavian Audiology,* 1975, *4,* 147−163.

Jerger, J., Mauldin, L., & Anthony, L. Brain-stem evoked response audiometry. *Audiology and Hearing Education,* 1978, *4,* 17−20; 24.

Katz, J., Basil, R., & Smith, J. A staggered spondaic word test for detecting central auditory lesions. *Annals of Otology, Rhinology and Laryngology,* 1963, *72,* 908−917.

Kirikae, I., Sato, T., & Shitara, T. Study of hearing in advanced age. *Laryngoscope,* 1964, *74,* 205−220.

Konig, E. Audiological tests in presbycusis. *International Audiology,* 1969, *8,* 240−259.

Konkle, D., Beasley, D., & Bess, F. Intelligibility of time-altered speech in relation to chronological aging. *Journal of Speech and Hearing Research,* 1977, *20,* 108−115.

Lynn, G., & Gilroy, J. Evaluation of central auditory dysfunction in patients with neurological disorders. In R. Keith (Ed.,), *Central auditory dysfunction.* New York: Grune & Stratton, 1977.

McCandless, G., & Parkin, J. Hearing aid performance relative to site of lesion. Paper presented at annual meeting of the American Academy of Otolaryngology, Las Vegas, Nev., September 1978.

Niemeyer, W. Problems of auditory prosthetic in age. *Electromedica,* 1968, *4,* 114−117.

Orchik, D., & Burgess, J. Synthetic sentence identification as a function of age of the listener. *Journal of the American Audiology Society,* 1977, *3,* 42−46.

Pestalozza, G., & Shore, I. Clinical evaluation of presbycusis on the basis of different tests of auditory function. *Laryngoscope,* 1955, *65,* 1136−1163.

Starr, A., & Achor, L. Auditory brain-stem response in neurological disease. *Archives of Neurology,* 1975, *32,* 761−768.

Sticht, T., & Gray, B. The intelligibility of time-compressed words as a function of age and hearing loss. *Journal of Speech and Hearing Research,* 1969, *12,* 443−448.

Dean C. Garstecki

16
Aural Rehabilitation for the Aging Adult

Aging is a dynamic series of biologic, social, and psychologic changes. Often these changes are subtle and may be manifested in the elderly adult as minor frustrations or as severe handicaps. Hearing impairment is most notable among the aging adult's handicapping sensory deficits. According to the Senate Committee on Aging ("Senate aging committee," 1968), 30 to 50 percent of the population age 65 and older suffer from a handicapping hearing impairment. Hull and Traynor (1977) report that presbycusis, the syndrome of problems relating to hearing loss due to aging, is present in as many as 60 percent of those age 65 years and older. Estimates of hearing impairment increase up to 90 percent (Chaffee, 1967) among institutionalized elderly adults, who make up approximately 25 to 33 percent of the entire elderly population (Hull & Traynor, 1975; Powers & Powers, 1978). It is also estimated that the number of people in this advanced age category will grow to exceed 30 million in the United States by the year 2000 (Brotman, 1977). The high incidence of hearing impairment in an ever-increasing elderly population suggests that the need for aural rehabilitation services for this group of people will escalate dramatically within the near future.

HEARING-IMPAIRED ELDERLY ADULTS

Most people who acquire a hearing impairment during the normal process of aging gradually adjust and learn to compensate for their loss. Initially, they find it beneficial to increase the volume control on their radio and television set. They may find it useful to have a receiver amplifier installed on their telephone. While they attempt to compensate for their loss through increased volume, they also complain about others not speaking as distinctly as they could. They find that they must ask others to repeat themselves more often. They miss the punch lines in jokes and confuse verbal directions, appointment times, and meeting places. They claim that they can hear, but they cannot understand, especially in noisy situations. They may have tried to use a hearing aid and abandoned it. Their attempts at maintaining auditory communication skills seem to meet with increasing failure. Without family counseling or therapeutic intervention, elderly adults may eventually begin to withdraw from situations in which they are expected to understand spoken messages.

Although similar types of hearing loss may exist among elderly adults, their ability to cope with and compensate for these deficits varies widely among individuals. Some people are more motivated and adept than others at solving problems relating to hearing loss. Harris (1977) classified hearing-impaired adults into three categories according to their level of motivation toward involvement in the rehabilitation process. The least responsible person is the "You-Fix-It" type. This person expects some other person to assume major responsibility for management of his or her problems. The "You-Fix-It" type seeks information, advice, and instruction. However, this person's actual role in the rehabilitation process is largely passive and progress is minimal. One who is interested in improving his or her present condition, but not at the present time, is the "Staller" type. This person wants information for prevention's sake and will collect information that may be of value at some future date. The Staller may make some progress in the rehabilitation process, but it is usually limited. The "Problem-Solver" type is the person who is most motivated toward improvement of his or her existing condition. Problem-Solvers seek, accept, and readily apply information that can assist them in understanding and managing their hearing-related problems and assist others in attaining positive changes. Compared with the other categories described, they make the greatest amount of progress in the shortest period of time. If one considers that these differences in motivation may exist not only within the groups of candidates for a rehabilitation program but also within any one elderly adult at some point in time during the rehabilitation process, then it is less difficult to explain why people with essentially the same chronological age and similar audiologic assessment results cope with their losses so differently. It is important, therefore, to take advantage of opportunities to promote positive action toward self-management of hearing problems.

Success in self-management of problems relating to hearing loss depends somewhat on the adult's ability to overcome hurdles that he or she is likely to meet in the rehabilitation process. Harris (1977) described certain "progressions and detours" that adults encounter in this process. Initially, they must learn to accept the fact that their hearing ability is gradually declining. They must learn to cope with feelings of anger and denial of existence of the problem. They may feel that others are not meeting their communication needs, are mumbling, or are inappropriately insisting that they seek professional assistance for dealing with their problem. Mixed with these emotions are feelings of frustration, embarrassment, depression, and self-pity. Eventually they may find it difficult to enjoy interpersonal communication as they did when their hearing ability was normal. Finally, they may feel that other people are beginning to turn against them. As they contemplate their situation, they may decide either to dwell on their present condition or to take action toward positive changes in their condition.

Once adults are self-motivated to make positive changes, they should be encouraged to follow through. They should see the physician, be fitted with a hearing aid, seek counseling, and take what-

ever steps are necessary to develop an improved self-image, feeling of self-worth, and ability to successfully engage in interpersonal verbal communication. As they begin to take constructive action toward their hearing health and communication problems, positive reinforcement will foster greater self-motivation toward participation in a rehabilitation program where they can begin to learn specific techniques for improving their communication skill. Through training they can begin to appreciate the influence of environmental factors, nonverbal communication cues, verbal cues, and understanding of the logical sequence of everyday conversation on their success in daily communication. They can gain confidence in taking responsibility for increasing the likelihood of successful communication.

EVALUATING THE NEED FOR AURAL REHABILITATION

Aural rehabilitation is the provision of service to hearing-impaired persons, and others concerned with hearing disorders, by appropriately trained professionals. Such service may include, but is not limited to (1) hearing evaluation, (2) hearing aid evaluation and orientation, (3) speech and hearing conservation, (4) assessment and remediation of speech, voice, and language disorders related to hearing impairment, (5) assessment and remediation of auditory, visual, and manual communication and linguistic skills, (6) measurement and modification of room acoustics, and (7) education and counseling of hearing-impaired individuals and significant other persons.

Thus, any elderly adult may find it beneficial to participate in at least some aspect of a rehabilitation program. However, the typical program participant is usually suffering from a hearing handicap. It may be that he has difficulty adjusting to the use of a hearing aid, understanding speech in noise, or coping with the problems relating to hearing loss.

Program participants can be identified in several ways. The elderly adult who is referred to an audiologist for assessment may gravitate to a rehabilitation program as part of the natural sequence of events in comprehensive audiologic care. Major referral sources include physicians, social workers, hearing aid dealers, senior activity center personnel, and representatives of retirement groups and agencies. Administrators, counselors, and activity directors of homes for the aged also are important referral sources. In addition, many elderly adults are self-referred or referred by a family member or close friend. Audiometric screenings conducted at community health fairs also serve to alert elderly adults to the need for professional care and may lead to their participation in a rehabilitation program. A "bridge club" effect often occurs as current program participants inform their families, friends, and relatives and they in turn tell others of the benefits to be derived from such service.

Audiometric Assessment

Once identified as a potential candidate for the program, specific rehabilitation needs must be determined. This may be accomplished by using audiologic–otologic assessment information and the client's own description of the problem. Audiologic assessment data provide information regarding the function of the auditory mechanism. Pure-tone audiometry results are used to describe the type and degree of hearing loss. Although the elderly adult tends to provide reliable pure-tone test data, several problems may be evidenced during the test procedure. The elderly adult is likely to exercise extreme caution in responding to test stimuli, thereby lengthening overall assessment time and increasing the likelihood of fatigue. Another common difficulty encountered in testing under headphone conditions is that elderly adults often demonstrate a high incidence of collapsing ear canals due to earphone pressure on the soft tissue of the pinna (Hull & Traynor, 1975; Zucker & Williams, 1977). The possibility of this occurring should be considered at all times and especially when air conduction test findings are poorer than bone conduction thresholds.

Elderly adults often prefer to use a verbal response instead of raising their finger or pushing a button in pure-tone audiometry. They also are motivated by positive verbal reinforcement. Each of these considerations, when applied, will facilitate the pure-tone assessment procedure, but with an increase in time required for the task. The outcome of the audiologic assessment of the elderly adult is often suggestive of the presence of a bilateral, symmetrical, sensorineural hearing loss with a gradually sloping audiometric configuration revealing a greater pure-tone sensitivity deficit in the higher frequencies.

Speech audiometry should also be incorporated in the audiologic assessment. This may require use of modified procedures for the elderly. As in pure-tone audiometry, responses may be slow and cautiously deliberated, necessitating the use of "live" rather than recorded test stimuli; this will negatively influence test–retest reliability. When confusion is demonstrated in understanding pure-tone test procedures, speech audiometry may precede pure-tone audiometry in the audiologic test battery. Speech reception thresholds should generally be expected to approximate pure-tone averages in the speech frequency range bilaterally. However, suprathreshold speech discrimination scores may be poorer than what might be predicted from pure-tone and speech reception threshold test results, a phenomenon referred to as "phonemic regression" (Gaeth, 1948). This suggests that the elederly adult's auditory deficit may be a complication of peripheral, sensorineural hearing loss along with higher-order auditory dysfunction.

Elderly adults have been noted to demonstrate pronounced deficits in difficult speech discrimination tests even when performing satisfactorily on routine speech discrimination tests (Bergman, Blumenfeld, Cascardo, Dash, Levitt, & Marguilies, 1976; Jerger, 1973). These results are suggestive of the central auditory system deterioration that is suspected in many adults. Findings from SISI, tone-decay, Bekesy, and loudness-balance testing (Martin, 1975) are generally unpatterned in this population, but useful in separating presbycusis from other life-threatening lesions. Impedance audiometry is challenging with the elderly in that structure changes in the pinna that normally occur with aging often result in an unusually large opening to the external auditory meatus. This opening must be sealed for assessment purposes. Once this is accomplished, normative impedance values can be applied to the elderly (Schow, Christenson, Hutchinson, & Nerbonne, 1978).

Because of their characteristic difficulty in understanding speech, compensatory procedures must be considered, the most common of which involves the fitting of a hearing aid. The hearing aid's primary function is to amplify sound and, therefore, in many instances, use of a hearing aid will not prove to enhance speech discrimination ability beyond what might be expected from an improvement in speech reception level. Some elderly adults actually find decreased listening efficiency with the use of a hearing aid.

A second way to compensate for reduced auditory function is through the use of vision. O'Neill (1954) stated that as competing noise levels increased (primary signal audibility decreased), the visual modality played a greater role in an individual's ability to understand speech. Neely (1956) found that auditory speech intelligibility can be improved by 20 percent through the use of visual speech cues. Binnie (1973) suggested that auditory–visual speech perception test scores may indicate how well people will be able to process everyday face-to-face communication. As is commonly known, however, the aging process also imposes a steady decrease in a person's visual efficiency. Schow et al. (1978) report that visual processing among the elderly may be reduced by anatomic changes in the sensory systems that decrease the ability to integrate information within one sense or from several senses. In addition, the elderly adult may demonstrate rigidity in responding and reluctance to alter original visual percepts.

Because of the likelihood of speech discrimination difficulty and limited ability to compensate for this problem through the use of a hearing aid and visual sensory input, the aural rehabilitation diagnostic battery should incorporate measures of ability to discriminate speech of varying linguistic complexity using auditory and auditory–visual sensory input modes in quiet and controlled noise backgrounds. To simulate varying common communication conditions, test stimuli should be presented with and without situational cues. These cues could include auditory background cues (i.e., environmental sounds related to the test stimuli), visual background cues (i.e., environmental scenes related to the test stimuli), and nonverbal cues (i.e., listener facial expression, posture, gestures, etc.). An organizational format for probing speech discrimination ability under varying conditions has been provided by Garstecki (1980). In his Speech Communication Profile, a grid (Fig. 16–1) is used for recording speech discrimination test scores obtained using stimuli of varying linguistic complexity. Results obtained using auditory and combined auditory–visual sensory input channels can easily be compared. Differences obtained in quiet and noise conditions and with and without situational cues can be noted for use in the development of a hierarchy of speech communication remediation goals.

Audiometric measures may be taken under the adult's normal listening mode and aided, if use of an aid is optional or just being considered. All of this information is critical for designing a client-centered rehabilitation program.

Self-assessment

It is also important to elicit the client's self-evaluation of his or her hearing handicap in planning the program. Properly directed, client interviews can yield important information relating to adults' understanding of their hearing impairments, motivation to do something about their problems, and prognosis for improvement. The interview approach is generally determined by the individual examiner. Generally, a nonauthoritarian, structured, open-ended questioning technique will prove to be effective with the elderly. As a group, they like to talk about their health problems with someone they perceive as being genuinely interested in them. The outcome of the interview should tell the examining audiologist what the client views as his or her major hearing-related problem. The interviewer should know what the client knows regarding treatment of hearing loss, and should be able to determine the impact that the hearing impairment has had on the client's everyday activities and how well the client has adjusted to the hearing loss. Through questions pertaining to the client's age at onset, mode of onset, and progression of the hearing loss, the audiologist can determine the client's motivation toward participating in a rehabilitation program. Is the client a "staller"? If the client has waited a long time before deciding to seek help, ask him why he waited. The answer to such questions may help determine the prognosis for successful self-management.

The client interview is a necessary first step in deciding whether or not elderly adults are candidates for aural rehabilitation programs. If they view themselves as needing more information relating to their hearing health or not as active in conversational situations as they would like to be, then an appropriate rehabilitation program should be designed for them. Once they have made a commitment toward participation in a program, further nonaudiometric evaluation of their hearing handicap should be conducted.

Hearing Handicap Scales

Hearing handicap scales can be used to gain valuable insight into the impact that hearing impairment has had on the clients themselves, their interaction with others, and in specific everyday communication situations. A variety of scales has been developed for eliciting this information from various hearing-impaired populations (Alpiner, Chevrette, Glascoe, Metz, & Olsen, 1971; Ewertsen & Nielsen, 1973; Giolas, Owens, Lamb, & Schubert, 1979; High, Fairbanks, & Glorig, 1964; Noble & Atherley, 1970). The scales that seem to have had greatest application to the elderly, either in standardized or modified form, include the Scale for Self-assessment of Hearing (High, et al., 1964) and the Denver Scale of Communication Function (Alpiner, et al., 1971). Another more recently developed scale, the Hearing Performance Inventory (Giolas, et al, 1979), also shows unusual promise for application to the elderly adult.

SCALE FOR SELF ASSESSMENT OF HEARING (SSAH)

The SSAH (High, et al., 1964) has two highly correlated forms ($r = 0.96$). Each form contains 20 questions covering four major content areas: speech perception, localization, telephone communication, and setting (multivoice and noise). Scoring is based on client ratings on a five-step continuum of relative frequency of occurrence ranging from "Almost always" to "Almost never." Cooperative clients can complete the form in a relatively short period of time, yielding information pertaining to particular rehabilitation needs. It illustrates difficulty that might be encountered by the elderly adult in everyday communication when (1) only auditory signals are provided (e.g., radio speaker), (2) combined auditory−visual signals, background noise, and situational cues are available (e.g., speaking with a bus driver), (3) auditory signal intensity is low (e.g., understanding a televised message at a 12-foot distance or understanding a whispered message), and (4) detecting warning signals (e.g., telephone ring, automobile horns). In all, the scale emphasizes assessment of the respondent's ability to communicate successfully in everyday conversation situations. Because the focus of elderly adults' rehabilitation programs is often centered on improving their communication skills, the scale provides the audiologist with information pertaining to the clients' interest in interpersonal communication, attitude toward and successful use of a hearing aid, ability to use visual speech perception and situational cues in everyday conversation, ability to stage-manage or manipulate the communication situation to their listening advantage, ability to communicate without visual or situational cues in quiet and in noise and to use auditory warning signals effectively. This information is critical in the development of client-centered remediation goals.

THE DENVER SCALE OF COMMUNICATION FUNCTION (DSCF)

The DSCF (Alpiner et al., 1971) consists of one form that uses a semantic differential continuum for rating reaction to 25 statements determining competence in four areas: communication with family members, the clients' feelings about their own ability as communicators, communication in social−vocational situations, and communication in general. The intent of the authors in developing this scale was to elicit the client's initial reaction to statements relating to common communication problems. A 15-minute time limit is imposed on the respondent. Client responses are recorded on a profile form for possible pre- and postremediation compari-

son of scores. Test−retest reliability has been found to be acceptable ($r = 0.729$), although, as with other scales, there is no guarantee that the client is answering the questions honestly.

DENVER SCALE OF COMMUNICATION FUNCTION FOR SENIOR CITIZENS LIVING IN RETIREMENT CENTERS (DSSC)

An interesting modification of the DSCF for use with the elderly was developed by Zarnoch and Alpiner (1977). Their Denver Scale of Communication Function for Senior Citizens Living in Retirement Centers (DSSC) is designed for presentation in an interview format. Seven major communication questions are posed, each followed by a Probe Effect and Exploration Effect series of questions. The Probe Effect questions are used to determine specific problem areas within the major item. Exploration Effect questions are used to determine how applicable a general question is to a particular respondent. An example of a major item and one question from the related Probe Effect and Exploration Effect series is shown in Figure 16−2.

The DSSC is useful for identifying specific problem areas for each respondent. One question is posed to survey each of the following areas: family communication, emotional reaction to hearing loss, communication with other people, general communication, self-concept, communication in group situations, and motivation toward participation in a rehabilitation program. The value of this modified scale lies in its comprehensive scope and brevity of administration time. It is a structured extension of the case history taking−audiologic assessment procedure that allows for effective identification and the evaluation of problems in communication.

HEARING PERFORMANCE INVENTORY (HPI)

The HPI (Giolas et al., 1979) has not yet had an adequate opportunity to withstand the test of time. However, several positive features of this scale should be noted. In a small number of elderly clients, this scale has already served to facilitate development of a relevant aural rehabilitation program. The inventory consists of one form containing 90 questions covering 6 major content areas: understanding speech, signal intensity, response to auditory failure, social communication, personal communication, and occupational communication. Responses are scored on a five-point continuum of relative frequency ranging from "Practically always" to "Almost never" and are obtained in about 20 minutes.

Name _____ Age _____ Date _____

1.0 Introductory Remarks
    1.1 Description of hearing loss:

    1.2 Description of hearing handicap:

2.0 Speech Audiometry
    2.1. Test Equipment and Conditions
        2.1.1. Audiometer:
        2.1.2. Test Stimulus:
        2.1.3. Stimulus presentation: _____ Tape _____ MLV
        2.1.4. Primary signal: _____ Rt. Spkr. _____ Left Spkr. _____ R & L Spkrs.
        2.1.5. Competing message: _____ Multi-speaker babble _____ Other _____
                                                             (specify)
        2.1.6. P/CM: _____ O db HL _____ Other — specify _____
        2.1.7. Primary signal presentation level: _____ 50 dB HL _____ Other — specify _____
        _____
        2.1.8. Listening condition: _____ Sound Field _____ Other — specify _____
        2.1.9. Listening mode: _____ Unaided _____ Aided
              2.1.9.1. Aid make:
              2.1.9.2. Aid model/style:
              2.1.9.3. Receiver type:
              2.1.9.4. Settings:
              2.1.9.5. Battery:
              2.1.9.6. Earmold:
              2.1.9.7. Aided Ear: _____ Right _____ Left _____ Both
    2.2. Test Findings
        2.2.1. SAT: A = _____
        2.2.2. SRT: A = _____
        2.2.3. Discrim. — Q: A = _____ A/V = _____
        2.2.4. Discrim. — N: A = _____ A/V = _____

3.0 Vision
    3.1 Binocular visual acuity: _____ (Snellen chart)
    3.2 Description of vision problem:

4.0 Sensory Input Channel Efficiency Rating
    4.1. Auditory Channel   (Intelligibility Rating)

	low				high	
4.1.1. Telephone conversation	1	2	3	4	5	NA
4.1.2. CB Radio conversation	1	2	3	4	5	NA
4.1.3. Walkie-Talkie/Intercom	1	2	3	4	5	NA
4.1.4. Public address system	1	2	3	4	5	NA
4.1.5. Radio broadcast	1	2	3	4	5	NA
4.1.6. Other _____	1	2	3	4	5	—

    4.2. Auditory-Visual Channel   (Intelligibility Rating)

	low				high	
4.2.1. One-to-one conversation	1	2	3	4	5	NA
4.2.2. Group conversation	1	2	3	4	5	NA
4.2.3. Lecture/Oral presentation	1	2	3	4	5	NA
4.2.4. Movie	1	2	3	4	5	NA
4.2.5. Theater	1	2	3	4	5	NA
4.2.6. Television program	1	2	3	4	5	NA
4.2.7. Other _____	1	2	3	4	5	—

(continued)

Figure 16-1 *(continued)*

5.0 Auditory Message Perception
    5.1. Descriptional of problem:

    5.2. Evaluation procedure (including description of test stimuli, competing message type, P/CM level, situation cues, etc.):

    5.3. Estimated level of message perception

5.3.1.	Running Discourse— Familiar Topic
5.3.2.	Running Discourse— Unfamiliar Topic
5.3.3.	Unrelated sentences
5.3.4.	Monosyllabic words

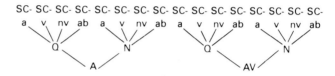

KEY: A = Auditory Channel; A/V = Auditory-Visual Channels; Q = Quiet Condition; N = Noise Condition; SC = Situational Clues (a = auditory; v = visual/picture; nv = non-verbal; ab = absent)

Fig. 16-1. Speech communication profile. (Reprinted, with permission, from Garstecki DC: Alternative approaches to measuring speech discrimination efficiency, in Rupp RR, Stockdell KG (eds.): Speech Protocols in Audiology. New York, Grune & Stratton, 1980, pp. 129-130.)

One primary advantage of this scale over the others described is that it includes questions that reflect the respondents' reactions to auditory failure. The scale provides questions that help determine whether negative reactions occur with specific types of people (e.g., friends versus strangers), under particular communication conditions (e.g., with individuals and/or in groups), or in selected situations (e.g., at a restaurant or play). In addition, the scale elicits information describing the type of behavior demonstrated in difficult communication situations (e.g., adjusts the hearing aid, asks for assistance, informs listener of loss, asks for repetition).

Scale items are categorized across and within major content areas. This is useful in determining common problems under various communication conditions. The organization of this scale facilitates the design of comprehensive rehabilitation program goals, provides prescriptive information for program implementation, and provides quantitative data for noting client progress in managing problems relating to hearing loss.

Besides using standardized hearing handicap scales to gain insight into the rehabilitative needs of elderly adults, it is also useful to probe critical incidents within the clients' communicative experiences and to determine how they perceive their state in life. Such probing might include asking for reaction to the

Item 4. Do you avoid communicating with other people because of your hearing problem?
        Yes _____ No _____

Probe Effect:
   c. Do you communicate during the social activities in the home?   Yes _____ No _____

Exploration Effect:
   b. What are your social activities in the home?

Fig. 16-2. Item four and sample probe effect and exploration effect questions. (Reprinted, with permission, from Zarnoch JM, Alpiner JG: The Denver Scale of Communication Function for Senior Citizens Living in Retirement Centers. Unpublished study, 1977.)

following types of statements and questions: (1) Think of a time when something unpleasant happened in connection with your hearing loss. What did you do to make the situation pleasant? (2) Tell me about a time when you mishandled a situation in which someone misunderstood your hearing handicap. (3) Tell me about a time when you were embarrassed by your hearing loss. (4) Why do you have a hearing loss? (5) What is it like to be hard of hearing? (6) How do others feel about your hearing loss?

Reactions to these and similar statements and questions can further the audiologist's understanding of the impact of hearing impairment on the elderly adult. By combining information from the audiologic assessment, client interview, and hearing handicap scales, the audiologist can paint a picture of the hearing-impaired adult's communicative competence and ability to deal with the present handicapping condition. This information establishes the groundwork for the development and implementation of the rehabilitation program.

AURAL REHABILITATION PROGRAM DESIGN

Once elderly adults have demonstrated an interest in seeking professional assistance for their hearing loss and the need for aural rehabilitation is verified by audiologic assessment data, speech communication profile scores, and self-reports of hearing handicap, then an appropriate remediation program can be designed.

Basic Considerations

To assist elderly adults in the self-management of their hearing related problems, an aural rehabilitation program must be designed to meet their self-perceived and real needs. Primary considerations in the development of such a program include several factors.

APPROACH

Clients must feel assured that the audiologist understands their problem and has their primary interest in mind in all rehabilitation procedures. Clients must feel confident that the audiologist is able to efficiently and effectively help them manage their problems.

The audiologist should focus on the clients' major problem and develop a solution to the problem that takes into consideration elderly adults' physical stamina and ability, personality, attitude toward themselves and others, attitude toward communication, problem solving ability, lifestyle, and reaction to failure. The audiologist should be highly familiar with the conditions of hearing-impaired adults' everyday communication problems as well as any other hearing-related difficulty.

The rehabilitation program should incorporate input not only from the managing audiologist but also close family members, spouses, friends, or any other person who might be regarded as a "significant other" by the client. Opportunity should be afforded for interaction with hearing-impaired age peers, successful graduates of the rehabilitation program, and specialists (physicians, social workers, psychologists, and so on) in the hearing health care professions. Consumer information should be made available through the above resources and shared, not only with the client, but with the family members.

Service staff and administrators of total-care facilities or homes for the aged may also benefit from involvement in the rehabilitation program. In-service training to improve communication with the elderly as well as to better understand the implications of hearing loss and its treatment, including consumer information, will be of value to these people.

GOALS

The long-range goal of the rehabilitation program is to develop the hearing-impaired adult's ability to self-manage problems relating to hearing loss. Specific short-range goals should be practically oriented. They should provide information to the client about the structure and function of the hearing mechanism, causes and treatment of aural pathology, interpretation and implications of hearing test results, and benefits and limitations in use of hearing aids and other sensory aids. This could be accomplished through lectures, demonstrations, and discussions.

The program goals also should be designed to inform the client about the dynamics of everyday communication, the communication cycle, and the influence of hearing impairment on this process. This would include consideration of barriers to effective communication, hints for stage-managing difficult communication situations, and consideration of special problems, such as the need to improve telephone communication strategies.

Procedures to improve the client's communication skills through use of audition and vision and, in some cases, use of manual communication, should be included. These should involve consideration of perceptual, linguistic, and "extra linguistic" or situational cues to message perception (Hodgson & Skinner, 1977). The client's use of residual hearing should be challenged. This includes consideration of hearing aid use and learning to listen under noisy conditions. Clients should be counseled regarding their attitude toward hearing aid use. They should be assisted in the selection, fitting, and use of an appropriate amplification system. They should develop optimal auditory communication skills through controlled exercises.

FORMAT

The rehabilitation program should be conducted in a pleasant, comfortable environment. The elderly client should have relatively easy access to the building and therapy room. The audiologist should use a room in which the "environment" can be controlled. That is, the lighting and ambient noise level should be either at optimal level or able to be manipulated for training purposes.

The program should be comprehensive in scope, offering information that will be of interest and use to each participant in each session. A passive admission policy (Luterman, 1967), in which there is no obligation to attend the program, will result in a group of more highly motivated clients. In other instances, in which fee for service is required, some clients may be motivated to participate in the program to take full advantage of their investment.

The program length may range from 10 to 20 weekly 2-hour sessions depending on the need and interest of the client. It may be useful to plan a 10-week short-term program for the majority population and an extended or "advanced" series of sessions for those who require extended or more intensive training and assistance. Session length should range from 45 to 60 minutes with time for socializing either before, during, or after the session. Opportunities for individual and group instruction should be provided with maximum group size limited to approximately eight hearing-impaired adults.

Program Emphases

In most cases, the program will emphasize three areas: improvement of communication skills, adjustment to the use of a hearing aid, and counseling in management of problems related to hearing impairment.

COMMUNICATION SKILLS

With the gradual onset of hearing loss in the normal process of aging, many elderly adults grow to enjoy the peacefulness afforded by loss of hearing. Others may use their hearing selectively, hearing what they want to hear when they want to hear it.

Many will blame their overall communication problems solely on hearing impairment. An early goal in the rehabilitation program is to motivate the clients to become active, full-time listeners. At the same time it may be beneficial to refresh their understanding of the normal communication cycle (Sanders, 1971) and how information perceived through an impaired auditory system can be supplemented by that received through other sensory receptors such as vision, taste, touch, and smell. Clients may begin to appreciate the value of attending to visual speech cues (lipreadng), facial expression, and body gesture as well as situational cues to message perception. Of course, the availability of supplemental cues will vary according to the communication situation. Some situations require "auditory-only" communication skill; others might be described as combined "auditory – visual" communication situations.

Auditory Communication. The term *auditory communication* refers to signal perception through use of audition alone. Examples of common auditory communication situations include telephone conversation, listening to a radio broadcast, and speaking with someone outside of your field of vision. Auditory commmunication is dependent on an auditory signal generator or human speaker, a spoken message code or language, a message transmission channel, and an auditory signal receiver or human listener. Factors that may negatively influence signal reception include hearing impairment, variation in message intensity level, acoustic properties of the message, and communication channel fidelity.

To design an appropriate remediation program, variables inherent in the client's difficult communication situations must be identified and isolated and then recombined in graduated steps to assist the adult in building satisfactory auditory communication skills. For example, for the client who demonstrates difficulty in telephone communication, several problem areas can be identified: message intensity, message fidelity, message content, and competing noise at the listener's station. Consideration should be given to the need for and feasibility of modifying any of these variables to improve telephone communication ability. Appropriate questions include the following:

1. Message intensity: Is it reasonable to expect the caller to increase his or her vocal intensity? Will amplification serve to improve signal reception? Will a telephone-receiver amplifier improve telephone communication, with or without a hearing aid?

2. Message fidelity: Will a change in hearing aid and/or telephone electroacoustic characteristics improve message clarity? How much does fidelity change when using telephone intercom systems versus local area transmission lines versus long distance transmission lines?

3. Message content: Does message perception improve with increases in linguistic content? What types of messages (names, numbers, etc.) are most frequently misperceived?

4. Message competition: Is the listener's telephone located in an acoustically and/or visually distracting location? What is the type, duration, nature, and level of auditory competition? What is the type, duration, and nature of the visual competition?

Answers to these questions will help determine which variables can be manipulated to maximize the elderly adult's success in telephone communication. Emphasis in rehabilitation is directed toward the selection and fitting of an appropriate amplification system, selection and installation of appropriate telephone communication equipment, modification of the listening environment, and development of proper telephone questioning strategies for use in difficult listening situations. Once the potential for successful telephone communication is improved through equipment and room modifications, communication skills are developed through a series of activities ranging from highly redundant message perception in quiet to message perception under the conditions commonly encountered in typical telephone communication situations.

Auditory−visual communication. Auditory−visual communication is the term used to describe the perception of messages through combined auditory and visual sensory modalities. A common example of auditory−visual communication is everyday conversation in which the listener can hear the speaker's message while watching his lip movements, facial expression, and body gestures and observe situational background cues. Other examples of auditory−visual communication include watching a television program and attending a play. In most instances, auditory and visual signals are transmitted simultaneously. Factors that influence auditory signal perception are the same as those discussed earlier. In addition, however, the listener's visual acuity and visual perception ability along with message visibility are important variables to consider.

Speech communication profile. To organize a communication remediation program, a Speech Communication Profile (Fig. 16−1) may be used. In section 5.0 of this profile, a grid is provided for recording standardized and/or experimental test data relating to communicative performance under varying types of listening conditions. In completing the grid, differences in message perception relating to changes in redundancy of information can be observed in terms of:

1. Linguistic content of the message: How does an increase in content change message perception?

2. Message audibility: How does message perception change when it is presented with a competing signal? What influence does noise type and signal to noise level have on message perception?

3. Sensory input: How does message perception change when auditory signals are combined with visual, nonverbal, and situational cues?

Although it is expected that greater success in message perception will be achieved under conditions of greatest redundancy of information and in quiet, the differences in performance across various conditions is of considerable prescriptive value. For example, in a study reported by Garstecki (1976), when elderly adults were asked to speechread CID Everyday Speech Sentences paired with related auditory and visual background cues, unrelated auditory and visual background cues, and without either auditory or visual background cues, the majority of the respondents demonstrated greatest success in visual speech perception when related cues were provided. Several exceptions were noted. Some subjects demonstrated undifferentiated performance across all conditions, some demonstrated best performance when no cues were provided, and some demonstrated undifferentiated high performance under absent and related cue conditions. These findings suggest that not all elderly adults are innately predisposed to use situational cues as an adjunct to visual speech perception. Some may require special training to comprehend the most highly redundant everyday communication. Their prognosis for improved visual communication will be dependent somewhat on their visual acuity and visual perception ability, which may show depreciation with age (Dublin, 1967).

Speechreading. Many elderly adults have misgivings about the benefits to be derived from lipreading (speechreading) lessons. They expect to be able to substitute visual speech perception for auditory speech perception. They must be informed of the value of watching the speaker while listening, but they must also learn to realize that there are many factors that deter complete understanding of speech through vision. For this reason lipreading is not practiced without voice in the rehabilitation program.

Most hearing-impaired elderly have some usable residual hearing ability that provides them with acoustic cues to speech perception in everyday communication. In simulating the everyday situation in the rehabilitation program environment, every attempt should be made to assist the client in using all sensory input modalities in combination with each other in message perception. One approach to structuring the rehabilitation program activities would be to order the exercises so as to promote the development of communication skills in a manner that initially guarantees success in practice while teaching concepts and strategies for successful communication in difficult situations. To do this one could structure a series of sessions using meaningful speech material that is graded in visibility. Binnie, Montgomery, and Jackson (1974) recommend that visual speech perception lessons be based on the presentation of homophenous sound categories that decrease in visibility by item: (1) bilabials /p, b, m/: (2) labiodentals /f, v/: (3) interdentals /ð, θ/: (4) rounded labials /ʃ, ʒ/; (5) linguals /s, z/; (6) linguals /t, d, n/; (7) rounded labial /w/ (Woodward & Barber, 1960); (8) lingual palatal /dʒ, tʃ/ (Bunger, 1961).

Another way to structure the program is to follow a progression of exercises in message perception beginning with conditions of greatest redundancy that incorporate use of familiar contextualized speech material presented under optimal listening and viewing conditions accompanied by related situational background cues. Factors contributing to message redundancy can be systematically varied to decrease the amount of redundancy of information provided to a level normally encountered by the adult in a difficult everyday communication situation. Some factors will be eliminated or held constant, while others will vary within limits of reason for the adult. For example, if the difficult communication situation is a social function where conversation takes place in a noisy, dimly lit room and nothing can be done to change the room conditions, these factors would be held constant in the remediation program activities. Remediation activities would emphasize use of stage-managing techniques to optimize the listener's communication opportunities and to develop skill in comprehension of predictive cues provided by reading facial expression, body gesture, and other nonverbal communication to supplement key-word recognition in understanding the general topic of conversation.

By structuring auditory-communication skill building according to an hierarchical system as provided by the Speech Communication Profile and/or the system proposed by Binne et al. (1974), rehabilitation of the elderly adult's communication skills can follow a logically progressing format that should be motivating in that, at least initially, some success is guaranteed. In addition, the practical value of planned activities is likely to be self-evident to the client.

Role-playing. A critical component of the rehabilitation program is the application of newly learned information to the communication process through role-playing. Role-playing activities can help develop appropriate strategies for the client's use outside of the security of the rehabilitation environment. These activities might be designed to increase awareness of the dynamics of the everyday communication process, to identify barriers to communication, and to develop appropriate strategies for increasing the likelihood of successful communication. Strategies that might be developed to improve everyday communication skills through role-playing might include: (1) letting visible speech movements supplement the audible aspects of everyday communication; (2) positioning oneself so that sun or room light is directed toward the speaker's face; (3) facing the speaker directly or sitting with your better ear toward the speaker; (4) using facial expression and body gesture cues to understand a message; (5) using situational cues to understand a message; (6) reducing competing noise by lowering the volume of a radio, turning off running water, lessening room echos, etc.; (7) educating others to the fact that natural speech is easier for you to comprehend than slowed or exaggerated speech articulation.

HEARING AID

Older adults should be encouraged to explore the possibility that a hearing aid may help improve their communication ability, especially under favorable listening conditions. Older adults are often skeptical about the values to be derived from hearing aid use. They expect the hearing aid to have the same effect on their hearing ability as eyeglasses have on correcting their vision problems. They are generally uninformed of the benefits and limitations of hearing aid use. Finally, they are suspicious of the motives of high-pressure hearing aid salespeople.

In order to assist the elderly adult in adjustment to hearing aid use, a variety of training sessions and listening exercises are incorporated into the rehabilitation program. The client is informed of the function of a hearing aid and familiarized with its component parts and general operation. Consideration is given to the probability of successful use of various types of hearing aid systems for different degrees and types of medically nonreversible hearing losses (Hodgson & Skinner, 1977). Rehabilitation program activities are designed to help the adult adjust to hearing aid use in a variety of situations. Listening activities include responding to speech discrimination test materials presented under controlled speech audiometry conditions. Test materials are presented with and without amplification in quiet and noise conditions. Selected hearing aids are also worn in various uncontrolled conditions to enable the client to make listening quality judgments and become acclimated to listening with the hearing aid. In this way, elderly adults actually participate in the decision-making process. Once an aid has been selected for purchase, they are assisted in procuring the aid and encouraged to have the aid and their performance with it monitored periodically.

The prognosis for successful hearing aid use by elderly adults may be determined by using a measurement scale designed by Rupp, Higgins, and Maurer (1977). This Feasibility Scale for Predicting Hearing Aid Use (FSPHAU) consists of 11 areas of concern in predicting the probability of an elderly adult's successful use of a hearing aid. These areas, in order of their relative weight from greatest to least, include motivation and mode of referral, magnitude of hearing loss, self-assessment of listening difficulties, age, manual finger and hand dexterity, financial resources, presence of a significant other person to assist, client's verbalization of the need for help, informal verbalization during the hearing aid evaluation, and visual ability. Each of these factors is rated on a one- to five-point scale with five indicating the most positive response. In regard to the above factors, the elderly adult will be most successful in hearing aid use if some of his motivation is self-generated rather than stemming from other individuals. There also is an inverse relationship between amount of hearing loss and benefit derived from hearing aid use. The better candidates generally demonstrate flat, gently rising or gently falling audiometric configurations with no greater than a moderately severe loss in sensitivity. More importantly, the higher the unaided speech discrimination ability, the greater the potential benefit from the use of an aid.

Older adults should be able to identify their difficult communication situations and know how to maximize their communication abilities in those situations. They must be able to operate the hearing aid and have the financial resources or access to financial assistance for covering the cost of an aid, a continuing battery supply, and occasional maintenance and repair. An important factor in the adjustment process is the understanding and support of a "significant other" person, one who is informed of the problems relating to hearing loss and hearing aid use by the

elderly adult. This should be a person with whom the elderly adult has daily contact.

COUNSELING

Inherent in the rehabilitation of hearing-impaired adults is extensive counseling of both the clients and their families. Many clients require counseling for purposes of motivating them to participate in a rehabilitation program. They may view themselves as not being worth the effort. Others may have difficulty accepting hearing impairment and may need counseling to reach a level of acceptance of their condition. Elderly clients must be apprised of the potential benefits to be gained from participation in a rehabilitation program and from hearing aid use. The family should understand the nature of hearing loss in the elderly and the benefits and limitations of hearing aid use. They must realize that, in some situations, the elderly may actually attend better without a hearing aid than with it. They also must realize that elderly family members may be frustrated, confused, angry, and embarrassed by their inability to hear and/or to use a hearing aid satisfactorily. They should understand the distinction between hearing impairment and senility in elderly adults. As part of the counseling activities of the rehabilitation program, hearing impaired adults, family members, and significant other persons may benefit from information on such topics as: (1) the nature of hearing loss and its treatment in an aging adult, (2) benefits and limitations of hearing aid use, (3) ways to improve interpersonal communication skills, (4) ways to conserve residual hearing ability, (5) sensory aids for the hearing-impaired, (6) telephone equipment for the hearing-impaired, (7) hearing aid dispensing regulations, (8) financial reimbursement for hearing health care through third-party payment, (9) experimental procedures for treating problems related to hearing loss ("implanted hearing aids," acupuncture, tinnitus maskers, etc.), (10) community services for hearing-impaired persons (otological care, audiological care, hearing aid dealer services, psychologic services, social services, counseling services, vocational placement services, telephones for hearing-impaired persons, captioned films, special church services, educational programs, etc.).

SUMMARY

An effort was made within this chapter to help prepare professionals who work with hearing-impaired elderly adults to understand some of the reasons for their actions and some of the procedures that rehabilitative audiologists may employ to help each one of them manage problems relating to hearing loss. In order to lay an appropriate foundation, discussion included a description of the incidence of hearing handicap among the elderly. The behaviors of hearing handicapped adults were reviewed with special emphasis on particular personality types and varying motivation toward self-management of hearing problems.

Determination of the need for aural rehabilitation was based on an expanded definition of the responsibilities of the audiologist in providing rehabilitation services. Suggestions for identification of candidates for aural rehabilitation were provided, along with a description of special considerations that might be applied in audiometric and nonaudiometric evaluation of hearing loss and its impact and hearing aid selection.

Rehabilitation programs that focus on the client's major problems with active participation of other persons were discussed. Program goals were stated to emphasize the importance of providing the client with educational information, direction in improving communication skills, and guidance in the selection and use of a hearing aid. Program format considerations for elderly clients were reviewed. As has been indicated, aural rehabilitation of the elderly adult may concentrate on improvement of communication ability. The communication process can be considered in terms of type of input modality as either auditory-only or auditory–visual combined. An example of a common auditory-only communication experience is a telephone conversation. The variables inherent in telephone communication were identified and consideration was given to modification of these variables for rehabilitation purposes. A commonly occurring auditory–visual communication experience is face-to-face conversation. Variables relating to message perception in this situation were identified and implications for training were reviewed. The discussion of communication skill remediation concluded with a list of strategies that might be employed in the communication process.

Another major concern in rehabilitation is ability of elderly adults to satisfactorily adjust to the use of a hearing aid. Prognostic indicators of successful adjustment were briefly reviewed with special consideration given to the importance of client self-motivation toward hearing aid use and support from the family or a significant other person. Finally, elderly adults' counseling needs were discussed as they relate to their own educational and psychological needs as well as those of their families and others.

REFERENCES

Alpiner, J., Chevrette, W., Glascoe, G., Metz, M., & Olsen, B. The Denver Scale of Communication Function. Unpublished study, 1971.

Bergman, M., Blumfeld, V. G., Cascardo, D., Dash, B., Levitt, H., & Marguilies, M. K. Age-related decrement in hearing for speech. *Journal of Gerontology*, 1976, *31*, 533–538.

Binnie, C. A. Bi-sensory articulation function for normal hearing and sensori-neural hearing loss patients. *Journal of the Academy of Rehabilitative Audiology*, 1973, *6*, 43–53.

Binnie, C. A., Montgomery, A. A., & Jackson, P. L. Auditory and visual contributions to the perception of consonants. *Journal of Speech and Hearing Research*, 1974, *17*, 619–630.

Brotman, H. B. Population projections. *Gerontologist*, 1977, *17*, 203–209.

Bunger, A. M. *Speechreading–Jena method*. Danville, Ill.: The Interstate Printers and Publishers, 1961.

Chaffee, C. E. Rehabilitation needs of nursing home patients: A report of a survey. *Rehabilitation Literature*, 1967, *18*, 377–389.

Dublin, E. B. *Fundamentals of neuropathology*. Springfield, Ill.: Charles C. Thomas Publishers, 1967.

Ewertsen, H. & Nielsen, B. Social hearing handicap index: Social handicap in relation to hearing impairment. *Audiology*, 1973, *12*, 180–187.

Gaeth, J. A study of phonemic regression associated with hearing loss. Unpublished doctoral dissertation, Northwestern University, Evanston, Ill.; 1948.

Garstecki, D. Situational cues in visual speech perception by geriatric subjects. *Journal of the American Audiology Society*, 1976, *2*, 99–106.

Garstecki, D. Alternative approaches to measuring speech discrimination efficiency. In R. Rupp & K. Stockdell (Eds.), *Speech protocols in audiology*. New York: Grune & Stratton, 1980.

Giolas, T., Owen, E., Lamb, S., & Schubert, E. Hearing performance inventory. *Journal of Speech and Hearing Disorders,* 1979, *44,* 169–195.

Harris, J. Adult aural habilitation: From the geriatric twenty's toward maturity. Paper presented at the California Speech and Hearing Association Conference, San Francisco, 1977.

High, W., Fairbanks, G., & Glorig, A. Scale for self-assessment of hearing handicap. *Journal of Speech and Hearing Disorders,* 1964, *29,* 215–230.

Hodgson, W., and Skinner, P. *Hearing aid assessment and use in audiologic habilitation.* Baltimore: Williams & Wilkins, 1977.

Hull, R. H., & Traynor, R. M. A communitywide program in geriatric aural rehabilitation. *ASHA: Journal of the American Speech and Hearing Association,* 1975, *17,* 33–34; 47–48.

Hull, R. H., & Traynor, R. M. Hearing impairment among aging persons in the health care facility: Their diagnosis and rehabilitation. *American Health Care Association Journal,* 1977, *3,* 14–18.

Jerger, J. Audiological findings in aging. *Advances in Oto-rhino-laryngology,* 1973, *20,* 115.

Luterman, D. A parent-oriented nursery program for preschool deaf children. *Volta Review,* 1967, *69,* 515–520.

Martin, M. *Introduction to audiology.* Englewood Cliffs, N. J.: Prentice-Hall, 1975.

Neely, K. Effects of visual factors on the intelligibility of speech. *Journal of the Acoustical Society of America,* 1956, *28,* 1275–1277.

Noble, W. G., & Atherley, G. R. The hearing measure scale: A questionnaire for the assessment of auditory disability. *Journal of Auditory Research,* 1970, *10,* 229–250.

O'Neill, J. J. Contributions of the visual components of oral symbols to speech comprehension. *Journal of Speech and Hearing Disorders,* 1954, *19,* 429–439.

Powers, J. K., & Powers, E. A. Hearing problems of elderly persons: Social consequences and prevalence. *ASHA: Journal of the American Speech and Hearing Association,* 1978, *20,* 79–83.

Rupp, R. R., Higgins, J., & Maurer, J. F. A feasibility scale for predicting hearing aid use (FSPHAU) with older individuals. *Journal of the Academy of Rehabilitative Audiology,* 1977, *10,* 81–104.

Sanders, D. A. *Aural rehabilitation.* Englewood Cliffs, N.J.: Prentice-Hall, 1971.

Sanders, D. A. Hearing aid orientation and counseling. In M. Pollack (Ed.), *Amplification for the hearing impaired.* New York: Gune & Stratton, 1975.

Schow, R. L., Christensen, J. M., Hutchinson, J. M., & Nerbonne, M. A. *Communication disorders of the aged.* Baltimore: University Park Press, 1978.

Senate aging committee launches investigation of hearing aids with two days of hearings before consumer interest subcommittee. *Washington Sounds,* 1968. Washington, D. C. (House Publication), *2,* 1968.

Woodward, M. F. & Barber, C. G. Phoneme perception in lipreading. *Journal of Speech and Hearing Research,* 1960, *3,* 212–222.

Zarnoch, J. M. & Alpiner, J. G. The Denver Scale of Communication Function for Senior Citizens Living in Retirement Centers. Unpublished study, 1977.

Zucker, K., & Williams, P. Audiological services in an extended care facility. Paper presented at the Annual Convention of the American Speech and Hearing Association, Chicago, 1977.

Barry A. Freeman

J. Stephen Sinclair

17

Hearing Aids for the Elderly

The American Speech and Hearing Association Committee on Rehabilitative Audiology (ASHA, 1974) suggested that the development of a comprehensive auditory management program for hearing-impaired persons should include the selection of an amplification system. The selection of an appropriate hearing aid facilitates the reception of speech sounds and enables hearing-handicapped persons to utilize those linguistic cues that can be perceived through audition.

It is estimated that the percentage of persons with potentially handicapping hearing impairments increases from 1.7 percent for the 18- to 44-year-old age group to 6.9 percent and 32 percent for the 45- to 64-year-old and 65-year and older groups, respectively (Schein & Delk, 1974). This oldest group constitutes approximately 11 percent of the current population of this country, and it is estimated that it will make up 20 to 25 percent of the population in 25 years. It is necessary, therefore, to recognize and assess certain aspects of a successful adult auditory rehabilitation program, of which amplification may be an integral part.

The purpose of this chapter is to provide an overview of the role of amplification in the rehabilitation of the hearing-handicapped adult. The information is organized in a format that parallels the decisions that must be made by both the client and the hearing health care professional throughout the rehabilitative program, as suggested in Figure 17−1.

The flowchart suggests that the initial responsibility for identifying a hearing handicap lies with the patient. The referral for audiological assessment may come from one of a number of sources, and the audiologist should determine if a hearing loss and hearing handicap exist. Appropriate recommendations can then be made for the patient. Specifically, this chapter presents those variables that must be considered for the selection of an appropriate amplification device and a successful hearing aid fitting.

CANDIDACY CONSIDERATIONS

Medical – Legal

The success of an auditory rehabilitation program requires that the etiology of the hearing loss and its associated handicapping factors be identified. Proper management of any hearing-impaired patient, therefore, should include the establishment of a medical diagnosis of the auditory pathology. In an attempt to secure medical management, the federal Food and Drug Administration (FDA) (*Federal Register*, 1977) has promulgated regulations governing the sale of hearing aids. These became effective on August 25, 1977, and are

based upon the recognition that an unnecessary or partially effective hearing aid device may be substituted for primary medical or surgical treatment, thus depriving the

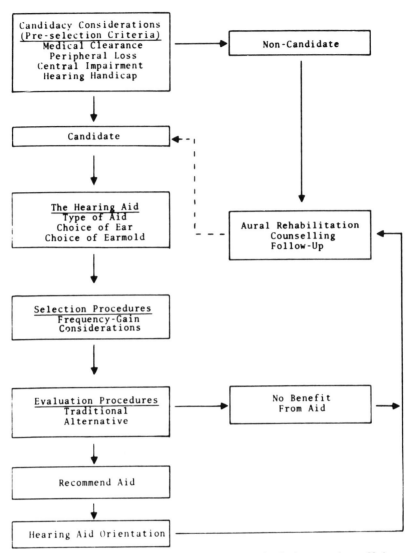

Fig. 17−1. Flowchart for determing hearing aid candidacy and selection procedures. If the person is considered a candidate for amplification, then hearing aids are selected for evaluation. An aid may or may not be recommended or the client may not be considered a candidate for amplification. In all instances, clients are referred for rehabilitation programs designed to help them overcome their handicap.

hearing impaired patient of benefit of appropriate medical diagnosis and care and resulting in a detriment to health (p. 9288).

The FDA has sought to overcome this problem and protect the consumer by requiring that the patient be informed of the recommendation for a medical evaluation prior to the sale of a hearing aid. In addition, the FDA has provided a list of seven warning signs (see Table 17−1) that can be used by the hear-

ing health care team to identify potential ear pathology for which the patient should seek prompt medical attention. The medical clearance, then, should be the initial step of the hearing health care management program. It should be used to secure a diagnosis and to determine whether a medical contraindication exists for amplification. However, associated psychologic, motivational, and peripheral and central pathologic factors that can interfere with successful rehabilitation also must be identified.

Table 17−1

Warning Signs of Potential Ear Pathology*

1. Visible congenital or traumatic deformity of the ear.
2. History of active drainage from the ear within the previous 90 days.
3. History of sudden or rapidly progressive hearing loss within the previous 90 days.
4. Acute or chronic dizziness.
5. Unilateral hearing loss of sudden or recent onset within the previous 90 days.
6. Audiometric air−bone gap equal to or greater than 15 dB at 500 Hz, 1000 Hz, and 2000 Hz.
7. Visible evidence of significant cerumen accumulation or a foreign body in the ear canal.
8. Pain or discomfort in the ear.

From the *Federal Register, 42* (31), 9286−9296, February 15, 1977.

*Hearing aid dispensers should advise prospective hearing aid users to consult a physician prior to dispensing an aid if any of these conditions exist.

Peripheral Hearing Loss

It is estimated that more than 90 percent of the adult patients seeking assistance for a hearing handicap have a sensorineural hearing impairment (Freeman, 1978; Sanders, 1978). The sophistication of medical and surgical intervention techniques have markedly reduced the need to provide amplification for the person with a conductive hearing loss. On occasion, the conductively hearing-impaired individual will require a hearing aid. A conductive loss of hearing is generally associated with good auditory discrimination and a wide dynamic range due to the intactness of the sensory and neural organs of the impaired ear. Thus, many of the problems that occur with an unsuccessful hearing aid fitting are not present for the conductively hearing-impaired person.

Sensorineural hearing loss, most frequently associated with aging, is termed *presbycusis* and presents a more difficult candidacy decision for amplification than occurs with a conductive hearing loss. This, in part, is due to a selective loss of acoustic information that may alter the reception of certain acoustic stimuli. The audiogram of a 70-year-old listener with a bilateral presbycusic type of sensorineural hearing loss is presented in Figure 17−2. With the spectrum of speech superimposed on this audiogram, it becomes apparent that the hearing loss is acting as a 2000 Hz low-pass filter with a 25 dB per octave slope. It may be expected that this person would have a problem recognizing higher-frequency consonant sounds (Fletcher, 1953). In addition, the average longer-term spectrum of speech (Figure 17−3) suggests that the energy of speech is greatest in the lower frequencies. Yet, most of the contextual information of speech is carried by the higher-frequency consonant sounds. The person with a high-frequency hearing loss thus may suffer the double penalty of having the greatest loss of hearing in those frequency regions that have the least energy available but carry a significant portion of the linguistic content.

In addition to the filtering effects of the hearing loss, presbycusis may be associated with a narrow dynamic range and an intolerance for amplified sound (Dix, 1968; Hood & Poole, 1966; Newby, 1972; Opheim & Flottorp, 1957). The dynamic range of hearing is defined as the difference between the threshold of audibility and the threshold of discomfort. Experimental evidence suggests that auditory discomfort levels for normal and cochlear-impaired ears are stable and should occur at approximately 90 to 110 dB SPL (sound pressure level), depending on the degree of hearing loss, instructions, and the psychophysical procedure used to measure it (Northern, 1978; Shapiro, 1979). Some writers have asserted that persons with a cochlear pathology, as in presbycusis, experience loudness discomfort levels at a lower intensity level than 110 dB SPL (Newby, 1972; O'Neill & Oyer, 1966).

Still unresolved, however, is the question of whether a reduced tolerance level has a physiologic or psychologic basis. If one accepts the contention that a low discomfort level for sound is a stable physiologic state (Schmitz, 1969), then one must also recognize that a hearing aid can cause continuous discomfort for persons with a narrow dynamic range. Persons with this problem may be poor candidates for amplification. The basis of this contention, in fact, has been used to justify the technological research that has focused on the development of hearing aid circuitry that can compress the amplitude of an incoming stimulus without altering its intelligibility. If, however, there is a psychologic basis for this reduced level of discomfort, then therapeutic approaches may be appropriate to increase tolerance for loud sounds. These approaches may include trial periods with amplification and formal auditory training lessons that are designed to increase acceptance of amplified sounds.

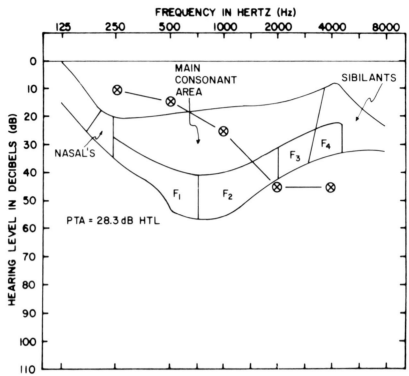

Fig. 17−2. Pure tone audiogram of a 70-year-old adult. The average loss of hearing in the speech frequencies (500−2000 Hz) is 28.3 db HTL bilaterally. Superimposed on the audiogram are the general spectra of speech. These are represented by the frequency regions where the nasal, consonant, and sibilant sounds and the first four formant regions (areas of concentrated sound energy) are located. The hearing loss at 2000 and 4000 Hz suggests that this person would hear some of the consonant and none of the sibilant speech sounds at normal conversational speech loudness levels.

Central Auditory Impairments

The detrimental effects of a peripheral hearing loss on the reception of acoustic stimuli may be complicated by a concurrent inability to adequately process linguistic information. Even if the sensitivity loss is remediated through amplification, there may still be a residual deficit in communication ability. Histologic evidence, for example, suggests that there is a generalized deterioration of the central auditory mechanism with advancing age (Appel & Appel, 1942; Bredberg, 1968; Brody, 1955; Ferraro & Minckler, 1977; Guild, 1932; Minckler, Jaeger, Ferraro, Powers, Grace, Campain, Metz, & Martin, 1977). Unfortunately, the clinical manifestations and the communicative handicap that may coexist from the central degeneration are poorly defined and may not be identified with traditional audiometric assessment techniques. The literature does suggest that older persons will have a disproportionate decrease in

discrimination ability as intensity of the stimulus increases, a phenomenon termed by Gaeth (1948) as phonemic regression. Similarly, older subject groups have difficulty recalling and repeating temporally altered linguistic material (Konkle, Beasley, & Bess, 1977; Korabic, Freeman, & Church, 1978). It also is not unreasonable to expect receptive problems other than a loss in the ability to discriminate speech stimuli. For example, poor auditory discrimination can coexist or be a by-product of an impairment of auditory memory (Freeman & Beasley, 1978). Deficits in auditory memory, therefore, may also contribute to a communication handicap.

The compound effects of peripheral and central auditory deficits may result in a marked communication problem and a tendency to withdraw from participation in communicative situations. Jones (1959) contended that people will pursue tasks that they do well but may avoid tasks that reflect weakness. Similarly, Alpiner (1967) remarked that the

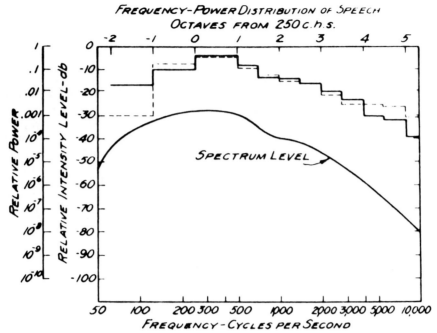

Fig. 17–3. Frequency–power distribution of speech. These measurements represent the sound pressures of speech as measured 30 cm from the talker's lips. The solid curved line is the overall spectra of speech. The horizontal solid bars represent the intensity levels in each octave band as the dB level below the average intensity for the speech of male speakers. The broken bars represent the intensity levels for female voices. (Reprinted by permission from Fletcher, H. *Speech and hearing in communication* (2nd ed.). New York: D. Van Nostrand, 1953. Copyright (1953) Bell Telephone Laboratories.)

least likely candidate for amplification is the poorly motivated, institutionalized elderly person, regardless of the degree of hearing impairment. It may be hypothesized that these persons make such poor candidates for amplification because of a psychologic and motivational state caused by the communication handicap. Hearing loss can result in defense mechanisms such as a denial of reality, withdrawal from social interaction, or other personality adjustment problems (Bolton, Cull, & Hardy, 1974). In the older population, a relationship exists between hearing loss and depression, marked suspiciousness, and paranoia. The hearing loss actually may be misinterpreted as senility or a mental abnormality. These conditions generally are not awarded social sympathy and may result in exclusion from social activities as well as withdrawal from communicative situations (Butler & Lewis, 1973). It is necessary, then, to identify those persons with a hearing handicap and to provide adequate auditory rehabilitation so that an interest and capability in communication can be maintained.

Hearing Loss and Hearing Handicap

The extent of a communication handicap and the need for amplification can be estimated through the use of the pure tone average (PTA) (Davis, 1970; Goodman, 1965; Newby, 1972; Sanders, 1978). This average comprises the hearing threshold levels at the midaudiometric frequencies of 500, 1000, and 2000 Hz. Berger and Millin (1971), for example, have used the PTA to predict the need for amplification according to the following scale:

1. A PTA of less than 40 dB hearing level (HL) is a minimal handicap and is borderline for amplification.
2. A loss averaging 40 to 85 dB HL should result in successful hearing aid use.
3. Losses of 85 to 100 dB HL suggest a marked handicap, but the individual can obtain some benefit from amplification.
4. A loss in excess of 100 dB HL results in a poor

candidate for a hearing aid due to the severity of the loss and degree of handicap.

The use of the PTA, however, as a means for determining amplification candidacy has certain limitations. First, it does not account for the contributions that frequencies above 2000 Hz may have in the discrimination of certain consonant sounds. Clinically, the PTA of the patient in Figure 17-2 would be 28 dB HL. According to the criteria presented by Berger and Millin (1971), the patient would not be a good candidate for amplification. Yet, the loss of the high-frequency information may be handicapping and could be compensated for by a hearing aid that selectively amplified the higher-frequency regions. Thus, the use of the PTA may tend to underestimate the hearing handicap and candidacy for amplification.

A second drawback to the use of pure-tone sensitivity as the sole criteria for hearing aid candidacy relates to an inability to predict speech discrimination scores from the pure-tone audiogram. Speech reception occurs at suprathreshold listening levels and in varying environmental conditions, making it a more complex acoustic event than tests for pure-tone sensitivity. Two individuals with identical pure-tone audiograms may present different speech intelligibility profiles. Since a primary goal of amplification is to improve speech communication, it is necessary to directly assess sensitivity to and suprathreshold understanding of a speech stimulus.

An underestimation of the benefits of amplification for individuals with a hearing loss in excess of 100 dB HL is a third disadvantage of the PTA. Ling (1976) noted an improvement in speechreading ability when low-frequency acoustic information was made available through amplification to severely hearing-impaired listeners. While the PTA of a patient may exceed 100 dB HL, there may be enough residual hearing below 750 Hz to justify a recommendation for a hearing aid evaluation. Furthermore, even the most minimal auditory contact with amplified sound patterns may help avoid psychologic problems of the elderly hearing-impaired (Ramsdell, 1970) and may heighten their awareness of environmental stimuli such as the sounds of doorbells or telephones and traffic patterns.

This is not to say that the pure-tone audiogram is dispensable in evaluating a person's hearing aid candidacy. The pure-tone data may be valuable in selecting the appropriate hearing aid frequency response, gain, and maximum output. As Ross (1978) noted, however, amplification often can be modified to fit individual needs, and no one should be ruled out as a candidate due to the degree or configuration of the pure-tone loss. This leaves the pure-tone audiogram as one of the several preselection criteria that must be used in defining hearing handicap and hearing aid candidacy.

While the hearing loss or deficit is defined by the results obtained on audiometric tests, the hearing handicap is determined by the communication deficit and associated problems of self-adjustment and social adjustment that may coexist or be a by-product of the loss of hearing acuity (Oyer & Frankmann, 1975). Thus, other hearing aid candidacy factors to be considered include social or vocational demands, motivation, manual dexterity, adaptability, and financial resources. These may be measured by scaled questionnaires (Alpiner, Chevrette, Glascoe, Metz, & Olsen, 1974; High, Fairbanks, & Glorig, 1964; Noble & Atherley, 1970; Rupp, Higgins, & Maurer, 1977; Sanders, 1975; Ward, Tucker, Tudor, & Morgan, 1977) but are too frequently determined in a busy clinical practice by highly subjective and unstructured interviews.

Davis (1970) defines hearing handicap as the disadvantage imposed by an impairment sufficient to affect one's "personal efficiency in the activities of daily living" (p. 263). An early effort to quantify the degree of hearing handicap and to predict hearing aid candidacy was made by Davis (1948) with the development of the Social Adaquacy Index (SAI). The SAI was a single value derived by comparing the interaction between the speech reception threshold (SRT) and the speech discrimination score. It was assumed that the SAI value represented the adequacy of hearing for everyday communication. Davis (1970), however, recommended abandoning the SAI, due to the poor standardization of the available recorded speech discrimination material and the questionable validity of using isolated monosyllabic words to predict communication abilities.

More recently, efforts have been made to identify hearing handicap by use of self-assessment questionnaires (High, Fairbanks, & Glorig, 1964; Noble & Atherley, 1970; Ward et al., 1977). These questionnaires generally elicit information pertaining to the loss of hearing sensitivity but have not correlated well to suprathreshold measures of speech intelligibility (Berkowitz & Hochberg, 1970; Jerger, Speaks, & Trammell, 1968; Peters & Hardick, 1974). Furthermore, they have not been designed to predict the psychologic or vocational dimensions of a hearing handicap, and thus, their value for predicting hearing aid candidacy is limited.

Another recent development has been the use of communication function profiles (Alpiner, 1978; Alpiner et al., 1974; Sanders, 1975). These are reportedly useful for identifying specific areas of communication problems, such as with the family or at work. These profiles have been used to plan rehabilitation programs and to assess an individual's success with amplification (Alpiner, 1978).

A more direct approach, the Feasibility Scale for Predicting Hearing Aid Use with Older Individuals, presented by Rupp, Higgins, and Maurer (1977), attempts to combine 11 prognostic indicators of hearing handicap into a single predictive value for success with amplification. The indicators include motivation, self-assessment of listening difficulty, magnitude of hearing loss, age, manual dexterity, and financial resources. These are evaluated on a six-point scale and each rating is weighted according to its assumed contribution to success with amplification. While the score and interpretation of this scale is subjective, it does allow for an organized assessment of many factors that may influence successful performance with a hearing aid. The correlation of the prediction score to the actual long-term use of amplification, however, is not well established.

In summary, a loss of hearing sensitivity is inadequate as a sole criterion for recommending amplification. The decision to obtain a hearing aid evaluation is multifaceted and includes information from the medical examination, the conventional hearing test, assessment of auditory tolerance levels, an estimate of central auditory dysfunction, and a determination of the handicap that may result from the physiologic impairments.

THE HEARING AID

A hearing aid is a device that facilitates the reception of sound by the listener (Olsen, 1977). This definition can be generalized to include a hand cupped behind the ear and an amplifier implanted on the neural pathway. Generally, though, it is an electronic device that converts acoustic energy into corresponding electrical energy, which, in turn, is converted back into acoustic energy via an electromechanical system that is coupled to the ear.

Electronic Components

The basic electronic components common to most hearing aids are the microphone, amplifier, receiver, and the power supply (Fig. 17–4). The microphone, which is usually either magnetic or electret, converts acoustic energy into electrical current while maintaining the waveform of the auditory stimulus. The amplitude of this current is increased by a battery-powered amplifier, the volume of which can be adjusted by the rotation of a volume control dial. When the amplified signal reaches the receiver, it is converted back into acoustic energy, which may be transmitted through a coupling system to the ear.

The last 25 years have seen many major innovations in hearing aid technology. This has resulted in improved acoustic fidelity, variability in frequency response modification, miniaturization of circuitry and power supply, greater acoustic gain and overall output level, development of output limitation circuitry, use of natural ear resonances and damping, increased instrument reliability and durability, and more cosmetic appeal and comfort (Berger and Millin, 1971). The hearing-impaired listener may be fit with any one of an array of hearing aid systems. Each system has its benefits and limitations, and the best choice for any individual is determined after evaluating numerous electroacoustic and psychoacoustic variables. The increasing number of amplification systems offers an opportunity for more hearing handicapped persons to be fitted successfully with an aid.

Electroacoustic Specifications

Several standard procedures have been developed for expressing the electroacoustic performance characteristics of hearing aids. The International Electrotechnical Commission (IEC), through IEC Publication 118 (IEC, 1959), and the American National Standards Institute, through ANSI S3.3–1960 (ANSI, 1960), specified methods for measuring the performance of hearing aids. Also, ANSI S3.8–1967 (ANSI, 1967) and the Hearing Aid Industry Conference (HAIC, 1961) recommended methods for the graphic display and expression of the performance data. Most recently, a new standard (ANSI S3.22–1976) recommends tolerances and methods for expressing hearing aid characteristics (ANSI, 1976; Lybarger, 1977; Kasten, 1978). This standard has been incorporated into the FDA regulations as the procedure for labeling the performance characteristics of hearing aids. Publication of the ANSI S3.22–1976 standard did not invalidate older measurement procedures, which differ substantially from the new ANSI standard. Therefore, any report of the electroacoustic characteristics of a hearing aid,

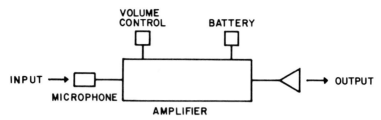

Fig. 17–4. Schematic representation of a simple hearing aid.

such as manufacturer specifications, should indicate the standard measurement technique.

False Notions

The technological advances that have been made with hearing aid systems make the predictability for successful auditory rehabilitation with a hearing aid less dependent on the type of hearing loss and more dependent on the individual's desire to wear amplification. Some misconceptions about who can benefit from amplification still exist (Freeman, 1978; Sanders, 1978) including:

1. Persons with a sensorineural hearing loss cannot wear a hearing aid.
2. Persons with a unilateral loss do not need a hearing aid.
3. Persons with poor auditory discrimination cannot wear a hearing aid.
4. Persons with a high-frequency hearing loss cannot wear an aid.
5. Persons with a severe loss of hearing cannot benefit from amplification.
6. Persons with a tolerance problem cannot wear an aid.
7. Persons with a mild hearing loss do not need an aid.

In the remainder of this chapter it will become evident that, despite some of the limitations of amplification devices, most persons desiring an aid can obtain benefit from one. Certain decisions, however, must first be made about the appropriateness of an aid for a client. These include selecting the type of hearing aid systems to be considered, identifying the ear to be fit, and choosing the appropriate earmold(s).

Amplification Devices

There are five categories of personal hearing aids that are currently available on the commercial market: earlevel, in-the-ear, body-type, bone conduc-

tion, and CROS (contralateral routing of signal) and its variations (Figs. 17–5 to 17–9).

EARLEVEL

The internal components of an earlevel instrument include the battery, amplifier, microphone, and receiver. A piece of tubing is generally used to connect the instrument to the ear coupler. Advancements in hearing aid technology and coupling materials have made it possible to build an earlevel instrument that, electroacoustically, can meet the needs of most hearing-impaired persons. The instrument may be small in size and cosmetically appealing. The small size, however, may be a deterrent for some clients with physical disabilities, such as paralysis or arthritis, in that they may have difficulty manipulating the controls of the instrument.

A variation of the earlevel instrument is the eyeglass hearing aid. The internal components of this system are housed within the temple of the eyeglass frame. Cosmetically, this hearing aid also may be appealing, but user complaints often include excessive weight of the eyeglasses, the inconvenience of not being able to wear one device without the other, and the inconvenience of losing access to both eyeglasses and the hearing aid if one is in need of repair.

IN-THE-EAR

Although these instruments were initially available only for persons with a mild loss of hearing, recent developments have led to the availability of an in-the-ear (ITE) instrument that, like the earlevel hearing aid, may electroacoustically meet the needs of adult hearing-impaired persons.

The ITE aid typically is custom made for the hearing-impaired person with its electrical components housed within the custom earmold (Preves & Hoke, 1978). The instrument's small size is a deterrent for persons who cannot manipulate the small external controls. The fact that the unit is custom

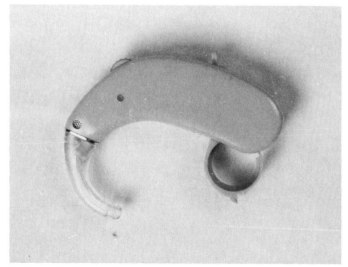

Fig. 17–5. Earlevel hearing aid (Courtesy of Siemens Hearing Instruments, Inc.).

made makes it difficult to assess a listener's performance with the aid prior to purchase. In addition, the earmold must fit properly to avoid acoustic feedback, and it is difficult to provide a loaner aid while the ITE aid is being repaired or modified. Regardless of these problems, the ITE aid has been gaining in popularity. HAIC reported that in 1965 the ITE aid comprised only 6.3 percent of the hearing aids sold in the United States (Kasten, 1972); in 1978, however, the market share of these aids increased to 29.5 percent (Pollack, 1980). This threefold increase in the use of ITE aids was complemented by an equivalent decrease in the sale of body-type hearing aids, a decrease in the sale of eyeglass aids, and an increase in the behind-the-ear instruments.

BODY TYPE

The body-type hearing aid typically is box-shaped and is carried on the body, attached to either an article of clothing or a special garment carrier. This type of aid differs from the earlevel and the ITE aids in that the receiver is external to the instrument but is attached to it by a cord. This greater separation between the receiver and the internal components makes it possible to generate more acoustic output than other types of instruments, while avoiding the problem of acoustic feedback. Although cosmetically more noticeable and thus less appealing to some persons, the controls of a body-type aid are easily accessible and, therefore, are less restrictive for a person with reduced manual desterity.

BONE CONDUCTION

The special case of the person who cannot wear a conventional device to couple the hearing aid instrument to the ear (e.g., stenotic ear canal, atresia, or chronic ear drainage) may require as the receiver a bone conduction oscillator placed against the mastoid process. This method of providing amplification normally is not desirable because of the output limitations of the bone conduction oscillator (Barry & Gaddis, 1977; Dirks, 1978) and the practical limitations of using an unstable coupling system.

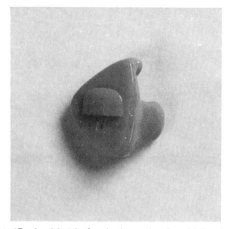

Fig. 17–6. Model of an in-the-ear hearing aid, in which components are housed within the earmold.

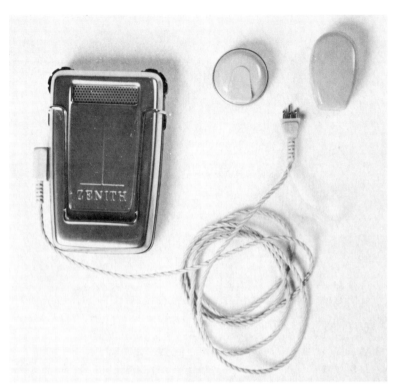

Fig. 17-7. Body-type hearing aid with a conventional and bone conduction receiver (Courtesy of Zenetron Inc., manufacturer of Zenith and Zenetron hearing aids.)

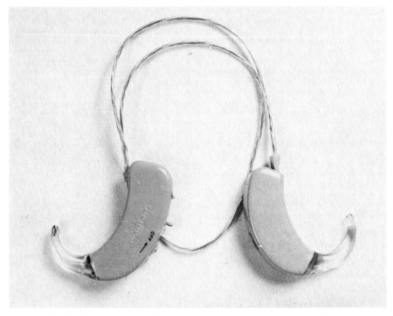

Fig. 17-8. Earlevel CROS hearing aid (Courtesy of Qualitone, Inc.).

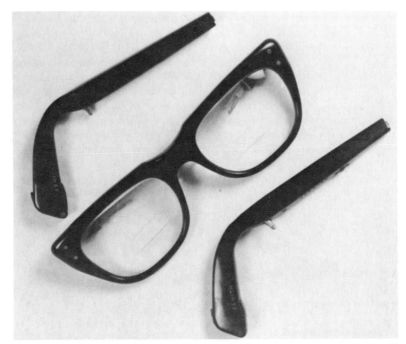

Fig. 17–9. Eyeglass binaural hearing aids with components housed within eyeglass temples (Courtesy of Zenetron Inc., manufacturer of Zenith and Zenetron hearing aids.)

CONTRALATERAL ROUTING OF SIGNAL (CROS)

The development of CROS amplification (Harford, 1966; Harford & Barry, 1965; Harford & Dodds, 1966; Wullstein & Wigand, 1962) has been beneficial especially to persons with a unilateral and/or high-frequency hearing loss. Basically, the CROS system provides the person with auditory stimulation in the impaired ear through a microphone that is fixed on that side of the head. The signal is routed to the contralateral ear providing improved auditory reception for an individual who otherwise might function with a unilateral hearing impairment. The numerous variations that have resulted since the inception of the CROS have led to the capability of selecting a hearing aid for persons with a large variety of types, degrees, and configurations of hearing losses.

Choice of Ear

The decision about which ear should be evaluated with a hearing aid may be resolved by using binaural amplification. The attributes of binaural hearing versus monaural listening are well described in the literature (Belzile & Markle, 1959; Briskey, 1972; Carhart, 1958; DiCarlo & Brown, 1960; Harris, 1965; Ross, 1977). For some persons, however, the auditory benefits from binaural aids may not outweigh the stigma or economic considerations involved in the purchase of two hearing aids.

Generally, the ear selected for amplification is the one that provides the least amount of distortion to the incoming signal, the ear with the widest dynamic range, and/or the ear with the greatest loss of sensitivity to auditory stimuli. These criteria assume that the better-hearing ear has thresholds that approximate normal hearing and can contribute to communication without amplification. If, however, the poorer ear is not a good candidate for amplification due, for example, to poor discrimination or a narrow dynamic range, then the better ear may be selected for the hearing aid or the person may be evaluated with a CROS amplification system.

The hearing threshold levels of most persons with a presbycusic type of hearing impairment are usually bilaterally symmetrical (Schuknecht, 1974). The choice of which ear to fit may be based on the preference of the listener, thus necessitating an evaluation and trial period with the aid on each ear. The person may find that in some situations the aid may be most beneficial when worn on the left ear, such as when talking on the telephone. Under different circumstances, such as when driving a vehicle, the aid may provide the most benefit when worn on the right ear. The final recommendation may be to make two earmolds and allow the individual to alternate the hearing aid.

The Earmold

The earmold is "a plastic insert device designed to conduct amplified sound from the hearing aid receiver into the ear canal with as much efficiency as possible" (Smith, 1977, p. 142). According to Lybarger (1972), there are four basic earmold systems:

1. In the conventional earphone system, the receiver from the hearing aid snaps directly into the earmold, thereby becoming an integral part of the coupling system.
2. The internal earphone system routes sound energy transmitted from a receiver that is internal to the hearing aid through a tube to the earmold.
3. The receiver earmold system is used for aids that have the receiver extended into the canal of the earmold, as in the in-the-ear hearing aid.
4. The open canal earmold is a coupling system that uses no more than a piece of tubing that projects into the external auditory meatus.

Each component of the earmold system such as the tubing, canal, and vent bore has its own acoustic characteristics of width, depth, and length that can significantly alter the response characteristics of the amplification system (Cox, 1979; Dodds & Harford, 1968, 1970; Hodgson & Murdock, 1970; Jetty & Rintelmann, 1970; Konkle & Bess, 1974; Northern & Hattler, 1970). The selection of an earmold must be considered one of the most important decisions in the hearing aid selection procedure. Electroacoustically, the earmold can alter the response characteristics of the amplification network. Therefore, selecting the appropriate acoustical variations of the earmold must be an integral part of the evaluation and fitting process. For the elderly, the comfort of the earmold is important. The rejection of a hearing aid by a hearing-impaired individual may not be a result of an adverse reaction to amplified sound, but rather may result from a poorly fitting earmold. That is, the mold may cause soreness to the ear or be uncomfortable. The making of an earmold for an elderly individual presents the unique problem of fitting an ear that is experiencing cartilagenous changes that may occur in the outer ear and external auditory meatus due to aging (Hull, 1978). In addition, an earmold

often is reported to give the client a plugged feeling and is rejected for that reason. This problem can be resolved by placing a small vent in the mold, thereby equalizing the pressure within the canal to outside air. Finally, placing the earmold in the ear and obtaining the necessary acoustic seal can be a frustrating task for any person. Proper instruction and counseling on earmold insertion can reduce many of the reasons for rejecting a hearing aid and maximizes the possibility of a successful hearing aid fitting.

SELECTION PROCEDURES

The selection of hearing instruments for clinical evaluation requires an understanding of the relationships between certain anatomical and physiological aspects of audition, handicap-deficit asymmetry, the electroacoustic response characteristics of amplification systems and their associated component parts, and the psychoacoustic correlates of the electroacoustic characteristics of the hearing aid. The formal hearing aid evaluation can commence only after decisions relevant to these factors have been made.

Frequency-Gain Considerations

Among the most important considerations for selecting a hearing aid for a hearing-impaired listener are the identification of those response characteristics that will be comfortable and provide a high quality of sound transmission. Three philosophical approaches or principles to selecting appropriate frequency-gain functions for an individual have been identified by Braida, Durlach, Lippmann, Hicks, Rabinowitz, & Read (1980):

1. The gain should increase in frequency regions in which the hearing loss increases so that aided hearing levels approximate normal response levels.
2. The gain should be selected independently of the type and degree of hearing loss.
3. The gain function should be minimized in those frequency regions in which the hearing loss is greatest and the dynamic range is narrow.

Proponents of the first principle (Brooks, 1973; Byrne & Tonnison, 1976; Fleming & Rice, 1969; Kemker, 1972; Martin, Grover, Worral, & Williams, 1976; Reddell & Calvert, 1966; Thompson & Lassman, 1969; Victoreen, 1960, 1973; Wallenfels, 1967; Watson & Knudson, 1940; Watson & Tolan,

1949) suggest that the ideal frequency-gain function may be obtained by either mirroring the pure-tone audiogram or by selecting a frequency response that matches a suprathreshold equal-loudness contour. Restoring the threshold curve to normal, as is suggested by mirroring the pure-tone audiogram, has been criticized for two reasons: First, individuals do not listen at threshold and, second, gain is likely to be greatest in frequency regions where the dynamic range is reduced. Selecting a response curve that approximates the equal-loudness contour, on the other hand, may have a different configuration and output level, but may typify the most comfortable listening level. For example, the typical presbycusic threshold hearing loss is more pronounced in the higher frequencies, but a suprathreshold response curve may be flatter than the one derived at threshold. Thus, the frequency response characteristic of a hearing aid for this hearing loss would be flatter if it were selected from the suprathreshold response rather than the pure-tone audiogram.

Davis, Hudgins, Marquis, Nichols, Peterson, Ross, & Stevens (1946), in the classic Harvard Report, first suggested the use of the second principle, namely, that the ideal gain may be selected independent of the hearing loss. They concluded that speech reception could be maximized for all hearing-impaired listeners by using either a flat frequency response or a response curve that had a 6 dB per octave high-frequency emphasis. Fletcher (1952), however, has noted that the functional gain of the hearing aids used by Davis et al. was different from the gain that was actually reported in their study. That is, they did not account for such variables as head diffraction and the resonant characteristics of the ear canal. In fact, Fletcher suggested that the flat response system functionally had a 6 dB per octave drop from 1000 Hz to 4000 Hz. Similarly, the system reported by Davis et al. as having a 6 dB per octave slope actually fell by 10 dB from 500 Hz to 250 Hz but was relatively flat from 500 to 8000 Hz. In addition to this criticism of the Harvard Report, Miller (1972) noted that most of the subjects used by the Harvard group had conductive hearing losses and were sophisticated hearing aid users. This does not represent the current population of elderly hearing aid users, who are often unsophisticated and have a sensorineural type of hearing loss (Sanders, 1978).

Pascoe, Niemoeller, and Miller (1974) have raised questions about the results of previous research with selective amplification. They suggested that many previous studies did not present accurate frequency-gain characteristics of the experimental amplification systems. They asserted that some researchers ignored the effects of the pinna, head diffraction, resonant characteristics of the ear canal, and associated variables that may alter the response of the hearing aid.

In their initial study, Pascoe et al. evaluated one presbycusic listener who had a bilaterally symmetrical, gradually downward-sloping, moderate sensorineural hearing loss. The subject's discrimination ability was measured in both quiet and noise. The results of the study suggested that, for this one subject, a flat functional gain response was superior to other experimental frequency response characteristics. More specifically, discrimination scores significantly decreased as amplification was reduced above 1500 Hz. Additionally, discrimination was significantly poorer for a coupler-determined flat frequency response that functionally had a gain function that was flat from 1000 to 1500 Hz, rose 19 dB between 1500 and 3000 Hz, and was again flat from 3000 to 6300 Hz. Discrimination was not degraded for those conditions in which low-frequency amplification was reduced. It would appear, then, that the selection of frequency-gain characteristics for this subject would be enhanced by determining the functional output of the amplification system.

In a followup to this project, Pascoe (1975) evaluated eight sensorineurally hearing-impaired elderly persons. The subjects listened to a closed-set word list in both quiet and noise through a master hearing aid that was adjusted to simulate five frequency response characteristics. The responses were defined both in terms of 2-cc coupler measurements and functional gain. Discrimination scores were consistently better with a response that functionally mirrored the sound-field audiogram. The lowest scores were obtained for a response that simulated "typical" hearing aids. The results suggested that, for this elderly population, mirroring the audiogram provided a distinct receptive advantage.

Alternative approaches to selecting a hearing aid independent of the audiometric configuration have been proposed but have not been applied specifically to an elderly population (Franklin, 1969, 1975; Harford & Fox, 1978; Martin & Pickett, 1970; Thomas & Pfannebecker, 1974; Thomas & Sparks, 1971; Skinner, 1976). Generally, the results seem to suggest that the frequency-gain function of hearing aids should emphasize frequency regions above 1000 Hz while maintaining a gain for conversational speech well within the comfort levels of the subject's dynamic range.

The third selection principle is based on the concept of decreasing the gain in the frequency regions that show the largest hearing loss. The premise here is that these regions will have the smallest dynamic range and thus the largest potential for internal distortion. Piminow (1963), for example, suggested that if a hearing loss exceeds 60 dB HL in a certain frequency region, then the amplification in this range should be minimized to reduce its contribution to an overall reduction in speech intelligibility. Similarly, Huizing, Kruisinga, & Taselaar (1960) suggested that atrophy of the central auditory system from either sound deprivation or aging can internally distort sound stimuli. They therefore recommended that speech discrimination be evaluated in varying preselected band-pass conditions. If the discrimination ability is poor in one particular band-pass condition, then this band would not be amplified. As applied to the elderly, this approach to selecting a hearing aid suggests that they must learn to discriminate speech by using those frequency regions in which the residual hearing is greatest. The other frequencies may not contribute to speech intelligibility.

Commonalities that can be found among the three philosophies of hearing aid selection include:

1. Elimination or reduction of low-frequency energy does not appear to be detrimental to speech intelligibility and, in many instances, can facilitate the reception of speech.
2. Mirroring the sound-field audiogram may provide optimum intelligibility of speech for elderly patients, but consideration must be given to the degree of high-frequency hearing loss and the subject's dynamic range of hearing.
3. Some consideration should be given to the potential detrimental effects of central auditory distortion. The literature has demonstrated that the elderly may have peripheral hearing loss that coexists with a central auditory processing impairment and that improving the frequency-gain characteristics will not necessarily resolve an impairment of speech intelligibility.

Future Directions

The physiologic and psychologic correlates of a narrow dynamic range of hearing in association with an intolerance for loud sounds has been suggested as a characteristic of a presbycusic hearing loss. It has been hypothesized, then, that the selection of a hearing aid for elderly hearing-impaired persons might be facilitated if there were an improvement of amplitude and frequency resolution techniques within hearing aids. Hearing aids then could amplify the impaired frequency regions without the discomfort or distortion that may be associated with the greater impairment and lower dynamic range of these frequency regions. It has become feasible, for example, for amplification systems to have electronic components that can amplitude-compress stimuli without distortion, thereby providing greater amplification to those frequency regions that have a narrow dynamic range of hearing. Compression systems are commercially available in the form of both peak limiting and automatic volume control (AVC). In peak limiting the sound is clipped at a predetermined output level. AVC systems, on the other hand, maintain a relatively constant input level that approximates the point of maximum speech intelligibility and comfort. Yet, there are inherent problems with each of these systems.

Braida et al. (1980) have suggested that a third system, which they term *syllabic compression*, may offer an undistorted and natural method of providing intelligible speech at comfortable listening levels. Syllabic compression is "concerned with altering the short-term intensity relations among speech elements" (p. 65) in an attempt to maintain a comfortable listening level. It has been reported that compression amplification systems clinically are not superior to conventional peak clipped systems (Caraway & Carhart, 1967; Kretsinger & Young, 1960; Lynn & Carhart, 1963; Rintelmann, 1972; Trinder, 1972; Vargo, 1977; Vargo & Carhart, 1972). Braida et al. (1980) suggested that this is due, at least in part, to the limited technological information that was available prior to 1970 when many of these studies were completed, and also to a lack of control by most researchers in fitting the amplification systems to the individual needs of their subjects. Villchur (1973) adds that the single-channel compression systems used in many studies were inadequate for the needs of a hearing-handicapped person.

Villchur designed a system to "restore normal loudness to each acoustical speech element of importance" (p. 1648). As he noted, this requires several compression channels, one for each frequency band. Utilizing this concept, Villchur demonstrated that speech intelligibility could be significantly improved while maintaining comfortable listening levels. This concept of multichannel compression systems is promising but needs study with subjects of varying degrees of hearing loss and audiometric configurations.

Technology also has facilitated the study of the effects that alterations of the frequency domain can have on speech intelligibility. Two of the methods under study are disproportionate and proportionate frequency shifting (Beasley & Maki, 1976).

Disproportionate frequency-shifted speech alters selected or single frequency bands of speech. The purpose is to shift those frequency regions that contribute to distortion and/or discomfort to a new frequency region that is, generally, lower and less impaired than the shifted region. Experimentation with disporportionate shifting, however, has not been fruitful. It has been suggested that this technique does not maintain the relatively invariant formant relationships of phonemes, thus making it difficult to linguistically encode the contextual information provided by the formant frequencies of speech. In an attempt to maintain these formant relationships, more recent research has focused on the use of proportionate frequency shifting (Beasley, Mosher, & Orchik, 1976; Bennett & Byers, 1967; Bennett & Linvill, 1975; Daniloff, Shriner, & Zemlin, 1968; Fairbanks, Everitt, & Jaeger, 1954; Mazor, Simon, Scheinberg, & Levitt, 1977; Shriner, Beasley, & Zemlin, 1969; Tiffany & Bennett, 1961; Zemlin, 1966). That is, the entire frequency spectrum is shifted proportionately and the acoustic relationships that are necessary for accurate perception of speech are maintained. A small number of studies have been carried out using proportionate frequency shifting techniques with the hearing-impaired, and these have met with limited success. Most of the investigations used prelingually hearing-impaired subjects, thus eliminating the potential linguistic advantages that a population with an acquired hearing loss would have in learning to process the frequency-altered stimuli. Further, the stimuli for these studies have been generated by equipment with limited frequency responses and/or inherent frequency distortion. Perhaps future research could take advantage of recent advances in computer technology to generate stimulus materials. These and other problems will need to be addressed prior to the development of frequency-shifted prosthetic devices. The potential benefits that may result from this technique, however, are still not defined, and more research is needed.

EVALUATION PROCEDURES

Traditional Procedures

The traditional and still widely practiced clinical evaluation of a person's performance with a hearing aid was first described by Carhart (1946). He rec-

ommended that four parameters of aided performance be assessed: effective gain, tolerance, and speech intelligibility measured in both quiet and noise. Each of these performance measures uses standardized, spondaic and phonetically balanced, monosyllabic word tests. Several hearing aids are evaluated clinically on the client and the aided results may be compared to the results obtained for an unaided test condition. The most appropriate hearing aid then can be selected from among the three to six that are employed with this procedure.

Alternative hearing aid evaluation procedures have been advocated, and although some are methologically divorced from the traditional procedure, the client is evaluated with the hearing aid gain adjusted to a subjectively determined most-comfortable-loudness (MCL) level. Shore, Bilger, and Hirsh (1960) suggested that the hearing aid gain be set at the client's unaided speech reception threshold (SRT), thus eliminating the subjective assessment of MCL. This gain, however, may exceed a comfortable listening level. The validity of the Shore et al. procedure is suspect in that it assumes that the client will wear the aid at this uncomfortable gain setting. More typically, however, the client will adjust the hearing aid to a comfortable listening level, and not necessarily to a higher listening level, which may or may not provide more intelligible speech. Thus, the aid should be evaluated clinically at the MCL.

In addition to evaluating each hearing aid at MCL, Carhart suggested that aids be assessed while set at the full-volume control rotation position. Currently, many clinicians forego this time-consuming portion of the traditional hearing aid selection procedure and, instead, may use the time to evaluate other hearing aids and/or to counsel the patient.

The traditional hearing aid evaluation procedure assessed auditory discrimination of speech using monosyllabic words in an open-ended response format. The words were presented in a white or sawtooth noise environment that was continuously varied until speech was barely intelligible. A more currently practiced modification of this procedure includes the assessment of speech discrimination presented with a competing message, either noise or speech, at a pre-established signal-to-noise ratio. More information and greater sensitivity to differences among hearing aids might be obtained by using closed-set monosyllabic rhyming tests (Owens & Schubert, 1977; Schwartz & Surr, 1979). The use of monosyllables, however, has come under criticism because of their insensitivity in predicting differences among hearing aids and because of a lack of face validity. Conversational speech is usually expressed by phrases or sentences; therefore, a communication handicap may not be assessed accurately by the use of single-word stimuli.

Several authors have addressed this problem and have used sentential stimuli to assess communication deficits (Beasley & Flaherty-Rintelmann, 1976; Freeman & Church, 1977; Jerger et al., 1968; Kalikow, Stevens, & Elliot, 1977; Kalikow, Stevens, Gerstman, & Morrison, 1976). Sentences simulate everyday communication tasks and place more stress on auditory processing than monosyllabic stimuli. The recall of sentential stimuli is more than a test of auditory discrimination. Other aspects of linguistic capabilities, including the ability to process temporal, syntactic, and semantic cues, are necessary to identify the stimuli.

Jerger and Hayes (1976) have used sentential stimuli to differentiate among various amplification systems. Their stimuli were approximations of real English sentences that were presented in conjunction with a competing message at several message-to-competition ratios. They noted that their technique created a more realistic listening situation than the presentation of monosyllabic words in either quiet or at a single signal-to-noise ratio. Although this procedure does appear to have great promise for the clinical evaluation of amplification systems, there is still a need to determine if sentential stimuli provide a more valid method of evaluating an individual's performance with a hearing aid than monosyllabic words.

Nontraditional Procedures

Alternative approaches, differing conceptually from the traditional hearing aid selection procedure, have been recommended as practical for clinical use (Jerger, 1967; Zerlin, 1962) but have not achieved widespread acceptance for use with an elderly population (Burney, 1972). Among the nontraditional selection procedures is the selection of an amplification system based on its electroacoustic performance characteriscics (Ross, 1975; Zink, 1972; Zink & Alpiner, 1968). In this procedure, the hearing aid is selected from manufacturer specifications or electroacoustic performance data obtained from the aid. This procedure can be economical because it eliminates the extensive traditional hearing aid selection process and requires less patient-contact time. This latter benefit may be most appealing for use with an elderly hearing-impaired person who may have financial limitations and/or a need for additional counseling.

The electroacoustic selection procedure, however, is based on four assumptions. First, it assumes that hearing aids that appear electroacoustically similar will provide equal benefit to the listener. Second, it requires that the response characteristics represented by the manufacturer's specifications are a valid representation of the stock hearing aid. Third, it assumes that the electroacoustic performance data are representative of the functional response characteristics of the hearing aid. Finally, it supposes that the hearing aid selection procedure is not important for all patients. At one time some of these assumptions may have been valid. They have not been tested formally with the elderly, however, and their validity for this population is thus still open to question.

In addition, technological advancements have made it possible to alter and selectively shape hearing aid response characteristics, but the psychoacoustic correlates of these changes are not well defined. This suggests that it is necessary to clinically evaluate elderly hearing-impaired persons with various amplification systems or response alterations prior to the recommendation of a hearing aid.

HEARING AID ORIENTATION

The role of the hearing health care professional does not end with the selection and fitting of a hearing aid. Every effort must be made to ensure that the hearing aid is functioning properly and that the patient is obtaining maximum benefit from amplification. Approximately 38 percent of hearing aid users are dissatisfied with their device (Rassi & Harford, 1968). Oyer, Freeman, Hardick, Dixon, Donnelly, Goldstein, Lloyd, & Mussen (1976) suggested that dissatisfaction may be related to inadequate counseling and follow-up of the hearing-impaired client. They found that many clients who did not return to audiology centers for hearing aid counseling were not aware that this service was available or were not motivated or encouraged to take advantage of the orientation programs. Perhaps this reflects the lack of an organized follow-up orientation program by the hearing health care professionals ("A conference on hearing aid evaluation procedures", 1967).

The hearing aid wearers and persons responsible for care of the elderly should have available information about the hearing aid and its component parts, including:

1. How to put the battery in its case properly and assure that external parts such as the earmold, tubing, and/or receiver are attached to the instrument properly.
2. How to put the hearing aid on and properly insert the earmold.
3. How to adjust the volume control and other external controls.
4. The name of the hearing aid manufacturer, battery type, battery life (both on the shelf and in the aid) and a place where replacement parts or service may be obtained.
5. The psychoacoustic limitations of the hearing aid and those communicative situations in which the aid will be the most and the least beneficial.
6. The importance of obtaining a hearing level assessment and otologic evaluation at least annually and preferably semiannually.
7. The necessity to avoid exposing the aid to excessive heat, moisture, hair spray, or perspiration; also, the fact that animals, especially dogs, are attracted by the scent that may emanate from hearing aids and will chew them if given the opportunity.
8. The importance of opening the battery compartment and removing the battery when the aid is removed for any length of time, such as at night. This assures that the aid is off and reduces the possibility of battery corrosion and leakage within the hearing aid.

The hearing aid is an electronic system that may be in need of occasional maintenance, even with proper care. To avoid unnecessary expenses, the hearing aid user should also know how to troubleshoot the hearing aid. The following points summarize troubleshooting for some of the most common hearing aid problems:

Squealing
The earmold may not be seated properly in the ear.
The tubing or nozzle on an earlevel instrument may be cracked and in need of replacement.
The receiver case on a body-worn hearing aid may be loose and in need of repair or replacement.
The hearing aid microphone may be seated near a reflecting surface such as a hat, wall, or article of clothing.
The hearing aid case may be loose or there may be internal squealing. This can be checked by closing off sound at the receiver. If there still is

squealing, then gently squeeze the case. If the squealing stops, then the case should be tightened. If it persists, then the aid may be in need of repair.

Uncomfortable earmold
The mold may have rough surface spots and be in need of buffing.
The helix may need to be removed, as it often is a source of irritation.
The earmold may be an improper fit and may have to be replaced.
The patient may have an allergic reaction to earmold material.
The earmold may need a vent to equalize the pressure in the external canal with outside air.

Intermittent, weak, or no sound
The earmold may not be properly seated in the ear.
There may be a weak battery. It is recommended that persons purchase a battery tester to monitor battery life.
If the instrument is a body aid, then check for a defective cord.
The earmold, tubing, or nozzle may be clogged with cerumen or a foreign object.
The battery contacts may need to be cleaned. The contacts can be cleaned with a rubber eraser and wiped clean with a cloth.
The tubing may be twisted.
The hearing levels of the client should be rechecked to rule out a change in the hearing threshold levels.

SUMMARY

In summary, an overview of those variables that interact in the selection process for amplification for the elderly have been presented. Generally, hearing aids are an integral part of a comprehensive aural rehabilitation program. The initial responsibility, however, for determining hearing aid candidacy and successful auditory rehabilitation lies with the hearing-handicapped individual, who must be properly motivated to try a hearing aid. Only then may the responsibility shift to the hearing health care professionals, who must assure that the hearing aid fitting is appropriate and that the patient is obtaining maximum benefit from amplification. Amplification can play an important role in auditory rehabilitation of elderly persons with an acquired communication handicap.

REFERENCES

Alpiner, J. Aural rehabilitation in the aged client. *Maico Audiological Library Series*, 1967, *4*, 9−12.

Alpiner, J. G. Rehabilitation of the geriatric client. In J. Alpiner (Ed.), *Handbook of adult rehabilitative audiology*. Baltimore: Williams & Wilkins Co., 1978.

Alpiner, J. G., Chevrette, W., Glascoe, G., Metz, M., & Olsen, B. The Denver Scale of Communication Function. Unpublished study, University of Denver, 1974. (Cited in Alpiner, J. G. Evaluation of communication function. In J. Alpiner (Ed.) *Handbook of adult rehabilitative audiology*. Williams & Wilkins, Baltimore, 1978).

American National Standards Institute. American standard methods for measurement of electroacoustic characteristics of hearing aids, S3.3−1960 (R−1971). New York, 1960.

American National Standards Institute. American standard methods for expressing performance, S3.8−1967 (R−1971). New York, 1967.

American National Standards Institute. American National Standard for specification of hearing aid characteristics. ASA STD 7−1976 (ANSI S3.22−1976). New York, 1976.

ASHA Committee on Rehabilitative Audiology. The audiologist: Responsibilities in the habilitation of the auditorily handicapped. *ASHA: Journal of the American Speech and Hearing Association*, 1974, *16*, 68−70.

Appel, F. W. & Appel, E. M. Intracranial variation in the weight of the human brain. *Human Biology*, 1942, *14*, 48−68.

Barry, S. J. & Gaddis, S. Physical and physiological constraint on the use of bone conduction speech audiometry. Paper presented at the Annual Convention of the American Speech and Hearing Association, Chicago, 1977.

Beasley, D. S., & Flaherty-Rintelmann, A. Children's perception of temporally distorted sentential approximations of varying length. *Audiology*, 1976, *15*, 315−325.

Beasley, D. S., & Maki, J. Time and frequency altered speech. In Lass, N. (Ed.) *Contemporary Issues in Experimental Phonetics*. New York, Academic Press, 1976.

Beasley, D. S., Mosher, N. L., & Orchik, D. J. Use of frequency shifted/time compressed speech with hearing impaired children. *Audiology*, 1976, *15*, 395−406.

Belzile, M., & Markle, D. M. A clinical comparison of monaural and binaural hearing aids worn by patients with conductive or perceptive deafness. *Laryngoscope*, 1959, *69*, 1317−1323.

Bennett, D. N., & Byers, V. M. Increased intelligibility in the hypacusic by slow play frequency transposition. *Journal of Auditory Research*, 1967, *7*, 107−118.

Bennett, I. M., & Linvill, J. G. A study of time domain speech compression by means of a new analog speech processor. *Journal of the Audio Engineering Society*, 1975, *23*, 713−721.

Berger, K. W., & Millin, J. P. Hearing aids. In D. Rose (Ed.,), *Otological assessment*. Englewood Cliffs, N. J.: Prentice-Hall, 1971.

Berkowitz, A. O., & Hochberg, I. Self-assessment of hearing handicap in the aged. *Archives of Otolaryngology*, 1970, *92*, 25−28.

Bolton, B., Cull, J. G., & Hardy, R. E. Psychological adjustment to hearing loss and deafness. In R. Hardy & J. Cull (Eds.), *Educational and psychosocial aspects of deafness*. Springfield, Ill.: Charles C. Thomas Publisher, 1974.

Braida, L. D., Durlach, N. I., Lippman, R. T., Hicks, B. L., Rabinowitz, W. M., & Reed, C. M. Hearing aids—A review of past research on linear amplification, amplitude compression, and frequency lowering. ASHA monograph #19. Rockville, Md., American Speech-Language-Hearing Association, 1980.

Bredberg, G. Cellular pattern in nerve supply of the human organ of Corti. *Acta Oto-laryngologica*, 1968, *Supplement 236*.

Briskey, R. J. Binaural hearing aids and new innovations. In J. Katz (Ed.), *Handbook of clinical audiology*. Baltimore: Williams & Wilkins, 1972.

Brody, H. Organization of the cerebral cortex: A study of aging in the human cerebral cortex. *Journal of Comparative Neurology*, 1955, *102*, 511−556.

Brooks, D. N. Gain requirements of hearing aid users. *Scandinavian Audiology*, 1973, *2*, 199–205.

Burney, P. A. A survey of hearing aid evaluation procedures. *ASHA: Journal of the American Speech and Hearing Association*, 1972, *14*, 439–444.

Butler, R. N., & Lewis, M. I. *Aging and Mental Health*, St. Louis: C. V. Mosby Company, 1973.

Byrne, D., & Tonisson, S. Selecting the gain of hearing aids for persons with sensorineural hearing impairment. *Scandinavian Audiology*, 1976, *5*, 51–62.

Caraway, B., & Carhart, R. Influence of compressor action on speech intelligibility. *Journal of the Acoustical Society of America*, 1967, *41*, 1424–1434.

Carhart, R. Tests for selection of hearing aids. *Laryngoscope*, 1946, *56*, 780–794.

Carhart, R. The usefulness of the binaural hearing aid. *Journal of Speech and Hearing Disorders*, 1958, *23*, 41–51.

A conference on hearing aid evaluation procedures. *ASHA Reports*, 1967, *2*.

Cox, R. Acoustic aspects of hearing aid–ear canal coupling systems. *Monographs in Contemporary Audiology*, 1979, *1*, 44 pp.

Daniloff, R. G., Shriner, T. H., & Zemlin, W. R. Intelligibility of vowels altered in duration and frequency. *Journal of the Acoustical Society of America*, 1968, *44*, 700–707.

Davis, H. The articulation area in the social adequacy index for hearing. *Laryngoscope*, 1948, *58*, 761–778.

Davis, H. Hearing handicap, standards for hearing, and medicolegal rules. In H. Davis & S. Silverman (Eds.), *Hearing and deafness*, New York: Holt, Rinehart, & Winston, 1970.

Davis, H., Hudgins, C. V., Marquis, R. J., Nichols, R. H., Jr., Peterson, G. E., Ross, D. A., & Stevens, S. S. The selection of hearing aids. *Laryngoscope*, 1946, *56*, 85–115; 135–163.

DiCarlo, L. M., & Brown, W. J. The effectiveness of binaural hearing aids for adults with hearing impairments. *Journal of Auditory Research*, 1960, *1*, 35–76.

Dirks, D. D. Bone conduction testing. In J. Katz (Ed.), *Handbook of clinical audiology*. Baltimore: Williams & Wilkins, 1978.

Dix, M. R. Loudness recruitment and its measurement with especial reference to the loudness discomfort test and its value in diagnosis. *Annals of Otology, Rhinology and Laryngology*, 1968, *77*, 1131–1151.

Dodds, E., & Harford, E. Modified ear pieces and CROS for high frequency hearing losses. *Journal of Speech and Hearing Research*, 1968, *11*, 204–218.

Dodds, E. & Harford, E. Followup report on modified earpieces in CROS for high frequency hearing losses. *Journal of Speech and Hearing Research*, 1970, *13*, 41–43.

Fairbanks, G., Everitt, W. L., & Jaeger, R. P. Methods for time or frequency compression–expansion of speech. *Transactions of IRE-PGA*, 1954, *AU-2*, 7–12.

Federal Register, 42 (31), 9286–9296, February 15, 1977.

Ferraro, J. A., & Minckler, J. The brachium of the inferior colliculus, the human auditory pathways: A quantitative study. *Brain and Language*, 1977, *4*, 156–164.

Fleming, D. B., & Rice, C. G. New circuit development concept in hearing aids. *International Audiology*, 1969, *8*, 517–523.

Fletcher, H. The perception of speech sounds by deafened persons. *Journal of the Acoustical Society of America*, 1952, *24*, 490–497.

Fletcher, H. *Speech and hearing in communication* (2nd ed.). New York: D. Van Nostrand, 1953.

Franklin, B. The effect on consonant discrimination of combining a low frequency pass band in one ear with a high frequency pass band in the other ear. *Journal of Auditory Research*, 1969, *9*, 365–378.

Franklin, B. The effect of combining low and high frequency pass bands on consonant recognition in the hearing impaired. *Journal of Speech and Hearing Research*, 1975, *18*, 719–727.

Freeman, B. A. Who is a candidate for a hearing aid? Presented at the symposium on *What the otolaryngologist should know about hearing aids*, E. A. R. Foundation, Nashville, 1978.

Freeman, B. A., & Beasley, D. S. Discrimination of time altered sentential approximations and monosyllables by children with reading problems. *Journal of Speech and Hearing Research*, 1978, *21*, 497–506.

Freeman, B. A., & Church, G. Recall and repetition of time compressed sentential approximations by normal hearing young adults. *Journal of the American Audiology Society*, 1977, *3*, 47–51.

Gaeth, J. A study of phonemic regression associated with hearing loss. Unpublished doctoral dissertation, Northwestern University, 1948.

Goodman, A. Reference zero levels for pure tone audiometry. *ASHA: Journal of the American Speech and Hearing Association*, 1965, *7*, 262–263.

Guild, S. R. Correlation of histologic observations and the acuity of hearing. *Acta Oto-laryngologica*, 1932, *17*, 204–207.

Harford, E. Bilateral CROS. *Archives of Otolaryngology*, 1966, *84*, 426–432.

Harford, E., & Barry, J. A rehabilitative approach to the problem of unilateral hearing impairment: The contra-lateral routing of signals (CROS). *Journal of Speech and Hearing Disorders*, 1965, *30*, 121–138.

Harford, E., & Dodds, E. The clinical application of CROS. *Archives of Otolaryngology*, 1966, *83*, 455–464.

Harford, E., & Dodds, E. Versions of the CROS hearing aid. *Archives of Otolaryngology*, 1974, *100*, 50–58.

Harford, E., & Fox, J. The use of high pass amplification with broad frequency sensorineural hearing loss. *Audiology*, 1978, *17*, 10–26.

Harris, J. D. Monaural and binaural speech intelligibility and the stereophonic effect based upon temporal cues. *Laryngoscope*, 1965, *75*, 428–446.

Hearing Aid Industry Conference. HAIC Standard Method of Expressing Hearing Aid Performance, New York, 1961.

High, W. S., Fairbanks, G., & Glorig, A. Scale for self-assessment of hearing handicap. *Journal of Speech and Hearing Disorders*, 1964, *29*, 215–230.

Hodgson, W., & Murdock, C. Effect of the earmold on speech intelligibility in hearing aid use. *Journal of Speech and Hearing Research*, 1970, *13*, 290–297.

Hood, J. D., & Poole, J. P. Tolerable limits of loudness: Its clinical and physiological significance. *Journal of the Acoustical Society of America*, 1966, *40*, 47–53.

Huizing, H. C., Kruisinga, R. J. H., & Taselaar, M. Triplet Audiometry: An analysis of band discrimination in speech reception. *Acta Oto-laryngologica*, 1960, *51*, 256–259.

Hull, R. H. Hearing evaluation of the elderly. In J. Katz (Ed.), *Handbook of clinical audiology*. Baltimore: Williams & Wilkins, 1978.

International Electrotechnical Commission. IEC recommended methods for measurement of the electroacoustical characteristics of hearing aids. Publication No. 118, Geneva, 1959.

Jerger, J. Behavioral correlates of hearing aid performance. *Bulletin of Prosthetics Research*, 1967, *10*, 62–75.

Jerger, J. & Hayes, D. Hearing aid evaluation. *Archives of Otolaryngology*, 1976, *102*, 214–225.

Jerger, J., Speaks, C., & Trammell, J. An approach to speech audiometry. *Journal of Speech and Hearing Disorders*, 1968, *33*, 318–328.

Jetty, A. J., & Rintelmann, W. F. Acoustic effects on speech audiometric scores using a CROS hearing aid. *Journal of Speech and Hearing Research*, 1970, *13*, 101–114.

Jones, H. E. Intelligence in problem solving. In J. E. Birren (Ed.), *Handbook of aging in the individual*. Chicago: University of Chicago Press, 1959.

Kalikow, D. N., Stevens, K. N., & Elliot, L. L. Development of a test of speech intelligibility in noise using sentence materials with controlled word predictability. *Journal of the Acoustical Society of America*, 1977, *61*, 1337–1351.

Kalikow, D. N., Stevens, K. N., Gerstman, H. L., & Morrison, R. The speech perception in noise tests: Description and clinical data. Paper presented at convention of the American Speech and Hearing Association, Houston, 1976.

Kasten, R. N. Body and over-the-ear hearing aids. In J. Katz (Ed.), *Handbook of clinical audiology*. Baltimore: Williams & Wilkins, 1972.

Kasten, R. N. Standards in standard hearing aids. In J. Katz (Ed.), *Handbook of clinical audiology*. Baltimore: Williams & Wilkins, 1978.

Kemker, J. F. The effect of five hearing aid evaluation procedures on speech discrimination. Paper presented at Convention of the American Speech and Hearing Association, San Francisco, 1972.

Konkle, D. F., Beasley, D. S., & Bess, F. H. Intelligibility of time altered speech in relation to chronological aging. *Journal of Speech and Hearing Research,* 1977, *20,* 108−115.

Konkle, D. F., & Bess, F. H. Custom-made versus stock earmolds in hearing aid evaluations. *Archives of Otolaryngology,* 1974, *99,* 140−144.

Korabic, E. W., Freeman, B. A., & Church, G. T. Intelligibility of time expanded speech with normally hearing in elderly subjects. *Audiology,* 1978, *17,* 159−164.

Kretsinger, E. A., & Young, N. B. The use of fast limiting to improve the intelligibility of speech and noise. *Speech Monographs,* 1960, *27,* 63−69.

Ling, D. *Speech and the hearing-impaired child: Theory and practice.* Washington, D.C.: Alexander Graham Bell Association for the Deaf, Inc., 1976.

Lybarger, S. F. Earmolds. In J. Katz (Ed.) *Handbook of clinical audiology.* Baltimore: Williams & Wilkins, 1972.

Lybarger, S. F. A profile of ASA STD7—1976. *Hearing Instruments,* 1977, *28,* 10−11, 36.

Lynn, G., & Carhart, R. Influence of attack and release in compression amplification on understanding of speech by hypoacusics. *Journal of Speech and Hearing Disorders,* 1963, *28,* 124−140.

Martin, E., & Pickett, J. Sensorineural hearing loss and upward spread of masking. *Journal of Speech and Hearing Research,* 1970, *13,* 426−437.

Martin, M. C., Grover, B. C., Worrall, J. J., & Williams, V. The effectiveness of hearing aids in a school population. *British Journal of Audiology,* 1976, *10,* 33−40.

Mazor, M., Simon, H., Scheinberg, J., & Levitt, H. Moderate frequency compression for the moderately hearing impaired. *Journal of the Acoustical Society of America,* 1977, *62,* 1273−1278.

Miller, M. H. *Hearing aids.* New York: Bobbs-Merrill, 1972.

Minckler, J., Jaeger, M., Ferraro, J., Powers, M. Grace, R., Campain, R., Metz, M., & Martin, S. The human auditory pathways, a quantitative study. *Brain and Language,* 1977, *4,* 152−155

Newby, H. A. *Audiology.* New York: Prentice-Hall, 1972.

Noble, W. G., & Atherley, G. R. C. The hearing measure scale: A questionnaire for the assessment of auditory disability. *Journal of Auditory Research,* 1970, *10,* 229−250.

Northern, J. L. Hearing aids and acoustic impedance measurements. *Monographs in Contemporary Audiology,* 1978, *1,* 1−23.

Northern, J. L., & Hattler, K. W. Earmold influence on aided speech identification tasks. *Journal of Speech and Hearing Research,* 1970, *13,* 162−172.

Olsen, W. O. Physical characteristics of hearing aids. In W. Hodgson & P. Skinner (Eds.), *Hearing aid assessment and use in audiologic habilitation.* Baltimore: Williams & Wilkins, 1977.

O'Neill, J. J., & Oyer, H. J. *Applied audiometry.* New York: Dodd, Mead & Co., 1966.

Opheim, O., & Flottorp, G. Meniere's disease. *Acta Oto-laryngologica,* 1957, *47,* 202−218.

Owens, E., & Schubert, E. Development of the California consonant test. *Journal of Speech and Hearing Research,* 1977, *20,* 463−474.

Oyer, H. J., Freeman, B. A., Hardick, E., Dixon, J., Donnelly, K., Goldstein, D., Lloyd, L., & Mussen, E. Unheeded recommendations for aural rehabilitation: Analysis of a survey. *Journal of the Academy of Rehabilitative Audiology,* 1976, *9,* 20−30.

Oyer, H. J., & Frankmann, J. P. *The aural rehabilitation process.* New York: Holt, Rinehart & Winston, 1975.

Pascoe, D. P. Frequency responses of hearing aids and their effects on the speech perception of hearing impaired subjects. *Annals of Otology, Rhinology and Laryngology,* 1975, (Suppl. 23), *84,* Part 2.

Pascoe, D. P., Niemoeller, A. F., & Miller, J. D. Hearing aid design and evaluation for presbycusic patient. *Journal of the Acoustical Society of America,* 1974, *55,* 461a.

Peters, G. M. & Hardick, E. J. The relationship between some measures of hearing loss and self-assessment of hearing handicap. Paper presented at annual convention of American Speech and Hearing Asso., 1974.

Piminow, L. The application of synthetic speech to aural rehabilitation. *Journal of Auditory Research*, 1963, *3*, 73−82.

Pollack, M. C. Electroacoustic characteristics. In M. C. Pollack (Ed.) *Amplification for the hearing impaired*. New York: Grune & Stratton, 1980.

Preves, D. A., & Hoke, M. L. Information and techniques used to design custom in-the-ear hearing aids. *Hearing Aid Journal*, 1978.

Ramsdell, D. A. The psychology of the hard of hearing and the deafened adult. In H. Davis & S. Silverman (Eds.), *Hearing and deafness*. New York: Holt, Rinehart & Winston, 1970.

Rassi, J., & Harford, E. An analysis of patient attitudes and reactions to a clinical hearing aid selection program. *ASHA: Journal of the American Speech and Hearing Association*, 1968, *10*, 283−290.

Reddell, R. C., & Calvert D. R. Selecting a hearing aid by interpreting audiological data. *Journal of Auditory Research*, 1966, *6*, 445−452.

Rintelmann, W. F. Effects of amplitude compresssion upon speech perception: A review of the research. *Scandinavian Audiology*, 1972, *1*, 127−134.

Ross, M. Hearing aid selection for the pre-verbal hearing impaired child. In M. Pollack (Ed.), *Amplification for the hearing impaired*. New York: Grune & Stratton, 1975.

Ross, M. Binaural versus monaural hearing aid amplification for hearing impaired individuals. In F. Bess (Ed.), *Childhood deafness: Causation, assessment and management*. New York: Grune & Stratton, 1977.

Ross, M. Hearing aid evaluation. In J. Katz (Ed.), *Handbook of clinical audiology*. Baltimore: Williams & Wilkins, 1978.

Rupp, R. R., Higgins, J., & Maurer, J. F. A feasibility scale for predicting hearing aid use (FSPHAU) with older individuals. *Journal of the Academy of Rehabilitative Audiology*, 1977, *10*, 81−104.

Sanders, D. A. Hearing aid orientation in counseling. In M. Pollack (Ed.), *Amplification for the hearing impaired*. New York: Grune & Stratton, 1975.

Sanders, J. W. The successful hearing aid user. *Otolaryngologic Clinics of North America*, 1978, *11*, 187−193.

Schein, J. D., & Delk, Jr., M. T. *The deaf population of the United States*. Silver Spring, Md.: National Association of the Deaf, 1974.

Schmitz, H. Loudness discomfort level modification. *Journal of Speech and Hearing Research*, 1969, *12*, 807−817.

Schuknecht, H. F. *Pathology of the ear*. Cambridge, Mass.: Harvard University Press, 1974.

Schwartz, D. M., & Surr, R. K., Three experiments on the California Consonant Test. *Journal of Speech and Hearing Disorders*, 1979, *44*, 61−72.

Shapiro, I. Evaluation of the relationship between hearing threshold level and loudness discomfort level in sensorineural hearing loss. *Journal of Speech and Hearing Disorders*, 1979, *44*, 31−36.

Shore, I., Bilger, R. C., & Hirsh, I. Hearing aid evaluation: Reliability of repeated measurements. *Journal of Speech and Hearing Disorders*, 1960, *25*, 152−170.

Shriner, T. H., Beasley, D. S., & Zemlin, W. R. The effects of frequency division on speech identification in children. *Journal of Speech and Hearing Research*, 1969, *12*, 413−422.

Skinner, M. W. Speech intelligibility in noise induced hearing loss: The effects of high frequency compensation. Unpublished doctoral dissertation, Washington University, 1976.

Smith, K. E. Earmolds and hearing aid accessories. In W. Hodgson & P. Skinner (Eds.), *Hearing aid assessment and use in audiologic habilitation*. Baltimore: Williams & Wilkins, 1977.

Thomas, I. B., & Pfannebecker, G. Effects of spectral weighting of speech in hearing impaired subjects. *Journal of the Audio Engineering Society*, 1974, *22*, 690−694.

Thomas, I. B., & Sparks, D. W. Discrimination of filtered-clipped speech by hearing impaired subjects. *Journal of the Acoustical Society of America*, 1971, *49*, 1881−1887.

Thompson, G., & Lassman, F. Relationship of auditory distortion test results to speech discrimination through flat versus selective amplifying systems. *Journal of Speech and Hearing Research*, 1969, *12*, 594–606.

Tiffany, W. R., & Bennett, D. N. Intelligibility of slow played speech. *Journal of Speech and Hearing Research*, 1961, *4*, 248–258.

Trinder, E. An attempt to correct speech discrimination loss in cochlear deafness by graded instantaneous compression. *Sound*, 1972, *6*, 62–67.

Vargo, S. W. Intelligibility of amplitude compressed speech in quiet: Normal and pathological hearing groups. *Audiology and Hearing Education*, 1977, *3*, 16–19.

Vargo, S. W., & Carhart, R. Amplitude compression: Speech intelligibility in quiet with normal and pathological hearing groups. *Journal of the Acoustical Society of America*, 1972, *53*, 327 (A).

Victoreen, J. A. *Hearing enhancement*. Springfield, Ill.: Charles C. Thomas Publisher, 1960.

Victoreen, J. A. *Basic principles of otometry*. Springfield, Ill.: Charles C. Thomas Publisher, 1973.

Villchur, E. Signal processing to improve speech intelligibility in perceptive deafness. *Journal of the Acoustical Society of America*, 1973, *53*, 1646–1657.

Wallenfels, H. G. *Hearing aids on prescription*. Springfield, Ill.: Charles C. Thomas Publisher, 1967.

Ward, P. R., Tucker, A. M., Tudor, C. A., & Morgan, D. C. Self-assessment of hearing impairment: Tests of the expanded hearing ability scale questionnaire on hearing impaired adults in England. *British Journal of Audiology*, 1977, *11*, 33–39.

Watson, N. A., & Knudson, V. D. Selective amplification in hearing aids. *Journal of the Acoustical Society of America*, 1940, *11*, 406–419.

Watson, L., & Tolan, T. *Hearing tests and hearing instruments*. Baltimore: Williams & Wilkins, 1949.

Wullstein, H. L., & Wigand, M. E. A hearing aid for single ear deafness and its requirements. *Acta Oto-laryngologica*, 1962, *54*, 136–142.

Zemlin, W. R. The use of bandwidth and time compression for the hearing handicapped. In E. Foulke (Ed.), *Proceedings of the First Louisville Conference on Rate Altered Speech*. Louisville, Ky.: University of Louisville, 1966.

Zerlin, S. A new approach to hearing aid selection. *Journal of Speech and Hearing Research*, 1962, *5*, 370–376.

Zink, G. D. Hearing aids children wear: A longitudinal study of performance. *Volta Review*, 1972, *74*, 40–41.

Zink, G. D., & Alpiner, J. G. Hearing aids: One aspect of a state public school hearing conservation program. *Journal of Speech and Hearing Disorders*, 1968, *33*, 329–344.

Section IV

Delivery of Speech, Language, and Hearing Services to Older Adults

EDITORS' INTRODUCTION

Problems in communication cannot be isolated from the context of society in general. The concern of the general population is probably best exemplified in the governmental programs that it is willing to support, and the most significant of such programs in recent years has been the provision of health care through Medicare and Medicaid. In that speech−language pathology and audiology are allied health professions, it is appropriate that the reader have a basic understanding of the growth and development of Medicare and Medicaid programs and the basic policies and procedures of these as they relate to the provision of speech and hearing services. Dowling (Chapter 18) has provided the historic perspective and basic outline of the Medicare and Medicaid programs. Although it is only an introduction in the area, nevertheless the reader should come away with a basic understanding of current policy, keeping in mind that government activities are subject to rapid change, thereby necessitating continued update by those who serve in the allied health professions.

''Consumerism'' is an area that has become a significant part of everday life in our society. Every area of endeavor has had consumer advocates, and probably the most controversial advocacy directly affecting the field of communication disorders has been the provision of hearing aids. Wood and Marlin

(Chapter 19) discuss the principal characters in this controversy, including the manufacturers, the dealers, the audiologists, the physicians, and, perhaps the lead character, the client. They provide the background from the consumer advocate position of the need for government intervention in order to change a delivery system that has been perceived to be not in the best interest of the consumer; they then provide the current status of such regulation and suggest the need for further change. As with any controversial issue, it is unlikely that all readers will agree with all of Wood and Marlin's positions and conclusions. Nevertheless, they do provide an excellent example of how older adults have become actively involved in issues that directly affect their quality of life.

Finally, Lubinski (Chapter 20) returns to the general issues related to the life long process of aging discussed by Knox (Chapter 1), as applied to home health care and institutional settings such as the so-called nursing homes. The provision of on-site services has become a public and, at times, volatile issue as a result of consumer and media activities, stimulated in large measure by increased knowledge through research in the health and social sciences and the development of programs based on this knowledge. Lubinski provides an overview of the legislative history in this area and the rationale for the need for further developments in the provision of speech and hearing services to older adults. Her approach to the topic encompasses the many specific points discussed in the previous 19 chapters, and her closing statement exemplifies the theme of this book, namely, that "The improvement of communication skills and opportunities of older individuals in all settings must be considered a right and not a privilege, a priority and not a by-product, and a reality and not an ideal."

Richard J. Dowling

18
Federal Health Insurance for the Elderly

The curricula of most of the best-regarded speech–language pathology and audiology training programs in the country, on analysis, suggest that proficiency in the delivery of speech, language, and hearing services depends exclusively on a practitioner's scientific and clinical training and his or her ability to translate the products of that training (i.e., scientific knowledge and clinical skills) into the delivery of services that are of a high quality. This view assumes a dualistic health care delivery world, composed only of service recipients and service providers, in which the former pay the latter directly for services rendered. But the real health care delivery world—the one that has predominated for the better part of two decades—is a tripartite world comprising, in addition to recipients and providers, "third-party" insurers or payers of health care service costs, who, under the banners of cost-effectiveness and quality assurance, impose standards of participation on recipients and providers alike.

A thorough understanding of the nature and roles of these standard-setting, bill-paying third parties is an ingredient of provider proficiency that is almost as essential as is the ability to render high-quality services. If the standards of third parties are not accommodated, provider bills will not be paid. If they are not accommodated, then providers, no matter how clinically able, cannot long survive in a competitive health care marketplace. And if there are no providers, there can be no services.

This chapter focuses on federal health care insurance for the elderly and is designed to provide the foundation for an understanding of the important role of third parties in today's health care delivery system. For two very significant reasons, the chapter could not find a more appropriate forum than this volume, the central theme of which is the improved delivery of speech, language, and hearing services to the communicatively disabled elderly. First, virtually all tripartite health insurance programs (whether designed for single individuals or groups and irrespective of the ages of program beneficiaries) are modeled on the federal government's program of health insurance, the principal beneficiaries of which are the nation's elderly citizens. An understanding of the federal program's requirements and mechanisms thus provides a substantial base on which can be built an understanding of all health insurance programs.

Second, elderly Americans constitute the most rapidly expanding segment of the national population. Life expectancy has increased dramatically during the last 40 years. According to the U.S. Bureau of the Census (1977, 1978), the average life expectancy at birth in 1940 was in the neighborhood of 63½ years, whereas today, life expectancy is 69 for men and 77 for women. Seventy-five percent of all infants born today will reach age 65 and, once there, will live an average of 16 more years, to age 81 (National Center for Health Statistics, 1978). The U.S. Census Bureau (1977) projects that by the year 2050, life expectancy will have increased another 3 years for men and another 4 for women, and this is a conservative estimate (Sheppard & Rix, 1977, pp. 62–63). In 1940, about seven percent of the U.S. population was 65 or older; today, the proportion is 11 percent, or 24 million people. After the year 2010, when the "baby boom" children of the late forties and early fifties become elderly, the percentage of elderly will soar. By 2030, about 18 percent of the population or some 55 million citizens will be 65 years of age or older (U.S. Bureau of the Census, 1978).

The composition of the elderly population will change, too (U.S. Bureau of the Census, 1970, 1978). In 1940, only 30 percent of older Americans were 75 years or older. By the start of the 21st century, they will make up nearly 45 percent of the nation's elderly population.

Elderly Americans already require more than a proportionate share of health care services. In the coming years, that share will grow as their numbers grow. Thus, the health care insurance program that serves as the model for other programs is likely as well to be the program most used by health care service recipients and providers.

The focus of this chapter on the federal government's health insurance program for the elderly will move from the general to the particular, beginning with a brief, general description of the program's evolution, then moving closer for a look at the purposes and principal components of its two major parts. Finally, the focus will narrow to an analysis of the aspects of federal health insurance, both existing and prospective, that relate directly to the health care needs of elderly Americans who are communicatively handicapped and to the providers of speech–language pathology and audiology services who must fill these needs.

THE MAKING OF MEDICARE/MEDICAID

When, in mid-1965, the United States Congress added the Medicare (Title XVIII) and Medicaid (Title XIX) titles to the Social Security Act of 1935 (U.S. House of Representatives, 1973, pp. 354–476), the event marked the end of a long and significant opening chapter in the saga of a nation at odds with itself over whether needed health care services should be available, as a matter of right, to its citizens.

The saga began nearly 70 years ago, when then former President Theodore Roosevelt first proposed a publicly supported, government-administered health insurance system for all Americans. The proposal languished during the twenties and most of the thirties, attracted strong and vocal advocates (i.e., labor unions, social liberals, and President Harry S. Truman) in the forties, and galvanized equally powerful opponents (i.e., organized medicine and fiscal social conservatives) in the fifties. In the early sixties, government-backed health insurance appeared high on the domestic agendas of the Kennedy and Johnson administrations, but in a version dramatically scaled down from the universally applicable program called for by Roosevelt and aggressively urged, 35 years later, by President Truman.

Presidents Kennedy and Johnson were political realists who recognized that, if they were to succeed at all in inaugurating a viable national program of health insurance, accommodation of the needs and interests of the program's two principal opponents was essential. Organized medicine, which is to say the American Medical Association, had begun organizing against what it termed "socialized medicine" during the Truman Administration and, in the dozen or so intervening years, had honed its lobbying, fund raising, and public opinion-making abilities into the sharpest interest group edge in the nation's capital. Congressional conservatives in both political parties worried publicly about the costs of a massive new health program and the bureaucracy it would inevitably spawn. They worried, too, about the price the separate states and their individual citizens would have to pay in terms of diminished independence when the federal government took control of so vital a service as the delivery of health care.

And so when the Kennedy–Johnson health care proposal went to Congress, it focused not on health insurance for all Americans, but on health care coverage for those Americans who most needed health care and who, in the absence of governmental intervention, were least able to afford it—the elderly and the poor. The part of the proposed program designed to be run solely by the federal government (i.e., Medicare for the elderly) would not be financed by tax dollars, but by a special trust fund that would operate in theory, at least, like most private insurance companies. Where the use of tax dollars was proposed (i.e., Medicaid for the poor and other socioeconomically disadvantaged citizens, including the aged), the responsibility for program structure and administration would be shared by the federal government and the governments of the separate participating states.

Architects of the proposal hoped for medicine's

support, and not without justification. After all, they reasoned, the new program would generate substantial new service delivery opportunities and a new source of substantial profit. But medicine stood firm: "Socialized medicine" was evil in the absolute, whether administered in large doses, affecting the nation's entire citizenry, or in small ones, affecting merely segments of the population. And medicine would continue to stand firm throughout the congressional debates on the proposal, even though a statutory prohibition against any federal interference in the practice of medicine was written into the first section (Section 1801) of the Medicare Title of the Social Security Act (U.S. House of Representatives, 1973, p. 356):

Nothing in this title shall be construed to authorize any Federal officer or employee to exercise any supervision or control over the practice of medicine or the manner in which medical services are provided, over the selection, tenure, or compensation of any officer or employee of any institution, agency, or person providing health services, or to exercise any supervision of control over the administration or operation of any such institution, agency, or person.

Program proponents had better luck with congressional conservatives, who continued to oppose on personal philosophical grounds any "federal takeover" of the health care system but who also were sensitive to changes in political winds and able to modify their political behavior accordingly. The ranks of union and social–liberal supporters of a federal health insurance program had grown dramatically during the years between the Truman and Kennedy–Johnson administrations. The elderly, the poor, and ethnic minority interests all had begun to organize national and local advocacy efforts and, by the time the 89th Congress convened in January 1965, their concerted support for the program was at least as strong as the opposition of organized medicine, their appeals at least as compelling. A sufficient number of congressional conservatives responded to these appeals and to the reality of overwhelming popular (i.e., voter) support for the Medicare/Medicaid legislation package to enable congressional passage by narrow House and Senate majorities.

When President Johnson signed the legislation into law as Public Law 89-97 on July 30, 1965, he committed the nation to the fulfillment of the proposition that needed health care services should and would be made available to some of its citizens as a matter of right. The significant first chapter in the saga of government-supported health care had ended.

The second would deal with whether the right to health care access should be extended to all Americans—not only to the elderly and the poor and otherwise socioeconomically disadvantaged, but to children and nonelderly adults as well.

Today, a decade and a half later, the opening pages of the second and likely final chapter have been written. Much has already been said—universally applicable National Health Insurance (NHI) has been rumored to be waiting "just around the corner" since 1970—and it appears that a good deal more has yet to be written before all Americans can avail themselves of a federally insured, federally regulated health care delivery system. We have yet to learn, for example, whether NHI will be made available with a single stroke to those not now covered by a federal program, or whether it will be phased in gradually over a period of years, covering children first perhaps (or persons facing "catastrophic" health care costs), then, some predetermined number of years later, expanding to cover adults through age 35, and finally, some several years thereafter, extending coverage to the remaining 36-to-64 age-group. Nor are we soon likely to know how NHI will be financed. Some call for total federal backing, using tax dollars or trust fund contributions to pay the bills. Others urge a joint public–private relationship, in which government would pay for "special" services (e.g., child care, catastrophic illness or injury care, and/or preventive services) and the private sector, operating in accord with minimum federal coverage criteria (and, possibly, cost standards), would pick up the rest with funds from group or individual insurance plans. Still others argue for a proscription against any federal financial commitment and for otherwise limiting government involvement to the establishment of non-cost-related regulations governing the eligibility of health service providers and setting minimum standard-of-care requirements.

The current odds are that the ultimate NHI legislative package will call for a gradual phasing in of coverage and that the financing burden will be divided into public and private proportions. But only time will tell what precise shapes the sentiment of Congress will take on these and related matters.

One shape is nearly certain, however: that health care services covered by NHI will be the same or nearly the same as the services that presently are covered by the existing federal health care financing program (especially those covered by Medicare) and the several services that Congress may choose to add to the program between now and the final enactment of NHI. Before we look at those services, paying special attention to those that relate to communicative disorders, let us look briefly at the difference between the Medicare and Medicaid programs and the general purposes and structures of each.

WHICH IS WHICH?

Both Medicare and Medicaid help pay the costs of health care. Both are important parts of the Social Security Act. Medicare is generally designed to serve persons who are 65 years of age or older and persons who, though not yet 65, are disabled. Medicaid is for the needy and medically indigent and for those who are also aged, blind, or disabled. Some people 65 years of age or older can benefit from both Medicare and Medicaid. That is, Medicare pays most (but not all) health care costs for program beneficiaries. Medicaid can pay what Medicare does not for people who are eligible for both programs.

Medicare is a federal program, administered by the federal government in a manner that is consistent from state to state and is found everywhere in the United States including the District of Columbia, Guam, Puerto Rico, and the Virgin Islands. Medicaid is a joint federal–state effort, in which states design their own individual programs according to broad federal regulations. State participation, however, is not mandatory. Thus, Medicaid varies from state to state, with programs in all U. S. jurisdictions but one—the state of Arizona.

Medicare provides "basic protection" against the costs of inpatient hospital care, post hospital extended care, and posthospital home health care. In addition, Medicare provides "supplemental protection" against the costs of physicians' services, medical services and supplies, home health care services, outpatient hospital services, and other services. All Medicaid programs pay for inpatient hospital care, outpatient hospital services, laboratory and x-ray services, skilled nursing home services, and physicians' services. In many states, Medicaid also pays for such services as dental care, home health care, eyeglasses, hearing aids, and other diagnostic, preventative, and rehabilitative services.

Medicare is an insurance program; money from trust funds pays the health care service bills of individuals insured under the program. Medicaid is an assistance program; money from federal, state, and local taxes pays the health care service bills of eligible persons. Medicare's "basic protection" is financed by separate payroll contributions; "supplemental protection" is financed by monthly premiums, half of which is paid by the insured person and the other half by the federal government. Medicaid is financed by federal and state contributions, with the federal government contributing at least half of a given state's Medicaid cost burden and the states paying the remainder, sometimes with help from the local governments within their respective jurisdictions.

Medicare and the federal government's participation in Medicaid are administered by separate bureaus (the Medicare and Medicaid Bureaus) of the Health Care Financing Administration, U.S. Department of Health, Education, and Welfare.*

THE A, B, AND C OF MEDICARE

Like Caesar's Gaul, Medicare *est omnis divisa in partes tres.* The first of these parts is called "Hospital Insurance Benefits for the Aged and Disabled" in Title XVIII (Chapter III, Title 20, Code of Federal Regulations) of the Social Security Act (U.S. House of Representatives, 1973, pp. 356–373), although the term "hospital insurance" is somewhat inaccurate in that it covers more benefits than those provided only in hospitals. It is commonly referred to as "Basic Medicare" or, beacuse it is contained in Part A of Title XVIII, "Part A Medicare."

Part A: Hospital Insurance

Part A is funded by hospital insurance taxes imposed by the U.S. Internal Revenue Code (1954) and is generally designed for necessary health care services that are covered by the program and provided by participating health care facilities. Facilities participating in Part A must meet standards designed to assure the provision of high-quality health care. They must agree not to charge the Medicare beneficiary for services paid for by Medicare and they must abide by the proscription of Title VI of the Civil Rights Act, which bars discrimination on the basis of race, color, or national origin.

Part A helps pay for covered services received by a program beneficiary who is an inpatient in a participating hospital or, if additional care is required after a hospital stay, is either an inpatient in a skilled nursing facility or a patient at home receiving services from a home health agency. Financing for Medicare's Part A is provided by means of a Hospital

*For more information, contact HCFA/DHEW, 6401 Security Boulevard, Baltimore, Maryland 21235.

Insurance Trust Fund, which contains the accumulated contributions of employees and their employers. These contributions are collected along with regular Social Security contributions from wages and self-employment income earned during an individual's working years. Additional financing is provided by a beneficiary's payment of a portion of hospital charges in each "benefit period" and different per-day amounts after certain periods of benefit use in hospitals and skilled nursing facilities. When a beneficiary is an inpatient, payments for up to 90 days are available for each benefit period. During the first 60 days, Part A pays for all but the first $160 for covered services. During the period beginning on the 61st day and ending on the 90th day, Part A pays all but $40 a day for covered services. So long as a beneficiary has paid the $160 in each benefit period, he will not be required to pay it again, even if he must return to inpatient status for a second time during the same benefit period. Of course, these dollar amounts are for 1979 and are reviewed annually. If hospital costs have changed significantly in a year's time, dollar amounts are adjusted accordingly. Further, Medicaid will pay what Medicare does not pay when the beneficiary is eligible for both Medicare and Medicaid coverage.

The benefit period concept is less complicated than it appears to be at first glance. Simply put, a benefit period is a number of consecutive days during which a beneficiary uses his Part A benefits. The beneficiary's first benefit period begins with his admission to a qualified hospital or skilled nursing facility. It ends when he has not been an inpatient of any hospital or other facility primarily providing skilled nursing or rehabilitative services for 60 consecutive days. A new period begins (and entitlement to full Part A benefits is renewed) when the beneficiary again enters a qualified hospital or skilled nursing facility.

If ever a beneficiary requires more than 90 days of Part A care in the same benefit period, he may draw from a lifetime reserve of 60 additional days. For each lifetime reserve day used, Part A pays for all covered services, except for $80 a day.

When a beneficiary is a bed patient in a covered hospital, Part A will help pay for the following:

1. Bed (a private room only if medically necessary) and board (including special diets)
2. Operating room charges
3. Nursing services
4. Medical social services
5. Drugs, biologicals, supplies, appliances, and equipment furnished by the hospital for use in the hospital
6. Laboratory tests, x-rays, and other radiology services
7. Other covered diagnostic or therapeutic items or services (including speech – language pathology and audiology diagnostic and therapeutic services) that are furnished by the hospital or by qualified providers who contract with the hospital

Part A will not help pay for such inpatient services and items as:

1. Private duty nurses
2. Personal comfort or convenience items furnished at the inpatient's request
3. Services not reasonable and necessary for the treatment of an illness or injury
4. Physician's services (Part B pays for these), and
5. Any extra charge for a private room, unless medically necessary.

Part A will also help pay for a variety of services required by the patient who no longer requires the level of care that hospitals provide, but who does require daily skilled nursing attention or other skilled rehabilitation care (e.g., speech – language pathology services). Providing the accommodation of certain requisites, Part A will pay for covered services provided in a participating skilled nursing facility during the first 20 days of care in each benefit period, and for all but $20 a day for up to 80 additional days in the same benefit period. The requisites are as follows:

1. A physician certifies that the patient needs daily skilled nursing care or other skilled rehabilitation services and orders such care.
2. The care, as a practical matter, can be provided only on an inpatient basis in a skilled nursing facility (i.e., home health care would not be appropriate).
3. The patient has had a medically necessary stay in a participating hospital for at least three consecutive days prior to admission in a skilled nursing facility.
4. The patient is admitted within a limited period of time (generally 14 days) after leaving the hospital.
5. The patient is admitted for further treatment of a condition for which he was treated in the hospital.

Should the patient leave a skilled nursing facilty and then, within 14 days, require readmittance to the same or another participating facility, he can continue to use his remaining extended care benefit days without a new 3-day hospital stay. Among the extended care services for which Part A will help pay are:

1. A semiprivate room (private where medically necessary) and all meals (including special diets)
2. Nursing and medical social services
3. Drugs, appliances, and equipment (e.g., wheelchairs, crutches) furnished by the facility
4. Physical and occupational therapy
5. Speech–language pathology services
6. Necessary medical supplies

Additional Part A payment assistance is available to the patient who, after a qualifying hospital or skilled nursing facility stay, requires continued care at home. Part A pays for this care when all of the following requirements are met:

1. A physician certifies that the patient is homebound and, within 14 days after discharge from a participating hospital or skilled nursing facility, establishes a home health care plan.
2. The required continuing care includes part-time skilled nursing care or physical therapy or speech–language pathology services.
3. The care is further treatment of a condition for which the patient received inpatient hospital or skilled nursing facility care.

Part A will pay for as many as 100 home health "visits" after the start of one benefit period and before the start of another, so long as the visits are made to provide necessary covered services and are furnished by a participating home health agency within a year after the patient's last covered hospital or skilled nursing facility stay. One visit is counted each time the beneficiary receives a covered health care service from a home health agency. If the beneficiary receives two different services on the same day (e.g., from a nurse and a speech–language pathologist), or if the beneficiary was the recipient of the same services twice on the same day (such as two calls by a speech–language pathologist) two visits would be counted.

Part A will help pay for the following home health services:

1. Part-time skilled nursing care
2. Physical therapy services
3. Speech–language pathology services; and, providing at least one of the above services is supplied:
    Occupational therapy services

Part-time home health aide services
Medical social services, or
Medical supplies and equipment

Part A will not pay for such home health services as full-time nursing care, drugs and biologicals, or delivered meals.

Part B: Medical Insurance

The second of Medicare's three parts is officially called "Supplementary Medical Insurance Benefits for the Aged and Disabled" (U.S. House of Representatives, 1973, pp. 373–397), but is referred to more commonly as "Supplementary" or "Voluntary Medicare," or the "Medical Insurance Program," or, because it is contained in Part B of Title XVIII, "Part B Medicare."

Part B is a voluntary program covering the costs of physicians' services and a selection of other services and items not covered under Part A. It is financed largely through monthly premiums from enrollees and matching contributions from the federal government. More specifically, a beneficiary pays a monthly premium (currently $8.20), which covers not more than half the cost of Part B protection for enrollees age 65 and older and amounts to considerably less than half the cost of protection for younger (i.e. disabled) enrollees. The premium rate must be reviewed annually and, if necessary, is increased in the month of July. The rate will never increase more than the percentage by which monthly cash benefits have been increased during the preceding 12-month period. Enrollees who delay "signing up" for Part B for a year or more after their eligibility for enrollment are required to pay an additional ten percent for each year they were eligible but not enrolled. The federal government pays all other costs of financing the Part B program.

Services provided under the program are also paid for through a beneficiary–government sharing arrangement in which the beneficiary pays the first $60 of "reasonable charges" plus 20 percent of any additional charges for a one-year period. Reasonable charges are determined by Medicare "carriers," organizations selected in each state by the Medicare Bureau of the Health Care Financing Administration to process Part B claims. These carriers (usually private insurance companies working under contract with the Medicare Bureau) are expected to take into account the customary charges made for similar health care services in a given locality. Further, there is but one $60 Part B deductible per year, not a separate deductible for each kind of covered service.

Part B pays 80 percent of the reasonable charges that exceed the initial $60.

The big payment item under Part B is physicians' service coverage, which, you will recall, is not reimbursable under Part A. Part B helps pay for physician bills for all covered services provided in the physician's office, a hospital, a skilled nursing facility, a clinic or group practice, a health maintenance organization, or in the beneficiary's home. Payment for covered services is made either to the physician on assignment or directly to the beneficiary. The physician accepts Part B payments on the condition that his total charge will not exceed the reasonable charge, that is, the deductible and coinsurance for covered services.

Physician services covered by Part B include:

1. All medical and surgical services provided by a doctor of medicine or osteopathy
2. Dental services involving surgery of the jaw or contiguous structures or the setting of fractures of the jaw or facial bones
3. The services of a podiatrist who is licensed by the state
4. The services of a licensed chiropractor in treating a subluxation of the spine by manual manipulation (the subluxation must be demonstrated by x-ray)
5. Such other services as are ordinarily and customarily furnished in a physician's office, including diagnostic tests and procedures (e.g., audiological evaluations), medical supplies, office nurse services, and drugs and biologicals that cannot be self-administered.

Part B will also pay 100 percent of the reasonable charges of radiologists and pathologists for radiology and pathology services received by an inpatient in a participating or otherwise qualified hospital. It will also help pay for ambulance transportation to a hospital, to a facility offering skilled nursing services, or from either of these settings to a beneficiary's home. Part B will not pay for:

1. Routine physical checkups and tests
2. The services of Christian Science practitioners and naturopaths
3. Routine dental or foot care
4. Cosmetic surgery (unless required as a result of accident or to improve the function or functions of a physical malformation)
5. Immunizations (unless directly related to an injury or immediate risk of infection, e.g., antitetanus injection
6. Eyeglasses and eye refractions and examinations

for prescribing, fitting, or changing eyeglasses, although it will cover corrective lenses required after a cataract operation
7. Hearing aids and examinations directly related to prescribing, fitting, or changing hearing aids.

Part B additionally will pay for covered services rendered to outpatients of participating hospitals and to homebound program enrollees. Reimbursement for outpatient services follows the usual Part B service-payment method, that is, Medicare pays 80 percent of the costs over and above the $60 deductible; the beneficiary is responsible for the remaining 20 percent. For home health services, Part B pays 100 percent of reasonable costs (once the $60 deductible is paid by the beneficiary) for up to 100 home health visits per calendar year. As indicated earlier, one visit is counted each time a beneficiary receives a covered service from a home health agency.

Among the outpatient services covered by Part B are laboratory services, x-ray and other radiology services, other diagnostic services (including diagnostic speech–language pathology and audiology services), emergency room or outpatient clinic services (including speech–language pathology services), such medical supplies as casts and splints, and drugs and biologicals that cannot be administered by the beneficiary. Home health services are covered by Part B only when:

1. A physician certifies that the beneficiary is homebound and in need of home health services.
2. The physician establishes and periodically reviews a home health service plan.
3. The beneficiary requires speech–language pathology services, physcal therapy, or part-time skilled nursing care.
4. The home health agency is a participating (i.e., certified by Medicare) agency.

In addition to the services rendered by practitioners who, for Medicare purposes, are considered to be physicians, Part B provides significant coverage of the outpatient services of two types of health care professionals who are not physicians, namely, physical therapists and speech–language pathologists. Coverage extends to these services when they are provided by or under arrangements (i.e., service-provision contracts) made by participating hospitals, skilled nursing facilities, home health agencies, public health agencies, rehabilitation agencies, and clinics. The Medicare program defines a rehabilitation agency as (Social Security Administration, 1976, p. 56):

An agency which provides an integrated multidisciplinary program designed to upgrade the physical function of handicapped, disabled individuals by bringing together as a team specialized rehabilitation personnel. At a minimum, a rehabilitation agency must provide physical therapy or speech pathology services, and a rehabilitation program which, in addition to physical therapy or speech pathology services, includes social or vocational adjustment services.

Under the Medicare program, a clinic is:

A facility established primarily for the provision of outpatient physicians' services. To accommodate this definition, an organization must meet the following test of physician participation: (1) the medical services of the clinic are provided by a group of physicians (i.e., more than two) practicing medicine together; and (2) a physician is present in the clinic at all times during hours of operation to perform medical services (rather than only administrative services).

Direct physician supervision of the delivery of physical therapy and speech pathology services is not required, but a physician must certify that the services were required as part of an overall plan of treatment developed by the physician while the beneficiary was under the physician's care. Beneficiaries are subject to the usual deductible and coinsurance amounts.

Part C: Medicare's Miscellaneous

Title XVIII's Parts A and B, with their definitions of the beneficiaries and benefits and their descriptions of the payment mechanisms that are respectively relevant, provide the basic framework for the Medicare program. It is the "Miscellaneous Provisions" of Part C (U.S. House of Representatives, 1973, pp. 397–445), however, that supply the program's nuts and bolts, that is, definitions of the kinds of health care services covered by both of the earlier two parts and of the varieties of health care institutions and professionals who may provide them. In section 1861 of Part C (U.S. House of Representatives, 1973, pp. 397–418), for example, appear the definitions of such terms as "spell of illness," "provider of services," "reasonable cost," and "arrangements for certain services"; for such provider types as "hospital," "skilled nursing facility," "home health agency," and "physician"; and for such services as "inpatient hospital services," "extended care services," "home health services," "physicians' services," "medical and other health services," and "outpatient physical therapy services" (which includes the definition of "speech pathology services," as per Public Law 92–603,

section 283[a]). Section 1862 of Part C (pp. 418–421) concerns exclusions from Parts A and B coverage (including "hearing aids and examinations therefor"). Sections 1863 and 1864 (pp. 421–423) deal with agreements between the Medicare program and state health agencies for the purposes of developing conditions of participation for providers of services and of determining compliance by providers with the conditions of participation. Section 1871 vests the Secretary of Health and Human Services with the authority "to prescribe such regulations as may be necessary to carry out the administration (p. 432)" of the Medicare program. Section 1877 (pp. 441–442) prescribes the penalties (i.e., fines and/or imprisonment) that may be imposed on providers who violate the terms and conditions of the Medicare law or the regulations developed under the authority of the law's section 1871.

Medicare-covered Speech and Hearing Services

For the purposes of the Medicare program, Parts A and B, speech–language pathology and audiology services are those speech, language, and hearing services that are rendered by a qualified provider to a Medicare beneficiary and that meet all of the following conditions. First, the services must be rendered according to a plan of treatment prescribed in writing by a physician, and the need for continued treatment must be recertified by the physician at 30-day intervals. Second, the services rendered must be directly and specifically related to the condition for which the beneficiary was hospitalized (under Part A) or for which the beneficiary is receiving Part B benefits. The services must be necessary to the treatment of that condition. Finally, the expected restoration potential must be significant in relation to the extent and duration of the speech–language pathology or audiology services required to achieve that potential.

A "qualified" speech and hearing service supplier is a speech–language pathologist or audiologist who, if practicing in a state where statutory licensure exists, holds a valid license for such practice and who either has been granted a Certificate of Clinical Competence* in the appropriate area(s) (i.e., speech pathology and/or audiology) by the American Speech–Language–Hearing Association, or has completed the academic and practicum requirements

---

*Requirements for certification can be obtained free from the American Speech–Language–Hearing Association, 1801 Rockville Pike, Rockville, Md. 20852.

for certification and is in the process of accumulating the necessary supervised work experience required for certification.

SPEECH PATHOLOGY

Under Part A, speech−language pathology services (called speech pathology and, less frequently, speech therapy in Medicare regulations) are available to beneficiaries who are hospital inpatients, inpatients in a qualified skilled nursing facility, or homebound and receiving services from a qualified home health agency.

In hospitals, speech−language pathology services may be provided by a qualified speech pathologist who either is a hospital employee or has contracted with a hospital to provide speech−language pathology services to inpatients. In the latter instance, the hospital bills the carrier for the services rendered and reimburses the speech pathologist according to the terms of the contract.

As with hospitals, speech pathology services provided in a qualified skilled nursing facility may be provided either by a speech pathologist who is employed by the facility, or, as is the more usual case, by a speech pathologist who contracts with the facility to provide services. The skilled nursing facility must have a written transfer agreement (dealing generally with the interchange of medical and other information) with the transferring hospital. A speech pathologist who has a contract with the transferring hospital cannot render services under that contract to a beneficiary who has been transferred to a skilled nursing facility; a separate hospital−nursing facility agreement is required.

Speech-language pathology services are available as a home health service to beneficiaries who have had a prior hospital confinement of at least 3 consecutive days. The service must be for further treatment for the condition for which the patient was hospitalized. Home health visits are limited to a total of 100 on all services available for each benefit period and can be made for up to 12 months after the beneficiary's most recent discharge from a hospital or skilled nursing facility. While both nonprofit and proprietary (i.e., for profit) home health agencies may participate in the Medicare program, Medicare regulations stipulate, for reasons clear to no one (not even the federal officials who must enforce the regulations) that a proprietary agency must furnish services through its employees only. Medicare Bureau officials have made clear, however, that they regard an individual speech pathologist under con-

tract with a proprietary agency as an employee of that agency.

Under Medicare's Part B, speech−language pathology services may be provided in a hospital's outpatient speech and hearing clinic; by a medical clinic, public health agency, or rehabilitation agency;* in a physician's office; or as a home health service. Recall that Part B covers as many as 100 home health visits a year without requiring the prior 3-day hospitalization required under Part A.

AUDIOLOGY

Like speech−language pathology services, some audiology services have been provided under Medicare's statutory authority since the program's inception. But unlike coverage of speech-related services, which was greatly expanded by Congress in 1972, the range of audiology coverage has not changed since Medicare's 1965 enactment. This is not to say that Congress does not intend to similarly treat audiology and speech pathology. Indeed, similar treatment was the congressional purpose in 1972. It was a purpose that was thwarted, however, by Congress's inability to differentiate between the two types of services.

It is the opinion of this writer—an opinion shaped by interchanges with the legislators and legislative staff personnel involved in the enactment of section 283(a) of Public Law 92−603 in 1972—that Congress believed that by expanding speech pathology benefits, it was also expanding audiology benefits. The Congress was aware in 1972 of the then 7-year-old proscription against Medicare coverage of "hearing aids and examinations therefor." Because it believed that aural rehabilitation was merely speech pathology (e.g., speechreading, speech conversation) plus hearing aid utilization, Congress thought that an expansion of speech pathology coverage would result in expanded coverage for all but amplification-related aural rehabilitation services as well.

All this is not to say that Medicare coverage of audiology services is not substantial. It is. Under Part A, for example, diagnostic and therapeutic audiology services requested by a physician are covered when provided to a hospital inpatient by an audiologist who

---

*An unpublished manuscript entitled *Guidelines for Speech and Hearing Facilities that Wish to Provide Outpatient Speech Pathology Services for Medicare Beneficiaries* is available at no cost from the Governmental Affairs Division of the American Speech−Language−Hearing Association, 10801 Rockville Pike, Rockville, Md. 20852.

is an employee of the hospital or by a nonemployee audiologist under contract with the hospital. An audiologist employed by the hospital also may provide audiology services for patients transferred to a skilled nursing facility, providing the hospital and the skilled nursing facility have a transfer agreement.

Under Part B, diagnostic audiology services are covered as "other diagnostic tests" (U.S. House of Representatives, p. 411) when a physician orders such testing for the purpose of obtaining additional information necessary for an evaluation of the need for (or appropriate type of) medical or surgical treatment. The tests must be performed by a qualified audiologist who is in private practice or on the staff of a speech and hearing facility that is not physician directed. A privately practicing audiologist must have obtained a billing number from the appropriate carrier. Note, too, that Medicare will not, under any circumstances, cover therapeutic audiological services rendered in the office of a privately practicing audiologist (nor either the therapeutic or diagnostic services rendered in the office of a privately practicing speech–language pathologist) (Stryker, 1976). Diagnostic and therapeutic audiology services also may be provided as a Part B benefit by an audiologist who is employed by a physician or in a physician-directed clinic, provided the physician is on the premises and supervises the audiological service delivery, and provided the services comprise an integral part of the physician's professional services.

Needed Medicare Improvements

As mentioned earlier, it is generally agreed by informed Washington observers of National Health Insurance developments that the health care services covered by the ultimately enacted NHI program will be the same or nearly the same as the services covered, at the time of NHI enactment, by the then existing federal health insurance program. If the services of speech–language pathologists and audiologists are to be represented optimally in the ultimate NHI benefits package, three major changes in the probable model for that package (i.e., Medicare) will be necessary.

1. Medicare currently requires that speech pathology services must be prescribed in writing by a physician who specifies the type(s) of speech pathology services to be rendered, their duration (i.e., the length of the period, up to 30 days, during which they are to be rendered), and their frequency (i.e., the number of times—per day or

week—they are to be rendered during the aforementioned period). The physician must certify the continued need for speech pathology services at 30-day intervals. The first change would replace the physician-prescription requirement with a physician-referral standard, under which a physician would merely refer a Medicare beneficiary to a qualified speech–language pathologist for needed services. The certification of need at 30-day intervals would still be required, but the type, duration, and frequency specifications would no longer be necessary.

2. Part B currently covers aural rehabilitation (i.e., therapeutic audiology) services only when those services are provided by a qualified audiologist who is employed by a physician or in a physician-directed clinic. The second change would (a) expand Part B coverage to aural rehabilitation services (including examinations designed to determine the need for and potential benefits of amplification) provided in service settings that are not physician directed (e.g., in a rehabilitation or public health agency, or as a home health service) and (b) apply to aural rehabilitation the services covered by Parts A and B using the physician-referral standard mentioned above.

3. Part B currently prohibits coverage of speech pathology and therapeutic audiology services provided in the office of a private practitioner. The third change would expand Part B coverage to such services, so long as the recipient of the services is referred to the private practitioner by a physician.

The first needed change, that is, from physician prescription to physician referral, is almost a surety, having already been passed by both Houses of Congress, though, unfortunately, in different congressional terms (U.S. Senate Report 93–553, 1973; U.S. House Report 95–1553, 1978). The change is under active consideration by the 96th Congress (U.S. Senate Bill 507, 1979), has merited the endorsement of both the U. S. Department of Health and Human Services and the major "carrier" of Medicare insurance, namely, Blue Cross ("Blue Cross Suggests Speech–Language Pathologists Role in treatment plan," 1978), and is not opposed by the principal representative of organized medicine (i.e., the American Medical Association). Proponents of the change, including physicians, have argued conclusively that physicians should not be required to specify in prescribed form the type(s), duration, and frequency of needed speech–language pathology services. Proponents rightly say that physicians generally are neither trained nor sufficiently experienced in the specifics of speech – language pathology care, and that, given the dramatic increases in malpractice claims and malpractice insurance rates, they are reluctant to detail service specifics with which they are not thoroughly familiar.

The second change, dealing with expanded coverage of aural rehabilitation services, appears to stand about an even chance of congressional enactment between now and the eventual adoption of a full NHI benefits package. The change was considered by the Ways and Means Committee of the U.S. House of Representatives during the 95th Congress ("Hearing Impaired 'Not Being Served' by Medicare Law," 1978) and is likely to be considered by both the House and the Senate during the 1979 – 1980 term of the 96th Congress. Congressional adoption of the proposed change will depend largely on the ability of proponents to overcome the opposition of a national otolaryngology association ("Mikva Bill 'Bad' in ACO's opinion; Dowling disagrees," 1978) and the shared concern of Congress and the Medicare Bureau that expanded aural rehabilitation coverage will cost more than the Medicare financing system can afford.

The third change, concerning Part B coverage of services provided in the office of a private practitioner, stands a less-than-even chance of congressional adoption. Both Congress and the Medicare Bureau maintain that the costs of such a coverage expansion would be prohibitive. If Congress can be convinced to amend Part B so as to include coverage of private office visits (and the likelihood is that it cannot), then it will do so only after instructing the Medicare Bureau to write and enforce regulations that are designed to severely restrict the coverage expansion. For example, in 1972, Congress expanded Part B physical therapy coverage to services provided in the office of a privately practicing physical therapist. Subsequent Part B regulations so severely restricted the scope of coverage ($80 per beneficiary, per year), however, as to render the expanded coverage virtually meaningless.

It might be suggested, and appropriately, that payment for hearing aids recommended by a qualified audiologist should be listed among the Medicare changes that might be advanced, in anticipation of National Health Insurance, by advocates for speech – language pathology and audiology. It is not listed (though it is being advanced by speech and hearing advocates), because it stands virtually no chance, now or in the foreseeable future, of congressional adoption. Congress realizes that the added coverage would seriously, perhaps critically, overburden the Medicare trust fund (U. S. Permanent Subcommittee on Investigations of the Senate Committee on Government Operations, 1975).

MEDICAID

Title XIX of the Social Security Act (U.S. House of Representatives, 1973, pp. 446 – 476), entitled "Grants to States for Medical Assistance Programs," provides for a program of health care assistance for certain low-income individuals and families. Popularly known as Medicaid (MediCal in the state of California), the program is financed jointly with federal and state funds, with the federal contribution ranging from 50 percent to 83 percent. It is administered by each participating state within broadly defined federal requirements and guidelines (Institute for Medicaid Management, 1978, Chapter II, Title 45 of the Code of Federal Regulations).

Medicaid is designed to provide health care assistance to the "categorically needy"—individuals who are eligible to receive cash payments under one of two Social Security Act welfare programs: Title IV – A, the program of "Aid to Families with Dependent Children" (AFDC), and Title XVI, the "Supplemental Security Income" (SSI) program for the aged, blind, and disabled. (The regulations for these programs are also in Chapter II, Title 45 of the Code of Federal Regulations, pp. 191 – 212, and 337 – 351, respectively.) In general, receipt of a welfare payment under either of these programs means automatic Medicaid eligibility. States may also provide Medicaid to the medically needy, that is, individuals who are aged, blind, or disabled, or members of families with dependent children and one absent, incapacitated, or unemployed parent, and who have enough income to pay for basic living expenses (that is, do not receive welfare payments), but who do not have enough income to pay for needed health care services.

Title XIX (Sections 1902(A) (13) (B) and 1905(A) (1)-(5), pp. 450 and 468, respectively) requires that the Medicaid programs of participating states must provide the following "basic services":

1. Inpatient hospital services
2. Outpatient hospital services
3. Laboratory and x-ray services
4. Skilled nursing facility services for individuals 21 years of age and older
5. Home health services for persons eligible
6. Nursing services
7. Physicians' services

8. Family planning services
9. Rural health clinic services
10. Early and periodic screening, diagnosis, and treatment (EPSDT) services for individuals under 21 years of age

In addition, states may elect to provide a variety of other services, including hearing aids, eyeglasses, drugs, dental care, and private duty nursing.

The states are empowered to change the benefit packages of their respective Medicaid programs at any time, providing the federal Medicaid Bureau is satisfied that a given state program remains within federal guidelines. Such alterations can be made to reflect the shifting sands of state politics, such as the desire of a governor or state legislature to expand or gradually limit health care for the poor or as a result of state budgetary problems. In recent years, inflation has been the bugaboo of most state programs, causing more than twice as many coverage reductions as coverage increases (Institute of Medicaid Management, 1978).

State programs are empowered also to determine the scope of services offered. They may limit the days of hospital care, for example, or the number of covered physicians' visits. States also may determine reimbursement rates for services, except for hospital care, in which case states either must accommodate the Medicare program's reasonable cost payment system or must win the Medicaid Bureau's approval of an alternate reimbursement system. Since mid-1976, states have been required to reimburse for skilled nursing facility and intermediate care facility services on a reasonable cost-related basis. (An intermediate care facility is defined generally as "a public institution [or distinct part thereof] for the mentally retarded or persons with related conditions," according to the Compilation of Social Security Laws, U.S. House of Representatives, 1973, p. 470).

States determine eligibility levels for their welfare programs and, because they do, exercise tremendous control over the income eligibility levels for Medicaid. Should a state opt to cover the medically needy, it can set the income level for eligibility at any point between the cash assistance level for an AFDC family (adjusted for family size) and 133⅓ percent of the payment to such an AFDC family. All these variations in benefits offered, groups covered, income standards, and levels of provider reimbursement mean that Medicaid programs vary greatly from state to state.

Medicaid operates as a vendor payment program. Payments are made directly to the provider of services and providers must accept the Medicaid reimbursement level as payment in full. Program beneficiaries in nursing homes are required to turn over any excess income to help pay for their care. Copayments may be required, as well.

About 18 percent of all state Medicaid program beneficiaries, or about four million Medicaid recipients, are "aged" (i.e., 65 years of age or older) with the result that about 40 percent of all Medicaid expenditures are for services rendered to persons 65 years of age or older (Institute for Medicaid Management, 1978). These persons also are covered by the Medicare program. In cases in which this dual coverage exists, most state Medicaid programs pay for Part B Medicare premiums, deductibles, and copayments, and for services not provided by Medicare. They do so by engaging in "buy-in" arrangements with the federal Medicare program, under which the federal program matches state payments for the Medicare premiums of categorically needy Medicaid beneficiaries. States themselves must pay the full premium payment costs for the medically needy. If a state does not buy into Part B coverage for elderly Medicaid beneficiaries, it cannot receive federal matching payments for services that would have been covered under Medicare if there had been a buy-in arrangement.

Forty-eight states and jurisdictions (including the District of Columbia, Guam and the Virgin Islands) have buy-in arrangements with Medicare; exceptions include Alaska, Louisiana, Oregon, Wyoming, Puerto Rico, and, of course, Arizona, which has no Medicaid program. According to the Medicaid Bureau, just over half of the four million elderly Medicaid recipients have payments made in their behalf for deductibles and coinsurance under buy-in arrangements.

With the substantial state-to-state variations in Medicaid programs and the frequency with which states increase or decrease their respective program benefits and otherwise modify the structures of their separate programs, an accurate listing in this volume of the speech and hearing benefits covered by the individual state programs is not possible. The surest way of learning the specifics of a given state Medicaid program, including a program's coverage of speech–language pathology and audiology services, is by direct, personal contact with the governmental agency that administers the program. To accommodate readers interested in doing so, the addresses of all state and U. S. territory Medicaid agencies are listed in Table 18–1.

Table 18-1
List of State Medicaid Agencies and Their Addresses

ALABAMA
Commissioner
Medical Services Administration
2500 Fairlane Drive
Montgomery, Alabama 36130

ALASKA
Director
Division of Public Assistance
Pouch H-07
Juneau, Alaska 99811

ARIZONA
No Medicaid Program

ARKANSAS
Director
Office of Medical Services
Division of Social Services
P. O. Box 1437
Little Rock, Arkansas 72201

CALIFORNIA
Director
Medical Assistance Division
Department of Health
714 P Street
Sacramento, California 95814

COLORADO
Director
Division of Medical Assistance
Department of Social Services
1575 Sherman Street
Denver, Colorado 80203

CONNECTICUT
Director
Bureau of Medical Care Administration
State Department of Social Services
110 Bartholomew Avenue
Hartford, Connecticut 06106

DELAWARE
Administrator
Medical Assistance Unit
Department of Health and Social Services
P. O. Box 309
Wilmington, Delaware 19899

DISTRICT OF COLUMBIA
Chief
Medical Assistance Division
Department of Human Resources
614 H Street, N.W., Room 708
Washington, D.C. 20001

FLORIDA
Administrator
Medical Services Program
Office of Social and Economic Services
Department of Health and Rehabilitative Services
1323 Winewood Boulevard
Tallahassee, Florida 32301

GEORGIA
Commissioner
Department of Medical Assistance
1010 West Peachtree Street, N.W.
Atlanta, Georgia 30309

GUAM
Director
Medical Care Service
Department of Public Health and Social Services
P. O. Box 2719
Agana, Guam 96910

HAWAII
Administrator
Medical Care Administration
Department of Social Services and Housing
P. O. Box 339
Honolulu, Hawaii 96809

IDAHO
Chief
Bureau of Medical Assistance
Department of Health and Welfare
State House
Boise, Idaho 83720

ILLINOIS
Director
Medical Programs Division
Department of Public Aid
316 South Second
Springfield, Illinois 62762

Table 18–1, continued.

INDIANA
Administrator
Medical Services Division
Department of Public Welfare
701 State Office Building
Indianapolis, Indiana 46204

IOWA
Chief
Medical Services Section
Department of Social Services
Lucas State Office Building
Des Moines, Iowa 50319

KANSAS
Director
Medical Services Section
Department of Social and Rehabilitation Services
State Office Building
Topeka, Kansas 66612

KENTUCKY
Director
Division for Medical Assistance
Department for Human Resources
Highway 127 South
Frankfort, Kentucky 40601

LOUISIANA
Administrator
Medical Assistance Program
Health and Human Resources Administration
P.O. Box 44065
Baton Rouge, Louisiana 70804

MAINE
Director
Division of Medical Assistance
Bureau of Social Welfare
Department of Human Services
State House
Augusta, Maine 04333

MARYLAND
Assistant Secretary for Medical Care Programs
Department of Health and Mental Hygiene
301 W. Preston Street
Baltimore, Maryland 21201

MASSACHUSETTS
Assistant Commissioner
Medical Assistance Division
Department of Public Welfare
600 Washington Street
Boston, Massachusetts 02111

MICHIGAN
Director
Bureau of Medical Assistance
Department of Social Services
300 South Capitol Avenue
Lansing, Michigan 48926

MINNESOTA
Director
Medical Assistance Program
Department of Public Welfare
690 North Robert Street
St. Paul, Minnesota 55155

MISSISSIPPI
Director
Mississippi Medicaid Commission
Room 313, Dale Building
2906 N. State Street
Jackson, Mississippi 39216

MISSOURI
Director
Medical Services
Department of Social Services
Broadway State Office Building
Jefferson City, Missouri 65101

MONTANA
Chief
Medical Assistance Bureau
Economic Assistance Division
Department of Social and Rehabilitation Services
P.O. Box 4210
Helena, Montana 59601

NEBRASKA
Chief
Medical Services Division
Department of Public Welfare
Fifth Floor
301 Centennial Mall South
Lincoln, Nebraska 68509

NEVADA
  Chief
  Medical Care Section
  Welfare Division
  Department of Human Resources
  251 Jeanell Drive, Capitol Complex
  Carson City, Nevada 89710

NEW HAMPSHIRE
  Director
  Office of Medical Services
  Department of Health and Welfare
  8 Loudon Road
  Concord, New Hampshire 03301

NEW JERSEY
  Director
  Division of Medical Assistance and Health
    Services
  Department of Human Services
  324 East State Street
  Trenton, New Jersey 08608

NEW MEXICO
  Director
  Medical Assistance Division
  Health and Social Services Department
  P.O. Box 2348
  Santa Fe, New Mexico 87503

NEW YORK
  Deputy Commissioner
  Division of Medical Assistance
  State Department of Social Services
  Ten Eyck Office Building
  40 North Pearl Street
  Albany, New York 12243

NORTH CAROLINA
  Director
  Medical Services Section
  Department of Human Resources
  325 N. Salisbury Street
  Raleigh, North Carolina 27611

OHIO
  Chief
  Division of Medical Assistance
  Ohio Department of Public Welfare
  30 East Broad Street
  Columbus, Ohio 43215

OKLAHOMA
  Director
  Medical Services Division
  Department of Institutions
  Social and Rehabilitative Services
  P.O. Box 25352
  Oklahoma City, Oklahoma 73125

OREGON
  Administrator
  Adult and Family Services Division
  Department of Human Resources
  417 Public Service Building
  Salem, Oregon 97310

PENNSYLVANIA
  Director
  Bureau of Medical Assistance
  Department of Public Welfare
  7th and Forester Streets
  Harrisburg, Pennsylvania 17120

PUERTO RICO
  Director
  Medical Assistance Program
  Department of Health
  P.O. Box 10037
  Caparra Heights Station
  Rio Piedras, Puerto Rico 00922

RHODE ISLAND
  Director
  Medical Care Program
  Department of Social and Rehabilitative Services
  600 New London Avenue
  Cranston, Rhode Island 02920

SOUTH CAROLINA
  Chief
  Medical Assistance Division
  Department of Social Services
  P.O. Box 1520
  Columbia, South Carolina 29202

SOUTH DAKOTA
  Administrator
  Office of Medical Services
  Department of Social Services
  New State Office Building
  Pierre, South Dakota 57501

Table 18-1, continued.

TENNESSEE	VIRGINIA
Director	Medical Director
Division of Medicaid	Bureau of Medical Assistance
Department of Public Health	State Department of Health
Cordell Hull Building	109 Governor Street
Nashville, Tennessee 37219	Richmond, Virginia 23219
TEXAS	WASHINGTON
Commissioner	Chief
Medical Programs	Office of Medical Assistance MS−LK−11
State Department of Human Resources	Health Services Division
John H. Reagan Building	Department of Social and Health Services
Austin, Texas 78701	Olympia, Washington 98504
UTAH	WEST VIRGINIA
Director	Director
Office of Medical Services	Division of Medical Care
Department of Social Services	Department of Welfare
150 West North Temple	1900 Washington Street, East
Salt Lake City, Utah 84110	Charleston, West Virginia 25305
VERMONT	WISCONSIN
Director	Director
Division of Medical Care	Bureau of Health Care Financing
Department of Social Welfare	Division of Health
State Office Building	Wisconsin Department of Health and Social
4 East State Street	Services
Montpelier, Vermont 05602	One West Wilson Street
	Madison, Wisconsin 53702
VIRGIN ISLANDS	
Director	WYOMING
Bureau of Health Insurance and Medical	Director
Assistance	Medical Assistance Services
Department of Health	Department of Health and Social Services
Franklin Building	Hathaway Building
Charlotte Amalie	Cheyenne, Wyoming 82002
St. Thomas, Virgin Islands 00801	

SUMMARY

The foundation for the preceding several pages is the conviction that a thorough understanding of the nature and roles of publicly and privately financed insurers of health care service costs is almost as important an ingredient of speech−language pathologist and audiologist proficiency as is the ability to render high-quality clinical services. This chapter is designed to provide the basis for such an understanding by focusing on the shape, the scope,

and the mechanisms of the federal government's program of health insurance for the elderly. This group is the most rapidly expanding segment of the national population and the segment that (notwithstanding the dramatic increase in its size) requires and uses more health care services, per capita, than any other population group. The chapter's primary focus has been the federal Medicare program—the health care insurer of all American citizens who are at least 65 years old. Medicare is the model for virtually all existing health insurance programs and policies and is the likely model for the health care benefit package that one day will be available to all Americans in National Health Insurance. The chapter should be read as the opening chapter of any area of new knowledge is read, that is, with the understanding that other chapters must follow and, one hopes, with the commitment to read them, to understand them, and to put the exercise to good use.

REFERENCES

Blue Cross suggests speech-language pathologist's role in treatment plan. *ASHA: Journal of the American Speech and Hearing Association,* August 1978, *20,* 647, 651.

Hearing impaired "not being served" by medicare law. *ASHA: Journal of the American Speech and Hearing Association,* 1978, *20,* 913.

Institute for Medicaid Management. *Data on the Medicaid program: Eligibility, services, expenditures for fiscal years 1966–78* (revised). Medicaid Bureau, Health Care Finance Administration, U.S. Department of Health, Education, and Welfare, 1978.

Mikva bill "bad" in ACO's opinion; Dowling disagrees. *ASHA: Journal of the American Speech and Hearing Association,* 1978, *20,* 409, 416.

National Center for Health Statistics, *Monthly Vital Statistics Report,* 1978, *12*(suppl. 2), 1.

Sheppard, H., & Rix, S. *The graying of working America.* New York: Free Press, 1977.

Social Security Administration. *Your Medicare handbook.* Publication No. (SSA) 76–10050, U. S. Department of Health, Education, and Welfare, 1976, 52–58.

Stryker, S. Procedures relating to Medicare and other third-party payments. *ASHA: Journal of the American Speech and Hearing Association,* 1976, *18,* 491–495.

U. S. Bureau of the Census, Demographic aspects of aging and the older populations in the United States. *Current Population Reports,* January 1978, Series P–23, No. 59, p. 26.

U. S. Bureau of the Census, *1970 census of population,* Vol. II: *Characteristics of the population.* Part I, "U. S. Summary." Table 39, pp. 1–93.

U. S. Bureau of the Census, Projections of the population of the United States, 1977 to 2050." *Current Population Reports,* July 1977, Series P–25, No. 704, p. 18.

U. S. House of Representatives. *Compilation of social security laws* (Vol. 1). Document No. 93–117 (Titles XVIII and XIX, as amended), 93rd Congress, 1st Session, 1973.

U. S. House of Representatives. *Medicare amendments of 1978.* House Report No. 95–1553, 95th Congress, Second Session, 1978, p. 17.

U. S. Internal Revenue Code, Sections 1301 (employer/employee taxes) and 1401 (self-employment taxes), 1954.

U. S. Permanent Subcommittee on Investigations on the Senate Committee on Government Operations. *Staff study of the state licensing laws and training requirements for hearing aid dealers.* October 1975, pp. 58–59.

U. S. Senate. *Report on the social security amendments of 1973.* Senate Report No. 93–553, 93rd Congress, First Session, 1973, pp. 66–67.

U. S. Senate. *Senate Bill No. 507,* 96th Congress, First Session, March 1, 1979.

Erica F. Wood

David H. Marlin

19

A Consumer Perspective: The Hearing Aid Delivery System

The last five years have seen a flurry of reform activities focused on the hearing aid delivery system. Consumer groups have investigated hearing aid dealer practices, Congressional committees have held hearings, and states have passed new laws regulating the industry. One federal agency has promulgated regulations and another is still in the rulemaking process. Studies have demonstrated that the hearing aid system has been fraught with conflict of interest and geared as much toward salesmanship and profit as health and hearing. This chapter will examine the current hearing aid delivery system, the rationale for reform, the legislative and regulatory response, and the issues that remain unresolved for the nation's millions of hearing-impaired consumers.

THE HEARING AID DELIVERY SYSTEM: PARTICIPANTS

The Hearing-impaired

Hearing loss is one of the most widespread chronic conditions in the United States. The National Center for Health Statistics has reported that there are 14.5 million persons in the United States who suffer from hearing problems (FTC Staff Report, 1978). This figure does not include the 1.2 million persons living in retirement homes or nursing homes, where the incidence of hearing impairments is estimated to be five times the rate in the general population.

The elderly weigh heavily in statistics on the hearing-impaired (FTC Staff Report, 1978). According to some estimates (FTC Staff Report, p. 20), approximately 30 percent of Americans over the age of 65 are hearing-impaired and as many as 90 percent of Americans in retirement homes and nursing homes have a significant hearing handicap. One survey (National Center for Health Statistics) of hearing-impaired persons reported that 55 percent of persons with a bilateral hearing loss were 65 years of age or older. The National Center for Health Statistics estimated that 40 percent of all hearing impairments are suffered by persons age 65 and over, and that 72 percent are suffered by persons age 45 and over. Moreover, the elderly are more vulnerable to sales abuses, both economically and psychologically. Most live on small, fixed incomes from Social Security and pensions and are rapidly losing the fight with inflation. In 1976, older households had half the income of their younger counterparts. In that year, some 3.3 million or a seventh of the elderly had incomes below the official poverty threshold, that is, $3,417 for an older couple and $2,770 for an older individual. Millions more clustered just above it. These same older households, while representing almost 11 percent of the population, accounted for about 29 percent of the personal health care expenditures in the U. S. (U. S. Senate Special Subcommittee on Aging, 1976).

Many older persons are isolated due to problems of health, transportation, and communication. Many

325

live alone and are particularly susceptible to the high-pressure tactics employed by salesmen who specialize in doing business at the home of the purchaser. Many have no one on whom to rely for consumer guidance. Less than one-half of those over 65 years of age have no more than an eighth grade education (U. S. Senate Special Committee on Aging, 1976). But even those with more formal training who did not grow up in an age of consumerism may not be on their guard in purchase situations and may not be ready to complain if subject to fraudulent selling techniques.

Elderly and other hearing-impaired persons may seek assistance from an audiologist, a physician, a hearing aid manufacturer, or a hearing aid dealer. Each is described briefly below.

Audiologists

Audiologists perform and evaluate the results of hearing tests that can be used to determine the need for a hearing aid as well as the most appropriate type of aid. They also provide counseling and rehabilitative services. Most audiologists practice in nonprofit community hearing and speech centers, hospitals, special clinics, or other rehabilitative settings. Some audiologists sell and dispense hearing aids as well.

Audiological training includes both formal academic courses and clinical experience. The American Speech−Language−Hearing Association has established professional standards for issuance of a Certificate of Clinical Competence in Audiology, specifically, a master's degree or the equivalent in audiology, including 300 hours of supervised clinical experience and 60 hours of academic course work, a 1-year internship in audiology, and the passing of a national examination. The Association has approximately 30,000 members, of which approximately 3,000 hold the certificate (FTC Staff Report, p. 105). An equivalency certificate also may be issued if an audiologist does not wish to belong to the Association. Twenty-nine states presently have audiologist licensure laws, which usually require a licensed audiologist to hold the Association's certificate or have a master's degree in audiology.

Physicians

A person experiencing a hearing loss may consult a family physician or general practitioner. While general practitioners may treat medical conditions that result in hearing impairment, they may have only minimal training in diseases of the ear and correction possibilities and may recommend consultation with an ear specialist. Physicians specializing in diseases of the ear are called "otologists," "otolaryngologists," or "otorhynolaryngologists," depending on whether they specialize only in the ear, in the ear and throat, or in the ear, nose, and throat, respectively. There are currently about 4,500 practicing medical ear specialists in the United States (FTC Staff Report, p. 102).

Hearing Aid Manufacturers

The hearing aid industry includes over 40 manufacturers who sell aids directly to retail hearing aid dealers, and about eight manufacturers control the largest portion of the sales volume (FTC Staff Report, p. 107). Manufacturers generally consider the retail sellers to be independent agents rather than franchises or representatives. They do, however, exert substantial influence on the dealers in advertising, prices, and sales policies. Manufacturers and distributors are represented by a national trade association, the Hearing Industries Association, which was formerly called the Hearing Aid Industry Conference.

Retail Hearing Aid Dealers

Hearing aid dealers test for hearing loss, fit and sell hearing aids, make earmold impressions, and clean and service hearing aids. They are currently the dominant participants in the delivery system. Most hearing-impaired persons first see the dealer when they are concerned about hearing loss and think perhaps an aid may help. Hearing aid dealers do most of the hearing testing and dispense most of the aids in the United States (FTC Staff Report, p. xxiii).

The retail hearing aid industry in the United States consists of approximately 5,600 hearing aid dealerships, employing between 10,000 and 17,000 sellers. Of these sellers, some 3,600 are members of the National Hearing Aid Society (NHAS) (FTC Staff Report, p. 197). NHAS has an optional certification program, requiring completion of a 20-week home-study course, passage of an examination, 2 years of supervised training, and good moral character. Approximately 2,300 of its members have been certified under this program.

RATIONALE AND NEED FOR REFORM

Consumer advocates contend that older and other hearing-impaired Americans do not receive effective hearing health care. They further submit that the current dealer-dominated hearing aid delivery system works poorly and offer this analogy: If your vision were poor, you would go to an ophthalmologist or an optometrist, get an eye examination and a prescription for eyeglasses, and then take this prescription to an optician who would grind the lenses according to the numbers on the prescription. But if your hearing is poor, you could—at least until the recent FDA regulations described below, which can be waived—simply walk in off the street to the office of a hearing aid dealer, receive a hearing test, and walk out after buying a $400 aid. In spite of the complexity of hearing loss, its acute effects, and the need for trained medical and audiological skills for diagnosis and treatment, no physician or audiologist traditionally had to be involved.

Some 70 percent of persons wearing hearing aids in this country have purchased them directly from a hearing aid dealer, without any medical or audiological consultation (Interdepartmental Task Force on Hearing Aids, 1975; Retired Professional Action Group, 1973). The disadvantages of this system are alarming; an inherent conflict of interest, lack of proper training, lack of proper equipment, and high cost.

Conflict of Interest

Hearing aid dealers play two potentially conflicting roles. On the one hand, they assess the consumer's need for a hearing aid, and, on the other hand, they seek to make a profit from the sale of a hearing aid. If they find that a consumer has no hearing loss, or cannot benefit from an aid, or would be better treated medically, they lose a sale. It has been contended that this dual role often results in the sale of a large number of unnecessary hearing aids (FTC Staff Report, 1978; National Council of Senior Citizens, 1975; Retired Professional Action Group, 1973).

The monetary motive is encouraged by the manufacturers' sales manuals. Some even suggest monthly sales quotas and provide instructions on good selling phrases, overcoming buyer objections, and getting in the customer's door. While only a small minority of dealers are unscrupulous, all are subject to the financial incentives to make a sale, further buttressed by industry pressure. Many primarily are businessmen and women and not health professionals, yet the evaluation and treatment for a hearing loss is a health problem requiring significant direction by health professionals.

Lack of Training

The hearing aid dealer normally lacks the training to be entirely responsible for a patient's hearing health care. Hearing and auditory processing is extremely complex, and learning to test appropriately and evalute hearing loss, let alone detect and diagnose ear disease, requires a rigorous training curriculum. Audiologists must have at least a master's degree, and physicians specializing in problems of the ear spend years in medical education and clinical training. Contrast this with the purely voluntary home-study course offered by the National Hearing Aid Society—a course pursued by only a small fraction of the nation's hearing aid sellers and widely criticized as superficial, inaccurate, and even "potentially dangerous" in causing prevention or postponement of adequate diagnosis and treatment (Percy Report, 1976).

Moreover, state law rarely provides for any formal educational requirements for dealers. In addition, state-mandated on-the-job training periods may in reality amount to little responsible supervision. Indeed, industry representatives have acknowledged that many salespersons are given only a few hours of training before selling aids on their own (FTC Staff Report, pp. 5646, 7054). Thus, while the dealer may well be sincerely interested in helping the consumer, the dealer normally is basically a tradesperson and not a skilled health practitioner.

Lack of Proper Equipment

Hearing aid dealers often lack the proper equipment to thoroughly evaluate hearing loss. Exhaustive testing with calibrated audiological instruments is essential in assessing the need for a hearing aid. Although some dealers have such equipment, most have only a portable audiometer and a master hearing aid, and often even this equipment is outdated and limited in function (FTC Staff Report, pp. 6231 ff, and 6275ff.). Further, dealers rarely own sound-level meters, which means that they cannot measure the presence and amount of background noise in the testing environment (FTC Staff Report, 1978). Even accurate instruments will not produce accurate results in a noisy environment. Testing should be done in a soundproof testing room, but too often dealers do not test in such an environment, particularly if they are testing in the consumer's home.

Hearing testing instruments are extremely sensitive and can easily go out of calibration, particularly as a result of high humidity, shock, vibrations while being transported, and exposure to dust. The equipment needed to accurately calibrate testing instruments is expensive, and often dealers do not own it. Federal Trade Commission records indicate that many sellers have never had their audiometer serviced (FTC Staff Report, p. F-237, fn. 1552). Many states, in fact, do not require calibration of equipment on a regular basis.

High Cost of Hearing Aids

The system of dealer evaluation is not one that saves money for the consumer. Without an accurate evaluation of hearing loss, the consumer may purchase a $400 aid that is useless, a difficulty that could have been avoided through proper audiological testing, costing perhaps $45 to $60. Since many older persons live on fixed, low incomes, an expenditure of several hundred dollars based on hope rather than accurate testing may prove financially crippling.

Even if the consumer genuinely needs an aid, the markups by the hearing aid industry are enormous. The parts in a $350 aid cost approximately $30, and the costs for labor, advertising, and promotion are about $45. The manufacturer sells the aid to a dealer for between $80 and $140, and the rest is dealer markup (Interdepartmental Task Force on Hearing Aids, 1975).

Sales Abuses

For several reasons, the dominant role of the hearing aid dealer in the delivery system bears critical scrutiny by advocates for the elderly and other hearing-impaired consumers. In 1973, the Retired Professional Action Group (RPAG), an organization funded by Public Citizen, Inc., undertook a pioneering study of hearing aid sales abuse. RPAG staff contacted over 1000 persons during the course of its investigations, including consumers, their families, dealers, manufacturers, physicians, ear specialists, audiologists, and federal and state officials. RPAG also conducted a special consumer study in Baltimore in which elderly volunteers had hearing tests by an audiologist, then visited hearing aid dealers throughout the city, compared the results, and reported on their experiences. RPAG became a catalyst and model for similar studies in other states (Public Interest Research Group in Michigan, 1973; Minnesota Public Interest Research Group, 1972), and the National Council of Senior Citizens (1975) conducted a study in the District of Columbia.

Meanwhile, Congressional concern mounted. Three Senate Committees (Subcommittee on Consumer Interests of the Elderly, U.S. Senate Special Committee on Aging, 1973; Subcommittee on Government Regulations, U.S. Senate Elect Committee on Small Business, 1975; Subcommittee on Investigations, U.S. Committee on Government Operations, 1975) held hearings on the hearing aid industry and each reconfirmed the inadequacies of hearing health care for hearing-impaired Americans, and particularly older Americans.

The federal executive branch amassed still further evidence. In May, 1974, the Secretary of Health, Education and Welfare established an Intradepartmental Task Force on Hearing Health Care. The Task Force submitted a comprehensive Final Report in July, 1975, supporting and further documenting the findings of Congress, RPAG, and other consumer groups, and making recommendations for federal action.

The Federal Trade Commission undertook perhaps the most extensive investigation to date. In June, 1975, it issued a proposed trade regulation rule on the hearing aid industry. The subsequent rulemaking proceeding produced a voluminous record of over 60,000 pages, including 11 weeks of public hearings in three cities, a presiding officer's report, and a lengthy staff report, as well as numerous exhibits, letters, and written comments. During the proceedings, the National Council of Senior Citizens was formally designated to represent consumers.

All of the studies revealed serious sales abuses including misevaluations and misfittings, misrepresentations, and high-pressure sales tactics.

MISEVALUATIONS AND MISFITTINGS

This scenario, recounted by an elderly Massachusetts woman for the Federal Trade Commission *Record*, has occurred all too frequently (NCSC Massachusetts Affadavit 24, FTC official transcript, p. 4441).

In June of 1974, a man called me from a hearing aid dealership and asked if he could come to the house to look at the hearing aid that I had. I agreed to let them come. Two men came and tested my hearing. They told me I needed two (2) new hearing aids. I signed their contract for the aids and paid them $839.

They delivered the aids to me, but they did not fit. I was very concerned because I spent so much money, but I could not use the aids. About a week later I called the company to complain and they came to see me. But they said I did not put them on right. I did not agree with this. I asked them for my money back, but I was refused. They came back five or six more times but still I could not use the aids. Each time I asked for a refund and each time I was told I could not have my money back.

. . . (I have) never used the aids. I still have them but they are no good to me for they do not help me at all.

The FTC staff noted that "the record in this proceeding is filled with reports of consumers who received no benefit from the purchase of a hearing aid" (FTC Staff Report, p. 51). Thus, the 1973 Retired Professional Action Group study in Baltimore found that 42 percent of visits to dealers resulted in recommendations for hearing aids when hearing professionals had determined previously that patients could not benefit from aids. A similar study by the National Council of Senior Citizens in Washington, D.C. in 1975 found that 3 out of 11 hearing tests by dealers (27 percent) led to recommendations of unnecessary hearing aids. It also found that most dealer testing results were inaccurate, showing recordings of greater than actual hearing loss in 7 out of 11 cases by as much as 2.6 dB. The Intradepartmental Task Force on Hearing Aids (HEW, 1975) estimated that 85 percent of persons who contact dealers directly are found "capable of being helped" by an aid; whereas in comparison, statistics for one Canadian province show that only 45 percent of persons who contact audiologists are diagnosed as needing a hearing aid (How to Buy a Hearing Aid, 1976). The U.S. and Canadian patient groups presumably were similar in that both were seeking help for a hearing problem. But the Canadian patients were diagnosed by professionals without a monetary motive in selling aids.

Misevaluations have been well documented. For example, hearing aids have been fitted and sold to consumers in the face of clear medical contraindications. At the FTC hearings, a number of witnesses reported aids being fitted on ears that were infected or draining (FTC Staff Report, p. 70). Placing an ear mold in the ear canal in such a case may exacerbate the infection. In addition, numerous witnesses and consumers have reported the sale of aids to persons with medically or surgically treatable ear pathologies. For instance, one elderly purchaser wrote to the FTC, "I've had a hearing aid for years, but don't even need one since my doctor examined my ears and removed a polyp from my right ear. . . . Never did the salesman for the aids ever examine my ears. The last hearing aid cost me $495. . . ." (FTC Staff Report, p. 54).

Epstein (1976) testified at the FTC hearings that he had seen about 20 patients a month who have worn or are wearing aids over ears that are surgically correctable. Kasden (1976) submitted a report that indicated that out of 2369 persons with otosclerosis, 1500, or 63.3 percent, were first seen by dealers who sold aids to 98.9 percent of them without telling them that medical or surgical treatment was available. Also, many persons have a hearing impairment that is neither medically correctable nor subject to benefit from amplification, but are nevertheless convinced to purchase aids. Aids are often sold to persons with normal hearing, as suggested by the RPAG study, PIRG reports, National Council of Senior Citizens study and the FTC proceedings. Examples from the FTC Record include that of an aid sold to the parents of a 12-year-old child with normal hearing (FTC Record, 1976, Section 8, p. 1346), a $379 aid sold to a consumer whose hearing for speech was "well within the normal limits for both ears," (FTC Record, Section 8, p. 8233, 1976), and two aids sold to a graduate student despite that fact that one ear had perfectly normal hearing (FTC, "Official Transcript," 1976, p. 278).

Finally, even if a person has a hearing loss that can benefit from amplification, he still may be sold an aid that is of little or no benefit. For example, an FTC witness testified that he had been sold one aid, and then a replacement aid, both fitted to his left ear, neither of which helped. Later audiological testing revealed that a completely different model should have been fitted to his *right* ear (FTC, "Official Transcript," 1976, p. 4858). Some consumers have reported being sold aids too weak for their hearing loss, while others suffer the pain and annoynace of an aid too powerful for their ear. The audiological staff of the Mayo Clinic collected a "bad fit" file and, in the first year and a half, counted 60 causes of grossly misfitted aids from all parts of the country (FTC Staff Report, 1978).

MISREPRESENTATIONS

Both in advertising and in direct contact with consumers, industry claims about hearing aid dealers and sellers, particular models of hearing aids, and hearing aids generally often have been misleading. The initial misrepresentation by hearing aid dealers and salesmen is often related to the fact that they are salespersons. Many have used an array of tactics (FTC Staff Report, 1978) to hide this fact, including ads resembling public service announcements and offering free hearing tests, professional-sounding business names such as "hearing center", "hearing clinic," or "hearing and speech center," offers of free hearing tests in the home by salesmen who do not state or imply that they are seeking to sell aids, and certificates, white coats, and occasionally even use of the title "doctor" to imply professional medical training.

Once in contact with the consumer, dealers may resort to misrepresentation about aids they are seeking to sell. For instance, the records of the FTC (Staff Report, 1978) show examples of claims that used aids were new, or that particular models were new, revolutionary, a breakthrough, or unique when they were not. In addition, claims were made that aids are tiny and inconspicuous without revealing that these small aids may not improve hearing as well as larger ones, and that aids are cordless, invisible, or require nothing in the ear or no tube, when this is not the case or when it is literally true but there were unstated disadvantages.

Finally, perhaps most harmful of all, dealers in too many instances have misrepresented the benefits of hearing aid use, including statements that aids will restore normal hearing, eliminate or greatly reduce background noise problems, or retard the progression of hearing loss. For instance, one elderly woman stated for the FTC record (FTC Staff Report, 1978) that a dealer came to her home, tested her hearing, and "told me I had lost quite a bit of hearing in my right ear and if I did not get an aid for that ear I would lose what little hearing I had left. He told me the aid would cost $509. Because I did not want to lose the rest of my hearing, I agreed to buy the aid . . ." (FTC Staff Report, p. 65).

HOME SALES AND HIGH-PRESSURE TACTICS

According to the FTC hearings (FTC Staff Report, 1978), 56 percent to 90 percent of hearing aid sales occur in the home. While industry representatives submit that home sales are a service to the elderly and homebound, they often serve as an opportunity to catch the consumer in a vulnerable situation in order to subject him to a sophisticated barrage of high-pressure selling tactics, resulting in rapid consummation of a sale, perhaps without the consumer fully recognizing that he or she had made a large commitment. Home visits are often unannounced. The prospective purchaser is surprised, unable fully to assess the qualifications of the seller, unprepared to confront the carefully planned sales pitch, and without an opportunity to talk with a doctor, audiologist, or knowledgeable friend or relative outside the seller's presence. The elderly are particularly susceptible. They are often lonely and eager to talk with sellers and may be awed by their apparent knowledge and background.

Dealers use a repertoire of calculated sales techniques geared to gain the confidence of the buyer and facilitate a sale, regardless of the consumer's need. These can include advertising free hearing tests, free booklets on hearing loss, free hearing aid replicas, or even free aids. Instead of receiving these promised items, the consumer will often find an eager salesman on his doorstep. They may use a third party as a selling influence or use a case history to detect a customer's particular weakness and to play on his or her emotions ("Do your grandchildren make fun of you because of your not hearing them correctly?"). Unscrupulous salespersons may speak softly when administering a hearing test and raise their voice when demonstrating hearing in the aided ear. They may use high-frequency word lists to test hearing loss and low-frequency word lists to test the aided ear. They may imply that the buyer will hear as well with the new aid as through the master hearing aid, although this may not be true. In fact, one manual suggests that when testing with a master aid, the seller should say, "Wouldn't it be nice to hear like this again?" Finally, sellers are adept at successfully closing a sale. The FTC staff finds that dealer closing techniques all "share one common purpose: They are designed to secure the customer's agreement to purchase without even permitting him to stop and seriously consider this difficult decision" (FTC Staff Report, 1978).

THE LEGISLATIVE AND REGULATORY RESPONSE

The deficiencies of the hearing aid delivery system and the attendant sales abuses described above call for governmental intervention to protect consumers, assure fairness, and encourage a reasoned, informed purchase decision. State legislatures, the U.S. Food and Drug Administration, and the Federal Trade Commission have responded to this need.

State Regulations

The first state regulation of hearing aid sales was an Oregon law enacted in 1959, requiring licensure of hearing aid dealers. This remained the only such state legislation until 1966, when the Federal Trade Commission proposed that the states enact licensure laws and developed a model act based on the Oregon statute. Although the hearing aid industry at first resisted these efforts, eventually the National Hearing Aid Society developed and promoted its own model statute, designed to increase the status of dealers through formal license procedures, but offering little relief for consumers. State legislatures began to enact hearing aid laws, usually adopting the

NHAS model. By 1978, 42 states had dealer licensure laws, four states and the District of Columbia had dealer registration systems, and Vermont governed hearing aid sellers by state health regulations. Illinois, Alaska, and Utah currently have no statutes or regulations.

Most of the laws are weak and hearing aid sales abuses have continued. Consumer advocates have criticized the state schemes as protecting the hearing aid seller rather than the hearing aid consumer (Retired Professional Action Group Report, 1973). They have concluded that the laws are deficient in requirements for dealer qualifications and training, medical and audiological clearance, consumer protection measures, and consumer-complaint procedures.

DEALER QUALIFICATIONS AND TRAINING

Generally anyone who is over 18 years of age, is of good moral character, and has a high school education can become a licensed hearing aid dealer by passing an examination administered by a state hearing aid board. The exams have often been criticized as an inadequate measure of competency. In 30 states those already selling aids when the law was enacted were ''grandfathered in'' without taking the exam. Several states require a trainee apprenticeship period, but none provides standards for supervision of the trainee. In fact, the trainee often begins to fit and sell aids immediately under a temporary permit, with no experience or training (FTC Staff Report, 1978; FTC, ''Official Transcript,'' 1976).

MEDICAL AND AUDIOLOGICAL CLEARANCE

A provision mandating medical and/or audiological evaluation prior to the purchase of an aid may remove the conflict of interest inherent in the delivery system. Currently only the District of Columbia, Hawaii, New York, Vermont, and West Virginia have prior medical clearance provisions that apply to all potential purchasers, with exceptions for replacement aids and persons who object to a medical examination on religious grounds. The D. C. statute prohibits sale of an aid without the written approval of an otolaryngologist after a medical examination and an audiological evaluation. Under New York law, recommendations may come from either an otorhynolaryngologist or an audiologist. Hawaii and West Virginia require approval of a licensed physician. Dealers in Vermont may not sell aids without a written statement from a physician, although the statement need not recommend purchase of an aid.

Minnesota initially had a provision prohibiting sale of an aid without a written recommendation from an audiologist, otolaryngologist, otologist, or licensed medical doctor, but the law was amended in response to dealer protest to permit persons under 60 years of age to waive the requirement.

In addition, statutes in six states require a prior medical evaluation when a dealer has notice of listed otologic symptoms, such as sudden or rapidly progressing hearing loss, dizziness, or active drainage from the ear. Connecticut, Florida, Maine, Minnesota, Pennsylvania, and Rhode Island prohibit sale in these cases without medical clearance, preferably by an ear specialist. Eleven other states require only that the customer be advised to consult a doctor. Customers who elect to purchase an aid without seeking professional advice must sign a waiver.

State laws generally are stricter with children. Twenty-five states require professional examination of a child before sale of an aid. Eight of these require both otological and audiological consultation. Four other states, namely, Ohio, Oregon, Washington, and Wyoming, also have medical clearance requirements for children, but permit a parent or guardian to waive this protection. Finally, nine states require the dealer to recommend professional approval before the sale of an aid for a child.

CONSUMER PROTECTION MEASURES

Consumers are especially vulnerable and sales tactics especially abusive in the home. Yet only seven jurisdictions, namely, the District of Columbia, Hawaii, Kentucky, Maryland, Michigan, New Hampshire, and New York, have restricted home solicitation of hearing aid sales.

An invaluable consumer remedy is the trial period and right to cancel which can be used to protect buyers from spending substantial sums on an aid not useful to them. Yet only ten states have enacted cancellation provisions for hearing aid sales. The District of Columbia, Connecticut, Kentucky, Maine, New Hampshire, and Vermont all grant at least a 30-day trial period, with specified cancellation charges. North Carolina, Washington, and Oregon allow cancellation only with a physician's statement that the aid is not beneficial.

CONSUMER COMPLAINT PROCEDURES

In most states the consumer subject to hearing aid sales abuse does not know where to seek assistance. State laws usually provide for a hearing aid dealer licensure board, but these are often dealer dominated and ineffective. In at least 25 states, dealers constitute a majority on the licensure board, and in most states, dealers make up at least half the panel. In many cases, the board is controlled by the dealer trade association. Fewer than half the state licensing statutes require consumer representation on the board.

While most licensure laws charge the board with receiving and handling consumer complaints, the majority do not specify any procedure for complaint handling, leaving dealer-dominated boards to devise their own methods. Many boards are hampered by meager budgets and little or no staff assistance. Moreover, consumers often are not aware of the boards' existence and function. Very few statutes require the purchase receipt to include information about how and where to file a complaint. Even when a complaint does reach the board, action is usually minimal, resulting in informal settlements or attempts to simply contact the parties and urge them to resolve their differences. Disciplinary actions are rare. Although penalties in the licensure statutes often include fines, imprisonment, and suspension and revocation of the license, these are seldom invoked (FTC Staff Report, 1978).

Because of the impotence of most state laws to protect hearing aid consumers, the Food and Drug Administration and the Federal Trade Commission have taken active roles in hearing health consumerism.

The Food and Drug Administration Regulations

On August 25, 1977, hearing aid regulations issued by the U.S. Food and Drug Administration became effective. The regulations provided for comprehensive consumer information on the use, care, repair, and limitations of hearing aids. They also contain a limited medical evaluation requirement.

CONSUMER INFORMATION

The FDA regulations require that each hearing aid manufacturing company develop a User Instructional Brochure, which must contain specific information on the use, maintenance, and repair of the aid; inform consumers that a hearing aid cannot restore normal hearing and cannot prevent or improve a hearing impairment; contain a warning that instructs dealers to advise medical consultation for customers who display seven signs indicating medical difficulties; include a notice to hearing aid users concerning the advisability of a prior medical evaluation; advise consumers to ask dealers about a trial period; and

contain certain technical data to assist in selecting, fitting, and checking the performance of aids.

All of this is useful consumer information. The regulations direct dealers to provide the brochure before a sale is made, to review its contents and to provide the consumer with an opportunity to read it. Monitoring and enforcement of this activity, however, is difficult. Further, the regulations do not stipulate at what point in the sales process this information is to be provided to the consumer. Thus, the sale may be essentially consummated when these items are reviewed. Finally, the brochure is necessarily lengthy and contains a plethora of facts, including complex technical data that may be difficult for the consumer to understand. Elderly persons with vision problems may not be able to read the fine print. In short, the valuable information may seldom reach its intended audience.

MEDICAL EVALUATION

The FDA regulations further provide that (U.S. Food & Drug Administration, 1977, pp. 420-421)

a hearing aid dispenser shall not sell a hearing aid unless the prospective user has presented to the hearing aid dispenser a written statement signed by a licensed physician that states that the patient's hearing loss has been medically evaluated and the patient may be considered a candidate for a hearing aid. The medical evaluation must have taken place within the preceding 6 months.

Anyone 18 years of age or older may waive the medical evaluation requirement if the dealer informs the buyer that waiver is not in his best interest, does not actively encourage the waiver, and affords the buyer an opportunity to sign a waiver statement. This waiver emasculates an already weak protection.

Consumer advocates were disappointed in the final version of the FDA regulations, which had been preceeded by lengthy debate and comment by both consumer and industry groups. However, the regulations at least provided a nationwide minimum of consumer protection that theretofore had not existed.

The Proposed Federal Trade Commission Rule

In 1975, the Federal Trade Commission published a Hearing Aid Industry Proposed Trade Regulation. The proposed rule contained a buyer's right to cancel after 30 days, as well as detailed provisions prohibiting misrepresentation and regulating abusive sales techniques. The Commission held extensive hearings on the proposed rule, drawing vigorous consumer and industry participation.

THE BUYER'S RIGHT TO CANCEL

The centerpiece of the proposed FTC rule was a trial period for the hearing aid purchaser. The rule required the seller to include in every contract or receipt pertaining to the sale of a hearing aid a provision giving the buyer the right to cancel a purchase or rental for any reason at any time within 30 days after receiving the aid. The proposed provision is a lengthy and comprehensive one, including a disclosure statement to inform buyers of their rights, a requirement that sellers inform buyers orally of their rights, and maximum cancellation charges.

The buyer's right to cancel was ardently debated throughout the rulemaking proceeding. The industry argued that (1) there was not a significant number of consumers who received no benefit from aids and who would have been helped by a trial period; (2) that a purchaser did not need to try out an aid in a variety of real-life situations; (3) that a trial period would be a disincentive to purchasers in making the necessary effort to learn to use an aid most effectively; and (4) that it would result in many returned aids that the dealers would have to sell or refurbish at great cost to them and ultimately to the consumer.

Consumer advocates, audiologists, and the FTC presiding officer and staff remained unpersuaded by these arguments. They pointed out that many dealers already offered trial periods and had not suffered economically. They submitted that only those dealers using little care in hearing evaluation and fitting and often selling unnecessary aids would be adversely affected. They felt that, whereas the rule as a whole might cause a slight additional cost for hearing aids and services, the risk to the consumer of buying an unnecessary hearing aid would be reduced. The presiding officer's report estimated that savings to consumers in preventing the purchase of unnecessary aids would total over nine million dollars (Shepherd, 1977).

PROHIBITED REPRESENTATIONS AND REQUIRED DISCLOSURES

The proposed rule set out specific prohibited representations concerning both hearing aid sellers and hearing aids, as well as mandating certain negative disclosures to offset advertisements that may mislead the unwary consumer.

Representations re Sellers The rule provided that "No seller shall make any representation to members of the consuming public without clearly and conspicuously disclosing that it is a seller of hearing aids." (FTL, "Hearing Aid Industry Proposed Trade Regulation," 1975, 440.8[a]). This requirement may be satisfied by a clear statement of the name of the seller's business if the name includes the term "hearing aid center" or other words that identify it with the sale of aids. Further, sellers may not misrepresent themselves as governmental or non-profit public service institutions through the use of terms such as "hearing clinic" or "speech and hearing center." They may not use the term "certified hearing aid audiologist"—a term the industry charged was legitimate, but which consumers submitted may imply clinical knowledge on the part of the dealers that they did not possess.

Representation re Aids The rule would prohibit a seller from representing "that any hearing aid will restore or help restore normal or natural hearing or will enable or help enable wearers to hear sounds normally or naturally" (PTL, "Hearing Aid Industry Proposed Trade Regulation," 440.9[a]). It also would prohibit sellers from claiming that hearing aids will stop or help to stop the progression of hearing loss. It particularly would prohibit expressions such as "delay may be harmful" or "act now before it's too late." Overwhelming evidence shows that no aid will halt or affect a progressive hearing loss. The prohibition would prevent the industry from threatening consumers with dire consequences if an aid is not purchased.

Finally, the rule would strike "puffing," a technique that is very effective on elderly and other hearing-impaired persons desperate for relief. It would provide that an aid may not be represented as new for more than one year from when it was first marketed. In addition, a statement that an aid is "unique, revolutionary, or special will be deemed to be a comparison to all other hearing aid brands and models," and must be documented with reliable scientific or medical evidence.

Negative Disclosure The rule would mandate that a claim that an aid will positively affect hearing capability must be presented accompanied by a statement that "many persons with a hearing loss will not receive any significant benefit from any hearing aid" (FTC, "Hearing Aid Industry Proposed Trade Regulation," 440.10[a]). It also would require that a representation that an aid will help a person understand speech in noisy or group situations must be accompanied by a statement that for many persons this will not consistently be so, and that a representation that two aids will help persons with a loss in both ears must be accompanied by a statement that many

persons with such a loss will receive no greater
benefits from two aids than from one.

PROHIBITED SELLING TECHNIQUES

The most debated of the rule's provisions regarding selling techniques is a section prohibiting
home visits to sell hearing aids without the prior written consent of the potential buyer. This consent must
"clearly and conspicuously state that such potential
buyer is aware that the seller may attempt to sell a
hearing aid during such a visit" (FTC, "Hearing Aid
Industry Proposed Trade Regulation," 440.7[b]).
The industry argued that this would prevent reputable
dealers from bringing genuine services to the
homebound who might not be able to seek help for
themselves. They suggested that if consumers had to
write for help, they might forego it forever, and thus
the section would be a step backward for the hard-
of-hearing.

But consumer advocates noted that a majority of
hearing aid complaints concerned in-home sales and
that elderly persons were particularly susceptible to
the in-home sales approach. While the proposed
section would not ultimately stop the dealer from
making house calls, at least consumers would not be
surprised and therefore might be better able to protect
themselves from high-pressure sales tactics.

UNRESOLVED ISSUES

The FDA regulations and the proposed FTC rule
together should provide a substantial, uniform level
of consumer protection for America's hearing-
impaired population. They are both necessary and
long overdue, but the two rulings are not sufficient.
A raft of unresolved issues still trouble consumer
advocates, including the weakness of the FDA clearance provision, the ramifications of the FDA regulations for state law, some deficiencies in the proposed
FTC protections, and the failure of Medicare and
often Medicaid to cover hearing aids and hearing
evaluations for aids.

The FDA Regulations: A Compromise of Consumer Interests

The preliminary HEW Intradepartmental Task
Force on Hearing Aids that preceded the FDA regulations emphasized the importance of professional
examination prior to purchase of an aid. Although the
regulations required that a consumer must have been

examined by a physician within 6 months before the
purchase of an aid, the regulations fell short of full
consumer protection in several critical respects. The
examination was to be by a physician rather than an
otologist or otolaryngologist, who has had advanced
training in special problems of the ear. Further, the
physician need only say the patient "may be considered a candidate for a hearing aid," not that he
recommends or prescribes a hearing aid. The strength
of the examination requirement was additionally
weakened by the waiver provision for persons 18
years of age or older. The waiver system easily may
be abused by dealers pressuring for a quick sale.
There is evidence that in states where a medical
examination can be waived, 40 to 50 percent of the
sales are made without medical examinations (U.S.
Department of Health, Education, and Welfare,
1978). Finally, the FDA regulations fail to require
audiological evaluations, leaving the hearing testing
to dealers and failing to take advantage of the training
of audiologists.

This last objection now requires a caveat. One
major benefit of substituting audiological for dealer
evaluation has been the prevention of conflict of
interest; audiologists generally have not sold aids for
profit, because the code of ethics of the American
Speech–Language–Hearing Association essentially
prevented it. In 1978, however, the Association
changed its code of ethics to allow audiologists to sell
aids for profit. The code still calls for objectivity,
consumer price information, dispensing aids as "part
of a program of comprehensive habilitative care,"
and establishing fees for services independent of
whether an aid is dispensed. Nonetheless, the code
change opens the door to possible consumer abuse,
even if by only a small minority of audiologists. It
adds a conflict-of-interest element that may make the
argument for prior audiological evaluation, although
a good one, necessarily less convincing that it was.

At the time the FDA rulemaking procedure was
initiated, a few states had taken bold steps to prevent
the sale of unneeded aids by requiring a prior medical
or audiological examination. Grass roots consumer
advocacy groups were pushing for stronger,
consumer-oriented hearing aid laws in several state
legislatures. When the FDA proposals were published in 1976, consumer advocates assumed they
could continue their efforts on the state legislative
front, despite their disappointment with the FDA
action. Consumers were lulled into foregoing a more
strenuous campaign against the FDA regulations by
the agency's specific assurance that "State and local
governments may impose more stringent conditions

for sale of hearing aids than are prescribed in . . . this section'' (804.421[a] (4) 41 Federal Register, 16763, 1976). Thus, it seemed that stricter state laws would be allowed to stand and that consumers could push for additional protection without interference by the federal government.

During the comment period for the proposed regulations, however, Congress passed the Medical Device Amendments Act of 1976 (Public Law 94–295, 90 Stat. 539). The Amendments mandate federal preemption of any state or local law ''which is different from, or in addition to'' FDA requirements with respect to medical devices, including hearing aids. The Amendments also allowed states to petition for exemption from the preemption effect of federal regulations, if the state requirement is ''more stringent'' or ''is required by compelling local conditions.'' (521[a] and [b] Medical Device Amendments to Federal Food, Drug, and Cosmetic Act).

Passage of the Medical Device Amendments meant, in brief, that gains in state hearing aid legislation could be preempted by the FDA requirements, thereby representing a serious potential setback in several states.

Senior citizen groups, consumer advocates and audiologists continued to argue that state and local policymakers should not be inhibited by preemption, since the Medical Device Amendments made specific provision for an exemption for ''more stringent'' requirements. They saw the application for preemption as merely a temporary procedural delay, not a barrier to enactment of strong state laws. However, in its regulations governing procedures for exemptions from preemption the FDA provides that the Commissioner may not grant an application for exemption if he determines that granting it ''would not be in the best interest of public health'' (43 Federal Register, 18667, May 2, 1978). In its proposed exemptions from preemption, the Commissioner denied exemption for state laws requiring audiological examination, reasoning that ''such a requirement would create an additional barrier to the receipt of hearing aids in parts of the country where audiological services are scarce . . .'' (43 Federal Register 33181, July 28, 1978), and would increase the cost of obtaining an aid. Yet states petitioning for exemption demonstrated persuasively that audiological services in their jurisdiction are not scarce and that audiological exams result in a cost savings to consumers. In addition, the FDA proposed to deny exemptions to state laws restricting the grounds for a waiver of medical evaluation.

The District of Columbia law, for instance, raises both issues. It requires an audiological evaluation and examination by a medical ear physician prior to the purchase of an aid. It allows waiver of this requirement only on religious or personal objections to medical evaluations. The FDA proposed to deny the D.C. law exemption from preemption on both counts (43 Federal Register 33183, July 28, 1978).

The FDA saga has been a trying one for hearing aid reform advocates. They submit that when Congress enacted the Medical Device Amendment in 1976, it never intended to lessen the extent of protection afforded to the public or to dilute state legislative drives for increased consumer protection. Yet that may be the result in dozens of states now reexamining their hearing aid laws but uncertain as to whether the reform effort would be worthwhile. Downey (1979) has provided a detailed analysis of the preemption issue.

The FTC Proposed Rule

The FTC has proposed potent and wide-ranging protection against hearing aid sales abuse. Nevertheless, a number of concerns about the rule merit further consideration. The proposed rule requires the seller to get the express written consent of a potential buyer prior to making a home visit. The voluminous FTC staff report, issued in September 1978, recommended that the requirement be modified to allow oral consent. Consumer advocates, including older Americans, supported the original proposal because of the inherent vulnerability of elderly consumers and the demonstrated tendency of home visits to lead to sales abuses. The telephone consent of older hearing-impaired consumers seems risky because they may not accurately hear or understand what is being told to them. Also, enforcement of an oral ''okay'' rule seems difficult at best.

Although the proposed rule requires prior consent for home sales visits, it does not prohibit unannounced home service visits. The National Council of Senior Citizens and other consumer groups have argued that the prior consent requirement should be extended to all seller visits to the buyer's home in order to minimize the use of service visits as subterfuges for new sales.

The FTC staff report recommended deleting several important disclosures in the proposed rule, namely, (1) that many persons will not benefit from hearing aids, (2) that many will not distinguish and understand sounds in noisy or group activities, and (3) that two aids will not necessarily provide more benefit than one. The staff feared discouraging already reluctant consumers from seeking help through hearing aids and reasoned that the right to cancel would provide a remedy against the raising of unrealistic expectations. Consumer representatives disagreed on grounds that the hearing-impaired know very little about the benefits and limitations of amplification devices, that hearing aid advertising has played on this ignorance, and that these disclosures are needed to enable consumers to make intelligent choices based on full information.

If buyers exercise their right to cancel, sellers must refund the purchase price less specified cancellation charges. The National Council of Senior Citizens and others, however, argued that the rule should disallow cancellation charges when a seller violates the rule's proscriptions. Sellers should not be compensated for sales induced by deceptive practices.

In the propsed rule, aids "prescribed" by an audiologist or physician and "identical replacement" aids are excepted from the cancellation provisions. The FTC staff, as well as consumer advocates, have recommended these exceptions be dropped. Experts agree that hearing aids, unlike eyeglasses, cannot be "prescribed" with complete accuracy, so that a trial period is necessary to insure benefit to the users. Users cannot be sure that a replacement aid will serve them as well as the initial aid and, therefore, need a trial period to thoroughly test the aid.

The hearing aid industry contended there was no need for the proposed FTC rule because of the issuance in 1977 of the FDA regulations. This argument overlooks the differing purposes of the two rules, as well as the deficiencies of the FDA rule and its effect on state hearing aid laws. The FDA's medical evaluation provision does not require the physician to recommend an aid or say the patient may be helped by an aid. That determination is still often in the hands of the hearing aid dealer. Indeed, a number of consumers who testified at the FTC hearing concerning misleading statements had in fact visited physicians before they purchased aids that did not help them. It is not easy to accept a diagnosis that one will not hear again.

In spite of its deficiencies, however, the FDA rule does provide some minimum standard of protection nationwide. The FTC could be supportive of FDA efforts by requiring an affirmative disclosure of the FDA medical evaluation provision to prospective buyers. The two rules could then work in concert and buyers would receive the protection of both through the coordinated efforts of the two agencies.

Finally, there is the question of enforcement.

The FTC staff argued that the buyer's right to cancel, with its required notices written in a clear "plain English" format, will be self-enforcing in that "Buyers will understand and be able to assert their own rights to immediate relief from undesirable hearing aid purchases" (FTC "Official Transcript," 1976). It remains to be seen whether this will occur. More difficult to enforce are the prohibitions dealing with oral conduct, because there will be no records on which to rely. Hearing-impaired consumers are notoriously reluctant to complain. Although the FTC staff pointed out that a number of states considered violation of an FTC rule to be a violation of their own consumer protection statutes, too few consumers, particularly older persons, know where or how to complain to state agencies.

Hearing Aids in Government Health Programs

Several federal agencies provide assistance in acquiring hearing tests and hearing aids. Veterans can get free diagnostic services and hearing aids through the Veterans Administration. This program is usually limited to veterans whose hearing losses are service-connected or to patients in VA medical centers. The Federal Rehabilitation Services Administration, working through state departments of vocal rehabilitation, assists persons whose hearing problems handicap employment. Help for children is available through a program of the Federal Maternal and Child Health Service, administered by state health departments or state crippled children's services.

But the giants in federal health programs are Medicare and Medicaid. Medicare is a health insurance program for the elderly sponsored by the federal government through the Social Security Administration. Medicaid is a joint federal–state assistance program designed to provide health care services to the poor. Briefly, Medicare covers hearing tests requested by physicians and leading to medical or surgical treatment. It does not cover hearing tests to determine the need for an aid or hearing tests for the selection of an appropriate aid. It does not cover the purchase of hearing aids, yet many senior citizens existing on meager Social Security payments simply cannot afford an aid. Thus elderly and consumer groups have advocated coverage of the cost of hearing tests by physicians and audiologists to determine the need for an aid and the purchase of an aid after proper professional evaluation.

Medicaid programs in about half the states currently offer assistance to income-eligible persons who cannot afford to buy an aid. The benefits and requirements differ from state to state and are constantly changing. Recent constraints on state budgets have caused several states to consider deleting coverage of hearing tests and hearing aids. States including hearing aids under Medicaid generally require prior physician evaluation and sometimes audiological evaluation. Consumers say these states should strengthen their standards to include prior examination by an audiologist and an otolaryngologist, and states that do not yet include aids under Medicaid should begin with this requirement. Finally, consumers point out that to ensure a uniform, high standard throughout the nation, the federal Medicaid regulations should be amended to direct that states require prior examination by both an audiologist and an otolaryngologist.

CONCLUSION

The hearing aid is a health device, but the hearing aid delivery system thus far has not reflected this basic tenet. Instead, it has been riddled with sales abuses alarming to the elderly and hearing-impaired community. Through the efforts of organized consumer and senior citizen groups, as well as interested state and federal policymakers, this is beginning to change. But consumers and governments must continue jointly to push for full protection for the nation's hearing-impaired population.

REFERENCES

Downey, M. Laboratories or puppets? The challenge of Federal pre-emption of state legislation. *ASHA: Journal of the American Speech and Hearing Association,* 1979, *21,* 7−11.

Epstein, S. Testimony on behalf of the National Council of Senior Citizens (NSCS). *FTC Transcript,* 1976, 4562−4622.

Federal Trade Commission (FTC) staff report. *Hearing aid industry staff report.* Final report to the Federal Trade Commission and hearing aid industry proposed trade regulation rule, Bureau of Consumer Protection, September, 1978.

Federal Trade Commission. Hearing aid industry proposed trade regulation. *Code of Federal Regulations,* 1975, *16,* 440ff.

Federal Trade Commission. Official transcript of proceedings before the Federal Trade Commission, Docket No. 215−244, Public hearings on proposed regulation rules: Hearing aid industry, 1976.

"How to buy a hearing aid," *Consumer Reports,* 1976, *41,* 348.

Intradepartmental Task Force on Hearing Aids, U.S. Department of Health, Education, and Welfare. Final report to the secretary on hearing aid health care, July, 1975.

Kasden, S. Testimony to Federal Trade Commission. *FTC Record,* 1976, sect. 5, 1282.

Minnesota Public Interest Research Group (MPIRG). Hearing aids and the hearing aid industry in Minnesota. November 13, 1972 (Available from MPIRG, 3036 University Avenue, Minneapolis, Minnesota, 55414).

National Council of Senior Citizens. Survey of hearing aid dealers in the District of Columbia. October, 1975.

Percy Report, *Staff study of the state licensing laws and training requirements for hearing aid dealers.* (Comm. Print). U.S. Senate Permanent Subcommittee on Investigations of the Committee on Government Operations, October 1975, pp. 58−59.

Public Interest Research Group in Michigan (PIRGIM). You know I can't hear you when the cash register is running: The hearing aid industry in Michigan. December 3, 1973 (Available from PIRGIM, 615 East Michigan Avenue, East Lansing, Michigan 48933).

Retired Professional Action Group. Paying through the ear: A report on hearing health care problems. *Public Citizen, Inc.,* Washington, D.C., 1973.

Shepherd, M.G. Report of the presiding officer on proposed trade regulations rule for the hearing aid industry, August 1, 1977. Federal Trade Commission, Public Record, 215–244.

U.S. Department of Health, Education, and Welfare. Oral hearing on exemption from federal pre-emption of state and local requirements on sale and labelling of hearing aids, October 31, 1978.

United States Food and Drug Administration, 21, *Code of Federal Regulations* 801. 420–421 (a) (1), 1977.

U.S. Senate Special Subcommittee on Aging, *Developments in aging: 1976.*

Rosemary Lubinski

20

Speech, Language, and Audiology Programs in Home Health Care Agencies and Nursing Homes

As individuals grow older they face a series of personal and social problems. There may be role adjustments associated with retirement, changes in the family constellation, illness, and the loss of a spouse. For many of the elderly there are reduced physical abilities, social influence, and contact with friends and family members. As these adjustments occur, older persons must rely more frequently on their own communication skills in order to remain independent and self-actualizing members of society. Communication becomes the crucial difference between isolation and social connectedness, between dependence and independence, and between withdrawal and fulfillment.

Effective communication for older persons involves the adequate production and reception of a message, congruity between the intent of the message sent and the message received, and a climate in which communication interaction is valued and reinforced. Successful communication gives older individuals knowledge about their environment, a sense of orientation toward their own roles and societal expectations, and a sense of usefulness and influence. In addition, communication serves a therapeutic role for the elderly in that through communication they may extend themselves beyond their immediate and often isolated surroundings, relieve loneliness, depression, and anxiety, strive toward self-realization during this phase of their life, and support other persons in a helping relationship. The value of

successful communication for older individuals is equally important for those who have adequate communication skills and for those with speech, language, and hearing disorders. Any factors that reduce the elderly individuals' ability or opportunity to communicate must be reduced or eliminated if successful communication is to be a reality for all aging persons (Lubinski, 1975, 1978, 1978–1979).

Speech–language pathologists and audiologists have traditionally viewed their role with the elderly as one of identifying and improving observable speech, language, and hearing skills. The communications disorders specialist has a variety of diagnostic and therapeutic roles with the elderly, particularly those in institutional facilities. According to Lubinski (1978):

> One role is an individual oriented role in which the communication disorders specialist focuses on the identification and remediation of specific speech, language and hearing disorders as they are usually defined. The second role is setting oriented, in which the communicologist directs his or her professional efforts toward the identification and correction of factors which contributed to the creation of handicapped communication environments (p. 5–6)

This chapter focuses on the traditional and innovative nature of diagnostic and rehabilitative services offered to older persons in their homes and in long-term care settings by communication disorders specialists. In order to implement quality service, the speech—language pathologist and audiologist need a broad background in aging, which this book seeks to provide. Further, the professional speech and language pathologist and audiologist must realize the close relationship between the type of delivery system and setting in which they work and the ultimate effect on the individual served. If we are to have a therapeutic effect, we need the knowledge, skills, and sensitivity to work with the older person and the environment in which he or she resides as a single entity. This chapter is based on the premise that in order to provide quality service, we must view the older person as not just a complex of speech, language, and hearing symptoms, but as a whole person who communicates in relation to his or her own skills, to the communication opportunities available, and to the reinforcement received for communicating.

HOME HEALTH CARE

About 95 percent of the elderly population in the United States live in the community, and most of these individuals reside in some form of family constellation. According to the Health Resources Statistics of the United States Department of Health, Education and Welfare (1976), about half of the persons age 65 and over live in the states of California, Illinois, New York, Ohio, Pennsylvania, Texas, and Florida. In addition, in the states of Florida, Arkansas, Iowa, Missouri, Kansas, Nebraska, South Dakota, Oklahoma, and Rhode Island, persons 65 years of age and older constitute at least 12 percent of the population. Further, statistics (U.S. Bureau of Census, 1970) indicate that of the noninstitutionalized elderly population, 83 percent of men and 59 percent of women live in a family situation. More than 30 percent live alone or with nonrelatives.

Many of the elderly who remain in the community or return to living in it need supportive or rehabilitation services. A relatively new alternative to providing health, rehabilitation, and social services to community-based elderly is through a home health care program. Brody (1977) defines a home health care program as

one that is centrally administered through coordinated planning, evaluation and follow up procedures, [and] provides for physician directed medical, nursing, social and related services to selected patients at home. Supportive medical services are here defined as nursing, physical, occupational and speech therapy aspects of home health care (p. 76).

The need for providing such services to individuals residing in the community was identified nearly 200 years ago when the poor were given home care by the Boston Dispensary starting in 1796. Even at that time, it was realized that home care reduced expense for sick persons and their families, allowed the family to play a supportive role in recovery, and hopefully did not humiliate the persons in need of care (Bergman, 1963). In 1945 Montefiore Hospital in New York City designed a program of home health care that has served as a model for many hospital-based home care programs.

The elderly are probably the largest group of individuals in need of receiving care through home health care agencies (Littauer, 1977). Brody (1977) estimated that one in three elderly persons in the community needs some form of service that can be provided through a home health care program. She stated that the number and complexity of physical, mental, and environmental problems of the elderly may overextend individual and family resources and necessitate community assistance.

The Scope of Home Health Care Services

The primary objective of providing home health care to the elderly is to help them function as effectively and independently as possible in their natural environment. Such services play a preventive role in attempting to keep the individual healthy and effective and forestalling further disabilities, dependence, and relocation to an institutional setting. In addition, home care is viewed as a means of reducing the cost of health and rehabilitation services to the individual, the family, and the community. Thus, it is possible to provide more beds in hospitals for the acutely ill and reduce the number of elderly in long-term care institutions. Littauer (1977) stated that home health care "reemphasizes the individualization of treatment and provides for continuity of services to the individual" (p. 38).

The essential services of home health care include the following: (1) medical, skilled nursing, laboratory, and diagnostic services, (2) maintenance or homemaker services, (3) legal, personal, and financial planning, (4) restorative therapies such as physical therapy, occupational therapy, speech therapy, and mental health counseling, and (5) home health aide services (Noelker & Harel, 1978). Home health agencies participating under the Medicare program must provide skilled nursing care and at least one other therapeutic service (Health Resources Statistics, 1976). The care given falls under various levels including concentrated or intensive, intermediate, and basic services. Intensive care involves concentrated, supervised, diagnostic and therapeutic services on an intermittent basis. Intermediate-level care and basic services are aimed at helping convalescent and chronically ill persons recover and maintain residence in their own homes. The home health care facility also links individuals and their families with other services available in the community. Frequently it is the home health care worker who informs individuals and their families about other services available in the community and the process whereby they may be obtained.

Home health care services are available from a variety of sources in the community. In 1974 there were about 2500 home health care programs in the United States. According to the Health Resources Statistics (1976), approximately 90 percent of these programs have been approved for Medicare funding and participation. Types of agencies providing this care include official health agencies administered by state, county, or local governments, visiting nurse associations, combined government and voluntary agencies, and hospital-based agencies. In discussing this type of service, O'Connell (1978) stated that in New York State, home health care is also included in public health nursing, county health departments, the county office for aging, family service programs, the American Cancer Society, and university speech and hearing centers. It should also be noted that some long-term care institutions, such as nursing homes, provide home health care through outreach programs supported by their facilities.

Funding for services received from home health care agencies is mandated and considered a priority service by the Older Americans Act (Title III). However, in 1975 only one percent of Medicare expenditures was directed toward home health care (Noelker & Harel, 1978). The use of home health care services to elderly persons is limited by such factors as eligibility requirements for service and limitations on the number of home visits permitted each individual per year. Even when state and local health agencies support these services, there are usually time and eligibility restrictions. Brody (1977) stated that Blue Cross and other insurance policies rarely reimburse for services given through a home health agency. Care should be taken in interpreting these findings because there are differences among states and among commercial carriers. A conservative conclusion, however, is that most home health care agencies seek support from Medicaid and Medicare in order to provide service.

Several types of individuals may be referred for or may seek home health care. Noelker and Harel (1978) investigated the client characteristics of participants in two programs in Cleveland, Ohio. One program, under the auspices of the Chronic Illness Center in that city, served a large group of older, widowed, isolated, chronically ill though ambulatory women who frequently had mental and behavioral disorders. In contrast, the clients served by the Visiting Nurses Association were considerably younger and exhibited more serious health problems and physical impairments associated with cerebral vascular accidents and cancer. Thus, home health care appears to offer services to a wide variety of homebound elderly persons differing in their degree of illness and dependence.

Speech, Language, and Hearing Services

Speech–language therapy and audiological services are provided by many home health care agencies. According to Health Resources Statistics (1976), about 20 percent of the total number of home health agencies in the United States provided speech therapy services in 1967. This percentage increased to 35 percent by 1975. Interestingly, speech therapy ranked fourth among services provided in 1975 as compared with nursing care, physical therapy, occupational therapy, medical social services, and home health aides services. Nursing care, physical therapy, and health aides services were provided by at least 70 percent of the agencies as compared to 35 percent of the agencies that offered speech therapy. Only occupational therapy and medical social services were provided by a smaller percentage of agencies. In a recent national survey of home health care agencies, Lubinski and Chapey (in press) found that speech and language services were available in 58 percent of the agencies responding. Results show that most home bound speech-language pathology programs are offered through visiting nurse associations. In addition, it appears that audiological services are available in only 5 percent of the programs.

The type of speech, language, and audiological services that may be offered by home health agencies includes diagnostic, therapeutic, counseling, and referral activities for clients and their families. Lubinski and Chapey (in press) found that speech-language pathologists in home health care spend about 60 percent of their time in direct therapy with clients in their homes, 12 percent in diagnosis, 7 to 10 percent in counseling, 12 percent in travel, and 4 percent in administrative duties. Their caseloads consist of 1 to 5 clients who are generally elderly individuals exhibiting aphasia, apraxia, or dysarthria. The speech-language pathologist providing this service tends to be employed part-time by the home health care agency, holds the Certificate of Clinical Competence from the American Speech-Language and Hearing Association, and is licensed in those states where it is available.

ADVANTAGES

The diagnostic and therapeutic roles of the speech—language pathologist in home health care programs are similar to those provided in a hospital or clinic. The difference lies primarily in direct contact with communication-impaired individuals and their families in their home environments. A major advantage of providing communication services in the home setting is that it facilitates the identification and perhaps reduction of environmental and interpersonal factors that may contribute to the communication problem. The speech—language pathologist may identify interpersonal forces that create communicative strain or that limit clients' opportunities to talk. For example, families may have unrealistic expectations for communication-impaired individuals and either exclude them from communication interaction or force them into situations with which they are not able to cope successfully.

The speech—language pathologist also has the advantage of providing therapy in the setting in which the client will be communicating. Therapeutic strategies are aimed at helping the individual attain communication effectiveness in that setting. Therapy content focuses on talking about people, objects, events, and relationships occurring in the home and the community. Therapy, therefore, can concentrate on those areas that are of immediate need to the client. For example, the physical props found in the natural context of the home are powerful, personal, and realistic stimuli for therapy.

Similarly, in homebound therapy clients and their families share in the responsibility for identifying areas of therapeutic focus and in the rehabilitation process. The communication disorders specialist can discuss therapy goals and procedures with family members who may assist in the therapy process. Since a family member is often in close proximity during the therapy session, direct and sometimes subtle, indirect modeling of communication strategies with the impaired person can be accomplished easily. The speech—language pathologist can demonstrate techniques that facilitate communication and ways to reinforce communication attempts by the client. Thus, the speech—language pathologist has an opportunity to observe the family member demonstrate therapy procedures and correct any misunderstandings the family member might have. This also allows the speech—language pathologist the opportunity to reinforce the family member for implementing and adapting therapy procedures and gaining insight into the communication problem.

Another advantage of speech and language therapy through home health service is that the speech—language pathologist has an increased opportunity to counsel the family. The therapist can provide counseling on a more personal basis with family members who may be frustrated with the communication-impaired person, angry, or guilty about their feelings toward the individual. The problems that the family member may be encountering in the home situation may be translated more realistically with the physical props available there. Service in the home makes the counseling role more vital and realistic to all involved.

One aspect of home visitations that is often overlooked is that families and clients can serve as hosts to the therapist. The role of sender and receiver of care becomes less rigid, and the clients have the opportunity to communicate with their families and the therapist in a more informal, social situation. Frequently, the therapist will be offered a refreshment, and during this time the stimulus-response aspect of therapy is eliminated. Grossman (1977) stated that communication in an informal natural setting facilitates therapeutic communication. He also added that "the opportunity to act as host . . . gives the client a feeling of reciprocity which at times makes it easier to accept help" (p. 81).

Speech and language services offered in the home present several other advantages. Since many of the clients are elderly and chronically ill, transportation is frequently a major reason for poor attendance at therapy sessions in a community hospital or clinic. The elderly person may be dependent on another family member or public transportation, which in turn may be hampered by weather, distance, illness, and inconvenience. The speech—language pathologist provides service in the client's own home, thereby reducing some of the impact of these factors. Communication services to those in rural settings who may lack any viable transportation are greatly facilitated through home health agency programs.

DISADVANTAGES

A number of problems face the communication disorders specialist who enters a client's home. There are logistical problems in that clients may live considerable distances apart and service to each client may be once or twice weekly. Distance, weather, and parking availability may delimit the number of therapy contacts per day and hence per week. Further, the speech–language pathologist may find the client ill or unable to participate in a session. While this time may be used for family counseling or administrative functions, it often creates inconvenience and a disrupted schedule. The speech–language pathologist also must carefully plan therapy materials to take into the home because clinic supplies will not be readily available. Only portable diagnostic and therapy materials can be used. This creates a problem for the audiologist, who at best can perform audiometric screening tests in the home with a portable audiometer and impedance bridge. Mobile audiometric test units, however, have become increasingly available in recent years (Alpiner, 1978).

Many of the advantages of providing speech and language therapy in the home can become disadvantages. For example, although the stimuli in the home can be real and useful therapy resources, for some clients the same stimuli can be distracting forces. Clients with perceptual and attention problems may be distracted by the myriad stimuli of the home including objects, people, and extraneous noises. Some clients work best in more structured, soundproof environments such as a clinic context. Further, while the family may also be a valuable resource in therapy, they also may disrupt sessions, answer for the client, or become emotionally upset by the therapy session. Some families may resent a therapist entering their home and become defensive about their care of the communication-impaired individual. Simply because the speech–language pathologist is a guest in the home, tactful and sensitive approaches to family involvement and counseling must be emphasized.

The family and the communication-impaired individual should be informed about the advantages of home therapy prior to the initiation of such therapy, and the objectives of therapy and the role of the family should be carefully outlined. The family may be less defensive if it realizes the important contribution it can make to the rehabilitation program. The family and the therapist can become a united force in helping the communication-impaired individual regain communication skills. Therapy can thus become an ongoing process rather than a fragmented effort.

One of the most pressing problems the communication disorders specialist faces is funding for providing the service in the client's home. There is a need for increased awareness by government agencies and insurance carriers that communication rehabilitation services in the home setting are crucial for the client living at home. Furthermore, these services should be available to a wide spectrum of communication-impaired individuals and their families. Funding and the number of sessions available to each individual should have wide latitude and be under the control of the communication disorders specialist. This professional thus has the responsibility of defining his or her role to the community at large. Many citizens, for example, are not aware that speech, language, and hearing diagnostic and rehabilitation services may be offered through home health care agencies. Community agencies and their physicians, nurses, and other professionals need to be aware of the communication problems homebound patients may have and know the procedures for referral to the communication disorders specialist.

Regardless of the problems encountered in providing speech, language, and hearing services through home health agencies, normally the advantages outweigh the disadvantages. It is quite possible that communication services in the home setting will become more readily available as the need for such intervention is defined. Each individual with a communication disorder has the right to a comprehensive spectrum of services offered by the speech–language pathologist and audiologist regardless of the setting in which he or she lives.

Nursing Home Care

When the family and the community can no longer meet the health, security, and maintenance needs of the aging and chronically ill individual in his own home, he or she is often faced with relocation to an institutional setting. The institutional setting may be called a home for the aged, nursing home, convalescent home, rest home, skilled nursing facility, or by a variety of other institutional names. In essence, these institutions provide congregate housing and medical and custodial care. The title of the institution generally defines the scope of nursing services available there. Geld (1964, p. 60) defined a home for the aged as a

voluntary, permanent, usually sectarian community . . . designed especially but not exclusively as a protective environment within a circumscribed single or multiple physical setting for that segment of our elderly population whose declining years are accompanied by physical, mental, economic and social deprivations.

Statistics

About 5 percent of the 22 million elderly persons in the United States live in institutional settings such as nursing homes. In 1971 (Health Resources

Statistics, 1976) there were over 1.1 million elderly persons in nursing homes and about 100,000 in mental institutions. A conservative estimate is that one person in five who is elderly will spend some time in a nursing home prior to death. Researchers also indicate that the 5 percent figure for institutionalized elderly persons is a gross underestimate (Ingram & Barry, 1977; Kastenbaum & Candy, 1973). Many of the institutionalized elderly are transferred to acute care hospitals when they are severely ill and often die there. Thus, the percentage of elderly in long-term care institutions is incorrectly reduced.

Prior to 1939 there were approximately 1200 institutions in this country that resembled a nursing home. However, by 1976 there were 23,000 nursing homes in the United States providing about 1,235,404 beds. There are three times as many nursing homes as general and surgical hospitals. Further, the number of long-term care facilities has increased between 1960 and 1970 by 140 percent. Indeed, the cost of this care has increased by 640 percent from $500 million in 1960 to close to $4 billion in 1973 (Health Resources Statistics, 1976; United States Senate Subcommittee on Long Term Care, 1974).

The rapid increase in the number of nursing homes may be due to a number of factors. First, the number of elderly persons is growing rapidly and steadily. According to the census figures used by the United States Senate Subcommittee on Long Term Care (1974), there are about 22 million persons 65 years of age or older in this country, of which about one third are at least 75 years of age. Further, those over 75 years represent the fastest growing of all population groups. In a study of population projections, Brotman (1977) estimated that by the year 2000 there will be close to 31 million old people in the United States constituting between 11 and 12.5 percent of the entire population. Brotman thus concluded that the older population was increasing at a faster rate than the younger population.

The number of older persons residing in institutions is also increasing. As individuals live longer they develop more chronic illnesses and require specialized, continuing care. Furthermore, as health care services become more pervasive and specialized, the traditional home for the aged assumes the genre of a nursing home.

Other factors contributing to the increase in nursing homes include the changes in family constellations (Health Resources Statistics, 1976) and family attitudes toward older family members, inflation in medical costs, and increased medical assistance programs for the aged. Such programs as those supported by the Social Security Act of 1935, the Social Security Act of 1965, and the Social Security Amendments of 1972 have changed the emphasis from complete payment for services by the individual to partial or complete funding by a government or outside agency. Furthermore, the family may perceive itself as no longer capable of caring for the medical needs of the older person. Community resources such as home health services may not be available or may be limited. The older individual then faces either no service, isolation, or relocation to a nursing home. For the majority of older persons relocating to a nursing home, this will be their final residence.

Types of Nursing Homes and Residents

The services offered in a nursing home range from the basic food, shelter, custodial, and health care provisions to social, medical, and rehabilitative services. However, nursing homes are generally classified according to the amount of continuous nursing care available. For example, a skilled nursing facility (SNF) provides full-time nursing services, and restorative therapies such as physical, occupational, and speech therapy are generally available. A second level of nursing home is the intermediate care facility (ICF), which provides fewer services, and the third level, residential care, is similar in nature to a home for the aged in that it provides minimal protective, custodial, and maintenance services for the relatively healthy older person. Many institutions contain several types of nursing facilities within one building. One wing or floor may be devoted to intensive care, while other areas may be assigned to those persons needing fewer servces.

The physical arrangement of a nursing home includes patients' rooms, bathrooms, communal areas such as day rooms, parlor areas, lounges, dining rooms, chapel and recreation areas, medical care areas, and facilities for rehabilitation therapies. While a number of homes still contain dormitory or multiple-occupancy style rooms, the trend is toward private and semiprivate rooms. Innovative facilities also contain efficiency apartments for single residents and apartment style accommodations for two to four residents. Generally, the patient's room is connected to a central nursing station by an intercom device, and the doors to patients' rooms are frequently kept open for visibility and hence accessibility to patients. Further, in most nursing homes, the patients' rooms are designed for maximum efficiency, and personal items must be kept to a minimum. Residents often display a few personal possessions such as family photographs, a television and/or radio, and personal mementos. Sandoz Pharmaceuticals (1975) published a manual entitled, *Positive Approaches to Selecting Alternative Living Arrangements for the Elderly,* which describes in detail the scope of the nursing home. Other discussions of the general characteristics of quality nursing homes (Anderson, 1974; Penchansky & Taubenhaus, 1965; United States Senate Subcommittee on Long Term Care, 1974; Winn & McCaffree, 1976) are also available.

At least three current resources delineate the characteristics of the nursing home population (Health Resources Statistics, 1976; Sourcebook on Aging, 1977; United States Senate Subcommittee on Long Term Care, 1974). The United States Subcommittee on Long Term Care (1974) defined the nursing home population as very old, female, widowed, alone, and white. The majority of persons in nursing homes are women who have an average age of 82 years and have been widowed. Most of these women come to the nursing home from their own homes. In fact, about 25 percent of the nursing home population formerly were housewives. About half have few relatives, most will remain in the nursing home for 1 to 2 years, and at least half will die there. According to the results of the Long Term Care Facility Improvement Study (1975) conducted by the Office of Nursing Home Affairs of Public Health Service, 52 percent of the patients in skilled nursing facilities have completed 8 years or less of schooling and only about 9 percent have attended college. Further, professional, technical, and managerial occupations are represented by about 8 percent of the residents, whereas unskilled and semiskilled represent about 51 percent. The vast majority of the patients retired from their jobs prior to admittance to the institution.

The residents within a nursing home generally exhibit a number of chronic illnesses. The United States Senate Subcommittee on Long Term Care (1974) found that the average patient in such a setting has four or more chronic illnesses, is nonambulatory, and takes four or five different drugs several times each day. The most frequent chronic illnesses among nursing home patients are cardiovascular disease, arthritis and rheumatism, diabetes mellitus, hypertension, senility, arteriosclerosis, stroke, and cancer (Zimmer, 1975). Other chronic illnesses exhibited by older persons in long-term care settings include diverticulosis, chronic lung disease, fractured hip, glaucoma, parkinsonism, blindness, paralysis and palsy not due to stroke, and chronic back problems (Vital and Health Statistics, 1973).

A significant number of older individuals in nursing homes also have mental or personality problems. According to the Senate Subcommittee on Long Term Care (1974) anywhere from 55 to 80 percent of the patients in long-term care facilities are mentally impaired. Zimmer (1975) in his study of health-related facilities and nursing homes in the Rochester, New York area indicated that about 53 percent of the patients in skilled nursing facilities were moderately confused and forgetful. When comparing the skilled nursing facility with the health related setting, however, he found less than one percent of the patients in either setting to be severely confused.

The types of clinical psychiatric problems patients in institutional settings may exhibit include simple deterioration, confusion, depression, paranoia, and neurosis (Bennett, 1975; Eisdorfer, 1977; Teeter, Garety, Miller, & Heiland, 1976). Weiner, Brok, and Snadowsky (1978) stated that a large percentage of aging institutionalized persons are senile (variously labeled chronic brain syndrome, organic brain syndrome, and senile dementia). The impairment results in "symptoms of deterioration such as confusion, disorientation, faulty recent memory, emotional lability, indifference, poor interpersonal relationships and apathy" (p. 58). These individuals may require custodial care, functional assistance in daily living, and restorative therapies.

The reasons why elderly persons relocate to a long-term care facility are simple to enumerate but complex when considered from the perspective of each individual. The decision to abandon a lifetime of personal possessions and familiar persons and places can be a shattering experience for individuals and their families. Zimmer (1975) found that older persons relocate to nursing homes because of their need for assistance with daily living, specific physical disabilities and frailty, mental status, and social reasons such as difficulty maintaining independent housing. More specifically, sensory losses of vision and hearing may create dangerous living conditions for the elderly in their own homes. For example, Beverley (1976) emphasized the important role of gradual sensory losses and their effects on mental status, personality, and independent living of older persons. Older individuals frequently participate in the decision to relocate to the nursing home. However, according to the Senate Subcommittee on Long Term Care many older people "regard the nursing home with fear and hostility and there are sharp increases in the death rate associated with transfer to nursing homes'' (1974, p. 17). The Senate Subcommittee on Long Term Care labeled this *transplantation shock* and Lawton and Jaffe (1970) called it the *relocation effect*. Ingram and Barry (1977) estimated that in 1972, one person in five who died in the United States and who was 55 years of age or older died in a nursing home setting. Bennett (1972) and Lieberman, Prock, and Tobin (1968) present summaries of the effects of institutionalization on older persons.

On entrance to the long-term care institution, older persons are classified according to their physical status (ambulation, medication, and nursing needs) and their behavior and adjustment (judgment, dependency, memory, and speech) (Waldman & Fryman, 1964). In many settings the patient is assigned to a room on a floor with other patients of similar mental and physical functioning. For example, there may be a floor or a section of the hospital for ambulatory patients who require minimal care, another area may be for the extremely senile, and another for those with progressive neurologic diseases such as Parkinson's disease or multiple sclerosis.

Staff

In order to provide health, maintenance, and custodial services to the geriatric patients in long-term care institutions, there are a variety of health care professionals as well as individuals who provide ancillary services. According to Health Resources Statistics (1976) there were about 650,000 full-time employees in nursing, personal care, and other homes in 1973. The staff in a nursing home can generally be subdivided into nine groups: administration, social service, medical, nursing, psychiatry, rehabilitation, food service, maintenance/housekeeping, and volunteers. The types of services offered in most long-term care settings include medical services, both preventive and therapeutic, personal care, rehabilitation, and recreation. Sandoz (1975) and Miller (1969) have outlined the numerous services performed within each of these programs.

The administrative staff generally includes the administrative director of the facility, the medical director, and their respective department heads. The role of this administrative staff is to plan and coordinate the entire functioning of the institution. The administrative director is responsible for regulatory policies, personnel and staffing, maintenance and safety, financial operations, public relations and reports, and evaluation of all aspects of the institution.

This individual is directly responsible to the governing body of the institution, which may be a board of directors, a partnership, or a proprietor (Miller, 1969).

The medical director is the other chief administrative officer within the facility. This individual supervises the entire medical, nursing, dietary, pharmacy, x-ray, laboratory, therapy, and social work services offered to the residents and their families. The medical director must be a physician and is the direct supervisor of the entire medical staff including the attending medical staff and the specialty physicians who either consult regularly or, in the case of large institutions, are on staff. In some nursing homes, residents may also be treated by their own physicians.

Also part of the medical staff is the nursing department. The nursing staff of a nursing home includes at least one licensed registered nurse, as well as licensed practical nurses, aides, and orderlies. Their primary functions are to provide for the daily health care of the residents, administer and monitor medications, and chart patient health and behavior changes.

Specialty services within the medical staff include laboratory, pharmacy, health records, and dietary staff, who provide for the health and food needs of the residents. The social service department consists of a social worker and staff who plan for new admissions, coordinate payment for services, and provide information, counseling, and referral for families and the institutionalized person. Rehabilitation services generally include physical therapy, occupational therapy, recreation therapy and speech—language pathology and audiology. Psychiatrists and/or psychologists may serve as consultants to the home and may provide continuing daily services depending on the philosophy, size, and financial status of the institution. Volunteers are also frequent adjuncts to nursing homes in a variety of departments and functions. The volunteer plays an important role in reducing isolation for the patients by stressing social adjustment, cognitive awareness, and mental state (Routh, 1970). Other support personnel are available in nursing homes including secretarial staff, housecleaning and maintenance personnel, accountants, and librarians. A chaplain is usually available to meet the religious needs of the patients.

Dobroff and Litwak (1977) stated that the function of all staff members is to ''articulate the partnership between the facility and the family'' (p. 32). While staff are assigned specific tasks, the ultimate goal is the comprehensive health care of the individual resident and the assurance of quality care to the family or other interested parties.

Problems Faced in Nursing Homes

While the goals for each program and staff member in a long-term care facility may be delineated explicitly in manuals and brochures, the implementation of services may be difficult. Problems facing nursing homes and other long-term care institutions include financial problems, employee/union difficulties, staff recruitment and turnover, government regulation, meeting the special needs of patients and families, and reducing the negative effects of institutionalization on individual patients.

Long-term care facilities face increasing costs in maintaining services presently offered and establishing new or innovative programs. Increases in payment from third-party sources often do not keep pace with inflation. According to the Sourcebook of Aging (1977) the average daily reimbursement from Medicare in 1976 was only $31 per day per person. Administrators are also faced with demands from staff for increased salaries and benefits and improved working conditions. The possibility of strike by staff members places the administration and patients in difficult positions, threatening the quality and maintenance of continued care for the institutionalized person.

Other problems facing nursing homes include the frequent turnover in employees, particularly those among the lower echelons. Further, the fulfillment of government regulations may become a priority for staff and administration resulting in the abandonment of new programs for which there is little allotment of staff, time, or financial support. Special programs that may be funded by short-term grants are frequently not supported by the nursing home when the research or demonstration funding is terminated.

A major problem to be faced by staff of nursing homes is the reduction or elimination of the negative impact of institutionalization on the aged. Ainsworth (1977) stated that "there are numerous potential threats to essential values when a person enters a home for the aged or a nursing home, any of which may create anxiety and increase physiological demands" (p. 19). Lieberman et al. (1968) describe the relocation effect to an institution as one that creates feelings of separation, rejection, loss, and despair. In some nursing homes there is an interest in the "distinctively human and individual problems of the institutionalized person above and beyond the technical

quality of service" (Kahana, 1973, p. 286). In these institutions it is realized that long-term care may result in negative psychologic, social, and cultural changes in the individual and may contribute to the development and exacerbation of both apparent and real medical conditions. Staff of institutions that ascribe to such an enlightened philosophy are caught in the trap of financial crisis and lack of staff time and commitment versus the need for humane treatment.

New Horizons in Nursing Home Care

There are new horizons in nursing homes despite financial and staff limitations. First, there is an increasing awareness that the needs of the geriatric person in an institution can be met in ways other than through the usual programs. Kahana (1973) suggested that one way to reduce the effects of institutionalization is to keep the individual in the community as long as possible. This may be accomplished through home care provided by the community and may include day care centers, senior citizens residences, and home care services.

Another approach to improving the quality of institutional life stems from the staff members' philosophy of institutionalization and aging. Kahana (1973) stated that some problems are due to "sheer senselessness or lack of sensitivity . . . others are inherent in the institutional model" (p. 284). Staff education prior to employment, continuing inservice education, and reinforcement for humane treatment are preventive and ameliorative approaches to staff sensitization and positive approaches to patient care.

Anderson (1974) indicated that other approaches to improved quality in nursing homes include licensure of staff members, financial incentives for rehabilitation of geriatric persons, and community control of nursing homes.

The United States Senate Subcommittee on Long Term Care (1974) identified four major areas for innovation in nursing homes. These included positive approaches to therapy and rehabilitation such as reality orientation, sensory training, and remotivation programs; improvements in the physical structure of buildings through improved architecture, design, and color; positive and innovative approaches to the education and utilization of employees such as sensitivity training, accident prevention programs, and continuing education for staff; and innovative activities or services such as self-government by patients.

Inherent in each of the innovative programs

sugested above is the philosophy that the older person entering a nursing home deserves quality care. This care involves the highest scientific and medical approaches to chronic illness and aging, and it involves the creation of a therapeutic milieu. The philosophy governing the care of the patients and the psychosocial environment in which the care is implemented are crucial to the maintenance and/or recovery of physical, psychologic, and emotional functioning of the older person. Enlightened staff of nursing homes seek to explore and expand the quality of the patients' entire life space.

THE SPEECH AND LANGUAGE PATHOLOGIST AND AUDIOLOGIST IN NURSING HOMES

National statistics (Long Term Care Facility Improvement Study, 1975) indicate that about one third of the patients in nursing home settings have speech and language problems and approximately the same number have a hearing impairment in one or both ears.

Statistics regarding the number of speech, language, and hearing handicapped among the elderly institutionalized population are scarce. In a study of characteristics of facilities and patients in long-term care facilities conducted by the Public Health Service Office of Nursing Home Affairs (Long Term Care Facility Improvement Study, 1975), it was estimated that in long-term care facilities about 68 percent of the patients can communicate their needs verbally. The remaining 32 percent reportedly have communication problems. Furthermore, when the speech and language disorders are defined, it is seen that 8.8 percent of the patients are dysarthric, 8.6 percent have language of confusion, and 8.7 percent refuse to speak. About 3.3 percent have aphasia. In regard to the hearing acuity of patients in long-term care settings, 67 percent have no impairment, 31.4 percent have impairment in one or both ears, and 1.5 percent are totally deaf. Speech and hearing problems rank second to visual impairment among skilled nursing home patients.

In a 3½-year study of 108 referrals to the speech pathology department in a skilled nursing facility in the Syracuse, New York area, O'Connell and O'Connell (1978) found that about 83 percent of the individuals had communication problems. O'Connell and O'Connell described the most common disorders to be aphasia, dysarthria, oral and verbal apraxia, laryngeal pathology, and confusion and impaired

memory. Further, she found that of those patients accepted for therapy, over 80 percent had multiple diagnoses including: aphasia and dysarthria (40 percent), aphasia and apraxia (25 percent), aphasia and confusion (25 percent), and dysarthria and confusion (5 percent). Of the aphasic individuals accepted for speech and language therapy, O'Connell found that 23.6 percent were considered mildly impaired, 13.3 percent were moderately impaired, whereas 44.7 percent were severely impaired and 18.4 percent were diagnosed as globally aphasic. The average number of treatment sessions for all patients serviced in the speech pathology department in this setting was 39 sessions spread over a period of about 4½ months. O'Connell further found that 95 percent of the individuals who were terminated from therapy were dismissed because of discharge from the facility, having reached a plateau in therapy or failed to profit from the treatment. Only about 5.6 percent of the patients were considered to have made substantial improvement, 24.1 percent showed moderate improvement, and 70 percent made slight or no improvement. O'Connell stated that "significant positive correlations were obtained between length and number of treatments and degree of change for communicative status" (p. 5)

The results of this study appear to indicate that the speech−language pathologist has a difficult role with the communication-impaired elderly population in a nursing home. For example, O'Connell and O'Connell found that as age increased the length of treatment and the degree of change decreased. This finding suggests that (1) our traditional rehabilitation efforts with the elderly may not be effective in this setting, (2) different techniques for measuring progress are needed, and/or (3) the goals of intervention with this population may need redefinition.

Traditional Role of the Speech−Language Pathologist

The traditional role of the speech−language pathologist in the nursing home is individual oriented. Speech-language pathologists and audiologists generally define their goals as identifying, diagnosing, and treating communication-impaired older persons and making appropriate referrals to other therapeutic and medical practitioners to alleviate associated problems. In some nursing homes, the speech−language specialist and audiologist also provide consultation to other disciplines. Inservice education is often given by these professionals and focuses on the symptomatology and remediation of the speech, language, and hearing problems of nursing home patients. In addition, inservice education highlights how those providing daily care can communicate more effectively with the communication-impaired individual.

In a national pilot study of speech, language, and hearing services available in 292 nursing homes across the country, Chapey, Lubinski, Chapey, & Salzburg (in press) found that in the 25 percent of the nursing homes responding to the survey, services, most frequently provided by speech pathologists in such settings included speech evaluations, articulation therapy, voice therapy, language therapy, speech screening, consultation with the family, hearing therapy, and fluency therapy. Treatment for dysphagia is seldom provided by the speech pathologist. Audiologists provide such services as audiometric screenings, complete audiometric evaluations, hearing aid evaluations and consultations, aural rehabilitation, and central auditory evaluations.

The results of this study indicate that the services of a full-time speech and language pathologist were available in only 3 percent of the responding nursing homes and part-time services were available in about 27 percent of the homes. Patients with communication problems were referred to a speech pathologist outside the nursing home in 24 percent of the respondents. Interestingly, 46 percent of the homes stated that they do not provide the services of a speech–language pathologist. Furthermore, audiological services by a part- or full-time audiologist appear to be available in only about 15 percent of the nursing homes responding, and 85 percent appear to provide no audiological services. In only 21 percent of the nursing homes did the speech pathologist screen all patients to identify possible communication problems. Sixty percent of the homes rely on referrals by other staff members to the communicologist, and in about 12 percent there are no procedures for screening or referring patients to a speech–language pathologist.

The results of this study combined with those of O'Connell and O'Connell (1978) present a gloomy picture of the speech–language pathologist's and audiologist's role and effectiveness in a long-term care setting. This, of course, is subject to interpretation. Generally, the studies can be considered pilot research into the area of services available and effectiveness of intervention. Larger numbers of respondents on a national scale would have to be obtained before the data were considered conclusive. The studies described, however, do appear to give strong indications of the trends in services available in nursing home settings. Further, the results of these studies do raise questions concerning the efficacy of our traditional role with the geriatric population in long-term care settings. Well-designed research of individual and group therapy relative to stimulus response, cognitive, and environmental approaches to intervention are needed.

The diagnostic role of the speech–language pathologist in the nursing home is somewhat different from that in a hospital or agency. As cited in the previous research by Chapey et al. (in press) communication screenings are sometimes available to all patients, but referral by nursing home staff is most common. The goal of differential diagnosis of speech and language problems from communication difficulties associated with hearing loss, chronic brain syndrome, and geriatric personality disorders can be a difficult task. Further, the multiplicity of physical, communication, psychologic, and emotional problems presented by one person and the overlay of years of institutionalization and/or isolation complicate the diagnosis. Identifying the cause of the problem becomes less crucial than delineating the symptoms and planning a feasible and effective therapeutic program.

The communication disorders specialist uses the traditional speech–language screening and diagnostic tests available in a nursing home. The specialist may be under time pressures to provide a quick diagnosis due, for example, to governmental regulations that have time restrictions. The standardized tests chosen may be determined by the length of time available for testing, the patient's communication and physical status, and the prerogative of the tester. Such tools as the Porch Index of Communicative Ability (Porch, 1971), the Boston Diagnostic Aphasia Examination (Goodglass & Kaplan, 1972), the Language Modalities Test for Aphasia (Wepman & Jones, 1961), the Minnesota Test for the Differential Diagnosis of Aphasia (Schuell, 1965), the Functional Communication Profile (Sarno, 1969), Examining for Aphasia (Eisenson, 1954), the Aphasia Language Performance Scales (Keenan & Brassell, 1975), and other standardized tests are frequently used.

None of these tests, however, are designed specifically for nursing home patients, and further, none focus directly on the communication needs of the institutionalized person. For example, these diagnostic tools do not evaluate the person's ability to verbally or nonverbally communicate health care or personal needs to the nursing home staff, nor do they describe how effective the individual is in interaction with staff, patients, or family members.

In addition to standardized language tests, some speech−language pathologists may use less formal approaches to define the cognitive, linguistic, and communicative abilities of patients (Chapey & Lubinski, 1979, in press; Chapey, Rigrodsky, & Morrison, 1977; Lubinski & Chapey, 1978; Lubinski & Chapey, 1980b; Muma, 1978). Similarly, standardized and informal procedures for identification and diagnosis of voice, articulation, and fluency problems are employed. When possible the speech−language pathologist tries to consult medical records, the family, and staff for other information that may contribute to an understanding of the problem. The goal of diagnosis is to identify those individuals who will profit most from intervention and to plan an appropriate program of rehabilitation.

The speech−language pathologist must also communicate the results of testing and therapy progress to other staff members and families. Information given to these persons must be clear, meaningful, and brief. Many nursing homes require that the speech−language pathologist and/or audiologist submit reports to the patients' charts, which are then available to all staff members. Furthermore, some nursing homes require that the reports follow the "SOAP" outline of subjective impressions, objective information, appraisal, and plan. The communication specialist will find that a brief jargon-free style of communication is necessary.

The audiologist also confronts a difficult problem with the hearing-impaired older institutionalized person. The older person in a nursing home may have had a hearing problem for a lengthy period of time, may have adjusted to a world of muffled sound, and possibly may have withdrawn from socialization. Further, some older people are resistant to participating in a hearing test, some may be confused and offer questionable responses, some may not understand and/or remember the instructions, and some may fatigue during a lengthy evaluation.

Other problems may be encountered after the diagnosis, once intervention is planned. If medical or surgical intervention is necessary, this may pose problems due to the individual's age and physical status. Amplification also presents a difficult area for the audiologist and/or hearing aid dispenser. Elderly patients in nursing homes have been a source for unscrupulous hearing aid salespersons, who sell them expensive and often inappropriate aides. Thus, nursing homes may include the communication disorders specialist as a consultant to or as a provider of sensory remotivation and reality orientation programs. These programs are aimed at the more regressed, less intact patients for psychosocial rehabilitation. The basis for both programs is effective communication among patients and staff members.

The use of the communication disorders specialist in such programs demonstrates the need for interdisciplinary approaches to rehabilitation of the older institutionalized person. The speech−language pathologist and audiologist are trained experts in communication and can provide information to and leadership for other professionals working in a long-term care setting. The speech−language pathologist and audiologist can work cooperatively with the other rehabilitation specialists including the physical, occupational, and recreation therapists as well as the nursing, medical, psychiatric, social work, and volunteer staff. Each individual who comes into contact with the elderly patient needs to know why the patient communicates as he or she does, the effects of communication problems on the total functioning of the individual, and how the staff members can communicate effectively with this person.

However, speech−language pathologists and audiologists face problems in implementing their diagnositc, therapeutic and consultative roles in a nursing home. The study of Chapey et al. (in press) identified ten problems these specialists encounter: cost of service, reimbursement for services, lack of space, lack of patient progress, lack of understanding of this specialist's role in the setting, not enough time allotted per patient for communication services, lack of equipment and materials, patient absenteeism, and lack of coordination of services. Individual speech−language pathologists and audiologists working in nursing homes may not face all of these difficulties and the impact of each problem may have differential effects on the functioning of the program. Unfortunately, a majority of respondents in the study indicated no plans for improving communication services to their patients and staff.

STRATEGIES FOR IMPROVING COMMUNICATION SERVICES

The speech−language pathologist and audiologist might improve the quantity and quality of their services in several ways. These items are suggestions and have not been subjected to the test of clinical research. They can, however, be considered guidelines for improved service.

One of the primary ways to improve the traditional diagnostic, therapeutic, and consultative roles of the speech−language pathologist and audiologist in a nursing home is through staff education. Staff education begins with informing the administration of the facility about the necessity of effective communication for all patients. The speech−language pathologist and audiologist need a strong, articulate rationale for the program. Further, this plan should be feasible within the particular institutional setting, adaptable, and have built-in steps for assessing progress and accountability. A plan presented to the administration might include a list of operational goals for the program, a succinct rationale based in the gerontologic and communication disorders literature, procedures and methods for all program phases, and techniques for assessing patient changes. In addition, such strategies as demonstration videotapes and/or audiotapes of diagnosis and therapy provide vivid and concrete examples of the program. Modest programs that are well designed and whose effects are measurable are more likely to gain acceptance, funding, and support than grandiose, impractical programs. Further, the communication disorders specialist might build into the total program demonstration and research projects for innovative approaches to intervention. When possible, other disciplines within the facility should be included to demonstrate coordination of services.

Inservice programs for staff members and for patients regarding communication disorders improve the image of the communication program and facilitate cooperation between the speech−language pathologist or audiologist and the staff. Once the patient leaves individual or group therapy sessions, the individual returns to daily life in the institution. The staff and other patients are the partners with whom the patient will interact. Both groups can facilitate or negate therapy carryover to conversational speech depending on their knowledge, sophistication, and attitudes. Lubinski (1975, 1978−1979) found that patients in a nursing home do not consider the communication-impaired as viable communication partners. In order for therapeutic endeavors to be meaningful, the communication-impaired person must have interested and willing partners and must be socially reinforced for communication attempts.

Staff and patient education might be conducted formally through a lecture format, or, perhaps more profitably, may be implemented in small group discussion and demonstration on the patients' floors. Communication-impaired patients might be paired with adequately communicating residents in therapy-like situations. This would provide both parties with

therapy and psychosocial benefits. Additionally, staff members and patients must also be reinforced for attempting to implement these suggestions.

Another strategy for improving communication services is that of enlisting the aid of families. Whereas all institutionalized elderly persons do not have close family members, many have relatives who can, if informed, play an important role in persuading administrators to support communication services. Family groups can become vital advocates for rehabilitation programs.

The speech−language pathologist and audiologist can also assume another role in the nursing home setting that might improve the quality of their service to all patients. This role is one whereby the communication disorders specialist directs his or her professional efforts toward identifying and remediating those aspects of the institution that create an environment devoid of communication opportunities. This role is oriented toward the environment in which communication occurs. Thus, the communication disorder specialist functions to improve the quality of the communication atmosphere for all patients in the nursing home.

THE COMMUNICATION-IMPAIRED ENVIRONMENT

On entering a long-term care setting, one frequently becomes aware that the communication occurring there is different than that in other settings. For example, a number of the patients sit silently in the communal areas such as the corridors, the day room, and around the nurses' station. Other patients may mumble to themselves, talk incoherently, and when they engage another in conversation, they may persevere on the same topic. Communication between patients and staff often focuses on daily care and the social amenities. Some individuals might argue, however, that this limited communication is a natural consequence of the disengagement process of aging whereby the elderly and society gradually disassociate. It is proposed that successful communication is a necessary ingredient for adjustment to a long-term care institution and that communication is desired by the institutionalized elderly.

Successful communication is not related to a particular length of utterance nor is it dependent on complex linguistic structures. Successful communication is the feeling of fulfillment gained when a message is sent and received. It is the awareness by older persons that their message is valued, that it is viewed as part of their social identity, and that it is giving them social connectedness with those in their environment. Successful communication allows older persons to remain active partners with their families, friends, and acquaintances. Successful communication means that older persons have the opportunity to transmit their most personal feelings and to relieve frustration within themselves and with others in their environment.

Successful communication occurs in a particular type of environment. It occurs in a climate that encourages interchange, that values and socially reinforces communication attempts and that minimizes the rules prohibiting communication. Lubinski (1978–1979) hypothesized that the institutional setting by its very nature affects the communication of older people and the staff involved in their care. Further, the nursing home may be considered an example of a communication-impaired environment and may contribute to the lack of meaningful communications among older persons in that setting.

Definition

A communication-impaired environment is defined as a setting in which there are few opportunities available for successful, meaningful communication. In such a context, individuals are not regarded as valued communication partners, their communication has little effect, and they perceive their own and others interactions as worthless. A communication-impaired environment has rules that govern where, when, to whom, and what kind of communication might occur. There is little variety in communication partners within the context and few or no opportunities to communicate with persons outside the setting. Furthermore, there are few reasons to talk and hence few topics of conversation. Communication centers on stereotyped, brief responses such as the social amenities of "How are you?" and "How's the weather?". People talk about what they are doing, feeling, and sensing. If the environment is static and unchanging, there will be few reasons to talk.

Another characteristic of the communication-impaired environment is that there are few places within the setting to have a private conversation. The residents of a nursing home are limited to a relatively small number of places where they might have a personal conversation that does not become the property of all. Conversations in public areas such as the day room, dining room, and hallways must be limited to neutral, guarded topics, because eavesdropping is common. Residents' own rooms can only be used for private conversations when roommates are not present. Indeed, residents do not perceive the nursing home setting as one in which they might find a confidant to exchange personal or intimate communication (Lubinski, 1975). This may be due, in part, to the lack of privacy in which trusted friendships might be developed and personal thoughts safely shared.

In a communication-impaired environment the administration and staff do not value or reinforce communication among the patients or between patients and staff members. Many staff members are overworked, poorly informed as to the importance of communication for older people, lacking in motivation and reinforcement for communicating with patients. Hence, staff members may concentrate primarily on providing health care and neglect the social aspects of communication. The therapeutic value of communication is taken for granted as a fruitful by-product of adequate health and custodial care. The administration is not willing to commit the personnel or the funds to create and maintain an atmosphere in which successful communication might flourish.

Another characteristic of the communication-impaired institution is that the patients themselves contribute to the limited communication opportunities. They are a weak group, demonstrating little cohesiveness and few or no initiating goals. Lubinski (1975) in her study of patient perception of communication in a long-term setting found that the patients feel they are unique from one another. They resist communication with other patients, whom they perceive as senile, dying, or seriously ill. Further, internal conflicts including minor thefts and arguments create discord.

Patients and staff also realize that there are rules governing communication that help to foster a communication-impaired environment. Staff and patients are reluctant to discuss the rules concerning talking, which appear subtly powerful and effective in delimiting communication. Examples of rules governing communication in a communication-impaired environment include the following: Patients should not talk loudly, should refrain from complaining or criticizing the institution or staff, should not talk after bedtime or have visitors during mealtime, and should avoid obvious eavesdropping. Patients consequently talk about neutral, safe topics such as social amenities, trivia, and the weather. These topics do not engender spontaneous, continuing conversations and result in a paucity of meaningful dialogue.

Another characteristic of the communication-impaired institution is the physical design of the setting. Shared rooms, corridors, and communal areas inhibit anything but the most general and impersonal conversations. In addition, the communal areas may have distractions such as noise, television, and traffic that also inhibit talking. Some residents may migrate to these communal areas so that they may observe the actions of the staff and the daily activity. Consequently they may refrain from talking, which would hamper their attention to these events.

The acoustical treatment of the facility in communal areas or the patients' own rooms does not encourage communication. Poor lighting and acoustics in potential communication areas restrict the effective transmission and reception of a message. Sensory losses among older people may require that communication areas be designed to enhance visual and auditory processing.

Every nursing home may not exhibit each of these characteristics of a communication-impaired environment. In some settings several of these criteria will be strongly manifested, whereas in others all the criteria will be present. The impact of the communication-impaired environment is undoubtedly individualized for each resident and staff member depending on their previous experiences and their present communication needs. The nursing home may be as restricting for the elderly individual who came to the institution from an isolated community setting as for one who lived in a stimulating home environment.

In spite of this dismal portrayal of communication in many institutional settings, strategies can be employed that may improve the quantity and quality of communication there. This is a new role for many communication disorders specialists. The first suggestion is to enlist the aid of the administration, the point from which institutional policy emanates and is endorsed. As stated previously, the administration may respond favorably to well-designed, innovative programs. The communication disorders specialist needs to define the communication needs of all patients within the setting, providing data about the frequency of their interaction, the quality of communication within the setting, and the patient and staff perception of communication. Administrators will be more likely to support the education of the staff and the initiation of a communication milieu philosophy if there is a demonstrated, documented need.

The speech−language pathologist and audiologist can function in an educational role with all staff members regarding the importance and impact of successful communication in an institutional setting. Education for staff members needs to be on a continuing basis, and practical suggestions for creating and maintaining interaction with all patients need to be provided. All suggestions must be easily incorporated in the daily routine of the setting, requiring little extra time, effort, or funding. It is far more profitable to offer suggestions that can be employed within existing programs and routines rather than to impose new programs.

Demonstration of effective communication with all patients can be accomplished through audio and video presentations, role playing, and live demonstrations. Each of these strategies makes the impact of communication deprivation more real for the staff members. The communication disorders specialist might determine with the aid of the appropriate staff one or two operational goals for the staff to try in the course of a week and at the end of that time review with them their progress and perceptions of changes in communication. This allows the staff members time to gradually change their own behavior, to become sensitive to the changes accomplished and to measure their own progress. Furthermore, it gives the instructor opportunity to reinforce staff members for attempting these changes. When problems arise, modifications can be made quickly and more easily. Continuing education for these goals should occur over a number of weeks or months and generally cannot be accomplished in a 1-hour session. The immediate goals are enhanced sensivity and behavior among the staff, hopefully resulting in long term philosophic changes in the staff's attitudes, knowledge, and skills in communicating with the aging institutionalized individual.

Other suggestions for the speech−language pathologist and audiologist include the evaluation of the physical setting. The goal is to identify and modify physical barriers to communication effectiveness. For example, simple changes in lighting and furniture arrangement can facilitate communication in communal areas. Window treatment that filters light naturally and group seating arrangements are simple ways to create a possible communication area. A modest investment in acoustical treatment of high-communication-traffic areas can also be beneficial; this work should be supervised by an acoustical engineer.

The communication disorders specialist might adopt one floor or one area of the institution to serve as a demonstration project and model to other staff members and patients. First, the communication disorder specialist should choose an area that has potential for improvement of communication, an area where at least a minimal amount of communication is occurring. Even minimal communication can be used to generate more interaction between patients and staff and between patients themselves. This can be done through the identification and matching of communication partners, through support of natural leaders among the patients, and through the development of a need to communicate. Older people will communicate if there is a reason and if this reason will help enhance their self-identity. The residents of a long-term care institution need a socially stimulating and reinforcing environment. There must be a balance of work and leisure activities that will serve as the basis for conversation. In addition, stimulation of the senses through color, taste, smell, movement, and texture aid in cognitive awareness and hence in communication.

The creation of a stimulating communication environment fits in well with the concept of a therapeutic community. Jones (1953) emphasized that in the therapeutic community patients and staff share in the government of the institution and in the functioning of treatment programs within the setting. Rosenstock, Goldman, and Rothenberg (1967) stated that the objective of milieu treatment is to regenerate social interaction, the skills for which may deteriorate with prolonged institutionalization.

Programs such as the ones advocated by Lubinski (1978) and sensory remotivation and reality orientation complement each other in the therapeutic community. For example, sensory training programs focus on reintegrating the regressed older persons into their environments through stimulation of the senses and improved communication and resocialization skills (Richman, 1969). Reality orientation programs (Taulbee & Folsom, 1966) are aimed at older persons who are moderately disoriented to their surroundings. The goal is to help individuals receive and transmit accurate information so that they can function successfully in their environment. In both programs, the need for and the development of successful communication skills is paramount. However, if these goals are to be realized, the communication climate of the institution must also be improved. Improving the older persons' sensory or communication skills in therapy will be worthless unless they live in an atmosphere that encourages communication and reinforces interchange among all the persons living and working there.

CONCLUSION

The focus of this chapter has been on the communication problems of older people at home and in the long-term care setting. In each context the communication problems affect not only individuals but those around them and the psychosocial structure of the setting. Communication and its disorders are inextricably related to the environment in which they occur.

Further, the traditional role of the speech–language pathologist and audiologist needs clear definition in both settings. In a day when financial and staff crises and government regulations dominate the provision of services, the communication disorders specialist needs a strong rationale for his or her program. Similarly, innovative programs such as the therapeutic communication community and research programs must be explicitly and behaviorly defined and have built-in accountability procedures. The improvement of communication skills and opportunities of older individuals in all settings must be considered a right and not a privilege, a priority and not a by-product, and a reality and not an ideal.

REFERENCES

Ainsworth, T. *Quality assurance in long term care.* Germantown, Md: Open Systems Corporation, 1977.

Alpiner, J. Community aural rehabilitation programs. In J. Alpiner (Ed.), *Handbook of adult rehabilitative audiology,* Baltimore: Williams & Wilkins, 1978.

Anderson, N. Approaches to improving the quality of long term care for older persons. *Gerontologist,* 1974, *14,* 519–524.

Bennett, H. Management of psychiatric conditions in the elderly. *Patient Management,* 1975, 40–45.

Bennett, R. Relocation studies. Discussion of papers presented at Symposium on Relocation of the Elderly, Gerontological Society Meetings, 1972.

Bergman, S. Background developments of home care. *Institute on coordinate home care: Selected papers.* Pittsburgh, Pa.: Montifiore Hospital Association of Western Pennsylvania, 1963.

Beverley, E. Nursing homes: Matching the facility to the patient's needs. *Geriatrics*, 1976, *31*, 100–110.

Brody, E. (Ed.). *Long term care of older people*. New York: Human Sciences Press, 1977.

Brotman, H. Population projections. Part 1: Tomorrow's older population (to 2000). *Gerontologist*, 1977, *17*, 203–209.

Chapey, R., & Lubinski, R. An empirical analysis of thought process intervention in adult aphasia. Paper presented at the Annual Convention of the New York State Speech and Hearing Association, 1979.

Chapey, R., & Lubinski, R. Semantic judgment ability in adult aphasia. *Cortex*, 1979, *15*, 247–255.

Chapey, R., Lubinski, R., Chapey, G., & Salzburg, A. Survey of speech, language and hearing services in nursing home settings. *Long Term Care and Health Services Administration Quarterly*, 1979, *3*, 307–316.

Chapey, R., Rigrodsky, S., & Morrison, E. The measurement of divergent semantic behavior in aphasia. *Journal of Speech and Hearing Research*, 1977, *42*, 287–295.

Dobroff, R., & Litwak, E. *Maintenance of family ties of long term care*. Rockville, Md.: United States Department of Health, Education, and Welfare, 1977.

Eisdorfer, C. Stress, disease and cognitive change in the aged. In C. Eisdorfer & R. Friedel (Eds.), *Cognitive and emotional disturbances in the elderly*. Chicago: Year Book Medical Publishers, 1977.

Eisenson, J. *Examining for aphasia*. New York: Psychological Corp., 1954.

Geld, S. Toward a definition of the modern home. In N. Leeds & H. Shore (Eds.), *Geriatric institutional management*. New York: G. P. Putnam's Sons, 1964.

Goodglass, H., & Kaplan, E. *Boston Diagnostic Aphasia Examination*. Philadelphia, Lea & Febiger, 1972.

Grossman, R. Social worker's viewpoint of home care. In E. Brody (Ed.), *Long term care of older people*. New York: Human Sciences Press, 1977.

Health Resources Statistics. U. S. Department of Health, Education and Welfare. Rockville, Md.: Health Resources Administration, 1976.

Ingram, D., & Barry, J. National statistics on deaths in nursing homes. *Gerontologist*, 1977, *17*, 303–308.

Jones, M. *The therapeutic community*. New York: Basic Books, 1953.

Kahana, E. The human treatment of old people in institutions. *Gerontologist*, 1973, *13*, 282–289.

Kastenbaum, R., & Candy, S. The 4% fallacy: A methodological and empirical critique of extension care facility program statistics. *International Journal of Aging and Human Development*, 1973, *4*, 15–21.

Keenan, J., & Brassell, E. *Aphasia Language Performance Scales*. Murfreesboro, Tenn.: Pinnacle Press, 1975.

Lawton, M. P., & Jaffee, S. Mortality, morbidity and voluntary change of residence by older people. *Journal of the American Geriatrics Society*, 1970, *18*, 823–831.

Lieberman, M., Prock, V., & Tobin, S. Psychological effects of institutionalization. *Journal of Gerontology*, 1968, *23*, 343–353.

Littauer, D. Principles and practices of home care. In E. Brody (Ed.), *Long term care of older people*. New York: Human Sciences Press, 1977.

Long term care facility improvement study. Washington, D.C.: Public Health Service Office of Nursing Home Affairs, 1975.

Lubinski, R. *Perception of oral–verbal communication by residents and staff of an institution for the chronically ill and aged*. Unpublished doctoral dissertation, Teachers College, Columbia University, 1975.

Lubinski, R. Geriatric communication in institutional settings. *Communicative Disorders: An Audio Journal for Continuing Education*, 1978, *3*.

Lubinski, R. Why so little interest in whether or not old people talk: A review of recent research on verbal communication among the elderly. *International Journal of Aging and Human Development*, 1978–1979, *9*, 237–245.

Lubinski, R., & Chapey, R. Constructive aspects of memory in adult aphasia. *Proceedings of the Clinical Aphasiology Conference.* Minneapolis: BRK Publishers, 1978.

Lubinski, R., & Chapey, R. Communication services in home health care agencies: Availability and scope. *Journal of the American Speech-Language-Hearing Association,* 1980a, in press.

Lubinski, R., & Chapey, R. Concept formation by aphasic adults using Rendler's universal-nonuniversal paradigm. *British Journal of Disorders of Communication,* 1980b, in press.

Miller, P. *The extended care facility: A guide to organization and operation.* New York: McGraw-Hill Book Co., 1969.

Muma, J. *Language handbook: Concepts, assessment, intervention.* Englewood Cliffs, N.J.: Prentice-Hall, 1978.

Noelker, L., & Harel, Z. Aged excluded from home health care. *Gerontologist,* 1978, *18,* 37–40.

O'Connell, P. Communication problems in the aging. Miniseminar presented at the Annual Convention of the New York State Speech and Hearing Association, April, 1978.

O'Connell, P., & O'Connell, E. Speech–language pathology services in a skilled nursing facility. Paper presented at the Annual Convention of the American Speech and Hearing Association, 1978.

Penchansky, R., & Taubenhaus, L. Institutional factors affecting the quality of care in nursing homes. *Geriatrics,* 1965, *5,* 591–598.

Porch, B. *The Porch Index of Communicative Ability.* Palo Alto, Calif.: Consulting Psychologists Press, 1971.

Richman, L. Sensory training for geriatric patients. *American Journal of Occupational Therapy,* 1969, *23,* 254–257.

Rosenstock, F., Goldman, M., & Rothenberg, R. Rehabilitation of the long-term patient: An action research program in milieu therapy. *Journal of Chronic Diseases,* 1969, *22,* 493–503.

Routh, T. *Choosing a nursing home.* Springfield, Ill.: Charles C. Thomas, Publisher, 1970.

Sandoz Pharmaceuticals. *Positive approaches to selecting alternative living arrangements for the elderly.* East Hanover, N.J., 1975.

Sarno, M. *The Functional Communication Profile.* New York: Institute of Rehabilitation Medicine, 1969.

Schuell, H. *The Minnesota Test for the Differential Diagnosis of Aphasia.* New York: Psychological Corporation, 1965.

Sourcebook on aging. Chicago: Marquis Academia Media, 1977.

Taulbee, L., & Folsom, J. Reality orientation for geriatric patients. *Hospital and community psychiatry,* 1966, *17,* 23–25.

Teeter, R., Garety, F., Miller, W., & Heiland, W. Psychiatric disturbances of aged patients in skilled nursing homes. *American Journal of Psychiatry,* 1976, *133,* 1430–1434.

United States Bureau of the Census. *Census of population: 1970, general population characteristics,* Final Report, PC(1)–B1. Washington, D.C., U.S. Government Printing Office, 1970.

United States Department of Health, Education and Welfare. *Facts about older Americans.* DHEW Publ. No. (OHD) 77–20006, 1976.

United States Senate Subcommittee on Long Term Care. *Nursing homecare in the United States: Failure in public policy.* Washington, D.C.: U. S. Government Printing Office, 1974.

Vital and health statistics—United States—1969. Chronic conditions and impairments of nursing home residents. DHEW, Series 12, No. 22, Rockville, Md., 1973.

Waldman, A., & Fryman, E. Classification of residents. In N. Leeds & H. Shore (Eds.), *Geriatric institutional management.* New York: G. P. Putnam's Sons, 1964.

Weiner, M., Brok, A., & Snadowsky, A. *Working with the aged.* Englewood Cliffs, N.J.: Prentice-Hall, 1978.

Wepman, J., & Jones, L. *The Language Modalities Test for Aphasia.* Chicago: University of Chicago Education–Industry Service, 1961.

Winn, S., & McCaffree, K. Characteristics of nursing homes perceived to be effective and efficient. *Gerontologist,* 1976, *16,* 415–419.

Zimmer, J. Characteristics of patients and care provided in health-related and skilled nursing homes. *Medical Care,* 1975, *13,* 992–1010.

Author Index

Subject Index